FOOD COMPONENTS TO ENHANCE PERFORMANCE

An Evaluation of Potential Performance-Enhancing Food Components for Operational Rations

Committee on Military Nutrition Research
Food and Nutrition Board
Institute of Medicine

Bernadette M.Marriott, Editor

National Academy Press
Washington, D.C.1994

NATIONAL ACADEMY PRESS 2101 Constitution Avenue, NW Washington, DC 20418

NOTICE: The project that is the subject of this report was approved by the Governing Board of the National Research Council, whose members are drawn from the councils of the National Academy of Sciences, the National Academy of Engineering, and the Institute of Medicine. The members of the committee responsible for the report were chosen for their special competences and with regard for appropriate balance. Part I of this report has been reviewed by a group other than the authors according to procedures approved by a Report Review Committee consisting of members of the National Academy of Sciences, the National Academy of Engineering, and the Institute of Medicine.
The Institute of Medicine was established in 1970 by the National Academy of Sciences to enlist distinguished members of the appropriate professions in the examination of policy matters pertaining to the health of the public. In this, the Institute acts under both the Academy's 1863 congressional charter responsibility to be an adviser to the federal government and its own initiative in identifying issues of medical care, research, and education. Dr. Kenneth I.Shine is president of the Institute of Medicine.
This report was produced under grant DAMD17-92-J-2003 between the National Academy of Sciences and the U.S. Army Medical Research and Development Command. The views, opinions, and/or findings contained in chapters in Parts II through VI that are authored by U.S. Army personnel are those of the authors and should not be construed as official Department of the Army positions, policies, or decisions, unless so designated by other official documentation. Human subjects who participated in studies described in those chapters gave their free and informed voluntary consent. Investigators adhered to U.S. Army regulation 70–25 and United States Army Medical Research and Development Command regulation 70–25 on use of volunteers in research. Citations of commercial organizations and trade names in this report do not constitute an official Department of the Army endorsement or approval of the products or services of these organizations. The chapters are approved for public release; distribution is unlimited.
Library of Congress Catalog Card No. 94-66363

International Standard Book Number 0-309-05088-X
Additional copies of this report are available from: National Academy Press 2101 Constitution Avenue, N.W. Box 285 Washington, D.C. 20055 Call 800–624–6242 or 202–334–3313 (in the Washington Metropolitan Area).

B454

Printed in the United States of America

The serpent has been a symbol of long life, healing, and knowledge among almost all cultures and religions since the beginning of recorded history. The image adopted as a logotype by the Institute of Medicine is based on a relief carving from ancient Greece, now held by the Staatlichemuseen in Berlin.

COMMITTEE ON MILITARY NUTRITION RESEARCH

ROBERT O.NESHEIM *(Chair),* Monterey, California

RICHARD L.ATKINSON, Department of Internal Medicine, Veterans Affairs Medical Center, Hampton, Virginia

WILLIAM R.BEISEL, Department of Immunology and Infectious Diseases, Johns Hopkins University School of Hygiene and Public Health, Baltimore, Maryland

GAIL E.BUTTERFIELD, Division of Endocrinology, Gerontology, and Metabolism, Stanford University School of Medicine; and Geriatric Research, Education, and Clinical Center, Veterans Administration Medical Center, Palo Alto, California

JOHN D.FERNSTROM, Department of Psychiatry, Pharmacology, and Neuroscience, University of Pittsburgh School of Medicine, Pennsylvania

JOEL A.GRINKER, Program in Human Nutrition, School of Public Health, University of Michigan, Ann Arbor

G.RICHARD JANSEN, Department of Food Science and Human Nutrition, Colorado State University, Fort Collins

ORVILLE A.LEVANDER, Vitamin and Mineral Nutrition Laboratory, U.S. Department of Agriculture, Beltsville, Maryland

GILBERT A.LEVEILLE, Nabisco Brands Incorporated, East Hanover, New Jersey

JOHN E.VANDERVEEN, Office of Plant and Dairy Foods and Beverages, Food and Drug Administration, Washington, D.C.

ALLISON A.YATES, College of Health and Human Sciences, University of Southern Mississippi, Hattiesburg

Food and Nutrition Board Liaison

JOHANNA T.DWYER, Frances Stern Nutrition Center, New England Medical Center Hospital, Boston, Massachusetts

Committee on Military Nutrition Research U.S. Army Grant Officer Representative

JAMES A.VOGEL, U.S. Army Research Institute of Environmental Medicine, Natick, Massachusetts

COL ELDON W.ASKEW, U.S. Army Research Institute of Environmental Medicine, Natick, Massachusetts (through February 21, 1994)

Staff

BERNADETTE M.MARRIOTT, Program Director

VALERIE McCADDON BREEN, Research Assistant

DONNA F.ALLEN, Project Assistant

FOOD AND NUTRITION BOARD

Staff

BERNADETTE M.MARRIOTT, Acting Director, Food and Nutrition Board
CATHERINE E.WOTEKI, Director, Food and Nutrition Board (through December 22, 1993)
MARCIA S.LEWIS, Administrative Assistant
SUSAN M.WYATT, Financial Associate

Preface

This publication, *Food Components to Enhance Performance,* is another in a series of reports based on workshops sponsored by the Committee on Military Nutrition Research (CMNR) of the Food and Nutrition Board (FNB), Institute of Medicine, National Academy of Sciences. Other workshops or symposia have included such topics as nutritional needs in hot environments, body composition and physical performance, nutrition and physical performance, cognitive testing methodology, and fluid replacement and heat stress. These workshops form a part of the response that the CMNR provides to the Commander, U.S. Army Medical Research and Development Command, regarding issues brought to the committee through the Military Nutrition Division of the U.S. Army Research Institute of Environmental Medicine (USARIEM) at Natick, Massachusetts.

FOCUS OF THE REPORT

Optimal job performance without compromising the health and well-being of employees is the goal of employers no matter what the field of endeavor. Intermittent or prolonged physiological and psychological stressors that employees bring to the workplace have an impact not only on their own performance but on that of those with whom they work and interact. The very significant effects of sleep deprivation on performance were clearly demonstrated in the recent report of performance decrements of medical interns and residents who needed to perform important medical tasks while on duty for extended periods of time, the Exxon Valdez accident, and similar military maritime accidents (National Commission on Sleep Disorders Research, 1993). The internal stressors an individual brings to his or her job are then compounded by the day-to-day physical and mental stresses of the job itself. Along with individuals engaged in the emergency and protective services in our communities—fire fighters, police, and emergency medical personnel—military personnel in combat settings endure highly unpredictable timing and types of stresses as well as situations that require continuing vigilance for hours or even days.

The U.S. Army has been led by concerns about individuals' abilities to avoid performance degradation and the need to enhance mental capabilities in highly stressful situations to an interest in devising military ration components that could enhance soldier performance. The Committee on Military Nutrition Research was asked to assist a collaborative developmental program between scientists at the U.S Army Research Institute of Environmental Medicine (USARIEM) and the U.S. Army Natick Research, Development and Engineering Center (NRDEC) by evaluating the performance-enhancing potential of specific food components. On the basis of recent research, the Army scientists specifically requested that the CMNR review and comment on the potential for tyrosine, other amino acids, complex carbohydrates, caffeine, carnitine, choline, and long-chain fatty acids to help sharpen an individual's performance under the strain of military missions. The committee was requested to indicate which if any of these food ingredients would offer the most promise for future research that would lead to the development of prototype ration components. Production of sufficient quantities of prototype rations to allow human testing of the effectiveness of such ration components in enhancing individual and unit performance in laboratory and controlled field settings could then proceed. The CMNR was asked to consider the research possibilities of each of the above listed food components and to also address six general questions about using food components to enhance performance in military combat settings. The questions that were posed to the committee are included in Chapter 1 of this report.

The views of military and nonmilitary scientists from the fields of neuroscience, nutrition, physiology, various medical specialties, and psychology on the most recent research concerning physical and mental performance enhancement in stressful conditions are included in this report. Although placed within the context of military tasks, the conclusions and recommendations presented in Chapters 1 and 2 of this report may have wide-reaching implications for individuals in any job setting.

HISTORY OF THE COMMITTEE

The Committee on Military Nutrition Research (CMNR) was established in October 1982 following a request by the Assistant Surgeon General of the Army that the Food and Nutrition Board of the National Academy of Sciences set up a committee to advise the U.S. Department of Defense on the need for and conduct of nutrition research and related issues. The committee's tasks are to identify nutritional factors that may critically influence the physical and mental performance of military personnel under all environmental extremes; to identify deficiencies in the existing data base; to recommend research that would remedy these deficiencies and approaches for studying the relationship of diet to physical and mental performance; and to review and advise on standards for military feeding systems. Within this context the CMNR was asked to focus on nutrient requirements for performance during combat missions rather than requirements for military personnel in garrison. (The latter were judged as not significantly different from those of the civilian population.)

Although the membership of the committee has changed periodically, the disciplines represented have consistently included human nutrition, nutritional biochemistry, performance physiology, food science, and psychology. For issues that require broader expertise than exists within the committee, the CMNR has convened workshops. These workshops provide additional state-of-the-art scientific information and informed opinion for the consideration of the committee in their evaluation of the issues at hand.

COMMITTEE TASK AND PROCEDURES

In May 1992, personnel from the USARIEM requested that the CMNR examine the current state of knowledge concerning the potential of a number of food components to enhance performance in military combat settings. This request originated from a Science and Technology Objective (STO) to prevent performance degradation of the soldier under the stress of sustained field operations as part of the overall initiative—"The Soldier as a System." This initiative recognizes the importance of all aspects of the soldier's equipment and person as important in moving toward enhanced capabilities necessary for the future (see Chapter 3; Army Science Board, 1991).

The committee was aware of the large volume and the diversity of quality of the scientific literature on the topic of performance enhancement. It decided that the best way to review the state of knowledge in this disparate area was through a workshop at which knowledgeable researchers could review published research with the committee. Such a workshop would enable the

CMNR to review the adequacy of the current research and to identify gaps in the knowledge base that might be filled by future research.

A subgroup of the committee met in May 1992, determined the key topics for review, identified speakers with expertise in these topics, and planned the workshop for November 1992. Invited speakers were asked to prepare a review paper on their assigned topic for presentation and publication and to make specific recommendations in response to several questions posed to them prior to the workshop. The CMNR also believed that it would be beneficial to include a review of earlier and ongoing military research. Scientists at USARIEM and NRDEC participated in the workshop, resulting in a well-rounded agenda.

At the workshop, each speaker gave a formal presentation, which was followed as time allowed by questions and a brief discussion period. The proceedings were tape-recorded and professionally transcribed. At the end of the presentations, a general discussion of the overall topic was held. Immediately after the workshop, the CMNR met in executive session to review the issues, draw some tentative conclusions, and assign the preparation of draft reviews and summaries of specific topics to individual committee members. Committee members subsequently met in a series of working sessions and worked separately and together using the authored papers and additional reference material to draft the summary and recommendations. The final report was reviewed and approved by the entire committee.

The summary and recommendations of the Committee on Military Nutrition Research constitute Part I of this volume, and Parts II through VI include the papers presented at the workshop. Part I has been reviewed anonymously by an outside group with expertise in the topic area and experience in military issues. The authored papers in Parts II through VI are ordered in this volume as they were presented at the workshop. These chapters have undergone limited editorial change, have not been reviewed by the outside group, and represent the views of the individual authors. Selected questions directed toward the speakers and their responses are included when they occurred to provide a flavor of the workshop discussion. The invited speakers were also requested to submit a brief list of selected background papers prior to the workshop. These recommended readings, relevant citations collected by CMNR staff prior to the workshop, and selected citations from each chapter are included in the Selected Bibliography (Appendix C).

ACKNOWLEDGMENTS

It is my pleasure as Chair of the CMNR to acknowledge the contributions of the FNB staff, particularly the excellent technical and organizational skills of Bernadette M.Marriott, Ph.D., the FNB program director for the CMNR. Her assistance in organizing the workshop and in bringing the proceedings to the point of publication is greatly appreciated. I wish to acknowledge as well the fine contributions by the workshop speakers and their commitment to participate and prepare detailed review papers on relatively short notice. The CMNR appreciates the assistance of COL Eldon W.Askew and others from the USARIEM, and Drs. C.Patrick Dunne and Irwin A.Taub of NRDEC for their assistance in identifying issues of concern to the military and obtaining the involvement of the military personnel who participated in the workshop. The assistance of Dr. Harris R.Lieberman in the planning and identification of participants is gratefully acknowledged. COL David Schnakenberg's scientific expertise and his historical knowledge of relevant military studies contributed significantly, as in the past, to the success of the workshop. The critiques of the anonymous reviewers and Food and Nutrition Board liaison member, Johanna Dwyer, in addition to comments by FNB director Catherine Woteki, provided helpful insights in the development of this final document. The editorial efforts of Michael Hayes are gratefully acknowledged. The assistance of Valerie Breen, CMNR research assistant, and Donna Allen, CMNR project assistant, in word processing, editing, and proofreading this report is greatly appreciated.

Finally, I am grateful to the members of the committee who participated significantly in the discussions at the workshop and in the preparation of the summaries of the proceedings. I also I want to thank committee members who participated in the initial planning of the workshop and those who drafted initial summaries of sections of this report. In particular, I want to thank former committee members Edward S.Horton, John A.Milner, and James G. Penland. The commitment of the members of this committee, who serve without compensation to provide sound, timely recommendations for consideration by the military, is commendable. It is a pleasure to work with this dedicated group.

ROBERT O.NESHEIM, *Chair*
Committee on Military Nutrition Research

REFERENCES

Army Science Board 1991 Soldier as a System. 1991 Summer Study Final Report. Assistant Secretary of the Army Research, Development and Acquisition. Washington, D.C.: U.S. Department of the Army.

National Commission on Sleep Disorders Research 1993 Wake up America: A National Sleep Alert, Volume 1: Executive Summary and Executive Report, submitted to the U.S. Congress and to the Secretary, U.S. Department of Health and Human Services, January 1993. Washington, D.C.

Contents

PART I

Committee Summary and Recommendations

PART I INCLUDES TWO CHAPTERS. Chapter 1 provides the background for the report. It describes the task presented to the Committee on Military Nutrition Research (CMNR) by the Military Nutrition Division, U.S. Army Research Institute for Environmental Medicine (USARIEM), U.S. Army Medical Research and Development Command; summarizes the relevant background material; and presents the committee's findings. The Army posed six questions to the committee; these questions are also listed in Chapter 1. In addition, Chapter 1 presents an overview of the relevant areas of concern, a review of the specific food components that the CMNR was asked to consider for their potential to enhance performance, and a summary of the committee's interpretation of the current scientific knowledge in these areas. Chapter 2 presents the committee's answers to the questions posed by the Army and its conclusions. Chapter 2 also includes the general and specific recommendations of the CMNR.

1

Introduction and Background

THE COMMITTEE'S TASK

The Committee on Military Nutrition Research (CMNR) of the Food and Nutrition Board (FNB), Institute of Medicine (IOM), National Academy of Sciences (NAS), was asked by the Division of Military Nutrition, U.S. Army Research Institute of Environmental Medicine (USARIEM), U.S. Army Medical Research and Development Command (USARMRDC), to review the potential for specific food components to enhance the performance of military personnel under the stress of field settings. The committee was thus charged with providing a thorough review of the literature in this area and with interpreting these diverse data in terms of military applications.

The committee was also asked to address six general questions that dealt with enhancement of performance.

1. Is enhancement of physical and mental performance in "normal," healthy, young adult soldiers by diet or supplements a potentially fruitful approach or are there other methods of enhancing performance that have greater potential?
2. The Army Science and Technology Objective (STO) states: By FY98 demonstrate a 10–15 percent enhancement of soldier performance in selected combat situations through the use of rations/nutrients that enhance caloric utilization and/or optimize the physiological levels of neurotransmitters. (Army Science Board, 1991).
   Is the level of enhancement identified in this STO reasonable with the current scientific knowledge?
3. Which food components, if any, would be the best candidates to enhance military physical and mental performance?
4. Should the mode of administration be via fortification of the food in rations, supplemented via a separate food bar or beverage component, or administered in a "vitamin pill mode"? Is palatability a significant issue in this type of supplementation?
5. Are there specific ethical issues that need to be considered with this type of research?
6. What regulatory issues must be considered with the types of food components that are being evaluated by the Army?

Within this context the CMNR was charged with specifically evaluating the potential of selected amino acids, carbohydrates, structured lipids, choline, carnitine, and caffeine to enhance performance. The committee was also asked to provide its recommendations regarding which, if any, of these compounds should be developed further within the current "Soldier as a System" initiative (Army Science Board, 1991).

The CMNR realized that there was a large amount of research—of variable quality—devoted to enhancement of performance. In addition, questions about dose levels, informed consent, time span, and timing of administration were raised with regard to the application and desired outcome within a combat setting. To help focus the objects of its report, the committee requested that the Army develop several scenarios that illustrated the hypothetical application of these food components. Seven scenarios written by Drs. Harris Lieberman and Mary Mays, USARIEM, are included in Appendix A.

To assist the CMNR in responding to these questions and developing their recommendations, a workshop was convened on November 16–17, 1992. This workshop included presentations from individuals familiar with or having expertise in cognition, endocrinology, exercise physiology, food engineering, food science, immunology, metabolism, neuropsychology, nutrition, nutritional biochemistry, performance psychology, and sports medicine. The invited speakers discussed their presentations with committee members at the workshop and submitted the contents of their verbal presentations as written reports. The committee met after the workshop to discuss the issues raised and the information provided. The CMNR later reviewed the written reports and drew on its collective expertise and the scientific literature to develop the summary, conclusions, and recommendations that appear in Chapters 1 and 2.

Terms Used in This Report

For the purposes of this report, the Committee on Military Nutrition Research defines the term *enhancement* to include both an avoidance of reduction in performance decrement during stress and improvement of performance above the baseline. Both physical and mental performances measured by a wide variety of tests are explored. Improvements over baseline performance and prevention of performance decrements during stress are admittedly widely different problems, but ones with similar overall military objectives. Possible approaches to each of these problems are also explored. *Ergogenic aid,* ("work-producing") is used to refer to any substance, whether in a food or not, that enhances physical performance.

Report Organization

This summary begins with an overview of the specific military issues and research that led to interest in performance enhancement. The committee then provides a summary of information related to nutrition and stress. This is followed by a review and interpretation of the available data on the food components proposed for consideration by the Army. Chapter 1 concludes with a discussion of the safety and regulatory aspects of performance-enhancing food components.

MILITARY RESEARCH ON NUTRITIONAL ENHANCEMENT OF SOLDIER PERFORMANCE

History and Current Research

The introductory chapter by COL Eldon W.Askew summarizes the interest of the Army in enhancing soldier performance (see Chapter 3). In the past, the focus for maximizing soldier performance has largely been on efforts to improve training, doctrine, and equipment, with little research emphasis on how the physical and cognitive abilities of individual soldiers may be enhanced through nutritional supplementation or design of rations. Military rations are designed in accordance with the nutritional standards established by the Military Recommended Dietary Allowances (MRDAs) (AR 40–25, 1985), which are intended to ensure that soldiers are receiving nutritionally adequate rations.

There has been a concern that the development of sophisticated equipment and the increasing demands that are made on the soldier, both physically in load carrying and in the cognitive abilities required to use the more sophisticated weaponry, place additional burdens on the nutritional needs of the individual. This has raised the question of whether soldier performance can be improved through design of special rations. USARIEM and the U.S. Army Natick Research, Development and Engineering Center (NRDEC), located at Natick, Massachusetts, share responsibility for implementing the new Science and Technology Objective (STO) that is principally directed at the sustainment or enhancement of soldier performance through the use of performance-enhancing food components (see description of this STO in question 2 on page 4). In this context, if soldier performance that may be reduced under the stress of sustained field operations could be sustained at preoperational levels, it would be considered an enhancement of performance.

COL Eldon W.Askew (Chapter 3) briefly summarizes the research that USARIEM has conducted in the past few years in three areas, dietary macronutrients (carbohydrates), nutritional pharmacology (caffeine), and nutritional neuroscience (tyrosine). These areas are reviewed in more depth in the chapters that follow (Chapters 15–17 and 20). Although some responses have been measured under carefully controlled laboratory conditions, the results have not always been transferable to field operations. The difficulty in obtaining precise measures in the field, the considerable variations frequently experienced among subjects, and the difficulty of actually duplicating conditions imposed either in the laboratory or in the field affect the outcome of this research.

The issues considered in the workshop and this report center around the identification of potential performance-enhancing nutrients or food components that may be used to supplement or improve the operational rations that already provide liberal allowances of nutrients as established by the MRDAs.[1] Soldiers who consume these military rations are thus presumed to be in a state of good nutrition.

[1] The Military Recommended Dietary Allowances (MRDAs) are being revised. The current edition is included in its entirety in Appendix B.

Design Issues for Rations

There are two primary tasks in meeting the objective of enhancing performance by using rations. The first requires the identification of food components that may, through prior research or consideration of metabolic pathways, appear to be candidates for evaluation. This task is further complicated by the need to design the appropriate environmental stresses and identify the physical and cognitive measures that may be sufficiently sensitive to evaluate their influence on performance.

The second requires the development of the appropriate delivery system to supply the components to the soldier in the proper amount and at the appropriate time.

Two introductory chapters (Chapters 4 and 5) by Irwin A.Taub and C. Patrick Dunne, of the Food Engineering Directorate, Natick Research, Development and Engineering Command (NRDEC), provide an excellent review of the complexity of developing operational rations for the military. These rations must meet special nutritional needs, be acceptable to the soldier, have sufficient shelf-lives under the storage time and conditions imposed for the ration system, and meet the safety and performance criteria established for the ration when used possibly 3 to 4 years after manufacture. The capability of NRDEC and the extent of the challenge this task presents are eloquently discussed in Taub and Dunne's chapters.

Biochemical Strategies and Issues

Biochemists may identify nutrients or food components that are important sources of energy or that function as metabolic regulators at the cellular level for which changes in the supply or concentration may affect metabolism at that site. However, in the complex functioning of the various tissues and organs and metabolic regulation, these cellular observations may not be transferable to performance enhancement of the individual. Therefore, it is important in selecting potential performance-enhancing components for study to carefully evaluate (1) the physiological basis for the potential performance enhancement at the functional site(s); (2) the potential for being able to deliver such a component through the physiological processes of digestion, absorption, and circulation; and (3) the delivery of the food component to the functional site at a concentration that will be effective and not adversely affect the complex interactions in the overall metabolism. With all of the complexities of human metabolism, it is important to carefully evaluate food components or nutrients as potential performance enhancers (physical and/or cognitive) on the basis of their demonstrated potential in studies on the functioning tissue or organ.

As discussed in the chapters by Drs. Dunne and Taub, the ration developers are acutely aware of these problems and are looking to the CMNR for guidance on the selection of components for evaluation in the appropriate food delivery systems.

PERFORMANCE ISSUES AND MEASUREMENT APPROPRIATE TO THE MILITARY

Physical Performance

The performance of physical tasks in any job setting requires the confluence of physiological and psychological processes. As discussed by James A.Vogel (Chapter 6), many of these processes and related factors can be viewed as potential targets for performance enhancement through ergogenic aids. Although experimental studies can focus on measurement of physical performance at levels ranging from the isolated muscle cell to the whole organism, the issue for the military is the performance of the soldier in physically demanding tasks, often under stressful conditions. Review of food components that may enhance physical performance through psychological factors that contribute to performance of all tasks, such as arousal, concentration, and motivation (see Dishman, 1989, for a review), will be reviewed in the following sections. In Chapter 6, Vogel focuses on the four categories of physiological factors that are involved in physical task performance: metabolic capacity, neuromotor control, energy substrates, and tissue homeostasis. The various physical performance tasks in the military involve several or all of these physiological categories,

> The physical task of firing a rifle is predominantly determined by neuromotor control factors, while that of running for long distances is predominantly determined by the other three groupings of factors (Chapter 6, p. 114).

Vogel contends that to evaluate the effectiveness of ergogenic aids, the specific target of action among these categories must be identified and then appropriately measured using well-validated techniques. A careful review of the most appropriate methodologies for each category is provided by James A.Vogel in Chapter 6. Evaluation of the effectiveness of any food component on performance would then optimally be tested in experiments that isolated the target categories in several stages: in a controlled laboratory setting, in a single field task, and as part of an operational scenario. Appendix A provides several scenarios that depict militarily relevant physical performance tasks in which ergogenic aids might prove effective.

Mental Performance

The issues of mental performance that are of concern to military personnel in a combat setting do not differ from those in a regular workplace, with the exception of the severity of the levels and types of stress superimposed on the situation. The ability to perceive, attend to, and respond appropriately to cues, as well as make appropriate decisions, and to remain vigilant are critical in military combat settings. These areas of cognitive performance also form the basis for many physical performance tasks, such as positioning and loading artillery shells or moving through a mine field. Laboratory studies in many settings have shown that well-trained personnel will typically sacrifice speed for accuracy in cognitive performance tests in stressful situations. Although in the workplace this may reduce monetary cost-effectiveness, in a field combat situation a significant decrease in speed of performance could be life-threatening.

Sleep deprivation is a major overlying factor that can further lead to performance degradation in the workplace (Commission on Sleep Disorders Research, 1993). This problem has long been recognized by the Army and thus has been the focus of laboratory and field research in military settings. In Chapter 7, Belenky et al. present a review of recent research on sleep deprivation and its effects on performance during continuous combat operations. Belenky et al. state that the "The ability to do useful mental work declines by 25 percent for every successive 24 hours awake" (p. 128). In laboratory and field studies, although psychomotor performance, physical strength, and endurance do not appear to be less affected by sleep deprivation, complex mental functions such as the ability to perceive and understand changing situations, adapt to changes, and plan alternative strategies are significantly degraded. For example, soldiers were able to maintain accuracy at fixed targets after 90 hours without sleep, but they exhibited poor performance with targets that appeared at random time intervals and in changing locations (Haslam and Abraham, 1987, see Belenky et al.; Chapter 7).

An extended, uninterrupted sleep (7-plus hours) appears to provide the best means of restoring cognitive performance. Sleep that is fragmented, however, has been shown to provide little recuperative value in terms of cognitive performance (Bonnet, 1987). Unfortunately, fragmented sleep—interrupted by noise, lights, and nearby movements—is more typical of combat settings than an uninterrupted rest. The trade-offs for commanders in allowing more sleep for their troops or making increased forward progress in an operation were addressed by McNally et al. (1989) through integration of experimental data from Thorne et al. (1983) into models of military performance under different conditions of sleep deprivation. The results indicate that restricting a unit's sleep is unproductive. The total output on any given task of units with mild to moderate sleep deprivation would be expected to drop as the days pass. During this time, the more complex reasoning and decision-based tasks would be expected to suffer the greatest decline in performance. In Chapter 7, Belenky et al. illustrate these types of problems with accounts of experiments using simulated artillery fire (Banderet et al., 1981) and after-action debriefings from Operation Desert Storm.

Preliminary data indicate that decrements in cognition-based performance are paralleled by decreases in glucose metabolism in specific areas of the brain (Thomas et al., 1988). The effects of dietary glucose supplements on performance enhancement under conditions of sleep deprivation have not been fully examined.

The scenarios in Appendix A provide additional direct examples of the types of cognitive performance changes that are of concern in military settings. Reduction in performance degradation through ingestion of food components that may affect neurotransmitters, more general neuronal excitability, or the specific brain regions involved in cognitive activities will be discussed in the sections that follow.

PROVIDING FOOD IN THE CONTEXT OF MILITARY COMBAT SETTINGS

Many contextual factors are influential in the amount and type of food that individuals consume. An individual's expectations (Cardello and Sawyer, 1992), the time of day (Kramer et al., 1992), the effort needed to obtain food (Collier, 1989; Engell et al., 1990), the amount and diversity of available food (Engell, 1992; Rolls et al., 1992), the appropriateness of the meal to the time of day (Birch et al., 1984; Kramer et al., 1992), food acceptability (Meiselman et al., 1988), food presentation (Cardello and Sawyer, 1992), and the dynamics of the social situation while eating (de Castro and Brewer, 1992; Goldman et al., 1991) all affect the amount eaten and what is selected. Since appropriate food intake is essential for performance, these contextual factors are recognized by the Army as important; however, the manner of food delivery in combat settings is necessarily constrained by the food engineering concerns that were previously described. As Meiselman and Kramer mention in Chapter 8, the long-term storage requirements for rations contribute to difficult demands for production as well as for the consumer. In addition, soldiers typically eat considerably less than the total ration that is provided for them (of the 3,900 kcal per day for moderate activity in a temperate climate, soldiers eat 2,000–3,000 kcal, on average). This reduction in intake does not appear to be related to food acceptance, since soldiers consistently give good ratings to military rations (see Chapter 8 for review). The stress of the training or combat situation is another mediating factor for consideration. Although a hungry individual may not eat if fearful, once eating does occur the level of intake will most likely be enhanced (Gray, 1987). Individual responses differ greatly, however, and although the "typical" response may be to reduce food intake under stressful conditions, some subgroups of the population increase food intake under the same conditions (see discussion in Chapter 8).

In Chapter 8 Meiselman and Kramer review the history, methodological approaches, and methodological issues related to research in food intake, contextual factors, and performance enhancement. In the military setting these authors point out that performance science has yet to resolve many methodological questions. Provision of food in a military setting and its impact on soldier performance are presented as complex multifactorial problems that require an initial resolution of the definition of performance. The authors refer to the military initiative that calls for soldier performance enhancement in the following five capabilities: lethality, mobility, command and control, survivability, and sustainment. Translating these capabilities into reliably measurable components of cognitive and physical performance that can be enhanced by food component intake in the context of military rations is no easy task. As discussed by these authors, not only will the contextual issues of food component provision require careful examination but new methodologies will most likely require development or refinement. In addition, physical and cognitive performance measurement need to be well-integrated—an area where there is little previous research.

In summary, although an individual's food intake in the military is influenced by the same set of factors that influence food intake in nonmilitary settings, the stress of military training or combat settings, the shelf life requirements, the packaging and delivery constraints of military rations, and the added performance capability demands result in a highly complex set of problems for performance enhancement. Research in this area will not only require careful attention to the issue of context in food item delivery—similar to standard military rations—but also to the integration of physical and cognitive performance measurement and most likely the development of new methodologies that would test the performance capabilities valued in soldier field settings.

STRESS AND NUTRIENT INTERACTIONS

The Central Nervous System

Primary neurotransmitters in the central nervous system include the monoamines dopamine, norepinephrine (NE), and serotonin (also called 5-hydroxytryptamine or 5HT). The catecholamine norepinephrine is believed to be an important neurotransmitter involved in the sleep-wake cycle, pain, anxiety, and arousal, whereas the indoleamine serotonin is thought to be important in many central processes, including pain perception, memory, appetite, thermoregulation, blood pressure control, heart rate, and respiration.

Tyrosine hydroxylation is the rate-limiting step in the synthesis of all major catecholamines including NE and dopamine, while serotonin is synthesized from tryptophan. Several lines of investigation have examined the effects of administration or manipulation of these or other precursors on various physiological functions and behaviors. Protocols have included acute (short-term, i.e, minutes to hours) manipulations as well as chronic (usually long-term -days to months- diet-related) administration.

Studies using acute paradigms have examined the behavioral consequences of altered neurotransmitter precursor availability and, hence, neurotransmitter synthesis. Alterations in brain amino acids and neurotransmitter levels are seen within 15–20 minutes after administration of amino acids such as L-tyrosine (TYR), or after feeding diets high in carbohydrates (CHOs) or protein to experimental animals (see Chapter 9 by John D.Fernstrom).

In addition, both serotonin and NE have been examined for their effects on macronutrient selection (see Chapter 13 by Richard J.Wurtman). In experimental animals pharmacological doses of NE (either central or peripheral administration) have been reported to enhance CHO consumption relative to protein or fat consumption, whereas central or peripheral administration of 5HT appears to inhibit CHO consumption while sparing protein and fat intake (see Blundell, 1986 for a review). In one example, with a two-diet choice (protein-rich versus CHO-rich), a small dose of 5HT introduced into the parventricular nucleus of experimental animals selectively suppressed the CHO-rich diet (Shor-Posner et al., 1986).

In Chapter 9, John D.Fernstrom reviews the biochemical basis underlying L-tyrosine (TYR) administration to counter stress. Results from several studies suggest that TYR administration enhances dopamine (DA) and NE synthesis in the brain and reverses deficient performance in rats and humans (Lehnert et al., 1984; Banderet and Lieberman, 1989). However, the author cautions that while TYR administration may increase transmitter (DA and NE) synthesis and release and may potentially affect brain functions, the exact consequences of TYR administration are unknown. Further study would be essential to understanding the usefulness of TYR or other pharmacological or nutritional agents that stimulate DA or NE release.

The studies of Levine and colleagues (Levine et al., 1990) further illustrate the effects of different types of stressful stimuli on increasing the activity of NE-containing neurons in the brain. Acute stress appears to have little effect on NE receptors in the brain. Chronic stress, however, is associated with increased NE synthesis and turnover (Stanford et al., 1984; Thierry et al., 1968). Chronic stress may also be associated with marked decrements in the number of activated beta receptors, in that a stress-induced increase in NE release by brain neurons via stimulation of beta receptors on target neurons and the production of second-messenger-mediated effects leads to beta receptor down regulation (Torda et al., 1981). The available evidence thus suggests that NE receptor responsiveness is changed following chronic stress and that these changes are different from those accompanying acute stress. Data also suggest that such changes are not uniform; i.e., NE receptors and subtypes as well as activity in different brain regions may differ. Therefore, agents such as TYR that enhance NE synthesis and release following acute stress may have different effects under chronic stress.

Stress also affects brain DA neurons, although there is some controversy whether all DA neurons or only some are activated by stress. Again, further research is needed to determine whether administration of TYR in animal models under acute stress stimulates DA synthesis and release and improves functioning. Stress also reportedly increases the brain levels of the major DA metabolite dihydroxyphenylacetic acid (DOPAC) (Dunn, 1988). There are few available studies on brain DA neuronal activity under chronic stress, but several suggest increased levels of DOPAC. Although one cannot determine at present whether DA receptor sensitivity is influenced by chronic stress, administration of TYR should stimulate DA receptor synthesis and release; this is again suggestive of enhanced performance.

Although stress does not influence the activity of the serotonin precursor neurons, stress does increase brain concentrations of the essential amino acid tryptophan (TRP)—possibly as a consequence of increased serotonin (5HT) synthesis and turnover. The mechanism responsible for the stress-induced increase in 5HT synthesis and turnover differs from those in DA and NE (see Fernstrom, 1990). In animals, with 5HT administration through a large dose of valine (or TYR), the stress-induced rise in brain TRP levels or the rise in brain 5HT may be blocked, with unknown consequences to brain function.

In summary, there are few studies that clearly define the catecholamine receptor responses to stress. In addition, there is marked diversity among the various catecholamines suggesting the need for additional animal studies to examine differences in acute and chronic stress on catecholamine receptors in particular brain regions, and their correlations with function.

Endocrine System Responses to Stress

A broad overview of endocrine system responses to military-type stresses is given by William R.Beisel (Chapter 10). Multiple endocrine responses are but one component of a complex of interacting responses that include close communications and coordination among the central nervous system (CNS), the endocrine system, and the immune system. Thus, molecular participants in these broad responses to stress include traditional hormones, neuropeptide mediators, and immunologically generated cytokines, all of which combine to induce the formation of secondary and tertiary molecular messengers within responding body cells.

Endocrine responses show different patterns, depending on the nature of the stress. Sudden or frightening forms of stress are likely to generate a typical "fight or flight" response, or "alarm reaction," manifested endocrinologically by the release of norepinephrine from CNS neurons and of epinephrine from the adrenal medulla and sympathetic nerve terminals. These two hormones, plus other neurotransmitters, initiate the well-known immediate responses to stress, including tachycardia, hyperventilation, sweating, and other sympathetic responses.

Typical military stresses generate endocrine responses that tend to be remarkably stereotyped in pattern, although they may vary with the form, duration, and severity of the inciting stress. Hormonal responses may also evolve longitudinally, over time, if stress is protracted. These hormonal responses are not simply "all out" but are carefully controlled by a variety of feedback loops.

Although Selye (1946) had theorized that an adrenocorticotropic hormone (ACTH)-induced production of adrenal glucocorticosteroids was the principal endocrine response to stress, subsequent findings revealed that the adrenals contributed only relatively small, brief portions of the overall panoply of endocrine responses. In fact, the adrenocorticoid component may consist of only a loss of the normal circadian rhythm of cortisol production, with the highest normal values which occur in the morning, being sustained throughout both day and night.

Pituitary responses to stress are initiated by the CNS action of neurotransmitters and immunologically generated cytokines, which lead to the CNS production of corticotropin releasing factor and other neurohormones. These, in turn, regulate the anterior pituitary gland production of ACTH, thyroid-stimulating hormone (TSH), growth hormone, and the gonadotropins. Pancreatic islet cell production of insulin and glucagon during stress may be stimulated by acute-phase cytokines (the interleukins IL-1 and IL-6 and tumor necrosis factor [TNF]).

As detailed in Chapter 10, comprehensive endocrine studies of military-type stresses have been performed in Ranger trainees of the Norwegian (see Opstad and colleagues 1980, 1981, 1982, 1983, 1984, 1985, 1990, 1992) and U.S. armies (Moore et al., 1992)[1]. These studies have documented a small adrenocorticoid response (with loss of circadian rhythm), an increased secretion of aldosterone and renin, and consistent large increases in plasma growth hormone values. In contrast, the production of thyroid and gonadal hormones was suppressed in these soldiers. The declines in prolactin and follicle-stimulating hormone were accompanied by sharp and sustained declines in levels of plasma testosterone and other gonadal androgens. These data are quite complete, with the exception of possible responses by neuroendocrine and intestinal hormones.

Although dietary factors certainly influence the endocrine system, there is no evidence that individual dietary components (other than carbohydrate) serve to alter the response patterns of the endocrine system to stress. Current evidence does not suggest that research initiatives along this line would be worthwhile. On the other hand, severe reductions in total dietary intake should be avoided during military stress, for starvation can initiate its own pattern of endocrine responses.

Attempts have been made by athletes to improve their strength, performance, and muscle mass by the prolonged use of androgenic steroids in pharmacological doses. But the adverse long-term medical consequences of such attempts far outweigh any short-term performance gains; this practice has now been outlawed by all major athletic groups.

In summary, despite the occurrence of stress-induced endocrine responses in military personnel, these responses are transient in nature. No hormonal manipulation of the endocrine system during military-type stress can be recommended.

Immune System Responses to Stress

A review of immune system responses to stress is also provided by William R.Beisel (see Chapter 10). Despite the paucity of data generated by sophisticated modern immunological methodologies, the available evidence indicates that military-type stresses do initiate a variety of responses in both innate (i.e., inborn, generalized, antigen-nonspecific) and adaptive (i.e., acquired, antigen-specific) immunity. Further, both arms of the adaptive

[1] Additional data on U.S. Army Ranger trainees were presented at a meeting of the Committee on Military Nutrition Research, Food and Nutrition Board, Institute of Medicine, National Academy of Science, in March 1993.

immune system (i.e., humoral immunity provided by specific antibodies generated by B lymphocytes, and cell-mediated immunity provided primarily by T lymphocytes) appear to be affected adversely by stress.

A large body of inadequately controlled data suggests that mental and emotional stresses may reduce cell-mediated immune system competence. Substantial data attest to the impairment of cell-mediated immunity, humoral immunity, and generalized innate immunity caused by generalized malnutrition or by isolated deficiencies of single essential micronutrients. A diet adequate in protein and energy and with adequate quantities of all essential nutrients provides the immune system with optimum protection.

In a study conducted at the Walter Reed Army Institute for Research (WRAIR), the month-long stress of Ranger training was accompanied by diminished humoral immunity (depressed antibody responses to standard vaccine antigens) (Moore et al., 1992). This finding confirmed in soldiers the substantial body of data showing impaired antibody production in animals subjected to various types of stress.

As detailed in Chapter 10, recent studies of cell-mediated immunity showed transient impairments of function during the course of Ranger training. Again, this result appeared to confirm, in humans, a large body of experimental data obtained in animals. These studies, however, contained no data on natural killer (NK) lymphocyte activities. Impairments of NK cell activities are caused by many forms of experimentally induced stress.

An important aspect of both innate and acquired immunity is the production (by lymphocytes, monocytes/macrophages, and many other body cell types) of cytokines with a wide range of actions. Cytokines include the various interleukins, interferons, colony-stimulating factors, cell growth factors, as well as tumor necrosis factor (TNF) and lymphotoxin. Many cytokines play an important role in stress responses, being responsible for initiating hormonal responses as well as acute-phase reactions, which in turn causes large nutrient losses (Beisel, 1991).

Acute phase reactions are important in military-type stresses such as infection, injury, or severe muscular exertion. These reactions include headaches, myalgia, arthralgia, fever, sleepiness, loss of appetite, loss of muscle protein, and an accelerated metabolism of stored body nutrients, all of which serve to reduce both physical and mental performance. Biochemical components of these cytokine-generated acute-phase reactions include the cellular production of prostaglandins, prostacyclines, leukotrienes, and nitric oxide, which, in turn, generate many of the accompanying symptoms. However, it is not known whether stress causes human cells to generate protective "stress proteins" in vivo; such information should be gathered initially in animals.

Decrements in military performance associated with cytokine-induced acute-phase reactions can by reduced, in part, by the prophylactic or therapeutic administration of common over-the-counter drugs (such as aspirin or ibuprofen) that block the formation of prostaglandins. In addition to reducing performance-impairing symptoms, such therapy appears to serve to reduce the destruction of muscle protein and the accelerated metabolism of stored body nutrients (see Beisel et al., 1968, 1974; Beisel, 1991).

In summary, impairments in humoral and cell-mediated immunity need to be defined more completely and more precisely, by using modern technologies, and their poststress duration must be delineated. Measurements of levels of key cytokines (IL-1, IL-6, and TNF) in plasma are needed during military-type stress to help define the potential usefulness of prostaglandin-blocking agents in the prophylaxis and therapy of stress-induced symptoms that interfere with optimal military performance.

Metabolic Responses to Stress and Activity

After abroad introductory analysis of the many complex factors implicated in metabolic responses to stress and physical activity, Edward S.Horton and William R.Beisel (see Chapter 11) focus the remainder of their chapter on the nutritional, endocrinologic, and physiological aspects of fuel metabolism needed to sustain physical and mental performance under a variety of stressful conditions.

These authors emphasize the fact that many different kinds of stress are involved in military performance and that the body's responses to these stresses are extremely complex, involving many separate systems. Acute and chronic stresses may call for widely different responses. Although adaptations to stress seem designed to aid in survival, some may be deleterious, a point to be considered when considering nutritional methods of enhancing performance.

Despite whatever stresses they face, soldiers must be able to think and act. Optimal performance requires optimal fuel metabolism—primarily glucose for the CNS and a mixture of glucose and fatty acids for muscle. Multiple levels of integration are involved in maintaining homeostasis of glucose and other fuels throughout periods of stress.

Under resting conditions, glucose uptake is mainly by noninsulin-dependent pathways in the CNS, blood cells, and kidneys, whereas only about one-third is used by insulin-dependent pathways, chiefly in skeletal muscles (which primarily burn fatty acids and some amino acids as their source of metabolic fuels). The blood glucose level remains quite constant, being supplied by hepatic glycogen and, to a smaller extent, by hepatic gluconeogenesis from glycerol, pyruvate, lactate, and amino acids. Fatty acids generated by lipolysis of body fat stores are the predominant source of energy.

Dramatic changes occur when exercise begins. Rapid increases in energy demands activate the sympathetic nervous system, which in turn stimulates both glycogenolysis within muscle itself and additional lipolysis in fatty tissues. Soon, blood flow to muscles is increased, and as more blood glucose is delivered, uptake of glucose by muscle is also increased.

These dramatic changes, however, are carefully regulated through at least five different mechanistic levels: hormone secretion, hormone integration, substrate availability, blood flow controls, and management of glucose uptake by cells. All of these controls are further influenced by the intensity of exercise, the duration of exercise, the antecedent diet, and the modifying effects of prior physical conditioning.

Leg muscle exercise on a cycle ergometer is accompanied by a progressive increase in glucose uptake, which is associated with increased blood flow and increased cellular uptake. Hepatic glucose production parallels demands, initially by glycogenolysis, and then by gluconeogenesis. Blood glucose will actually increase initially during brief high-intensity exercise. As exercise continues, however, fatty acid dependency is increased, and after several hours, fatty acids become the predominant fuel. With prolonged, exhaustive exercise, the liver cannot keep up with glucose needs.

Activation of the sympathetic nervous system is the key initiating factor, which leads in turn to stimulation of muscle cell glycogenolysis, fat cell lipolysis, and activation of both the adrenal cortex and medulla. The adrenal response gives rise to both cortisol and epinephrine and, thus, secondarily to an increase in hepatic glucose output. The epinephrine also stimulates glucagon secretion while inhibiting that of insulin.

Norepinephrine concentrations rise proportionally to the intensity of exercise, once it is above half of maximum. Insulin values actually fall during exercise, whereas the glucagon values increase slowly, responding both to the intensity and the duration of exercise and to the rising catecholamine concentrations.

Animal studies have shown that the falling insulin-to-glucagon ratio stimulates hepatic glucose production. On the other hand, a falling insulin-to-norepinephrine ratio activates lipolysis and mobilizes fatty acids. Pancreatic clamp techniques have demonstrated the effects of individual hormones, with others held constant. Glucagon increases cause prompt increases in arterial blood glucose, primarily because of enhanced hepatic glycogenolysis. Epinephrine also increases arterial blood glucose, but more slowly, acting to stimulate both glycogenolysis and gluconeogenesis in the liver and lipolysis in the periphery. On the other hand, the effects of norepinephrine are primarily in the periphery, releasing substrates that slowly lead to enhanced hepatic gluconeogenesis. Cortisol alone seems to play little role in acute hepatic glucose production.

This increase in glucose turnover during stress is generally related to increased hepatic production, but factors such as blood flow to skeletal muscle and changes in the cellular uptake of glucose are also involved. Certain neurotransmitters, when injected into the third ventricle of dogs, cause responses that mimic many of the initiating and counterregulatory hormonal responses and glucostimulatory effects of stress. Similar experimental studies in dogs with alloxan-induced diabetes demonstrate the need for permissive amounts of insulin to obtain a stress-related increase in peripheral glucose utilization.

Studies of glucose utilization in skeletal muscle during stress have also involved the carrier-mediated pathways of glucose transport across cell walls, producing evidence that insulin and the contraction stimulus of exercise exert independent effects for increasing glucose transport into muscle cells. Additional research is needed in the areas of peripheral glucose uptake.

More research is also needed to understand the initiating CNS and sympathetic nervous system role, and the actions of various neurotransmitters and their receptors in stimulating and maintaining the hepatic production of glucose during exercise-related military stresses.

POTENTIAL PERFORMANCE-ENHANCING FOOD COMPONENTS

Physical Performance Enhancement

A broad overview of food components that may optimize physical performance is provided by John L.Ivy (Chapter 12). Ivy divides such ergogenic aids into five categories: (1) mechanical, (2) psychological, (3) physiological, (4) pharmacological, and (5) nutritional. The line between the last two categories is difficult to draw, especially from a regulatory point of view, since foods and drugs are regulated quite differently. This difficulty is of particular relevance to the subject of this report, since food components will fall into classifications either as nutritional or pharmacological ergogenic aids. The general rule is that a nutrient consumed at a level reasonably comparable to a dietary level and acting via the known mechanism for that nutrient would be considered a nutritional aid. In contrast, when nutrients are consumed at levels much greater than dietary levels and have physiological effects clearly different from their known nutritional roles, they are usually considered to be acting via a pharmacological route. However, from a legal or regulatory perspective, the distinction between the "foods" and "drugs" may be less clear, as described by John E.Vanderveen (Chapter 23). In addition, food compo nents that are not nutrients but that have pharmacological effects may pose complications, for example, the inhibition of insulin secretion caused by mannoheptulose found in avocados (Simon et al., 1972). Ivy, in his review, considers five mechanisms by which a variety of foods and derivatives of food products may act as ergogenic aids. These are (1) acting as central or peripheral stimulants, (2) increasing the storage or availability of limiting substrates, (3) acting as a supplemental fuel source, (4) reducing or neutralizing metabolic by-products, and (5) enhancing recovery.

The prime example of a central stimulant found in food beverages is caffeine, as discussed elsewhere in this report (Chapter 20). Another example is branched-chain amino acids (BCAAs). It has been hypothesized that supplementation with BCAAs might delay the fatigue associated with endurance exercise by preventing a rise in brain serotonin levels. However, data are not available to confirm this hypothesis. Still another possibility is the facilitation of excitation-contraction at the neuromuscular junction by choline. The utility of choline supplementation is considered in more depth in Chapter 19.

The ergogenic aid most used to increase the storage and subsequent availability of a limiting substrate is carbohydrate. The well-known procedure to accomplish this is by exercise-stimulated glycogen depletion and then feeding a high-carbohydrate diet. Storage of increased levels of muscle glycogen results. Another possibility is phosphate loading, which has been reported to increase maximal oxygen uptake, possibly via an increase in the blood concentration of 2,3-diphosphoglycerate. This has the effect of increasing tissue oxygen extraction.

Carbohydrate also can act as a supplemental fuel source during exercise. This topic was considered extensively in an earlier CMNR report (Marriott and Rosemont, 1991). Other possible approaches to increasing aerobic endurance via a supplemental fuel source considered by Ivy include elevating plasma-free fatty acid levels via either consumption of a high-fat meal or secondary to the lipolytic effect of caffeine, consumption of a combination of pyruvate and dihydroxyacetone, or consumption of medium-chain triglycerides (see also Chapter 18).

A decrease in muscle pH during exercise is believed to limit physical performance; thus, buffering this pH change makes physiological sense. Consumption of sodium bicarbonate has been demonstrated to increase cycling duration at 90 percent $\dot{V}_{O_2\,max}$ by reducing acidosis (Sutton et al., 1976). Dichloroacetate has been reported to lower blood lactate concentrations in animals and humans (Carraro et al., 1989; Schneider et al., 1981). Ivy also emphasizes that body heat during exercise limits physical performance, and hence, water can be considered one of the most important ergogenic aids. To enhance recovery after physical activity, water and carbohydrate are both needed, as emphasized also in the previous CMNR workshop proceedings on fluid replacement and heat stress (Marriott and Rosemont, 1991).

In summary, data from a wide range of studies on the effects of ergogenic aids indicate that there are a variety of foods and food products that act through one of five known mechanisms to improve athletic performance. Acting to increase both storage and availability of a limiting substrate and as a supplemental fuel source, data on the athletic performance enhancement of carbohydrates are most compelling. Physical tasks performed in the military occasionally mirror the short-term intensive bursts of activity studied in athletic competitors. However, most research with carbohydrate supplementation has been conducted in prolonged continuous moderate exercise such as marathon running or situations that do not readily compare to the exercise demands of military combat.

Food Components that May Enhance Mental Performance

Various foods and food components have been evaluated for their behavioral effects in animals and humans, including protein and carbohydrate (CHO), caffeine, and several amino acids such as tryptophan, tyrosine, and phenylalanine. Since the dosages of these cognitive enhancers are far greater than those available in foods, many investigators believe that these substances should be classified as pharmacological agents rather than nutritional supplements and that their safety as well as their efficacy in these separate formulations have not been demonstrated.

In one well-designed, well-controlled experiment, tyrosine was given to male volunteers exposed to an acutely stressful environment (Banderet et al., 1987). Behavioral, cardiovascular, and endocrine measures were taken using a double-blind, placebo-controlled crossover design with each subject participating twice in three experimental conditions, combinations of cold (15°C) and hypobaric hypoxia (4,200 or 4,700 m) and a control condition. Tyrosine ameliorated many of the adverse consequences of the environmental stress and improved vigilance while lessening anxiety.

In general, to demonstrate nutrient or neurotransmitter effects on mood and performance, it is critical to use well-designed, specific tests. Improved performance may best be demonstrated with monotonous vigilance tests of long duration (Lieberman, 1989). In addition, dose-response functions should be convincingly demonstrated. Mood tests should include a range of possible affective responses such as depression and anxiety as well as behaviors including estimates of sleepiness and vigor. Differences in functioning can also be examined under experimental conditions ranging from neutral to extremely stressful or painful.

Presently, there are many unresolved issues. It is critical to select appropriate methods to examine the somewhat subtle effects of these nutrients on behaviors. Whether these nutrients can be used as sedatives or stimulants, antidepressants, or antistress agents will have major practical consequences. Further research is thus desirable.

Nutrients on Neurotransmitter release

A discussion of issues relating nutrients and neurotransmitter release and behavioral consequences can be found in Wurtman (1988). Chapter 13 of this report, also by Richard Wurtman reviews the history of much of the research relating nutrients to brain function and the reverse (i.e. brain function to food/ nutrient choices). The major hypothesis in this area of research is that metabolic events occurring outside the brain and primarily occurring as consequences of eating behavior (e.g., amount, frequency, and type of macronutrient) can affect the levels of neurotransmitter precursors and thus guide the selection of nutrients in the next meal(s). With "normal" feeding, brain tryptophan levels and serotonin synthesis undergo variation. This variation itself reportedly produces differences in food choices such as that following an overnight fast (e.g., CHO-rich breakfast versus protein-rich breakfast).

The theory that serotonin is part of a feedback loop in the control of diet selection has led to much scientific debate. Experimental data suggest that neither the control of macronutrient intake nor diet-induced changes in neurochemistry are easily demonstrable or robust (Holder and Huether, 1990). In contrast, supporters maintain that the diet-induced changes in brain neurochemistry (e.g., serotonin or 5-hydroxytryptamine [5HT]) are meaningful and are involved in the process of food/macronutrient selection (see Blundell, 1986; Booth 1987; Booth et al, 1986; Garattini et al., 1986).

In particular, concern has been voiced as to the mechanism whereby contextual and sensory differences in food components can be meaningfully separated from macronutrient content. Note is made of the absence of a metabolic/neurochemical mechanism: "Neurochemistry or indeed neuroanatomy, unconnected to any account of how sensory information could be used to direct behavior towards the diets in a manner that achieves nutrient-oriented selection, leaves the feedback idea as a magical incantation, not a scientific hypothesis" (Booth, 1987, pp. 195–196).

Fernstrom (1987) reported that although it appears possible to relate protein and CHO intake to effects on the serum tryptophan/large neutral amino acid ratio and, thus, to brain tryptophan levels and serotonin synthesis in fasting rats in a single-meal situation, such a relationship does not exist in chronic stress studies. Additionally, the use of anorectic agents such as fenfluramine does not provide convincing data for a suppression of CHO intake rather than total food intake. Some investigators are hopeful that the dietary self-selection paradigm will help to untangle this area if proper controls are available to determine differences in taste, smell, and texture.

Another area of scientific controversy has been the role of brain serotonin in excessive CHO snacking. Consumption of CHO-rich foods has been related, in animals and humans, to increases in the synthesis and release of brain serotonin and a decrease in the CHO content of a subsequent meal. An increase in the central uptake of the precursor tryptophan is the mechanism that has been presented. This increase in central serotonin level and decrease in CHO intake are not seen with protein intake.

One aspect of this hypothesis that has been extensively discussed is the concept of CHO craving. Rats have been reported to modify food choice (thereby diminishing their CHO intake) as a consequence of pretreatment with CHO snacks or pharmacological agents, facilitating serotoninergic neurotransmission (Wurtman and Wurtman, 1979). A question has been how well CHO-rich versus fat-rich foods are characterized in these discussions. (Amounts in grams versus calories represent markedly different total percentages, and thus, CHO-rich foods are frequently rich in other nutrients, fat in particular.) It is also unclear whether CHO cravers prefer sweet CHOs primarily. According to the feedback loop theory, the response of serotoninergic neurons to food-induced changes in the relative concentration of plasma amino acids allows for a special "sensor" role in nutrient choice (Wurtman, 1983, 1988).

CHO cravers have been suggested to show enhanced mood and reduced depression following CHO consumption. This decreased depression has been interpreted as a consequence of the food-induced changes in central serotonin levels (Lieberman et al., 1986b). In addition, it has been suggested that obese CHO cravers treated with an anoretic agent, D-l fenfluramine (which increases serotonin activity) decrease CHO snacking. Such drugs have also been considered in the treatment of several "affective" disorders, for example, seasonal affective disorders [SADS] (O'Rourke, 1989), premenstrual syndrome (PMS) (Brzezinski et al., 1990), and smoking cessation (Spring et al., 1991). However, the general conclusion seems to argue for further specification of CHO cravings and cravers.

The animal data are most convincing for fasted single meal situations. Most experimental evidence from the food choices of free-living human subjects suggests high daily variability. Meals following extended fasts such as breakfast may be high in protein (eggs, fish) as well as CHO. Although subjects confined to the hospital (Wurtman and Wurtman, 1989) showed relatively less variability, the food intake records and food frequency data suggest greater variability in CHO and fat. Also unresolved is how this sensor mechanism might work and the interrelationships between brain and plasma levels.

In summary, there are insufficient data at this time to determine whether the neurotransmitter effects discussed in this section can be utilized to improve performance in military settings. It is unclear whether CHO or protein bars would promote sleep or decrease hunger thereby improving concentration in high-stress conditions. It is also unclear whether the ingestion of CHO is regulated by animals or humans to produce or control such differences. The use of pharmacological agents at varying doses might allow examination of the interrelationship between CHO consumption and brain serotonin levels. However, regulation is difficult to demonstrate, especially with marked variations in food intakes dependent on time of day, choices available, amounts, etc.

SPECIFIC FOOD COMPONENTS

Tyrosine

Tyrosine is a nonessential dietary amino acid because it can be synthesized in vivo from the essential amino acid phenylalanine and because protein synthesis continues normally even if tyrosine is absent from the diet. However, tyrosine is recognized to be a physiologically important precursor of the catecholamine neurotransmitters dopamine, norepinephrine, and epinephrine. The physiological consequences of changes in concentrations of these neurotransmitters raises intriguing possibilities that expanded intakes of tyrosine beyond that typically present in the diet may alter a host of reactions and biological responses.

In Chapter 15, Harris R.Lieberman describes the results of human and animal studies which evaluated the effects of tyrosine supplements on mental performance under stressful conditions was evaluated. This and other evidence demonstrate that catecholaminergic (CA) neurons play a key role in the regulation of arousal level and anxiety. The primary hypothesis for these studies is that the function of CA neurons is dependent on the concentrations of the catecholamine neurotransmitters, which in turn are dependent on the supply of the precursor tyrosine. Further, it is hypothesized that under stress, the concentration of tyrosine is limited by its supply, which can be enhanced by large dietary supplements. In studies conducted with rats, administration of single doses of tyrosine in amounts of 200–400 mg/kg of body weight reduced the adverse effects of acute stresses such as cold and hypobaric oxygen (Rauch and Lieberman, 1990). The decline of core body temperature due to cold stress was reduced, whereas normal behavioral responses were restored. Specifically, swimming time in the cold was improved by tyrosine, as was spatial learning and memory in a water maze under conditions of hypobaric oxygen. Other beneficial effects of tyrosine in rats under stressful conditions also were described by Lieberman.

Only a few studies have been reported in which single supplements of tyrosine were given to human subjects. These also are described by Lieberman (Chapter 15). Using a double-blind crossover design (100 mg of tyrosine per kg of body weight given orally versus placebo, human subjects at USARIEM were exposed to a combination of 4 hours of hyperbaric oxygen (4,200 or 4,700 m) and cold (15°C) (Banderet and Lieberman, 1989). Mood and mental performance were assessed using a battery of standardized behavioral tests. These adverse environmental conditions resulted in impaired cognitive performance, headache, lightheadedness, nausea, and general malaise. Tyrosine significantly reduced the severity of these symptoms, and improved functioning believed to be regulated by catecholaminergic neurons such as vigilance, alertness, and anxiety. In other studies at the U.S. Air Force Armstrong Laboratory (Dollins et al., 1990), the subjects who were given 100 mg of tyrosine per kg and exposed to lower-body negative pressure simulating gravitational stress, exhibited reduced adverse cardiovascular symptoms in comparison with controls. In these Air Force studies, the total dose of tyrosine administered to a 70-kg man would be 7 g. This compares to estimated phenylalanine and tyrosine intakes from 100 g of protein per day of 4 and 3 g/day, respectively.

Additional studies on the effect of tyrosine in reducing cognitive deficits resulting from cold stress were reported by Stephen T.Ahlers and colleagues (Chapter 16). In studies carried out in an environmental chamber at the Naval Medical Research Institute, administration of 150 mg of tyrosine per kg of body weight completely reversed cold-induced memory loss using the delayed matching-to-sample (DMTS) test. This controlled study in the laboratory chamber was followed by a study under field conditions. After a day in which all the military personnel performed maneuvers in the cold (−20°C), half of the subjects were given 75 mg of tyrosine per kg, and the other half a placebo. Subjects given tyrosine also performed substantially better on the DMTS memory test under field conditions.

In summary, the studies reviewed suggest strongly that single doses of tyrosine can ameliorate some of the adverse effects of stress on cognitive performance in both animals and humans. The results are consistent with the hypothesis that under stress, the substrate supply of tyrosine to the brain may limit the synthesis of the catecholamine neurotransmitters norepinephrine, dopamine, and epinephrine. Many more studies are needed to confirm these findings under a greater variety of stressful conditions. In addition, the safety of such large single doses of tyrosine has not yet been demonstrated. Further, data are lacking concerning the beneficial (or harmful) effects in humans of long-term administration of tyrosine supplements, as might be needed in continuous combat operations.

Carbohydrates

As discussed by John L.Ivy (Chapter 12), an important role has been demonstrated for carbohydrates in sustaining or enhancing physical performance. The role or potential role of dietary carbohydrate in other aspects of performance is considered by Spring and colleagues in Chapter 17. Target behaviors of relevance to the military were defined as mood and performance, with emphasis placed on sensorimotor and cognitive performances.

Spring et al. rightly consider mood, even though it is difficult to measure and even more difficult to quantify, to be an underrated outcome. Mood changes, including the motivation to undertake difficult tasks, are particularly important under stressful conditions such as combat. Stressful situations can unmask performance deficits that are not apparent under nonstressful conditions. In contrast, motivation, interest, and effort can increase functional capacity and overcome performance deficits caused by physiological conditions such as undernutrition. In a study cited by the authors, Gambian road workers subjected to calorie deprivation sufficient to cause significant weight loss nonetheless produced as much work output as nondeprived workers (Diaz et al., 1991). The authors explained these results as being derived from a strong motivational effect based on a monetary reward.

The role of carbohydrates in fatigue also is considered by Spring et al. (Chapter 17). Fatigue is defined as

> (1) weariness from bodily or mental exertion; (2) a cause of weariness, labor, exertion; (3) *physiological,* temporary diminution of the irritability or functioning of organs, tissues, or cells after excessive exertion or stimulation; and (4) *mechanical,* the weakening or breakdown of material subjected to stress. (Random House, 1982).

The ability of carbohydrate supplements to prolong endurance during exercise clearly is related to preventing fatigue in a physiological sense (definition 3 above). The sense in which the word *fatigue* is used by Spring et al. relates to definition (1) i.e., weariness from bodily or mental exertion. It might better be called *perceived fatigue* since it may or may not correlate with physiological indicators. Nevertheless, as emphasized by Spring and her colleagues, when fatigue is perceived to be present, whether for physiological or psychological reasons, performance can be reduced.

The experimental model discussed by the authors is the measurement of subjective mood feelings postprandially following high-carbohydrate or high-protein meals. Both breakfast and lunch are considered. High-carbohydrate, low-protein lunches increased reported fatigue more than did higher-protein lunches. Breakfast of any macronutrient composition reduced fatigue compared with that in the baseline state. Protein-rich breakfasts reduced fatigue to a greater extent than did protein-poor, carbohydrate-rich breakfasts. Whether for breakfast or lunch, on a weight-for-weight basis, protein is reported to be more satiating than carbohydrate, an effect of possible importance in military situations.

The well-described effect of carbohydrate in increasing the tryptophan (TRP)/large neutral amino acid (LNAA) ratio in plasma is considered to be a possible mechanism for postprandial effects of carbohydrate on perceived fatigue. It has been reported that as little as 4 percent protein in the diet can prevent the elevation in the TRP/LNAA ratio caused by carbohydrate (Teff et al., 1989). Consistent with these data is the fact that the fatiguing effect of carbohydrate is most reliably seen when the meals contain less than 4 percent protein. In addition, considerable individual variation is encountered in these types of experiments, and from a military standpoint any practical utility is difficult to discern. The third, or physiological, definition of fatigue can also be a factor of major importance in military stresses involving severe or prolonged muscular exertion. Muscle fatigue, typified, for example, by the performance declines during the last stages of prolonged sprints or marathons, is associated with the buildup of lactic acid and other metabolic products of carbohydrate, amino acid, and fatty acid substrates used by the exercising muscles.

Also considered by Spring et al. (Chapter 17) are effects of carbohydrate on cognitive performance, which is affected differently by carbohydrates at breakfast, at lunch, or in snacks. However the reported effects are variable and not very robust. For example, even skipping breakfast altogether has only weak and inconsistent effects on cognitive performance in young children, adolescents, and adults. When performance differences were observed following meals varying in macronutrient composition, cognitive performance was better after higher-protein breakfasts (Spring et al., 1992).

Typically, it is observed that tasks involving cognitive performance including vigilance, reaction time, sorting, and arithmetic show steady improvement during the day, although the pattern is interrupted temporarily by a postlunch slump (see discussion in Chapter 17). Cognitive performance declines after lunch with bigger declines associated with bigger lunches. In addition to the number of calories, protein-poor meals have been reported to elicit larger decreases in cognitive performance than protein-rich meals (Lieberman et al., 1986a). Negative effects of skipping lunch were reported to be modest in a laboratory setting and somewhat more robust in a field setting involving prolonged highway driving. In another setting, Kanarek and Swinney (1990) reported that a late afternoon calorie-rich snack enhanced performance compared with performance after consuming a low-calorie diet soda. No differences were observed between a confectionery-type snack and yogurt when both contained at least 25 percent protein.

In summary, meals containing protein and carbohydrate have more beneficial effects than meals that are nearly protein-free. However, any behavioral effects seen are time and context dependent. Snacks have utility in enhancing performance between meals. Spring and colleagues emphasize that research on diet and behavior has tended to overemphasize simple cognitive/sensorimotor measures, and insufficient attention has been given to more subtle characteristics such as the motivation to undertake important activities and the ability to cope with stress and exhibit sociability.

Glucose

Data suggesting that administration of glucose enhances working memory during cold stress are reviewed by Stephen T.Ahlers and colleagues (Chapter 16). Previous studies reported in the literature and cited by the authors suggest that glucose administration can improve both long-term and working memory. Ahlers et al. evaluated the effect of glucose administration on the cold-induced impairment of working memory in rats using the delayed matching-to-sample (DMTS) test. Doses of glucose between 10–100 mg/kg of body weight substantially blocked the impairment of accuracy in matching in the test caused by cold exposure. Initial data reported by Belenky et al. (Chapter 7) demonstrated a decrease in brain glucose metabolism accompanying sleep deprivation-induced decrements in cognitive performance (Thomas et al., 1988).

In summary, there are tantalizing hints that glucose administration during cold stress and after sleep deprivation, such as could be accomplished with a candy bar, has some potential to improve memory and performance on cognition-based tasks. Much more work is needed to explore this possibility.

Structured Lipids

An overview of the performance enhancement potential of structured lipids is provided by Ronald L.Jandacek (Chapter 18). Structured lipids are defined as fats that are synthesized from mixtures of long- and medium-chain fatty acids. Structured lipids are therefore differentiated from typical dietary fats by the presence of significant amounts of medium-chain fatty acids (i.e., fatty acids containing 6 to 10 carbon atoms). Jandacek reviews the digestion, absorption, and metabolism of long- and medium-chain fatty acids because any possible performance enhancement potential for structured lipids depends on differences in the way long- and medium-chain fatty acids are handled by the body.

A major demonstrated advantage of structured lipids in enteral and parenteral nutrition is through the provision of essential fatty acids and a high caloric density with a small osmotic load. These nutritional advantages of structured lipids have been demonstrated most notably under conditions of stress such as trauma, burns, and infection. Although such nutritional support has clear military importance, it is not closely relevant to the subject of this report.

The possibility that structured lipids might have performance-enhancing potential is based on the hypothesis that glycogen utilization during exercise might be spared by the rapid oxidation of the medium-chain fatty acids present in structured lipids. Medium-chain fatty acids in the diet are delivered directly and rapidly to the liver via the portal circulation. They appear to be preferentially oxidized compared to long chain triglycerides. It is further postulated that following metabolism in the liver, the ketone bodies that are produced, acetoacetate and ß-hydroxybutyrate, would be delivered to the muscle, sparing glycogen utilization. Unfortunately the studies published to date, as reviewed by Jandacek, do not support the hypothesis.

In summary, although structured lipids have an important role to play in enteral and parenteral nutrition, their potential for enhancing physical and mental performance, especially in a military setting, is low.

Choline

Choline is an essential component of the human diet that is important for the normal functioning of all cells (Zeisel, 1988). Choline and choline-containing compounds are critical for a wide variety of metabolic processes within the body, including acting as a messenger within the cells and as neurotransmitters in the nervous system, controlling muscle contraction, providing methyl groups in a variety of intracellular reactions, as a component of triglyceride transport, and participating in the immune response.

Functions of Choline

Perhaps the best-known function of choline is as a component of acetylcholine, an important neurotransmitter. A small fraction of dietary choline is acetylated to acetylcholine by the action of acetyltransferase, an enzyme present in the terminals of cholinergic neurons in the brain and periphery. Acetylcholine in the brain is intimately associated with memory. Acetylcholine acts as a signaling agent in muscle by transmitting the neural signal across the neuromuscular junction. The availability of acetylcholine in the peripheral nerves and muscles affects muscle function. Deficiency of choline in the diet decreases the conduction velocity of nerve transmission and produces earlier fatigue.

Choline is critical for signal conduction in a number of tissues. Choline-containing phospholipids act as vital elements in signaling across cellular and intracellular membranes. Agents from outside the cells stimulate hydrolysis of phosphatidylinositides, and the resulting protein phosphorylation cascades are a major mechanism for transmitting messages into the interior of cells. Phosphatidylcholine and sphingomyelin and their metabolites play a role in this by serving as mediators and modulators of transmembrane signaling. Hundreds of messengers have been identified as mediated by the hydrolysis of phospholipids (e.g., insulin, norepinephrine, serotonin, vasopressin, thrombin, growth factors, and cytokines).

Choline is critical for lipid metabolism because phosphatidylcholine is a component of very low density lipoproteins (VLDLs). VLDLs are the major vehicle for transporting the triglycerides synthesized in the liver. Adequate choline must be available for the liver to form VLDLs, or triglyceride accumulation in the liver occurs.

Choline's role in methyl group metabolism is through its metabolite, betaine, which serves as a methyl donor in the formation of methionine from homocysteine. Choline metabolism is linked to folate and vitamin B_6 metabolism, the other major mechanism for methyl group donation. Disturbances in folate or methionine metabolism result in changes in choline metabolism and vice versa.

Dietary Choline and Choline Deficiency

Free choline or choline-containing esters are present in a wide variety of foods in the diet, and the usual intake of such compounds by humans is probably about 700–1000 mg per day. There is no recommended dietary allowance for choline for humans, but intakes of 500 mg/day result in decreased plasma choline and phosphatidylcholine concentrations. The human body (reference 70-kg man) contains about 500 mg of free choline and 30 g of choline esters. Diets deficient in choline produce liver dysfunction within 3 weeks, resulting in massive triglyceride accumulation in the liver and increases in plasma concentrations of liver enzymes. Dietary deficiency of choline also produces changes in muscle conduction velocity on electromyography, and choline-deficient animals are more sensitive to the effects of administered acetylcholine. Finally, choline is the only single nutrient for which dietary deficiency is associated with the development of cancer. Choline-deficient rats have an increased incidence of hepatocellular malignancy and are much more sensitive to the effects of administered carcinogens.

Potential Areas of Clinical and Military Interest

Choline should be of interest to the military for several reasons, relating to its diversity of functions in the body. Soldiers who are active in the field frequently are given high calorie meals. Although studies have shown that the average calorie intake actually decreases in the field, those soldiers who increase their caloric intakes may be at risk of developing liver abnormalities, particularly fatty liver. This phenomenon can be prevented by adding choline or choline-containing products to the diet. Likewise, injured individuals who require total parenteral nutrition (TPN) may develop liver function abnormalities, since choline in TPN formulas is present only as phosphatidylcholine in the lipid emulsion. Malnourished soldiers who are given high-calorie TPN formulations may require extra choline (such as lecithin supplements) to prevent hepatic steatosis and liver function abnormalities.

Choline deficiency reduces muscle performance, and there is evidence that choline supplements may enhance performance. Supplementation (2.8 g) with dietary choline during a 20-mile (32-km) run prevented the drop in plasma choline concentrations usually seen and improved run time by 5 minutes (Sandage et al., 1992). Additional placebo-controlled, randomized, double-blind trials are needed to determine whether choline supplementation will enhance the performance of military personnel in the field.

Choline supplementation enhances memory and reaction time in animals, particularly aging animals, and enhances memory in humans (Bartus et al., 1980; Meck et al., 1989). The mechanisms of this are unclear, but increases in dendritic spines in the cerebral cortexes of aging mice suggest that choline may alter the anatomy of brain cells (Bertoni-Freddari et al., 1985; Mervis et al., 1985). An increase in muscarinic receptor density in the brain also has been suggested, as has acetylcholine content. Alterations in brain function may occur via changes in phospholipid biosynthesis that alter brain membrane composition and structure. These observations suggest that research should be done to determine whether choline supplementation enhances intellectual performance in the field.

Since choline and vitamin B_6 are critical for methyl group metabolism and folate metabolism and acts as a messenger for some growth factors, protein synthesis is dependent on adequate choline status. Wound healing is delayed in choline-deficient animals. Additional research is indicated to determine whether choline supplementation enhances wound healing in injured soldiers, particularly in injured individuals who are malnourished. Also, since choline deficiency alters the immune response, this may affect wound healing and recovery from injury or illness in the field.

In summary, basic studies to evaluate the mechanisms of action of choline in altering signal transduction may point the way to future clinical studies on improvement of both muscle and intellectual performance. Some studies of injury and injury in malnourished individuals would better be done in animals initially.

Caffeine

The literature on the effects of cafeine on behavior, performance, and health is extensive and somewhat contradictory (for reviews see for example Bergman and Dews, 1987; Graham, 1987; Hughes et al., 1988; Jarvis, 1993; Smith et al., 1994a,b). David Penetar and colleagues (Chapter 20) present a new study on the effects of caffeine on cognitive performance, mood, and alertness in human subjects who had been sleep deprived, and summarize current knowledge about the use of such supplements. Caffeine is known to exert its central nervous system-mediated effects by blockade of adenosine receptors. Its stimulant effects when compared with those of other drugs such as amphetamines are weak, but most studies to date suggest that it tends to delay sleep, reduce the deterioration of performance associated with fatigue and boredom, and decrease steadiness of the hands, particularly when performance is already partially degraded on repetitive, nonintellectual tasks.

Less well understood are the effects of caffeine in reversing changes caused by sleep deprivation. To clarify these issues, three doses of caffeine (150, 300, and 600 mg/70 kg of body weight) were assessed among normal healthy males after 2 days of sleep deprivation. Cognitive performance, mood, alertness, vital signs, serum caffeine concentrations, and plasma catecholamine levels were also assessed.

Cognitive performance was measured using a computerized assessment battery. Choice reaction time (for 8 hours), sustained attention (for 10 hours), and logical reasoning (for 12 hours) significantly improved after caffeine administration, although tests of code substitution and immediate and delayed recall were unaffected.

Mood was assessed by ratings on a profile of mood states questionnaire. Significant increases in vigor were reported for 2 hours after taking the dose, with decreases in fatigue and confusion. Also, significant improvements in mood for 2 hours postdose were reported on visual analog scales for increased alertness, confidence, energy level, and talkativeness and decreased sleepiness. However, anxiety and jitteryness/nervousness also increased. At 12 hours postadministration, ratings for increased energy levels, decreased sleepiness, and jitteryness/nervousness remained elevated.

Alertness, assessed by the modified multiple sleep latency test, also improved for 4.5 hours after caffeine administration, with alertness returning to 50 percent of rested levels when the highest doses were used. Oral body temperature remained elevated for 12 hours and blood pressure (diastolic) for one hour, but neither heart rate nor systolic blood pressure were elevated.

It was concluded that large doses of caffeine reversed sleep deprivation-induced degradation in cognitive performance, mood, and alertness without serious side effects. These data were consistent with those represented in most other studies reviewed. Therefore, Penetar et al. (Chapter 20) recommended that caffeine be included in rations at 250 mg per tablet and that it be made available to soldiers for maintaining performance during specific military operations. The authors did not study individuals with habitually high levels of caffeine ingestion; it would be useful to determine whether the effects of the doses of 300–600 mg noted in this study were as pronounced in individuals with markedly higher levels of typical intakes.

Sustaining optimal soldier performance is recognized to depend on other measures as well. The first is training, so that tasks can be performed with a minimal level of cognitive effort, cross-training so that individuals can substitute for each other, developing and adhering to appropriate work and rest cycles, exerting wise leadership so that unnecessary demands are not placed on subordinates, and modification of systems to minimize errors. Second, enforcing sleep discipline so that the sleep-deprived individual sleeps as much as he or she can and in as a hygienic manner as possible.

The relationship between caffeine intake and health outcomes particularly cancer incidence, cardiovascular disease (CVD), and effects on fertility, and pregnancy and child outcome, has been the focus of many studies. While data from individual studies has been contradictory, reviews tend to conclude that there is no significant association or negligible/transient effects relating moderate caffeine consumption and cancer, CVD, fertility, and osteoporosis (see for example AMAC, 1984; Cooper et al., 1992; Gordis, 1990; Joesoef et al., 1990; Johansson et al., 1992; Lubin and Ron, 1990; Olsen, 1991; Rosenberg, 1990; Schairer et al., 1986; Wilson et al., 1989). However, reports continue to demonstate that caffeine intake causes an elevation in blood pressure (Smith et al., 1994a,b). Although the blood pressure elevation produced by caffeine has been interpreted as transient and within the range produced by typical activities (HHS, 1988; Myers, 1988), blood pressure bears monitoring in any future studies of performance enhancement with caffeine supplementation. Recent reports that assessed the safety of caffeine consumption during pregnancy have continued to produce conflicting information (Eskenazi, 1993; Infante-Rivard et al., 1993; Mills et al., 1993). These data indicate that high levels of caffeine intake (>300 mdg/d) potentially increases the risk of spontaneous abortion and intrauterine growth retardation during pregnancy (Mills et al., 1993). The risk to pregnant women of low levels of caffeine intake is uncertain. Further, women often do not realize they are pregnant and/or do not receive prenatal care until after the time period when most spontaneous abortions occur. Should the Army pursue further research in performance enhancement using caffeine products, these health issues must be carefully considered.

In summary, continued research on the mechanisms for the evident effects of caffeine on cognitive performance, mood, and alertness and how these may be enhanced in combination with other dietary measures is warranted. Of particular interest is how to maximize positive effects when performance is already degraded. Individual differences, expectancy, and placebo effects need further elucidation. In the meantime, practical applications of demonstrated effects in ration planning may be in order.

Carnitine

In Chapter 21 Peggy R.Borum reviews the current evidence on whether administration of carnitine enhances physical performance. Carnitine, (ß-hydroxy-τ-trimethylammonium butyrate) is a minor nitrogenous compound in muscle that plays a critical role in energy metabolism. Carnitine functions as a transportable high-energy compound that can be reformed without the use of ATP. It acts as a storehouse of high energy compounds, stimulates fatty acid oxidation, transports acyloenzyme A (acyl-COA) across membranes, prevents the accumulation of lactate, and stimulates carbohydrate and amino acid utilization. These functions have led to the hypothesis that supplementation of free carnitine, acetylcarnitine, or propionylcarnitine theoretically might enhance the oxidation of fatty acids during exercise, thus sparing the use of muscle glycogen, delaying the onset of fatigue, and enhancing exercise performance. Today, research is hindered by the lack of a simple method that permits measurement of the various acylcarnitines in large numbers of samples.

Originally, carnitine was called vitamin B-T because it was essential for a mealworm; present evidence is that it is not a vitamin for healthy humans, and there is no Recommended Dietary Allowance for it (National Research Council, 1989). In humans, a rare inborn error of carnitine metabolism is associated with muscle fatigue. Carnitine deficiency may also occur secondary to other pathologies. Most Americans consume 50–100 mg of carnitine per day in their diets, with some eating three times that amount. Carnitine appears to be safe, but there is little evidence that more is better in normal individuals.

Clearly, carnitine is important metabolically in the exercising muscle. However, existing studies of carnitine supplementation differ in their reported effects, depending on the training or conditioning of the subject; the intensity of exercise; and the type, dose, timing, and route of supplement administration employed. The forms of carnitine used in supplementation studies vary. Most investigations have used free carnitine, but the uptake of the various acylcarnitines as opposed to free carnitine may differ from organ to organ. In studies of carnitine supplements on exercise performance, the amounts used are several times higher than usual dietary intakes of the substance. The absorption of pharmacological doses of carnitine may differ from that of lower doses. The time between carnitine supplementation and exercise has also varied in studies to date. The intensity of exercise also alters muscle metabolism, and it appears to affect carnitine metabolism in muscles. In addition, physical training alters many aspects of muscle metabolism, including that of carnitine.

Few changes are observed with low-intensity exercise, but with high-intensity exercise after the point at which elevated plasma lactate concentrations are first observed and below the individual's maximal work capacity, the free carnitine concentration decreases and the short-chain acylcarnitine concentration increases (Hiatt et al., 1989). These changes persist into recovery after exercise. In contrast to muscle, changes in the type and amount of carnitine in plasma are relatively slight during or after exercise (Hiatt et al., 1989). Training affects nutrient utilization in muscle during exercise, and these changes include increased free fatty acid oxidation during prolonged exercise. There is evidence in isolated intact mitochondria in human muscle preparations that pyruvate oxidation increases when L-carnitine is present in the medium and that it decreases when either inhibitors of pyruvate or carnitine are added (Uziel et al., 1988). Human subjects performing maximal exercise tests on bicycle ergometers have been studied with 2g supplements of L-carnitine or placebos, and increases in both plasma lactate and pyruvate levels with maximal exercise were lower after carnitine administration throughout the trial, with greater or equal work accomplished, although returns to baseline concentrations of lactate were the same in both groups (Siliprandi et al., 1990).

Other evidence in humans suggests that carnitine supplementation may modestly increase the use of fatty acids during exercise. Carnitine supplementation may preserve the available coenzyme A pool. Carnitine supplementation prior to exercise increases work output in maximal exercise tests in some, but not all, studies (Oyono-Enguelle et al., 1988; Vecchiet et al., 1990). Exercise may also alter metabolic compartmentalization of carnitine and acylcarnitine in muscle during and after exercise, with free carnitine falling and short-chain carnitine rising (Decombaz et al., 1992). However, in the same study, which did not employ carnitine supplementation, there was little evidence that endurance conditioning had an effect on skeletal muscle carnitine concentrations, nor were there correlations between total carnitine concentration in muscle at rest and finishing time or between muscle carnitine and maximal aerobic power or duration of training. In another study, following carnitine supplementation for 5 days, the ratio of acylated to free carnitine increased from preexercise values during exercise and remained elevated for 40 minutes postexercise (Soop et al., 1988).

In summary, while carnitine functions as a transportable high energy compound that can be reformed without the use of ATP, carnitine supplementation has not been demonstrated to improve physical or mental performance in well-nourished individuals. Basic research on the effects of various forms of carnitine in exercise may be in order. These will be facilitated by the development of simple methods that permit measurement of various acylcarnitines in large numbers of samples. There is no conclusive evidence to date that carnitine supplementation is helpful in enhancing physical performance during exercise. The status of carnitine research is such that, at present, no recommendation to increase levels of carnitine in rations are called for.

SAFETY AND REGULATORY ASPECTS OF POTENTIAL PERFORMANCE-ENHANCING FOOD COMPONENTS

Safety of Amino Acids

Military rations exceed the RDAs for protein and the protein source provides an adequate intake of the essential amino acids. Therefore, the supplementation of military rations with amino acids at the usual range of dietary intakes would not be expected to improve performance. Amino acid intakes at several times the usual dietary intakes must be evaluated for safety as well as effects on performance. Several of the chapters address the use of tyrosine supplements to enhance performance. Such use is pharmacological rather than nutritional and therefore presents different concerns with regard to safety. In Chapter 22, Timothy J.Maher discusses the recent issue associated with supplements of L-tryptophan. In this incident, the occurrence of eosinophilia-myalgia syndrome (EMS) was associated with the use of L-tryptophan supplements. It was subsequently shown that the induction of EMS was associated with one or more impurities in one particular product and was not the result of L-tryptophan ingestion per se. Nonetheless, this experience raised safety concerns about the use of amino acid supplements specifically and more generally the use of all nutrients as supplements at physiological levels. It is clear that these types of supplements must be highly purified before they can be considered safe for use. The safety of amino acid supplements has been the subject of a recent review by the Life Sciences Research Office (LSRO) of the Federation of American Societies of Experimental Biology (Anderson and Raiten, 1992).

Much research has been published on the important nutritional roles of amino acids as the essential building blocks for proteins and as precursors of other physiologically important compounds such as hormones and neuroactive peptides. These needs are normally met by the quantities of amino acids supplied by ingested foods and are presented to the body as a mixture of many amino acids. These levels of exposure are generally recognized as presenting no safety concerns. However, amino acid supplements, particularly methionine and lysine, can provide much greater quantities of single amino acids, which raises the potential of direct toxic effects or the possibility of creating "imbalances" of amino acids that could have deleterious consequences.

Amino acid supplements proved to be a boon in poultry and swine production by permitting the upgrading of low-quality plant proteins to allow for maximal growth rates. In these circumstances the exposure levels were of the same order of magnitude as expected from normal diets, and the likelihood of toxicities or imbalances was nil. More recently, over-the-counter (OTC) availability of amino acid supplements and their potential use in pharmacological quantities have created concern. The LSRO report (Anderson and Raiten, 1992) reviews in detail the literature on animal and human studies that can shed light on the safety of supplements. It is clear from the LSRO report that many amino acids can have toxicological effects, that there is a paucity of information to establish safe use levels for individual amino acid supplements, and that there is adequate evidence to raise concern about certain vulnerable population groups.

One of the amino acids that was discussed at length during this workshop and that forms the basis for this report is tyrosine, which was reported to have beneficial effects in response to stress by virtue of its role as a precursor for catecholamines. Tyrosine appears to be well tolerated by rats consuming a high-protein diet, but in animals fed low-protein diets, a distinct syndrome is observed involving cataracts, skin lesions, and histopathological changes (Anderson and Raiten, 1992).

In summary, the available evidence, while inadequate to establish safety, does raise concerns about the indiscriminate use of amino acid supplements. These data make it clear that before advocating any use of supplements, appropriate safety studies should be conducted. The LSRO, in its report (Anderson and Raiten, 1992), has proposed a two-tiered approach to animal testing for individual amino acids or mixtures of amino acids. Human clinical studies were also recommended by LSRO, again involving a two-tiered approach (see Anderson and Raiten, 1992). These recommendations represent a sound starting point for establishing the safe use of amino acid supplements.

Regulation of Food Components by the U.S. Food and Drug Administration[1]

The considerations for the approval of food additives are well developed by John E.Vanderveen in Chapter 23. The most important consideration is the demonstrated safety of the material in question. The general approach to demonstrating safety is delineated in the U.S. Food and Drug Administration's (FDA) Red Book[2]. A further consideration is the matter of whether the uses considered during the CMNR workshop in November, 1992 represent usage as a "food" or as a "drug." Different regulations control each class of materials. Further, if a substance is classified as a "drug," then not only must safety be demonstrated but data showing efficacy must also be presented.

It would seem critical for the military to follow the same requirements that the FDA would require for general use in the civilian population. Therefore, in considering any of the materials that have been discussed as agents capable of enhancing performance, it is important to recognize that none of these materials has been demonstrated to be "safe," notwithstanding the fact that all of these agents exist in natural foods. Importantly, the proposed uses (to enhance performance) require exposure levels that are in excess of what would be consumed in foods.

It would seem that the intended uses as performance enhancers, with the exception of candy bars or CHO supplements, would classify the compounds in question in the drug category. The testing requirements are not necessarily more stringent for a drug, in fact, as noted by John E.Vanderveen, a drug classification permits a benefit-risk consideration that is not possible for a food category consideration. Thus, it would be necessary to generate data demonstrating minimal risk from the expected exposures and data clearly demonstrating a benefit from the proposed doses.

---

[1] The views expressed in this section reflect the policy of the Food and Drug Administration at the time of the CMNR workshop in November, 1992. In the future, the policy may be revised to meet legislative mandates or public health needs.

[2] This document is currently under revision. On March 29, 1993 the FDA issued a notice (58 FR 16536) announcing the availability for comment of a draft revision of *Toxicological Principles for the Safety Assessment of Direct Food Additives and Color Additives Used in Food.*

SUMMARY

The increasing sophistication of weapon systems and the complexity of military operations place heavy demands on the soldier to effectively use these systems in military operations. Although thorough training can prepare the individual for effective use of these systems, these sophisticated weapons and the associated training do not eliminate and, in fact, may not reduce the physical demands on the individual soldier in combat. Also, although computers and other information processing aids may help the soldier to process information for effective decision making, the consequences of errors in cognition are multiplied. Therefore, maintaining or enhancing physical and mental performance of the individual engaged in combat is an important objective and deserves a major effort in the identification and evaluation of systems for delivery of those components that pass the rigorous tests for enhancing performance. Although the November 1992 workshop and this report form a good starting point in the selective evaluation of nutrients or food components, it is important that there be a continuing evaluation of the basic nutrition, biochemical, and neuroscience research literature to further identify possible candidates for evaluation. In the following chapter, the CMNR discusses the specific evaluation of the nutrients or components covered in this workshop and makes recommendations for their evaluation. Future research recommendations are also presented.

REFERENCES

AMAC American Medical Association's Council on Scientific Affairs 1984 Cafffeine labeling, a report on the safety of dietary caffeine. JAMA 252:803–806.

Anderson, S.A., and D.J.Raiten, eds. 1992 Safety of Amino Acids Used as Dietary Supplements. Bethesda, Md.: Life Sciences Research Office.

Army Science Board 1991 Soldier as a System. 1991 Summer Study Final Report. Assistant Secretary of the Army Research, Development and Acquisition. Washington, D.C.: U.S. Department of the Army.

Banderet, L.E., and H.R.Lieberman 1989 Treatment with tyrosine, a neurotransmitter precursor, reduces environmental stress in humans. Brain Res. Bull. 22(4):759–762.

Banderet, L.E., J.W.Stokes, R.Francesconi, D.M.Kowal, and P.Naitoh 1981 Artillery teams in simulated sustained combat: Performance and other measures. Pp. 581–604 in Department of Health and Human Services National Institute for Occupational Safety and Health Report 81–127: The Twenty-Four Hour Workday: Proceedings of a Symposium on Variations in Work-Sleep Schedules, L.C.Johnson, D.I.Tepas, W.P Colquhon, and M.J Colligan, eds. Washington, D.C.: U.S. Government Printing Office.

Bartus, R.T., R.L.Dean, J.A.Goas, and A.S.Lippa 1980 Age-related changes in passive avoidance retention: modulation with dietary choline. Science 209:301–303.

Beisel, W.R. 1991 Nurition and infection. Pp. 507–542 in Nutritional Biochemistry and metabolism, 2nd ed., M.C.Linder, ed. New York: Elsevier.

Beisel, W.R., B.B.Morgan, Jr., P.J.Bartelloni, G.D.Coates, F.R.DeRubertis, and E.A.Alluisi 1974 Symptomatic therapy in viral illness. A controlled study of effects on work performance. J. Am. Med. Assoc. 228:581–587.

Beisel, W.R., R.F.Goldman, and R.J.T.Joy 1968 Metabolic balance studies during induced hyperthermia in man. J. Appl. Physiol. 24:1–10.

Bergman, J., and P.B.Dews 1987 Dietary cafeine and its toxicity. In J.Hathcock (ed.) Nutritional Toxicology. New York: Academic Press.

Birch, L.L., J.Billman, and S.S.Richards 1984 Time of day influences food acceptability. Appetite 5:109–116.

Blundell, J.E. 1986 Serotonin manipulations and the structure of feeding behaviour. Appetite Supl. 7: 39–56.

Bonnet, M.H. 1987 Sleep restoration as a function of periodic awakening, movement, or electroencephalographic change. Sleep 10:364–373.

Booth, D.A. 1987 Central dietary "Feedback onto nutrient selection": Not even a scientific hypothesis. Appetite 8:195–201.

Booth, D.A. E.L.Gibson, and B.J.Baker 1986 Gastromotor mechanism of fenfluramine anorexia. Appetite Suppl. 7:57–69.

Cardello, A.V., and F.M.Sawyer 1992 Human dietary responses to covert manipulations of energy, fat, and carbohydrate in a midday meal. Am. J. Clin. Nutr. 56:36–43.

Carraro, F., K.Samuel, J.I.Rosenblatt, and R.R.Wolfe 1989 Effect of dichloroacetate on lactate concentration in exercising humans. J. Appl. Physiol. 66:591–597.

Cooper, C., E.J.Atkinson, H.W.Wahner, W.M.O'Fallon, B.L.Riggs, H.L.Judd, and L.J.Melton 1992 Is caffeine consumption a risk factor for osteoporosis? J. Bone & Min. Res. 7:465–471.

de Castro, J.M., and E.M.Brewer 1991 The amount eaten in meals by humans is a power function of the number of people present. Physiol. Behav. 51:121–125.

Decombaz, J., B.Gmuender, G.Sierro, and P.Cerretelli 1992 Muscle carnitine after strenuous endurance exercise. J. Appl. Physiol. 72:423–427.

Diaz, E., G.R.Goldberg, M.Taylor, J.M.Savage, D.Sellen, W.A.Coward, and A.M.Prentice 1991 Effects of dietary supplementation on work performance in Gambian laborers. Am. J. Clin. Nutr. 53:803–811.

Dishman, R.K. 1989 Psychology of sports competition. Pp. 129–164 in Sports Medicine, A.J.Ryan and F.L.Allman, Jr., eds. New York: Academic Press.

Dollins, A.B., L.P.Krock, W.F.Storm, and H.R.Lieberman 1990 Tyrosine decreases physiological stress caused by lower body negative pressure (LBNP). Aviat. Space Environ. Med. 61:491

Dunn, A.J. 1988 Stress-related elevation of cerebral dopamergic systems. Ann, N.Y. Acad. Sci. 537: 188–205.

Engell, D. 1992 Sensory influences on meal consumption. Rose Marie Pangborn Memorial Symposium. August 2–6, Jarvenpaa, Finland.

Engell, D., F.M.Kramer, S.Luther, and S.Adams 1990 Sensory influences on food intake. Presented at the Society for Nutrition Education 1990 Annual Meeting, Anaheim, Calif.

Eskenazi, B. 1993 Caffeine during pregnancy: grounds for concern? JAMA 270:2973–2974.

Fernstrom, J.D. 1987 Food-induced changes in brain serotonin synthesis: Is there a relationship to appetite for specific macronutrients? Appetite 8:163–182.

Fernstrom, J.D. 1990 Aromatic amino acids and monoamine synthesis in the central nervous system: Influence of the diet. J. Nutr. Biochem. 1:508–517.

Food and Drug Administration 1982 Toxicological Principles for the Safety Assessment of Direct Food Additives and Color Additives Used in Food. Washington, D.C.: U.S. Department of Health and Human Services.

Goldman, S.J., C.P.Herman, and J.Polivy 1991 Is the effect of a social model on eating attenuated by hunger? Appetite 17:129–140.

Garattini, S., T.Mennini, C.Bendotti, R.Invernizzi, and R.Samin 1986 Neurochemical mechanism of action of drugs which modify feeding via the serotoninergic system. Appetite Supl. 7:15–38.

Gordis, L. 1990 Consumption of methylxanthine-containing beverages and risk of pancreatic cancer. Cancer Letters 52:1–12.

Graham, D.M. 1978 Caffeine-Its identity, dietary sources, intake and biological effects. Nutr. Rev. 36: 97–102.

Gray, J.A. 1987 The Psychology of Fear and Stress. Cambridge: Cambridge University Press.

Hiatt W.R., J.G.Regensteiner, E.E.Wolfel, L.Ruff, and E.P.Brass 1989 Carnitine and acylcarnitine metabolism during exercise in humans. Dependence on skeletal muscle metabolic state. J. Clin. Invest. 84:1167–1173.

Holder, M.D., and G.Huether 1990 Role of prefeedings, plasma amino acid ratios and brain serotonin levels in carbohydrate and protein selection. Physiol. Behav. 47:113–119.

Hughes, J.R., S.T.Higgins, W.K.Bickel, W.K.Hunt, J.W.Fenwick, S.B.Gulliver, and G.C. Mireault 1991 Caffeine self-administration, withdrawal, and adverse effects among coffee drinkers. Archives Gen. Psychiatr. 48:611–617.

Infante-Rivard, C., A.Fernandez, R.Gauthier, D.Michele, and G.E.Rivard 1993 Fetal loss associated with cafeine intake before and during pregnancy. JAMA 270:2940–2943.

Jarvis, M. 1993 Does caffeine intake enhance absolute levels of cognitive performance? Psychopharmacology 110:45–52.

Joesoef, M.R., V.Beral, R.T.Rolfs, S.O.Aral, and D.W.Cramer 1990 Are caffeinated beverages risk factors for delayed conception? The Lancet 335:136– 137.

Johansson, C., D.Mellstrom, U.Lerner, and T.Osterberg 1992 Coffee drinking: a minor risk factor for bone loss and fractures. Age and Aging 21:20–26.

Kanerek, R.B., and D.Swinney 1990 Effects of food snacks on cognitive performance in male students. Appetite 14:15–27

Kramer, F.M, K.Rock, and D.Engell 1992 Effects of time of day and appropriateness on food intake and hedonic ratings at morning and mid-day. Appetite 18:1–13.

Lehnert, H., D.K.Reinstein, B.W.Strowbridge, and R.J.Wurtman 1984 Neurochemical and behavioral consequences of acute, uncontrollable stress: effects of dietary tyrosine. Brain Res. 303:215–223.

Levine, E.S., W.J.Litto, and B.L.Jacobs 1990 Activity of cat locus coeruleus noradrenergic neurons during the defense reaction. Brain res. 531:189–195.

Lieberman H.R. 1989 Cognitive effects of various food constituents. In Handbook of the Psychophysiology of Human Eating. R.Shepherd, ed. (Chap.11). New York: John Wiley & Sons.

Lieberman, H.R., B.Spring, and G.S.Garfield 1986a The behavioral effects of food constituents: Strategies used in studies of amino acids, protein, carbohydrate and caffeine. Nutr. Rev. 44 (May suppl):61–69.

Lieberman H.R., J.J.Wurtman, and B.Chew 1986b Changes in mood after carbohydrate consumption among obese individuals. Am. J. Clin. Nutr. 44:772–778.

Lubin, F. and E.Ron 1990 Consumption of methylxanthine-containing beverages and the risk of breast cancer. Cancer letters 53:81–90.

Marriott, B.M., and C.Rosemont 1991 Fluid Replacement and Heat Stress. Report of the Committee on Military Nutrition Research, Food and Nutrition Board, Institute of Medicine. Washington, D.C.: National Academy Press.

McNally, R.E., A.M.Machovec, D.T.Ellzy, and S.R.Hursh 1989 SAOC Contract No. MDA903–99-D-1000: Evaluation of Sleep Discipline in Sustaining Unit Performance. McLean, Va.: Science Applications International Corporation.

Meck, W.H., R.A.Smith, and C.L.Williams 1989 Organizational changes in cholinergic activity and enhanced visuospatial memory as a function of choline administered prenatally or postnatally or both. Behav. Neurosci. 103:1234–1241.

Meiselman, H.L., E.S.Hirsch, and R.D.Popper 1988 Sensory, hedonic and situational factors in food acceptance and consumption. Pp. 77–87 in Food Acceptability, D.M.H.Thomson, ed. London: Elsevier Applied Science.

Mervis, R., L.Horrocks, P.Demediuk, L.Wallace, D.R.Meyer, S.Beall, K.Caris, and E.Naber 1985 Neurobehavioral effects of chronic choline-containing diets on the adult and aging C57BL/6NNIA mouse brain. Ann. N.Y. Acad. Sci. 444:469–470.

Mills, J.L., L.B.Holmes, J.H.Aarons, J.L.Simpson, Z.A.Brown, L.G.Jovanovic-Peterson, M.R. Conley, B.I.Graubard, R.h.Knopp, and B.E.Metzger 1993 Moderate cafeine use and the risk of spontaneous abortion and intrauterine growth retardation. JAMA 269:593–597.

Moore, R.J., K.E.Friedl, T.R.Kramer, L.E.Martinez-Lopez, R.W.Hoyt, R.T.Tulley, J.P.DeLany, E.W.Askew, and J.A.Vogel 1992 Changes in soldier nutritional status and immune function during the Ranger training course. Technical Report No. T13–92. Natick, Mass.: U.S. Army Research Institute of Environmental Medicine

Myers, G. 1988 Effects of caffeine on blood pressure. Archives Int. Med. 148:1189–1193. National Commission on Sleep Disorders Research

1993 Wake up America: A National Sleep Alert, Volume 1: Executive Summary and Executive Report, submitted to the U.S. Congress and to the Secretary, U.S. Department of Health and Human Services, January 1993. Washington, D.C. 76 pp.

National Research Council 1989 Recommended Dietary Allowances, 10th Edition. A Report of the Subcommittee on the Tenth Edition of the RDAs, Food and Nutrition Board, Commission on Life Sciences, Washington, D.C.: National Academy Press.

Olsen, J. 1991 Cigarette smoking, tea and coffee drinking and subfecundity. Amer. J. Epidemiol. 133:734–739.

Opstad, P.K. 1992 Androgenic hormones during prolonged physical stress, sleep, and energy deprivation. J. Clin. Endocrinol. 74:1176–1183.

1991 Alterations in the morning plasma levels of hormones and the endocrine responses to bicycle exercise during prolonged strain. The significance of energy and sleep deprivation. Acta Endocrinol. (Copenhagen) 125:14–22.

Opstad, P.K., and A.Aakvaag 1981 The effect of a high calorie diet on hormonal changes in young men during prolonged physical strain and sleep deprivation. Eur. J. Appl. Physiol. 46:31–39.

1982 Decreased serum levels of oestradiol, testosterone, and prolactin during prolonged physical strain and sleep deprivation, and the influence of a high calorie diet. Eur. J. Appl. Physiol. 49:343–348.

1983 The effect of sleep deprivation on the plasma levels of hormones during prolonged physical strain and calorie deficiency. Eur. J. Appl. Physiol. 51:97–107.

Opstad, P.K., A.Aakvaag, and T.O.Rognum 1980 Altered hormonal response to short-term bicycle exercise in young men after prolonged physical strain, caloric deficit, and sleep deprivation. Eur. J. Appl. Physiol. 45:51–62.

Opstad, P.K., D.Falch, O.Øktedalen, F.Fonnum, and R.Wergeland 1984 The thyroid function in young men during prolonged exercise and the effect of energy and sleep deprivation. Clin. Endocrinol. 20:657–669.

Opstad, P.K., O.Øktedalen, A.Aarvaag, F.Fonnum, and P.K.Lund 1985 Plasma renin activity and serum aldosterone during prolonged physical strain. Eur. J. Appl. Physiol. 54:1–6.

Oyono-Enguelle, S., H.Freund, C.Ott, M.Gartner, A.Heitz, J.Marbach, F.Maccari, A.Frey, H.Bigot, and A.C.Bach 1988 Prolonged submaximal exercise and L-carnitine in humans. Eur. J. Appl. Physiol. 58:53–61.

Random House 1982 The Random House College Dictionary. New York: Random House.

Rauch, T.M., and H.R.Lieberman 1990 Pre-treatment with tyrosine reverses hypothermia induced behavioral depression. Brain Res. Bull. 24:147–150.

Rolls, B.J., A.E.Andersen, T.H.Moran, A.L.McNelis, H.C.Baier, and I.C.Fedoroff 1992 Food intake, hunger, and satiety after preloads in women with eating disorders. Am. J. Clin. Nutr. 55:1093–1103.

Rosenberg, L. 1990 Coffee and tea consumption inrelation to the risk of large bowel cancer: A review of epidemiologic studies. Cancer Letters 52:163–171.

Sandage, B.W., R.N.Sabounjian, R.White, and R.J.Wurtman 1992 Choline citrate may enhance athletic performance. Physiologist 35:236a.

Schairer, C., L.Brinton, and R.Hoover 1986 Methylxanthines and benign breast cancer. Amer. J. Epdemiol. 124:603–611.

Schneider, S.H., P.M.Komansky, M.N.Goodman, and N.B.Ruderman 1981 Dichloroacetate: Effects on exercise endurance in untrained rats. Metabolism 30:590–595.

Selye, H. 1946 General adaptation syndrome and diseases of adaptation. J. Clin. Endocrinol. & Metab. 6:117–230.

Shor-Posner G., J.A.Grinker, C.Marineaux, O.Brown, and S.F.Leibowitz 1986 Hypothalamic serotonin in the control of meal patterns and diet selection. Brain Res. Bull. 17:681–689.

Siliprandi, N., F.Di Lisa, G.Pieralisi, P.Ripari, F.Maccari, R.Menabo, M.A.Giamberardino, and L.Vecchiet 1990 Metabolic changes induced by maximal exercise in human subjects following L-carnitine administration. Biochim. Biophys. Acta 1034:17–21.

Simon, E., G.Frenkel, and P.F.Kraicer 1972 Blockage of insulin secretion by mannoheptulose. Isr. J. Med. Sci. 8:743–752.

Smith, A., A.Kendrick, and A.Maben 1994a Effects of breakfast and caffeine on cognitive performance, mood, and cardiovascular functioning. Appetite 22:39–55.

Smith, A., A.Maben, and P.Brockman 1994b Effects of evening meals and caffeine on cognitive performance, mood and cardiovascular functioning. Appetite 22:57–65.

Soop, M, O.Bjorkman, G.Cederblad, L.Hagenfeldt, and J.Wahren 1988 Influence of carnitine supplementation on muscle substrate and carnitine metabolism during exercise. J. Appl. Physiol. 64:2394–2399.

Spring, B., R.Pingitore, M.Bourgeois, K.Kessler, and E.Bruckner 1992 The effects and non-effects of skipping breakfast: The results of three studies. Presented at the Annual Meeting of the American Psychological Association, Washington, D.C.

Stanford, C., M.Fillenz, and E.Ryan 1984 The effect of repeated mild stress on cerebral cortical adrenoceptors and noradrenaline synthesis in the rat. Neurosci. Lett. 45:163–167.

Sutton, J.R., N.L.Jones, and C.J.Toews 1976 Growth hormone secretion in acid-base alterations at rest and during exercise. Clin. Sci. 50:241–247.

Teff, K.L., S.N.Young, L.Marchand, and M.I.Botez. 1989 Acute effect of protein or carbohydrate breakfasts on human cerebrospinal fluid monoamine precursor and metabolite levels. J. Neurochem. 52:235–241.

Thierry, A.M., F.Javoy, J.Glowinski, and S.S.Kety 1968 Effects of stress on the metabolism of norepinephrine, dopamine, and serotonin in the central nervous system of the rat. I. Modifications of norepinephrine turnover. J. Pharmacol. Exp. Ther. 163:163–171.

Thomas, M, H.Sing, G.Belenky, D.Thorne, T.Balkin, D.Penetar, D.Redmond, J.Norcross, P.Newhouse, H.Mayberg, H.Holcomb, B.Sadzot, R.Dannals, J.Links, and H.Wagner 1988 Positron emission tomography measurement of human regional cerebral glucose utilization following 48 hours of sleep deprivation. Soc. Neurosci. Abstr. 14:48.

Thorne, D.R., S.G.Genser, H.C.Sing, and F.W.Hegge 1983 Plumbing human performance limits during 72 hours of high task load. Pp. 17–40 in Proceedings of the 24th DRG Seminar on the Human as a Limiting Element in Military Systems. Toronto: Defence and Civil Institute of Environmental Medicine.

Torda, T., I.Yamaguchi, F.Hirata, I.J.Kopin, and J.Axelrod 1981 Mepacrine treatment prevents immobilization-induced desensitization of beta-adrenergic receptors in rat hypothalamus and brain stem. Brain Res. 205:441–444.

U.S. Department of Health and Human Services 1988 The Surgeon General's Report on Nutrition and Health, Washington, D.C.: U.S. Government Printing Office.

Uziel, G., B.Garavaglia, and S.Di Donato 1988 Carnitine stimulation of pyruvate dehydrogenase complex (PDHC) in isolated human skeletal muscle mitochondria. Muscle Nerve 11:720–724.

Vecchiet, L., F.Di Lisa, G.Pieralisi, P.Ripari, R.Menabò, M.A.Giamberardino, and N.Siliprandi 1990 Influence of L-carnitine administration on maximal physical exercise. Eur. J. Appl. Physiol. 61:486–490.

Wilson, P.W.F., R.J.Garrison, W.B.Kannel, D.L.McGee, and W.P.Castelli 1989 Is coffee consumption a contributor to cardiovascular disease? Insights from the Framingham Study. Arch. Int. Med. 149:1169–1172.

Wurtman, R.J. 1983 Behavioral effects of nutrients. Lancet 1:145–147.

1988 Presynaptic control of release of amine neurotransmitters by precursor levels. NIPS (Am. Physiol. Soc.) 3:158–163.

Wurtman, J.J., and R.J.Wurtman 1979 Drugs that enhance central serotoninergic transmission diminish elective carbohydrate consumption by rats. Life Sci. 24:895–904.

Zeisel, S.H. 1988 Vitamin-like molecules. Pp. 440–452 in Modern Nutrition in Health and Disease, M. E.Shils and V.R.Young, eds. Philadelphia: Lea & Febiger.

2

Conclusions and Recommendations

CONCLUSIONS

As stated in Chapter 1, the Committee on Military Nutrition Research (CMNR) was asked to respond to six specific questions dealing with the potential for food components to enhance performance for military personnel in combat settings. The committee's responses to these questions appear below. The committee further reviewed the current knowledge base regarding specific categories of food components that were identified by Army scientists as having potential to enhance performance in light of the classification of ergogenic aids and the mechanisms of action as discussed by John Ivy (Chapter 12). Substances that may optimize physical performance are frequently referred to as ergogenic aids (Chapter 12). These may be divided into five categories: (1) mechanical, (2) psychological, (3) physiological, (4) pharmacological, and (5) nutritional. The mechanisms by which foods or food components may act as ergogenic aids as discussed by Ivy are (1) acting as central or peripheral stimulants, (2) increasing the storage or availability of limiting substrates, (3) acting as a supplemental fuel source, (4) reducing or neutralizing metabolic by-products, and (5) enhancing recovery. Each food component was also reviewed in light of the time frames and military scenarios drawn up by Army scientists (see Appendix A). The recommenda tions and conclusions drawn about the potential for these food components to enhance performance are included in the specific committee recommendations that follow.

GENERAL CONCLUSIONS

General Concepts of Performance Enhancement

The first consideration in maintaining or enhancing performance is to endeavor to insure that troops are in a well-hydrated, rested and well-nourished state-including optimal amounts of all essential micronutrients, plus the best in military training, both physical and mental, in advance of anticipated periods of stress. Under these circumstances performance is unlikely to be improved in the absence of the imposition of military operations which impose physical or mental stress.

Obviously battlefield situations are not free of stress. Under these conditions troops are frequently deprived of sleep, apprehensive, haven't eaten sufficient food to meet their energy expenditures, dehydrated to varying degrees and exposed to environmental extremes of heat, cold, altitude, etc. which impacts on their physical and mental state. Given these conditions, enhancement of performance is more likely to be restoring performance to non-stressed baseline than to improvement over that expected from well-nourished and well-rested troops. The military Science and Technology Objective (STO) of enhancing performance by 10–15 percent is more realistic in short term enhancement of performance under stress than to obtain super performance from troops in a well-fed, well-rested state.

While some of the food components considered in this report may be used at usual dietary levels (caffeine, carbohydrate) others are likely to be at levels of intake that may be considered pharmacological. These components may be provided in operational ration items designed to be used at specific times and provide short-term enhancement through increased vigilance, reduced feeling of fatigue, improved mental state, etc. The enhancement capability of a component likely will have a threshold which must be met to have a benefit and will also likely have a "wear out" when the stimulus can no longer overcome the adverse effect of the stress. In researching the effectiveness and safety of these pharmacological components it will be important to determine these levels and time periods to evaluate both safety and efficacy.

It is also noted that some of these helpful nutritional effects may be maximized by the additional use of conventional over-the-counter drugs that block the intracellular formation of stress-induced prostaglandins, which contribute importantly to many symptoms and the ill effects of stress.

Food Components or Nutrients that Offer Potential to Enhance Performance

The following food components have potential for enhancing performance under certain circumstances that may be encountered in military operations.

- **Carbohydrates.** The role of carbohydrate as a fuel source for extended physical activity is well-known. Increased storage of glycogen prior to extended physical performance through consumption of high-carbohydrate meals and consuming carbohydrates during an extended physical activity as a means of increasing performance is well established. Studies with soldiers in military activities are less clear but likely relate to the more intermittent nature of the physical activity, in comparison with the extended moderate-to high-level physical activities of athletic competition. The value of carbohydrate supplementation in extending physical performance is usually demonstrated after 60–90 minutes of continuous activity at 60 to 70 percent of maximal oxygen uptake $\dot{V}_{O_2\ max}$. Moderate to heavy physical activity of a lesser time period followed by rest or reduced activity does not usually demonstrate a value for carbohydrate supplementation during the activity.

  The potential role for carbohydrates in affecting such behaviors as mood, performance, and satiety, with emphasis placed on sensorimotor and cognitive performance as discussed in Chapter 18, is worthy of further consideration. Mood changes that may affect motivation to operate under stressful conditions are an important consideration. These stressful situations, such as combat, may unmask performance deficits that are not apparent under nonstressful conditions. It also should be emphasized that meals containing protein and carbohydrate demonstrate more beneficial effects than meals that are nearly protein-free. The behavioral effects seen are usually time context dependent. Snacks (providing combinations of protein and carbohydrate) may have utility in enhancing performance between meals. Research in evaluating the benefits of supplemental carbohydrates on performance should include the more subtle evaluations of motivation and coping in addition to the simple cognitive and sensorimotor measures.

  Evaluation should be made of the potential performance-enhancing benefits of supplemental carbohydrate and carbohydrate-containing snacks on physical and cognitive performance, including mood and motivational effects.

- **Caffeine.** Caffeine exerts its central nervous system-mediating effects by blocking adenosine receptors. Its stimulant effects when compared with those of other drugs such as amphetamines are weak, but most studies to date suggest that caffeine tends to delay sleep and reduce the deterioration of performance associated with fatigue and boredom. Caffeine at higher doses reverses sleep deprivation-induced degradation in cognitive performance, mood, and alertness—important considerations in extended military operations in subjects who report low levels of caffeine intake. The principal side effects include nervousness/jitteryness and decreased sleepiness, which may persist for several hours.

Caffeine definitely should be considered in developing performance-enhancing rations or ration components. Caffeine is safe as a component of food at doses required to overcome sleep deprivation and has been included in diets in coffee and many soft drinks. Since many soldiers may not normally drink coffee, a mechanism for including caffeine in another ration component that can be selectively used when the situation requires should be evaluated. It appears that doses of 300–600 mg/70-kg person will achieve the desired stimulus in those nonhabituated to caffeine; additional research needs to be conducted to determine the effects of this level of caffeine in those with higher habitual intakes.

- **Tyrosine.** The amino acid tyrosine is the precursor of the neurotransmitters dopamine, norepinephrine, and epinephrine. Under highly stressful conditions, the availability of tyrosine may be rate limiting for the synthesis of these neurotransmitter products. The observation that the functioning of catecholaminergic neurons can be precursor dependent is the basis for the hypothesis that tyrosine will mitigate the adverse effects of acute stress, because such neurons regulate, in part, the behavioral, cardiovascular, and neuroendocrine consequences of stress.

  A series of studies in animals has demonstrated that the performance decrement observed in highly stressed animals can be restored by tyrosine supplementation. Studies in humans as well as animals suggest that the amino acid tyrosine may have beneficial effects on humans that are subject to acute stressors. The adverse effects of hypoxia, cold, body negative pressure, and psychological stress have been reduced by treatment with tyrosine. Research is needed to define methods of administration and the effective and safe levels of tyrosine required.
- **Choline.** Choline and choline-containing compounds are critical for a wide variety of processes within the body, including acting as a messenger within the cells and as neurotransmitters in the nervous system controlling muscle contraction, providing methyl groups in a variety of intracellular reactions, acting as a component of triglyceride transport, and participating in the immune response. The best-known function of choline is as a component of acetylcholine, an important neurotransmitter.

  Free choline and choline-containing esters are present in a wide variety of foods in the human diet. The usual intake is estimated to be in the range of

200–1,000 mg per day. There is no Recommended Dietary Allowance (RDA) for choline in humans, but intake of 500 mg/day results in decreased plasma choline and phosphatidylcholine concentrations. Diets deficient in choline produce liver dysfunction within 3 weeks, resulting in massive triglyceride accumulation in the liver and abnormalities of plasma levels of liver enzymes.

There is evidence that diets low in choline reduce muscle performance. Dietary choline supplementation of individuals with normal intakes during a 20-mile (32-km) run improved the run time by 5 minutes and prevented the drop in plasma choline levels normally associated with the run. Placebo-controlled, randomized, double-blind trials are needed to determine whether choline supplementation will enhance performance of military personnel undergoing rigorous activity in the field.

Choline supplementation enhances memory and reaction time in animals, particularly aging animals, and enhances memory in humans. Although the mechanisms for this are unclear, there are indications of alterations of the anatomy of brain cells. Carefully controlled laboratory studies with human subjects may suggest field studies to evaluate cognitive performance enhancement in stressful field situations.

With the diversity of functions of choline in the body, there is ample reason for interest in reviewing its possible value in maintaining or enhancing performance of the soldier. Since choline is a normal constituent of many foods and can safely be used at the high usual levels of intake, it is worthy of evaluation to determine whether it may enhance either the physical or the cognitive performance of soldiers who are functioning in a stressful environment.

Other Food Components of Theoretical Importance but Low Probability of Improving Performance

On the basis of a review of information presented at the workshop and review of background materials, it is concluded that the following materials have some theoretical importance but offer a very low probability of demonstrating an improvement in performance under conditions anticipated in military operations.

- **Carnitine.** Carnitine is important metabolically in exercising muscle. Carnitine functions as a transportable high-energy compound that can be reformed without the use of ATP. It acts as a storehouse of high-energy compounds, stimulates fatty acid oxidation, transports acylcoenzyme A (acylCoA) across membranes, prevents the accumulation of lactate, and stimulates carbohydrate and amino acid utilization. These functions have led to the hypotheses that supplementation of free carnitine, acetylcarnitine, orpropionylcarnitine theoretically might enhance the oxidation of fatty acids during exercise, thus sparing the use of muscle glycogen, delaying the onset of fatigue, and enhancing exercise performance.

Most Americans consume 50–100 mg of carnitine per day, with some consuming three times that amount. Carnitine appears to be safe, but there is little evidence to suggest that higher amounts are beneficial to healthy individuals. Carnitine has been extensively researched, and at this time there is no conclusive evidence that carnitine supplementation is helpful in enhancing physical performance during exercise.

Its importance metabolically in exercising muscle indicates that research on its use should be followed. It is not recommended for consideration in military ration development at this time.

- **Structured lipids.** Structured lipids are defined as fats that are synthesized from mixtures of long- and medium-chain fatty acids. Therefore, they are differentiated from typical dietary fats by the presence of medium-chain fatty acids (5–10 carbon atoms). Their potential as a performance-enhancing ingredient is based on the hypothesis that glycogen utilization during exercise may be spared by the rapid oxidation of the medium-chain fatty acids. Since the medium-chain fatty acids in the diet are delivered directly and rapidly to the liver via the portal circulation, their metabolism in the liver produces the ketone bodies acetoacetate and ß-hydroxybutyrate, which would circulate to the muscle and be oxidized, sparing glycogen.

  The nutritional advantages of structured lipids have been demonstrated mostly in individuals with such stresses as burns, trauma, and infection. Research to date has not supported the hypothesis that the supplements of structured lipids will spare glycogen utilization during exercise, which is more closely related to the objective of enhancing physical or mental performance during military operations. In the absence of new data that demonstrate potential in this area, the inclusion of structured lipids in rations or food components for improving performance is not recommended.

ANSWERS TO THE QUESTIONS POSED TO THE COMMITTEE

The committee has answered the six questions posed by the Army in light of the general conclusions described above. These answers are further elaborated in the recommendations that follow.

1. Is enhancement of physical and mental performance in "normal," healthy, young adult soldiers by diet or supplements a potentially fruitful approach, or are there other methods of enhancing performance that have greater potential?

Emphasis should be given to making sure that troops are adequately hydrated and fed prior to military operations. There is little evidence from current nutrition research to suggest that soldiers already consuming nutritionally adequate rations as specified in the Military Recommended Dietary Allowances (MRDAs) will show significantly improved performance when nutritional supplements are added (as differentiated from pharmaceutical levels of some food components). Troops going into operational situations are presumably in good physical condition and have been consuming adequate amounts of military rations to meet their nutrient needs. Individual vitamin and mineral supplements are unlikely to improve performance under these circumstances. Soldiers who have been deprived of adequate food intake for a period under the pressure of military operations would likely benefit from receiving additional food to overcome the caloric deficit before entering another operation. Similarly, if they have been deprived of adequate sleep or rest because of extended physical activity, an opportunity to sleep or physically rest would help restore performance to normal levels.

Stimulants such as caffeine may help in the short term to overcome the effects of physical and mental fatigue when continuous operations are required.

2. The Army Science and Technology Objective (STO) states: By FY98 demonstrate a 10–15 percent enhancement of soldier performance in selected combat situations through the use of rations/nutrients that enhance caloric utilization and/or optimize the physiological levels of neurotransmitters. (Army Science Board, 1991).

Is the level of enhancement identified in this STO reasonable with the current scientific knowledge?

The Army Science and Technology Objective (STO) of demonstrating a 10–15 percent enhancement of performance through specific ration or nutrient consumption by Fiscal Year 1998 is overly optimistic, particularly if this is expected as enhancement over the level achieved by normal, well-fed, physically fit soldiers. However, if enhanced performance is defined as restoring or preventing all or part of the decrease in performance that is usually encountered over extended field operations, then there may be opportunities to achieve this objective.

Current studies of troops in extended field operations show that troops tend to reduce food intake, lose weight, and in some instances dehydrate.

Overcoming these deficits is more likely to maintain performance. Since only modest dehydration will result in reduced performance, ensuring adequate fluid intake offers the best opportunity to overcome potential performance deficits. Adequate food intake to meet caloric needs also will help maintain high levels of performance. Under conditions of extended moderate physical activity, carbohydrate supplementation to maintain muscle glycogen levels can extend the ability to perform at this activity level. Simply eating frequent meals may accomplish this. Stimulants such as caffeine may also temporarily maintain physical and cognitive performance.

3. Which food components, if any, would be the best candidates to enhance military physical and mental performance?

Food components that would help provide energy sources to large muscles would be most likely to enhance or maintain performance. The proper use of carbohydrate supplements for persons engaged in continuous, moderate physical activity over at least 1.5 to 2 hours has the ability to extend the time to exhaustion. Caffeine has also been demonstrated to improve physical and cognitive performance. Tyrosine may also benefit cognitive performance under certain circumstances. Choline has shown some possible benefit in improving performance over extended periods of physical activity. Studies with marathon athletes need to be carefully reviewed relative to these applications to military operations. Soldiers in military operations seldom are required to perform at a similar continuous level of physical activity and over the extended time period as athletes in marathon events.

4. Should the mode of administration be via fortification of the food in rations, supplemented via a separate food bar or beverage component, or administered in a "vitamin pill mode"? Is palatability a significant issue in this type of supplementation?

The answer to this question depends not only on what food component or individual nutrient is under consideration but also on issues of safety and efficacy that have not yet been addressed. Depending on the circumstances, carbohydrate supplements can be delivered effectively in either beverages or snack bars. Caffeine is currently widely consumed either in beverages or in pill form, as a means of enhancing wakefulness and alertness. It could easily be added to snack bars or food items, but because of adverse reactions to caffeine in some individuals as well as religious proscriptions, this would be less desirable. It is premature to answer the question for individual nutrients such as tyrosine, tryptophan, and choline. Their effectiveness depends on large increases in plasma levels and is reduced when consumed as part of a normal meal containing protein and carbohydrate. Conversely, their safety is likely to be highest when these substances are consumed as supplements to a meal. The safety of these substances as single supplements when given in large enough doses to be effective has not yet been demonstrated.

5. Are there specific ethical issues that need to be considered with this type of research?

The ethical issues depend upon the nature of the enhancement. When the safety of the use of the ration is not an issue, informing the soldiers about the ration and its purpose should suffice.

If the component(s) is used at a pharmacological level, the criteria for evaluating the safety of the component as a drug should be met. Soldiers should be informed of its benefits, and possible side effects and should be educated concerning its condition of use. Research needs to proceed through proper stages of safety and efficacy evaluation before trials on large numbers of troops are conducted. Issues related to ethnicity, gender, and religious beliefs need to be considered, and evaluation and follow-up on any reported adverse or side effects must be conducted.

The best guidelines for this research would be U.S. Food and Drug Administration (FDA) guidelines for research on proposed new drugs.

6. What regulatory issues must be considered with the types of food components that are being evaluated by the Army?

The considerations for the approval of food additives are well developed by John E.Vanderveen in Chapter 23. The most important consideration is the demonstrated safety of the material in question. The general approach to demonstrating safety is well spelled out in the FDA's Red Book (Food and Drug Administration, 1982). A further consideration is the matter of whether the uses considered during this workshop represent usage as a "food" or as a "drug." Different regulations control each class of materials. Further, if a substance is classified as a "drug," then not only must safety be demonstrated but data showing efficacy must also be presented.

It would seem critical for the military to follow the same requirements that the FDA would require for general use of a component in the civilian population. Therefore in considering the components other than caffeine and carbohydrates that have been discussed as agents capable of enhancing performance, it is important to recognize that none of these materials has been demonstrated to be "safe," notwithstanding the fact that all of these agents exist in natural foods at levels required for potential effects. Importantly, the proposed uses (to enhance performance) require exposure levels that are in excess of what would be consumed in foods.

It would seem that the intended uses as performance enhancers would classify the compounds in question in the drug category. The testing requirements are not necessarily more stringent for a drug; in fact, as noted by

Dr. Vanderveen, a drug classification permits a benefit-risk consideration that is not possible for a food category consideration. Thus, it would be necessary to generate data demonstrating minimal risk from the exposures expected and data clearly demonstrating a benefit from the proposed doses.

RECOMMENDATIONS

General

1. On the basis of data presented at the workshop, the Army's prior selection of carbohydrate, caffeine, and tyrosine as food supplements that may enhance performance is fully justified. It is recommended that research with all three should continue.
2. The utility of caffeine in reversing the degradation in cognitive performance, mood, and alertness associated with sleep deprivation that has been widely explored at USARIEM and elsewhere is well understood. It is recommended that future research with this compound explore and attempt to categorize individual differences in responses to caffeine as well as the issue of expectancy and placebo effects.

Recommendations Regarding Food Components Proposed by the Army

On the basis of the papers presented by the invited speakers, discussion at the workshop, and subsequent committee deliberations, the Committee on Military Nutrition Research recommends the following:

1. The following components have clearly demonstrated their ability to enhance performance under appropriate simulated conditions and should be evaluated in appropriate delivery systems.

Caffeine. Caffeine functions as a weak stimulant that, in low doses, tends to delay sleep and reduce the deterioration of performance associated with fatigue and boredom. At higher doses caffeine reverses the sleep deprivation-induced degradation in cognitive performance, mood, and alertness. The long experience with the use of coffee suggests that caffeine is *safe* at levels required to achieve the desired effects, and its effects are reversible over time. **The primary issues that need to be answered in providing caffeine are the appropriate carrier that should be used to provide the supplement and the amount required to achieve the desired benefit in those both**

habituated and nonhabituated to it. Since it would not be desirable to inhibit sleep when operations permit, the timing and availability of the caffeine-containing food component should be evaluated.

Carbohydrate. Carbohydrate is an important fuel source and is particularly important for enhancing extended continuous physical activity. The potential role for carbohydrate in affecting such behaviors as mood, performance, and satiety relating to sensorimotor and cognitive performance has not been as thoroughly evaluated. Many studies have been carried out with carbohydrate supplements, with the major emphasis on physical performance. **The committee recommends that this line of research at USARIEM should be continued. However, emphasis should be shifted to the effect of the macronutrient composition of meals and supplements on the affective domain, including such aspects as mood, perceived fatigue, and motivation.** Hedonic properties and the timing and setting of meals and supplements are important variables to be considered, as are food preferences and aversions related to race, ethnicity, geography, and gender. Carbohydrate-containing snacks, which also provide sufficient protein, should be evaluated as a means of overcoming fatigue and improving mood and performance. Research to evaluate the performance-enhancing potentials of such products should be conducted not only as a means of potentially improving performance in the short term but also as an aid in overcoming some of the caloric deficits usually noted for troops in field operations. It is also suggested that the possibility of providing caffeine in such a product may define a product that could be used in a particularly stressful time to enhance performance.

2. The following components are suggested for further research on the basis of their importance in energy metabolism and/or neurotransmitter actions in the body.

Choline. On the basis of its diverse functions in the body, both in physical performance and in cognitive function, and limited studies demonstrating potentially improved performance in extended physical activity, in cognitive function in animals and humans, and its relative safety, the committee believes that choline should be evaluated for its performance enhancement potential. **The committee recommends that choline should be added to the list of food supplements that have potential to enhance performance and that are being evaluated at the U.S. Army Research Institute of Environmental Medicine (USARIEM).** It is suggested that carefully controlled laboratory studies with human subjects be conducted initially, the results of which may suggest field studies that could be used to evaluate enhanced physical and/or cognitive performance under stressful field conditions.

Tyrosine. Research has demonstrated that tyrosine may be rate limiting for the synthesis of neurotransmitter products under highly stressful conditions. Animal studies and limited human studies have demonstrated that tyrosine may have beneficial effects in overcoming the adverse effects of acute stressors. These data are encouraging and demonstrate that additional research should be conducted under carefully controlled conditions to further define when tyrosine may be beneficial in reversing acute stress. The research with tyrosine currently being carried out at both USARIEM and the Naval Medical Research Institute is exciting. **The committee recommends that this research be expanded, with more emphasis placed on safety, interactions with ration consumption, stress, and field studies.** Data are required on the safety of tyrosine use at levels required for efficacy. Since the effect of tyrosine appears to be pharmacological, the FDA protocols for demonstrating safety and efficacy should be considered. Evaluation of the proper method of delivering an effective dose of tyrosine to affected troops would also be required.

3. The following compounds have a low probability of enhancing performance through their use in military rations.

Carnitine. Because of its importance metabolically in exercising muscle, research in the exercise physiology literature should be monitored, but carnitine is not recommended for consideration in performance enhancement ration development and evaluation by the military until it is demonstrated that carnitine supplementation over that normally supplied in usual military rations has some value.

Structured lipids. There are no data to support the fact that structured lipids spare glycogen utilization during exercise and therefore support improved performance. It is recommended that structured lipids not be further evaluated as a performance-enhancing component of operational rations.

Specific Recommendations

Tyrosine. Although tyrosine has been demonstrated to reverse the effects of certain acute stressors, some critical issues remain to be addressed before it can be recommended for use in enhancing the performance of acutely stressed military personnel. These issues, as outlined by Harris R.Leiberman (Chapter 15), are as follows:

1. demonstrating the generalizability of tyrosine effects across a wider range of stressors,
2. establishing a dose-response function for tyrosine's beneficial effects,
3. determining whether tyrosine has efficacy in chronic stress paradigms,
4. determining the safety of tyrosine administration,
5. assessing the risks and benefits of acute versus chronic administration of tyrosine, and
6. determining the most appropriate method for providing tyrosine supplementation.

Choline. Both clinical and basic research into choline and its effects on the body may have relevance for the military. Several clinical studies are obvious:

1. studies to determine whether choline supplementation enhances endurance and muscle performance, and
2. studies to determine whether choline supplementation enhances intellectual performance and whether this alters performance of soldiers in the field.

Carbohydrate supplements. Since carbohydrate supplements have been shown to enhance performance in athletes performing at moderate to heavy levels of physical activity for extended periods of time, it is desirable to evaluate various military operational scenarios to determine whether and when a carbohydrate supplement would be advantageous. Suggested areas are:

1. continuous load carrying at 50–70 percent maximal oxygen uptake for 1–2 hours without resting, and
2. sleep-deprived states when moving into simulated-combat situations.

Another possible area of research would be to determine the amount of protein needed in relation to carbohydrate to prevent the "perceived fatigue" effect reported with carbohydrate intake.

Other Areas that Offer Research Potential

- While tryptophan was extensively used by many individuals, serious saftey concerns led to its being banned from use. Depending upon federal regulatory guidelines, tryptophan may at some point offer research potential in the area of sleep promotion. Issues of mode of administration and dose would be areas of significant concern for military research with tryptophan.
- Laboratory research indicates heightened self report of fatigue after ingestion of high-carbohydrate, low-protein supplements. Studies of carbohy

drate/protein ratios in supplements also offer research potential for sleep promotion.

- Limited data from laboratory studies suggest that the buffering effects of sodium bicarbonate ingestion on muscle pH changes during physical exercise offer potential for further research.
- Glycerol is another substance that, although not specifically covered in this workshop, may warrant further investigation as a dietary supplement to enhance performance.
- Likewise, while not specifically discussed in the CMNR workshop, there are reports that carbohydrate supplementation is beneficial in improving performance at high altitude.
- Although this report has emphasized the specific isolated food components identified by the U.S. Army, and thereby focused recommendations regarding these components on a component-by-component basis, further research would need to include careful investigations of the interactions among any components as well as the interactions of regular dietary levels of caffeine and carbohydrates with performance-enhancing food components.
- Symptoms that frequently occur during stress (including headaches, myalgias, somnolence, and reduction in food intake) contribute importantly to decrements in performance. Carefully controlled studies should be considered during military-type stresses of the ancillary use, prophylactic and/or therapeutic, of common, symptom-treating, over-the-counter drugs that block the cytokine-induced intracellular production of prostaglandins, that is, drugs such as aspirin or ibuprofen. Prostaglandin blockade with such drugs could not only reduce symptoms to improve performance but could also have the ancillary nutritional benefits of improving appetite and reducing the hypermetabolic loss of body nutrients and muscle protein known to be associated with prostaglandin release.

AREAS FOR FUTURE RESEARCH

The Committee on Military Nutrition Research recognizes the potential value for performance enhancement in combat settings and suggests a number of areas for future research within the military. The CMNR believes that the military services, through their pool of volunteer personnel, offer an excellent and often unique opportunity to generate research data and statistics on the nutrition, health, and stress reduction in service personnel. These findings can be directly applied to improving both the health and the performance of military personnel and those of the general U.S. population.

1. Much of the research needed to establish the safety of large doses of tyrosine and potentially choline needs to be carried out with rats. Amino acid, neurotransmitter, and metabolite levels need to be measured in specific brain nuclei, and many other animal studies are needed including gross and microscopic pathologies in both short-and long-term experiments. Possibly this could be accomplished through the Army funded neuroscience research at the Pennington Biomedical Research Center, Baton Rouge, Louisiana, in support of the human studies at USARIEM.
2. Performance, including cognitive, emotional, and physical aspects, is of crucial importance to all service branches. **It is recommended that an interservice committee be established to coordinate and facilitate research and development activities in this area.**
3. **A final general recommendation is to focus nutrition/ performance research on diet/stress/immune function relationships in both acute and chronic situations.** It would be desirable to relate the research, at least in part, to researchable issues raised by the two Ranger studies. Immunological studies should include studies of humoral immunity, cellular immunity, and plasma cytokine concentrations before, during, and after the period of stress.

The Committee on Military Nutrition Research is pleased to participate with the Division of Nutrition, U.S. Army Research Institute of Environmental Medicine, U.S. Army Medical Research and Development Command, in programs related to the nutrition and health of U.S. military personnel. The CMNR hopes that this information will be useful and helpful to the U.S. Department of Defense in developing programs that continue to improve the lifetime health and well-being of service personnel.

REFERENCES

Army Science Board 1991 Soldier as a System. 1991 Summer Study Final Report. Assistant Secretary of the Army Research, Development and Acquisition. Washington, D.C.: U.S. Department of the Army.

Food and Drug Administration 1982 Toxicological Principles for the Safety Assessment of Direct Food Additives and Color Additives Used in Food. Washington, D.C.: U.S. Department of Health and Human Services.

PART II

Background and Introduction to the Topic

IN PARTS II THROUGH VI the papers from workshop are included in the order in which they were presented. The chapters have undergone limited editorial change, have not been reviewed by an outside group, and represent the views of the individual authors. Selected questions directed toward the speakers and their responses are included to provide the flavor of the workshop discussion. The invited speakers were requested to submit a brief list of selected background papers before the workshop. These recommended readings, relevant citations collected by CMNR staff before the workshop, and selected citations from each chapter are included in the Selected Bibliography (Appendix C).

Part II includes three chapters. The interest of the Army in enhancing soldier performance and the research recently conducted at the United States Army Research Institute of Environmental Medicine (USARIEM) that centers on three areas—dietary macronutrients (carbo-hydrates), nutritional pharmacology (caffeine), and nutritional neuroscience (tyrosine) are summaried in the first chapter. The next two chapters, present a review of the complexity of developing operational rations for the military.

3

Nutritional Enhancement of Soldier Performance at the U.S. Army Research Institute of Environmental Medicine, 1985–1992

Eldon W.Askew[1]

INTRODUCTION

The purpose of the workshop on which this volume is based is to provide focus and direction to the joint Science and Technology Objective (STO), responsibility for which is shared by the U.S. Army Research Institute of Environmental Medicine (USARIEM) and the U.S. Army Natick Research, Development and Engineering Center. The thrust of this STO is to sustain and enhance soldier performance in environmental extremes through performance-enhancing food components. Integral to this objective is the prevention of performance degradation (the preservation of pre-deployment performance capability), especially under the stress of sustained field operations at

[1] Eldon W.Askew, Chief, Military Nutrition Division, U.S. Army Research Institute of Environmental Medicine, Natick, MA. 01760–5007

environmental extremes (U.S. Department of the Army, 1991). This research is necessary to move the soldier of today toward enhanced capabilities in the future. The U.S. Army refers to this overall initiative as *The Soldier as a System* (U. S. Department of the Army, 1991) and recognizes the importance of the individual items and equipment that the soldier wears, carries, or consumes (U.S. Department of the Army, 1991).

The U.S. Army has always been interested in the enhancement of soldier performance. Until recently, however, this concept primarily encompassed efforts to improve training, doctrine, and equipment, with relatively little emphasis on food as a tactical weapon. The advent of the concept of sports nutrition and the documentation by the scientific community of the influence of nutrients on physical and mental performance have pointed the way toward the application of sports nutrition and nutritional neuroscience strategies to military scenarios. The U.S. Army Research Institute of Environmental Medicine has investigated the application of some of these sports nutrition and nutritional neuroscience principles on soldier performance at high altitudes, in the cold, in the heat, and in conjunction with load-bearing work.

The purpose of this brief chapter is to review what the Army has accomplished in the area of nutrition and performance research conducted at the U.S. Army Research Institute of Environmental Medicine from 1985 to 1992 and to provide a new starting point for further research on the science and technology objective. The other chapters presented in this volume will assist the Army in determining additional avenues of research through their reviews of the current status of nutrition and performance enhancement research in general. It is hoped that this information will permit the Army researchers to focus their efforts on potentially fruitful avenues of research.

Nutrition and performance research at the U.S. Army Research Institute of Environmental Medicine (USARIEM) has focused on three general areas:

- dietary macronutrients (carbohydrate),
- utritional pharmacology (caffeine), and
- nutritional neuroscience (tyrosine).

METHODOLOGY

The data presented in this chapter consist of means±standard deviations. Significant differences ($P<0.05$) are noted, but only concise descriptions of the experimental designs are given. The reader is referred to the references for additional experimental design details.

MACRONUTRIENT AND PERFORMANCE RESEARCH AT USARIEM

USARIEM scientists have conducted a number of studies on the performance enhancing aspects of dietary carbohydrate. These research efforts are in the following areas:

- carbohydrate and work at high altitude,
- carbohydrate and thermoregulation in the cold,
- carbohydrate and work in the heat,
- carbohydrate and load-bearing work, and
- carbohydrate and marksmanship.

Carbohydrate and Work at High Altitude

The influence of liquid carbohydrate (CHO) supplements on work performance at high altitudes has been investigated in two USARIEM studies (Askew et al., 1987). These two studies differed principally in the manner in which they measured work performance. A study conducted at the summit of Mauna Kea (4,100 m) evaluated CHO-supplemented and non-supplemented soldiers runn-ing for 2 h/day for the first 4 days of exposure to high altitude (Askew et al., 1987). The performance measure was the total distance run during a 2-hr period (70 percent maximal oxygen uptake $\dot{V}_{O_2\ max}$ at sea level) each day for 4 days. Consumption of the supplement or a placebo beverage was voluntary, but average consumption was about 200 g of CHO per day in addition to that obtained from the diet. The supplemented group ran at an average rate of 12.0 ±0.8 km/2 h whereas the non-supplemented group ran at an average rate of 10.7 ±0.5 km/2 h. This difference was significant at $P< 0.05$.

A second study measured the time that it took a group of test subjects to hike the length of the Barr Trail from an elevation of approximately 305 m to the summit of Pikes Peak (4,300 m) (Baker et al., 1990, Smith et al., 1993). The total distance was 21.7 km and the total time (in minutes) required to hike this route was recorded. The test was conducted before and after 3 weeks of acclimation to high altitude, and the test subjects received approximately 300 g of CHO per day in the form of a liquid glucose polymer supplement. The control group received a placebo drink containing no CHO. Under the conditions of the study, there was no significant difference in hiking times at the beginning or end of the 3-week altitude exposure period, although the carbohydrate supplement did significantly increase total dietary carbohydrate intake (Baker et al., 1990).

Carbohydrate and Thermoregulation During Cold Exposure

Neufer et al. (1988) and Young et al. (1989) investigated the influence of cold exposure on the rewarming response after hypothermia and thermoregulation during immersion in cold water. Neufer et al. (1988) fed test subjects 120 or 600 g of CHO per day and studied the effect of mild hypothermia on the rewarming response of these two groups. They found that the low muscle glycogen levels associated with the low dietary carbohydrate intake did not impair the rewarming time during passive rewarming and suggested that individuals suffering from mild hypothermia rewarm spontaneously despite significant muscle CHO depletion. This study thus provided little evidence for a critical role of CHO in the rewarming process.

Young et al. (1989) studied the influence of high or low muscle glycogen levels produced by a combination of exercise and diet (low-carbohydrate diet, 15 percent CHO; high-carbohydrate diet, 65 percent CHO) on thermoregulation during immersion in cold water. The treatments produced muscle glycogen levels of 144±124 and 543±53 mmol of glucose per kg of dry tissue. There was, however, no significant difference between the low- and high-carbohydrate treatment groups in the shivering response, metabolic rate, or maintenance of body core temperature during this experimental exposure to the cold. Young et al. (1989) concluded that the thermoregulatory response to cold stress was not impaired by a substantial reduction in muscle glycogen levels. Apparently, other metabolic substrates such as fat can adequately fuel the heat-generating response when muscle glycogen stores are low. This study did not, however, establish whether there is some minimal muscle glycogen level that is obligatory for sustaining muscle metabolism during this experimental exposure to the cold.

Carbohydrate and Work in the Heat

Rose et al. (1987) examined the thermoregulatory and hydrational status of men during sustained work in a hot (37°C), dry (20 percent relative humidity) environment. They studied 11-heat acclimated young men engaged in 24 h of sustained, 45-min bouts of treadmill walking (1.56 m/sec) interspersed with 15-min rest periods each hour. The subjects consumed either a nutrient solution (24.8 g of CHO, 24 mEq of sodium per liter) or a placebo solution to maintain a constant body weight during the period of sustained activity. Subjects consumed approximately 700 ml (17.4 g CHO/h) of the test solution per hour during the period of sustained activity. Only 2 out of 11 subjects were able to complete a full 24-h period of sustained activity. Although these two subjects happened to receive the nutrient solution, the mean endurance times for those receiving the placebo control and nutrient solutions (16±3 versus 17±4 h) were not significantly different. Likewise, there was no significant difference in metabolic rate, plasma volume, fluid intake, sweat rate, plasma glucose concentration, or skin or rectal temperature. There was also no significant difference in the gastric emptying rates of the test or placebo solutions (Levine et al., 1991). The relatively low level of carbohydrate used in the study may account for the lack of an anticipated ergogenic effect; however, it is also possible that the nature of the sustained work test chosen for this study contributed to the lack of sensitivity to carbohydrate. Foot and leg soreness, chafing, blistering, and heat rash, rather than exhaustion were the main reasons for terminating the sustained treadmill walking.

Carbohydrate and Load-Bearing Work and Marksmanship

Moore, R.J. et al. (1991) studied the effects of low (250 g), moderate (400 g), and high (550 g) carbohydrate diets on load-bearing work and perceived exertion. Tharion and Moore (1993) also studied laser marksmanship[1] as a function of the carbohydrate content of the diet in this same study. A total of 13 test subjects in a double-blind, repeated-measures experimental design each consumed three test diets for three 5-day study phases: Phase 1: 250 g CHO diet; Phase 2:400 g CHO and Phase 3:550 g CHO in the same order for all subjects. In terms of work, all phases consisted of days 1 to 3, road marching (19 km/day) while carrying 45-kg packs; day 4 encompassed treadmill running without a pack and metabolic measurements related to the lactate threshold; and on day 5, test subjects carried a 45-kg load while walking until exhaustion at 5.6 km/h on a treadmill set at a 5 percent grade. Subjects rested for 10 min during each hour during the 30–194-min march. Relative perceived exertion (Borg scale) readings were recorded at regular intervals throughout the test period. Laser marksmanship determinations were begun within 5 min following the treadmill walk to exhaustion. Marksmanship accuracy was measured by the tightness of the shot group (area, mm^2 of the shot group). Accuracy was better maintained in subjects on a higher level of carbohydrate intake, but the results did not reach statistical significance. Although the study provided some suggestion of a beneficial effect of carbohydrate on perceived exertion and possibly fine motor coordination, it suffered from a relatively small sample size, precluding definitive conclusions or generalization of the data.

The results are listed in Tables 3–1 and 3–2. The results of the study thus indicated that while there was no significant effect of diet on endurance, the localized perception of the degree of difficulty of the work was greater for those on the low-carbohydrate diet.

NUTRITIONAL PHARMACOLOGY (CAFFEINE RESEARCH)

The ergogenic effect of caffeine during cycle ergometer work at a simulated high altitude in an altitude chamber (Fulco et al., 1989) as well as during marching on the Pikes Peak Barr Trail (King et al., 1993) has been studied by scientists at USARIEM. Caffeine has also been evaluated as an agent to enhance human performance of tasks that require a high level of vigilance (Lieberman et al., 1993).

Fulco et al. (1989) studied the effect of a placebo or caffeine (4 mg/kg) on the endurance times of eight test subjects on a cycle ergometer (80–85 percent $\dot{V}_{O_2\ max}$) at sea level, after 1 h of simulated altitude (4,300 m) exposure (acute altitude exposure), and after 2 weeks at the summit of Pikes Peak (4,300 m). At sea level, there was no significant effect of caffeine on the mean endurance time to exhaustion (26.3±11.9 versus 27.5±15.6 min). During

TABLE 3–1 Influence of Carbohydrate on Endurance and Perceived Exertion During Load-bearing Work

	Grams of Dietary Carbohydrate		
Parameter	250	400	550
Endurance time min*	117±32	120±41	144±29
Relative perceived exertion†	18.0±1.8	16.5±0.8	16.7±2.1

NOTE: Data from subjects completing at least 110 min of load-bearing work (*n*=6).

* No significant differences, $P>0.05$.

† Lower extremity rating. The relative perceived exertions for groups receiving 400 and 550 g were significantly less ($P<0.05$) than those for the group receiving 250 g of CHO.

SOURCE: Adapted from Moore et al. (1991).

[1] Laser marksmanship is shooting done with a real weapon (AR-15) equipped with a laser device that fires a laser beam when triggered, instead of live ammunition. The strike of the laser beam upon the target is recorded electronically.

TABLE 3–2 Influence of Carbohydrate on Marksmanship Before and After Load-bearing Work

	Shot Group Tightness (mm^2) for Groups Receiving the Following Grams of Dietary Carbohydrate		
Time	250	400	550
Before	50.7±19.2	48.0±27.0	38.9±20.2
After	54.9±27.9	46.0±19.6	40.2±16.0
Before versus after	NS	NS	NS

NOTE: There were 11–13 test subjects per treatment group. The subjects shot 10 shots as rapidly as possible without sacrificing accuracy. NS indicates not significant. The term "shot group tightness" is a measurement of marksmanship accuracy that refers to the area, mm^2, of the shot group.
SOURCE: Adapted from Tharion and Moore (1993).

acute altitude exposure in the altitude chamber, the mean endurance time of the caffeine treated group increased 54 percent relative to that of the placebo group (22.8±6.9 versus 35.0±10.7 min; $P<0.01$). Following 2 weeks of altitude exposure on Pikes Peak, the mean endurance time of the caffeine-treated group was increased 24 percent compared with that of the placebo group (30.5±14.5 versus 38.7±46.1 min); however, this difference was not significant at $P<0.05$. Caffeine was effective in significantly reducing the perception of effort at 10 min of exercise during the acute altitude exposure.

King et al. (1993) recently tested the effect of a similar dose of caffeine (4 mg/kg) on the hiking times of eight test subjects hiking the Barr Trail (21.7 km) to the summit of Pikes Peak (4,300 m). They could not find a significant difference between the placebo and the caffeine-treated groups (272±37 versus 264±22 min; $P>0.05$).

Lieberman et al. (1993) studied the effect of caffeine on vigilance in 20 test subjects receiving doses ranging from 32 to 256 mg of caffeine. The placebo group received no caffeine. All doses of caffeine significantly improved the number of correct detections on a Wilkinson auditory vigilance task Wilkinson (1969). The results obtained after administration of a 256-mg dose of caffeine are shown in Figure 3–1. These scientists also studied the effect of a single 200-mg dose of caffeine or a placebo on the mean number of correct detections in 10-min time blocks over 12 successive 10-min time blocks.

Caffeine significantly increased the number of correct detections throughout the 120-min test period. The results of the work of Lieberman et al. (1993) and Fulco et al. (1989) show that caffeine can increase physical and mental performance under carefully controlled laboratory conditions; they do not, however, show that a similar effect will be present under field conditions.

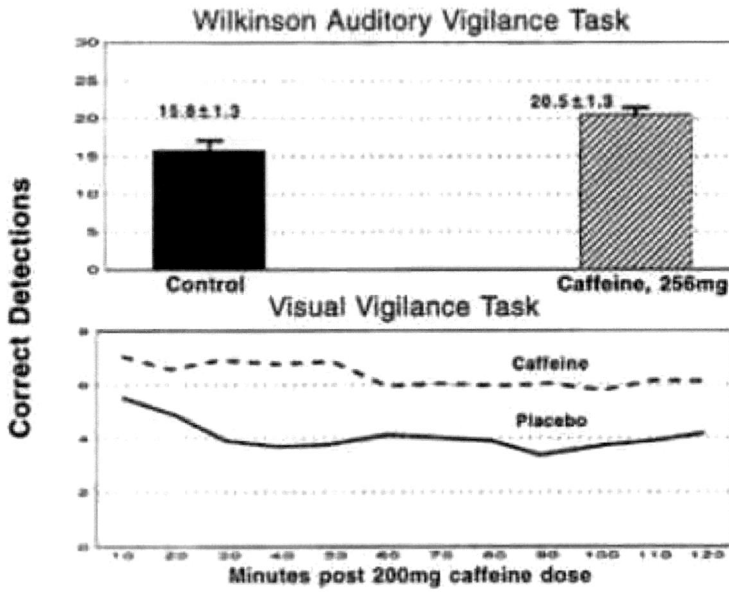

FIGURE 3–1 Influence of caffeine on auditory and vigilance tasks. The differences between the caffeine and control groups were significant ($P<0.05$). SOURCE: Adapted from Lieberman et al. (1993).

NUTRITIONAL NEUROTRANSMITTER RESEARCH (TYROSINE)

Tyrosine is a large neutral amino acid and is a precursor of the neurotransmitters norepinephrine and dopamine, which are secreted by catecholaminergic neurons during stressful situations. Some of the behavioral effects of acute stress may result from the depletion of norepinephrine and/or dopamine. Banderet and Lieberman (1989) studied the effect of tyrosine administration (100 mg/kg in two divided doses) on the protection of humans from the adverse consequences of a 4.5 h exposure to cold (15°C) and simultaneous simulated high-altitude chamber exposure (4,700 m). They employed a double-blind, placebo-controlled crossover design and found that tyrosine significantly decreased some measurements of symptoms, adverse moods, and performance impairments. Since these were a rather specialized set of testing circumstances, the authors cautioned that further research should be accomplished to determine whether tyrosine would be beneficial under other stressful (for example, field) circumstances. Further discussion concerning this particular study can be found in Chapter 15.

CURRENT USARIEM NUTRITION AND PERFORMANCE ENHANCEMENT RESEARCH

The U.S. Army Research Institute of Environmental Medicine is currently engaged in research employing glycerol to achieve hyperhydration at high altitude and in the cold to combat altitude- and cold-induced diuresis and dehydration. Glycerol is also being investigated as an agent for use in the prevention of high-altitude cerebral edema. Future work is planned to determine whether glucose electrolyte beverages may have a beneficial effect on hydration status and performance of military tasks in the heat.

SUMMARY

Most of USARIEM's work on dietary methods to enhance performance has centered around carbohydrate, caffeine, and tyrosine, and recent work has focused on glycerol. Caffeine and tyrosine have shown considerable promise of performance enhancement of military tasks; however, the positive results obtained with these two compounds have come from carefully controlled laboratory tests, not measurements of soldiers performing military field tasks. Indeed, most of the carbohydrate research and the portion of the caffeine research that was done under field conditions has failed to demonstrate a positive significant impact. This is perhaps due to the rather large amount of experimental "noise" associated with conducting performance tests in the field. It appears that field tests of physical performance require more closely controlled experimental testing conditions, larger numbers of test subjects, or both. Most of the USARIEM field studies employ 6–12 test subjects per treatment group. Subject availability, attrition, or manageability (logistical) aspects usually result in this final number of participants in field studies.

As this brief review illustrates USARIEM has been actively exploring the diet-performance interface between soldiers and their environment for the past 7 years and intends to increase its efforts in this direction in the future. The information gained from the chapters in this volume will help investigators at

USARIEM focus their research efforts on these and other nutrients that might prove to be beneficial to soldier performance enhancement.

REFERENCES

Askew, E.W., J.R.Claybaugh, G.M.Hashiro, W.S.Stokes, A.Sato, and S.A.Cucinell 1987 Mauna Kea III: Metabolic Effects of Dietary Carbohydrate Supplementation During Exercise at 4,100 m Altitude. Technical Report No. T12–87, (AD A180 629). Natick, Mass.: U.S. Army Research Institute of Environmental Medicine.

Baker, C.J., R.W.Hoyt, T.E.Jones, C.S.Fulco, and A.Cymerman 1990 Dietary considerations of a carbohydrate supplement at high altitude. FASEB J. 4:A567.

Banderet, L.E., and H.E.Lieberman 1989 Treatment with tyrosine, a neurotransmitter precursor, reduces environmental stress in humans. Brain Res. Bull. 22:759–762.

Fulco, C.S., P.B.Rock, L.A.Trad, M.S.Rose, V.A.Forte, Jr., P.M.Young, and A.Cymerman 1989 Effect of Caffeine on Endurance Time to Exhaustion. Technical Report No. T17–89, (AD A212 069). Natick, Mass.: U.S. Army Research Institute of Environmental Medicine.

King, N., C.S.Fulco, C.J.Baker-Fulco, S.Muza, T.Lyons, and A.Cymerman 1993 Field Trial of Caffeine on Physical Performance at Altitude: An Attempt to Overcome the Challenge. Technical Report No. T8–93, (AD A264 260). Natick, Mass.: U.S. Army Research Institute of Environmental Medicine.

Levine, L., M.S.Rose, R.P.Francesconi, P.D.Neufer, and M.N.Sawka 1991 Fluid replacement during sustained activity in the heat: Nutrient solution vs. water. Aviat. Space Environ. Med. 62:559–564.

Lieberman, H.R., B.J.Fine, J.L.Kobrick, and J.D.E.Gabrieli 1993 Effects of caffeine on mental performance and mood: Implications for aircrew members. In Nutrition and Metabolic Disorders and Lifestyle of Aircrew Advisory Group for Aerospace Research and Development Conference Proceedings, No. 533. Oslo, Norway: specialized printing services (SPS), Loughton, U.K.

Moore, R.J., J.F.Patton, E.W.Askew, and R.P.Mello 1991 Effects of dietary carbohydrate intake on perceptual responses to prolonged load carriage exercise. FASEB J. 5:A1657.

Neufer, P.D., A.J.Young, M.N.Sawka, and S.R.Muza 1988 Influence of skeletal muscle glycogen on passive rewarming after hypothermia. J. Appl. Physiol. 65:805–810.

Rose, M.S., R.P.Francesconi, and L.Levine 1987 Effects of a NBC (Nuclear, Biological and Chemical) Nutrient Solution on Physiological and Psychological Status During Sustained Activity in the Heat. Technical Report T25–87, (AD A188 175). Natick, Mass.: U.S. Army Research Institute of Environmental Medicine.

Smith, S.A., R.W.Hoyt, W.J.Tharion, C.S.Fulco, T.E.Jones, and A.Cymerman 1993 Effect of acclimatization to 4300 m on Piles Peak Hill climb performance. P. 314 in Hypoxia and Molecular Medicine, J.Sutton, C.Houston, and G.Coates, eds. Burlington, Vt.: Queens City Press.

Tharion, W.J., and R.J.Moore 1993 Effects of carbohydrate intake and load-bearing exercise on rifle marksmanship performance. Technical Report No. T5–93, (AD A262 333). Natick, Mass.: U.S. Army Research Institute of Environmental Medicine.

U.S. Department of the Army 1991 The Soldier as a System Army Science Board Final Report. Washington, D.C.: Assistant Secretary of the Army for Research Development and Acquisition.

Wilkinson, R.T. 1969 Some factors influencing the effect of environmental stressors on performance. Psychol. Bull. 72:260–272.

Young, A.J., M.N.Sawka, P.D.Neufer, S.R.Muza, E.W.Askew, and K.B.Pandolf 1989 Thermoregulation during cold water immersion is unimpaired by low muscle glycogen levels. J. Appl. Physiol. 66:1809–1816.

4

Optimizing the Design of Combat Rations

Irwin A.Taub[1]

INTRODUCTION

As Operation Desert Storm demonstrated, success on the battlefield depends on superior tactics, high-tech advanced equipment, and high-performing troops who can, under very stressful conditions, properly use the equipment to achieve the tactical objectives set for them. High performance, in turn, depends on the soldiers having—besides good training and suitable protective clothing—nutritionally optimized combat rations.

Accordingly, it is the responsibility of the food and behavioral scientists at the U.S. Army Natick Research, Development and Engineering Center (referred to as Natick), working closely with the nutritionists and physiologists at the U.S. Army Research Institute of Environmental Medicine, to optimize the design, processing, and storage of combat rations. If this responsibility is discharged properly, soldiers will consume these rations more completely, they will enjoy them more, their morale will be boosted, and they will ingest special constituents that will help them to perform well even under unusual circumstances and in many different battlefield situations.

[1] Irwin A.Taub, Food Engineering Directorate, U.S. Army Natick RD&E Center, Natick, MA 01760–5018

This chapter highlights the factors crucial to designing combat rations and puts into perspective the related research in food science and technology that underlies the development of such rations.

OPTIMIZATION CONSIDERATIONS

Six major factors must be taken into consideration in optimizing combat ration design.

Performance enhancement is the key factor and was the focus of the workshop on which this volume is based. Its relevance is self-evident, and more detail on related research is given below.

Caloric densification is extremely important for situations in which a soldier must have highly compact rations that are also easy to handle. These rations have many calories packed into a very small volume. Some of the components have a caloric density of about 7 kcal/mL. The dairy bar is illustrative.

Component preservation is the basis for providing shelf-stable operational rations in the field. The components must be microbiologically stable, which can be achieved either by destroying all the pathogenic and spoilage microorganisms or by inhibiting their growth. Moreover, even after accomplishing that, one must ensure that the food remains biochemically, physically, and chemically stable. It should have the same structure and appearance after 3 years of storage at a nominal temperature of 27°C (80°F) as it had when it was first produced.

Heating and cooling of such rations is an important consideration, because hot food and appropriately cool beverages affect morale and proper food and water intake.

Unless there is *consumer acceptance* of the food, it will not be consumed and nutrition could be compromised. Meeting all of the nutritional requirements is predicated upon consumption of the entire ration. Satisfaction with the ration contributes as well to the social well-being of the soldier.

Lastly, *quality monitoring* by using time-temperature integrators is also important. It makes it possible to ensure that, despite high temperature stresses over long storage periods, the food has the intended attributes and nutrients at the time of consumption.

Details on rations and the research relating to the six factors that are crucial to designing combat rations appear elsewhere (Beard, 1991). Only the work done at Natick on component preservation and on the heating of rations that would not generally be familiar is discussed here, primarily by reference to the combat rations currently under development.

SELF-HEATING INDIVIDUAL MEAL MODULE

A conceptually new self-heating ration is called the self-heating individual meal module (SHIMM) (Figure 4–1). In many ways it is similar to the Meal Ready-to-Eat (MRE) and has some of the MRE components, including the pouch bread, which remains stable and does not become stale even after 3 years of storage, and the Desert Chocolate Bar, which will not melt in one's hands. What clearly distinguishes this ration from the MRE is the placement of the entree item in a polymeric tray that has an integral heater capable of being activated by the pull of a tab. The entire component is actually a two-tray system, with the upper tray containing the separately processed food nested within the lower tray containing the chemical heating system. The high quality and familiar appearance of the components, the convenience of the tray-plate configuration, and the flameless, nonpowered heating contribute to the entree's and the SHIMM's appeal.

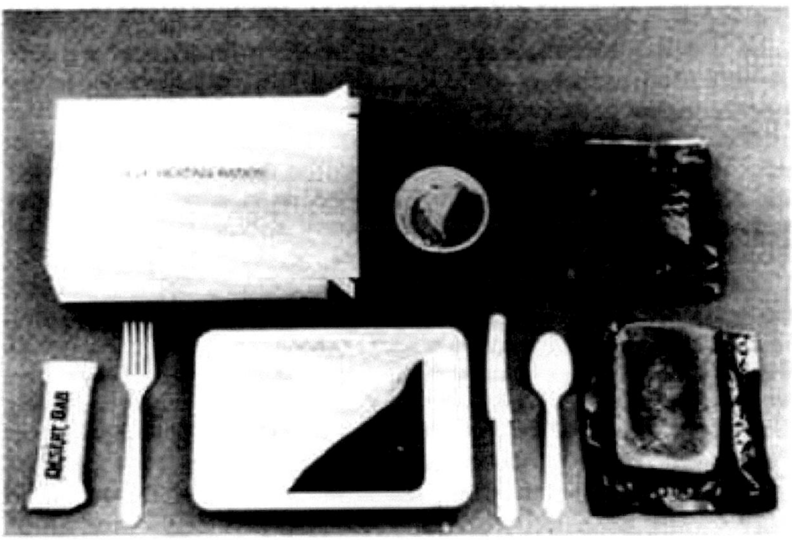

FIGURE 4–1 Demonstration version of a self-heating individual meal, with the contents of the upper and lower packages (shown glued together) displayed separately. The upper package contains the entree, such as the Salisburg steak shown here; the lower package contains the remaining items, including the utensiles. The lids for the entree and fruit cup have been pulled back, and the pouch bread has been removed from its protective packaging.

Component Preservation

With regard to preserving the components so that this combat ration is shelf-stable, all contaminating microorganisms, the pathogenic and spoilage microorganisms, must be destroyed. Two strategies are currently available: irradiation sterilization and thermal sterilization. Irradiation would be particularly suitable for whole-meat food items; thermal processing is used for casseroles, gravy-based items, and vegetables in a brine solution.

In the case of processing by irradiation, the meat is first precooked to a medium rare state to inactivate proteolytic enzymes and to make it ready to eat. It is put into a flexible pouch or a metal container, the air inside the container is evacuated to eliminate the oxygen, and the container is then hermetically sealed. The food components are then frozen and subjected to a high dose of irradiation, equivalent to destroying 12 decades of *Clostridium botulinum.* (Destruction of a hypothetical population of 10^{12} *botulinum* spores is the basis for the commercial sterility of irradiation processed and thermally processed packaged foods.)

The irradiated beefsteak shown in Figure 4–2, although used by U.S. astronauts, has not yet been approved for general use in the United States. Over the last 3 years it has been used in South Africa by the South African Army, with very favorable results. Investigators are working toward a generic clearance of this technology by the U.S. Food and Drug Administration so that it can be applied to the production of similar high-quality entree items.

More conventionally, an entree item formulated as a stew or with some gravy to conduct the heat would be subjected to thermal processing. In the case of the Salisbury steak shown in Figure 4–3, the container has a thin cross section, so a whole-meat item could be thermally sterilized without significant overprocessing and without the associated degradation in quality.

Various other thermal sterilization techniques are being explored, including ohmic and microwave heating. With ohmic heating, the passage of an electrical current through the food produces the high temperature needed to destroy the microorganisms; with microwave heating, the microwave energy is absorbed by the water in the food, which increases the water's temperature, and the heat is transferred from the water to the other constituents. In both cases, the intention is to achieve a high-temperature, short-time exposure, thereby killing the microorganisms but retaining the nutrients and other quality factors of the food.

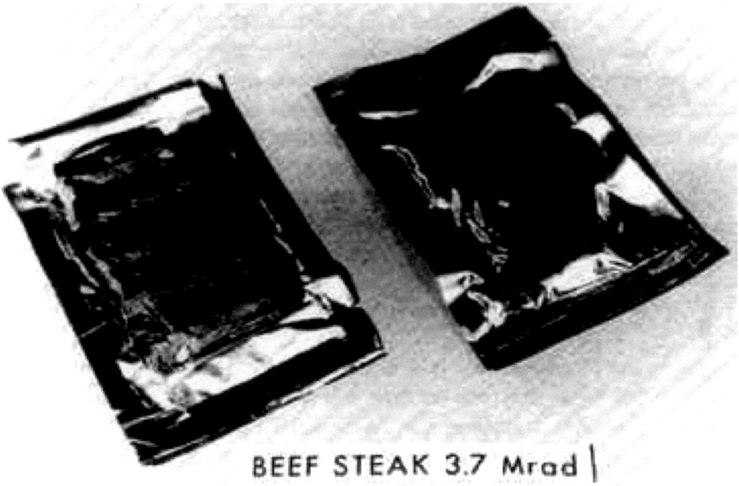

FIGURE 4–2 Irradiated beefsteaks, shown as packaged on the right and as removed from the package on the left.

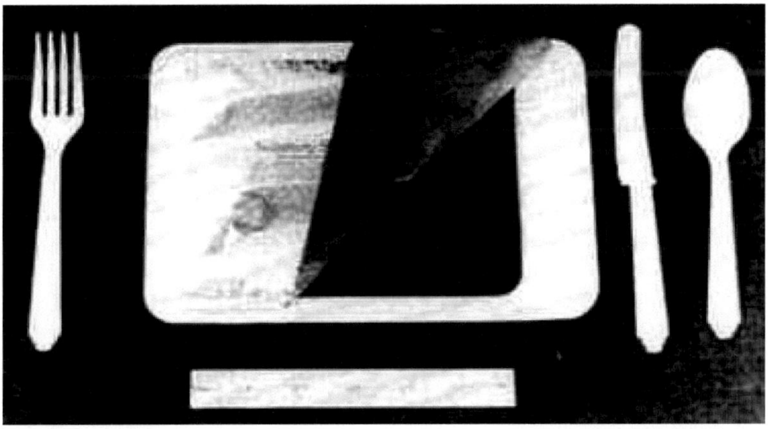

FIGURE 4–3 Demonstration version of the self-heating individual meal entree, a Salisbury steak, with the lid pulled back and a 6-inch rule placed alongside for comparison. Note the pull tab on the right front corner. Source: Courtesy of Don Pickard, Food Engineering Directorate, U.S. Army Natick Research Development and Engineering Center, Natick, Mass.

Self-Heating

With regard to heating the food prior to consumption, the SHIMM utilizes a chemical heating pad—a magnesium-iron material that is embedded in a high-density polyethylene matrix and that is activated by water. The pad is about one-half the length of the lower tray, which also holds a polymeric bag with the activating solution (Figure 4–4). Upon pulling the tab, the soldier rips open the bag, the water comes into contact with the pad, a chemical reaction immediately takes place, and heat is generated. Within 10 min, the soldier has a hot meal.

Consumer Acceptance

With regard to acceptance, it is crucial that the customers (i. e., military personnel) like what they see so they will want to consume the ration. To ensure that favorable reception, the developers of the meals follow a simple principle espoused by behavioral scientists: When receiving the ration, soldiers should perceive a benefit, both nutritionally and gastronomically. Consequently, if there is going to be a positive association with the ration, the visual presentation becomes very important.

Such considerations have been and are being made both in connection with the SHIMM and by further modifying the MRE. One experimental version of a modified MRE is called the FieldBreak (Figure 4–5). Not only is the meal bag colorful and attractive in name and appearance but so are the individually packaged components. It is assumed that the soldier will associate this military food with a well-liked commercial product, which will very likely increase his or her interest in, and consumption of, the ration.

NUTRITIONAL ENGINEERING FOR PERFORMANCE ENHANCEMENT

As indicated initially, the foremost consideration is to nutritionally engineer combat rations to contain performance-enhancing components. Inherent in such efforts is the assumption that there is a fundamental connection between performance and nutrition. Accordingly, a performance-nutrition response surface can be constructed as a guide to ration design.

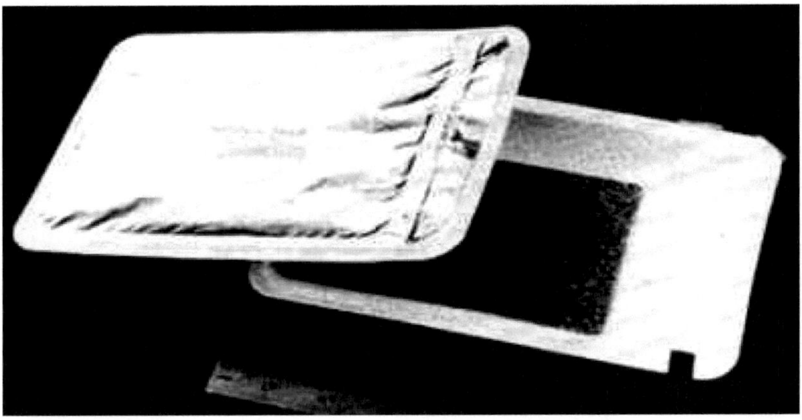

FIGURE 4–4 Demonstration version of the self-heating individual meal entree, with the upper tray separated from the lower tray to show the chemical heater and the polymeric bag with the activating solution. Source: Courtesy of Don Pickard, Food Engineering Directorate, U.S. Army Natick Research Development and Engineering Center, Natick, Mass.

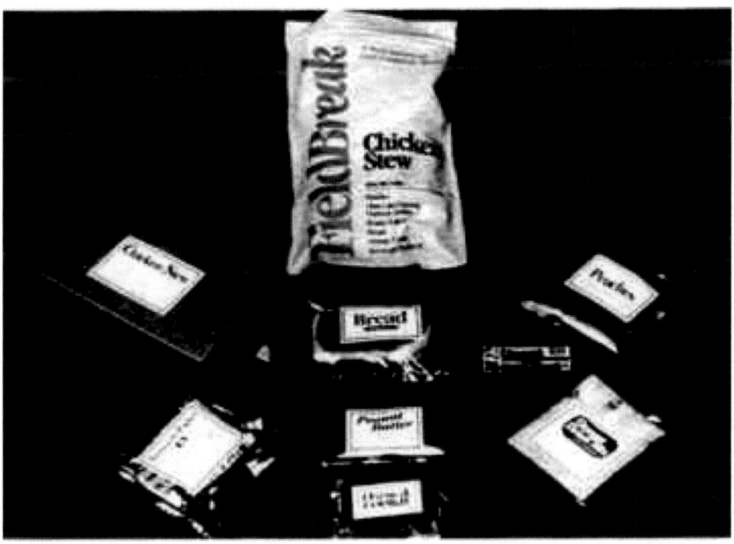

FIGURE 4–5 Proposed version of the Meal Ready-to-Eat, renamed FieldBreak, in commercial-style packaging for the meal bag and for the individual components, displayed separately. Source: Courtesy of Joan Kalick, Solider Science Directorate, U.S. Army Natick Research Development and Engineering Center, Natick, Mass.

Basic Performance-Nutrient Concept

To put the basic performance-nutrient concept into perspective, a hypothetical performance-nutrient response surface is shown in Figure 4–6. It plots performance along the *z* axis, running from 0.5 to 1, where 1 is the "ideal," however it is defined. Any type of physical or cognitive performance can be normalized in this way and then correlated with particular nutrients. In this case, performance is plotted against the amount of carbohydrates in the ration (along the *x* axis) as well as against the total number of calories (along the *y* axis). It is important to note that as one increases the caloric content, the ration package gets heavier; at constant calories, as one increases the carbohydrate content, the package not only gets heavier but it also becomes disproportionately bulkier because of the replacement of the more energy-dense lipids.

These concerns are relevant to optimizing the weight and bulk of rations without compromising performance. Consequently, if an actual surface determined through experimentation looked like the one in Figure 4–6—and some results already obtained (see Chapter 3) imply that it would—then design decisions would be based on the relatively flat portion of the response surface, the flatness indicating approximately comparable performance. A ration with fewer calories and adequate, but not superfluous, carbohydrates would lead to suitable performance while maintaining the weight and bulk of the ration.

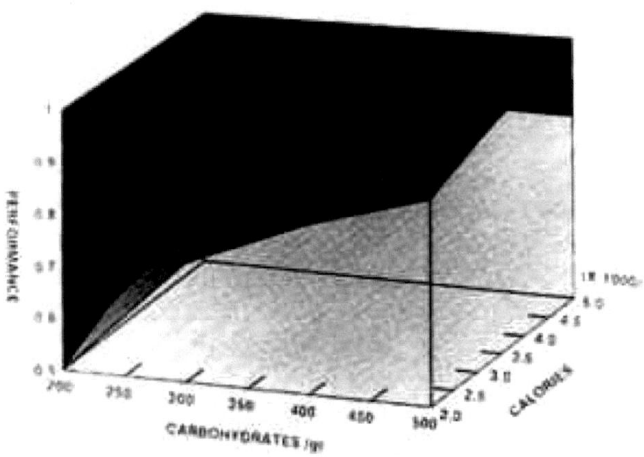

FIGURE 4–6 Hypothetical response surface showing the dependence of an unspecified performance index on total carbohydrates and total calories.

Several kinds of nutrients for which there could be a positive link with performance are being considered. They are as follows:

- Macronutrients
- Carbohydrates (type and total)
- Lipids
- Metabolic acids
- Carnitine
- Pectin
- Neurotransmitter precursors
- Tyrosine
- Phosphatidylcholine

The macronutrients, particularly the carbohydrates, are crucial. There is interest in not only total carbohydrates but also in the type of carbohydrates. If the delivery of glucose to the bloodstream could be modulated through a judicious selection of complex carbohydrates, then physical endurance might be extended. The rate and extent of carbohydrate conversion, as reflected perhaps in the glycemic index, will form the basis for future experimentation. Various metabolic acids are important as well, since these may influence carbohydrate and lipid utilization.

Precursors to neurotransmitters, such as tyrosine and phosphatidylcholine, are potential performance-enhancing ingredients. The work of Banderet and Lieberman (1989) has already shown that tyrosine can reduce the severity of the symptoms of high-altitude sickness among susceptible individuals. Zeisel (1990) has suggested that choline is an essential nutrient and has also indicated that muscle function and mental alertness could be improved by increasing the amount of phosphatidylcholine in the diet. The potential importance of choline to performance is evidenced by data from marathon runners (Conlay et al., 1986).

The formulation of rations with optimum levels of such ingredients and without compromising the quality of the food or its acceptance is a fundamental challenge for food technologists.

Goal Programming

The design of diets that can be used experimentally to determine the performance-nutrient link—and, ultimately, to design optimal rations containing the desired nutrients—requires the mathematical approach of goal programming (Hintlian, 1990).

For this purpose investigators use LINDO, which stands for Linear Interactive aNd Discrete Optimization. The illustrative equation in Table 4–1 shows the *objective function* that must be minimized. LINDO allows one to impose many kinds of constraints on minimizing this function, so that more than just nutrient composition is taken into account.

Experimental Diets

In using LINDO in connection with the study described by Askew (see Chapter 3) on assessing the influence of total carbohydrates on performance, the level of carbohydrates in each diet had to be fixed, while the levels of protein and fat were allowed to deviate about specified target values. Moreover, the experiment required three isocaloric diets of 3,200 kcal each, with each providing 250, 400, or 550 g of carbohydrates per day. Consequently, for the diet intended to contain 550 g of carbohydrates per day in each of four daily menus, the protein and fat levels were allowed to deviate minimally from target values of 90 g for the former and 116 g for the latter.

Since the acceptance of the diet might be compromised by the presence of too many similar components from among those being used to establish the menus, the following constraints on meal composition were imposed: at least one entree, no more than two fig bars, at least one cereal bar, and no

TABLE 4–1 Illustrative Equation for Minimization of the Objective Function for Obtaining a Diet with Fixed Carbohydrates and Targeted Levels of Fat and Protein within Specified Constraints

Objective Function
Minimize:+n(fat)+p(fat)+n(prot)+p(prot)
Such that:
CHO=550 (or 400 or 250 g/day)
Prot=90+n(prot)−p(prot)
Fat=116+n(fat)−p(fat) (or 182 or 249 g/day)
Cereal Bar≥1
Entree=1
Fig Bar≤2
CHO from beverage≤250 g

NOTE: CHO, carbohydrate; prot, protein; n and p, negative and positive deviations, respectively, of the protein and the fat.

more than 250 g of maltodextrin (M 500) from the beverages. These are constraints on the number of units of each component, consistent with the integer solutions computed.

The actual computation involves equations for each nutrient, whether fixed or targeted, taking into account the contributions of individual components to the total, as is illustrated for carbohydrates (Table 4–2). These components with carbohydrates, as illustrated for were configured as food bars, dried items, or baked products. Each has a very specific weight of, for example, 30, 40, or 70 g. Since the solution is constrained to be an integer solution, the program will select none, one, or multiples of each component and will provide a set of optimized solutions, taking the percent carbohydrates into account. These range from 2.1 percent in the beef jerky, to 17.7 percent in the fruit chew, to 50 percent in the cornflake bar, and to 79.7 percent in the strawberry oatmeal bar. The total was to be 400 g in the illustration shown in Table 4–2. A specific constraint was to limit the overall selection to only two flavors of each of the different types of components. Similar computations were made for the diets that contained 250 or 550 g of carbohydrates per day.

For the study described by Askew (see Chapter 3) on assessing the effect of total carbohydrates on performance, the program generated four different daily menus for each of the three carbohydrate levels. A sample menu for Day 1 served to the study group receiving 250 g of carbohydrates is outlined in Table 4–3. Three meals (breakfast, lunch, and dinner) and two snacks (in

TABLE 4–2 Objective Function for Carbohydrates Showing the Contributions to the Total Carbohydrates of Individual Components Whose Weights are Selected in the Optimization Procedure

Objective Function for Carbohydrates
Minimize: *n*(fat)+*p*(fat)+*n*(prot)+*p*(prot) CHO: 30.2 bludst+32.4 chchdst+28.5 apcndst+25.5 pecdst+30.4 chhvdst+44.8 shwt +43.4 wheats+44.5 branf+41.3 life+45.4 grnut+50.0 crnflk+17.4 cocbev+2.1 beefjy +17.7 frchew+4.7 crml+78.1 oatmbs+79.7 oatsw+78.2 oatapcn+24.9 crcxcw +36.5 sfchw+39.8 sgvchw+29.1 chchchw=400 Constraint: Only one or two flavors allowed

NOTE: prot, protein; *n* and *p*, negative and positive deviations, respectively, of the protein and the fat; CHO, carbohydrate. The abbreviations of the food items are replaced in the equation with the weights of those components available for use, and the coefficients represent the percent carbohydrates in each of the components. Illustrative of these abbreviations are the following: crnflk=corn flake bar; beekjy=beef jerky; frchew=fruit chew; and oatsw=strawberry oatmeal bar.

TABLE 4–3 Sample Menu for the Optimized Experimental Diet Providing 250 g of Carbohydrates on Day 1 of a 4-Day Menu

Meal and Food		Weight (g)
Breakfast		
Life cereal bar		30
Nut dairy bar		40
Cocoa bar		30
Beverage		13
Lunch		
Creamed chicken chowder bar		47
Bacon and cheese shortbread		25
Smokecraft Slim Jim		46
Almond fig bar		30
Beverage		13
Dinner		
Chicken and rice entree		70
Seafood chowder bar		47
Fried onion shortbread		25
Infused flat bread		50
Almond dairy bar		40
Beverage		13
Snacks		
A.M.:	Cocoa bar	30
	Coconut Bear Valley bar	20
	Beverage	13
P.M.:	Cheese shortbread	25
	Vanilla dairy bar	40

the morning and afternoon) were served. The breakfast included a yogurt-based dairy bar, which could be rehydrated to a regular yogurt consistency. The lunch was Spartan compared with that obtained at fast-food outlets, but it included a chicken chowder, a Slim Jim, and a fig bar. More conventionally, the dinner included a very tasty seafood chowder, a well-liked chicken with rice entree, a flat bread (which was infused with lipid to increase calories), and an almond bar for dessert. Although three dairy bars were on the menu, no flavor was duplicated. The adjustable carbohydrates, however, were obtained by using a flavored maltodextrin-based beverage containing 13 g of carbohydrates four times a day. The fixed weight of each component was used, representing one unit of the particular configuration; none was broken into smaller units.

Tailored-Ration System

The goal-programming approach can be applied to designing rations as well. It is particularly suited to the concept of a tailored ration system in which the rations are optimized for various situations that might require different nutrients. The idea is to assemble a situation-specific ration by combining a core module of 1,500 kcal with other supplementary modules. As schematically outlined in Figure 4–7 for four situations, one could add to the core module the following tailored supplements: a hot weather supplement (HWS) for the desert; a cold weather supplement (CWS) for the arctic; a high altitude supplement (HAS) for mountainous terrains; and a snack food supplement (SFS) for general use. The tailored ration shown in Figure 4–7 is for the standard temperate environment.

The modules would be combined to provide the total number of calories and any special nutrients needed for each situation. Two core modules for standard use would provide 3,000 kcal (Figure 4–8). In the case of the arctic situation, the CWS alone would have 3,000 kcal, so the total number of calories associated with one CWS and one core module would be 4,500 kcal. In the case of the high-altitude situation, the HAS could be designed with appropriate calories and with high tyrosine-containing components to meet the needs posed by the low-oxygen and, possibly, low-temperature conditions.

The prototype core module with its components is shown in Figure 4–9. Totaling 1,500 kcal, it could have an entree such as the dehydrated pork and rice, the MRE pouch bread, a meat stick, two compressed cereal bars, two maltodextrin packets (which would be configured as a bar rather than as the powder shown in Figure 4–9), and a dairy bar. Despite having a high caloric density of 6.8 kcal/mL with 56 percent of the calories coming from lipids, the dairy bar is a very popular, highly rated item that can be eaten as is or made into a pudding. It exemplifies components that can be made to meet stringent nutritional needs and still meet stringent consumer expectations.

Depending on what is ultimately learned and confirmed about the link between performance and nutrients, specific ingredients would have to be formulated into suitable components that could be optimally combined into rations appropriate to military situations.

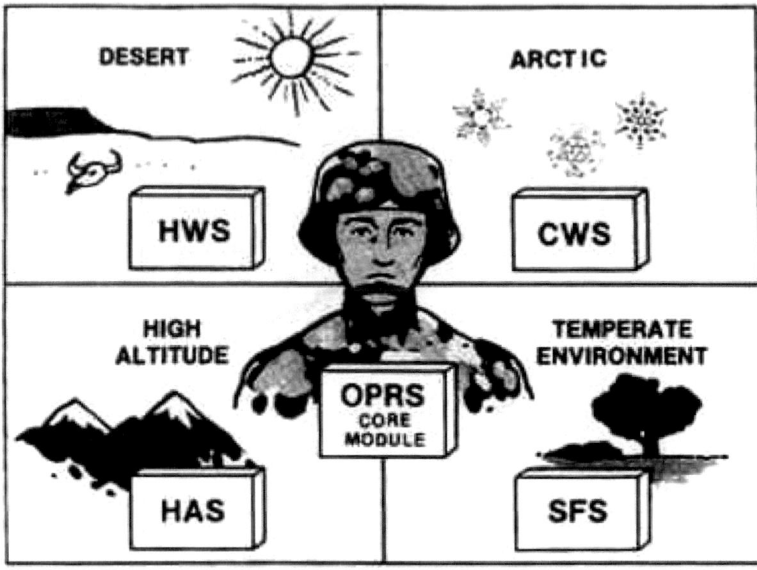

FIGURE 4–7 Schematic representation of the tailored ration concept showing the situation-specific hot weather supplement (HWS), cold weather supplement (CWS), high altitude supplement (HAS), and snack food supplement (SFS) that can be combined, as appropriate, with a core module designed for standard situations.

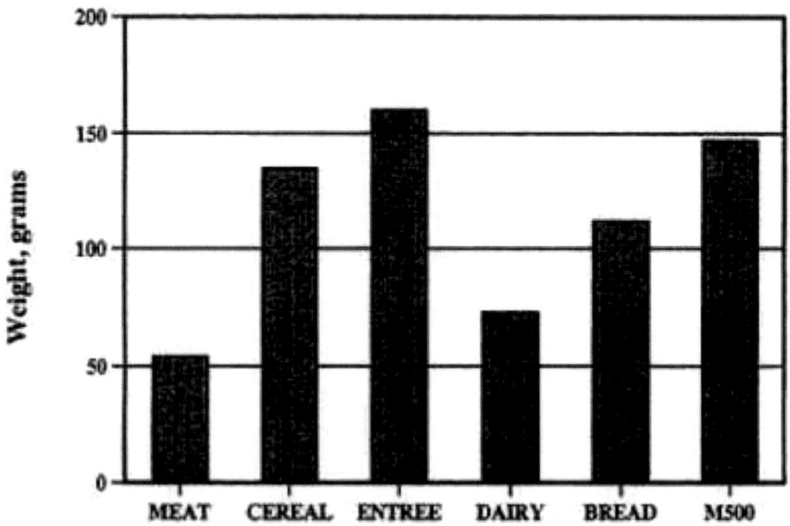

FIGURE 4–8 Weight distributions among the components tailored for use in two core modules for standard use, totaling 3,000 kcal. M500, maltodextrin.

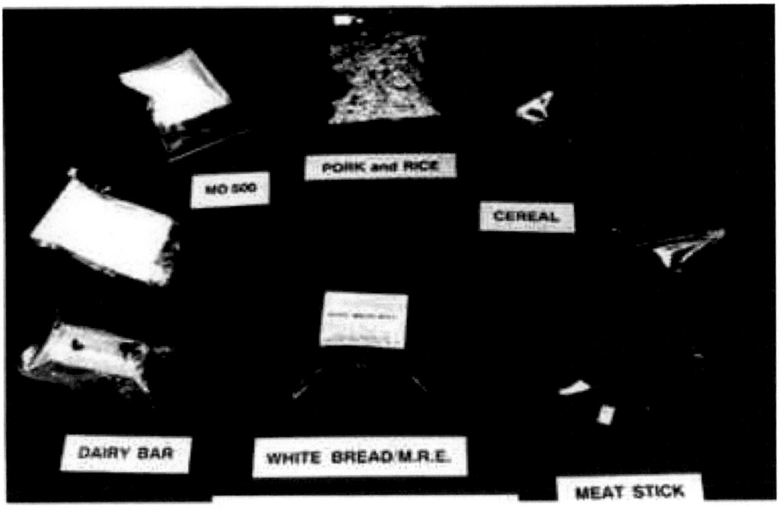

FIGURE 4–9 Demonstration version of the core module components, which total 1,500 kcal. Except for the Meal Ready-to-Eat (MRE) bread, all are dry components, and many are compressed into bars to reduce their volumes. MD 500, maltodextrin.

SUMMARY: THE CHALLENGE

As the foregoing indicates, the task for food technologists can be thought of as the *performance-nutrient challenge.* After the nutritionists and physiologists select the ingredients of greatest potential—those that would have a positive effect on performance—the food technologist would have to ensure that the related ration components are formulated and processed in a compatible and acceptable manner, that these ingredients can tolerate long-term storage, that they can survive digestion and remain physiologically active, and that they can be delivered in a modulated manner to the targeted physiological sites.

If the challenge can be met, then the combat rations will not only contain performance-enhancing nutrients and related constituents, but these nutrients will also be optimally available at the time of consumption and will be fully consumed. The overall goal is to go beyond that challenge so that soldiers who consume such rations will recognize and experience the performance benefits of extended endurance and heightened alertness.

REFERENCES

Banderet, L.E. and H.R.Lieberman 1989 Treatment with tyrosine, a neurotransmitter precursor, reduces environmental stress in humans. Brain Res. Bull. 22:759–762.

Beard, B. 1991 Hot meals in a hot spot: How we feed our troops in Saudi Arabia. Food Technol. 45:52–56.

Conlay, L.A., R.J., Wurtman, K.Blusztajn, I.L.G.Coviella, T.J.Maher, and G.E.Evoniuk 1986 Decreased plasma choline concentrations in marathon runners. N. Engl. J. Med. 315:892.

Hintlian, C.B. 1990 Use of math programming techniques to design experimental diets and military rations. In Abstracts of the IFT (Institute of Food Technologists) Annual Meeting. Chicago: 169.

Srzezinski, A.A., J.J.Wurtman, R.Gleason, T.Nader, and B.Laferrere 1990 D-fenfluramine suppresses the increase calorie and carbohydrate intakes and improves the mood of women with premenstrual syndrome. Obstet. Gynecol. 76:296–301.

Zeisel, S.H. 1990 Choline deficiency. J. Nutr. Biochem. 1:332–349.

5

Biochemical Strategies for Ration Design: Concerns of Bioavailability

C.Patrick Dunne[1]

INTRODUCTION

This chapter presents a strategic overview that shows how some modern technologies and biochemistry interact with nutrition and physiology research efforts in the design and development of future ration systems. These ration systems will enhance the performance of troops under stressful battlefield conditions.

Investigators are seeking detailed information to fill the knowledge gaps in the optimum nutrition concept postulated by Walter Mertz, among others (Mertz, 1981). The curve shown in Figure 5–1 is a simplification of a multidimensional response surface. The Committee on Military Nutrition Research has been seeking some definitions of the optimum nutrition plot on the *y* axis that will measure a response in terms of performance on a military-related task. Most current nutritional standards are historically based on the avoidance of deficiency. Animal nutrition standards may be based on the experimental measurement of growth. Also, one must take with caution the

[1] C.Patrick Dunne, Food Engineering Directorate, U.S. Army Natick RD & E Center, Natick, MA 01760–5018

oversimplification of a curve such as the one shown in Figure 5–1 for a single nutrient, in that it overlooks several types of nutrient-nutrient interactions; the presence or absence of any other nutrient may shift the optimum curve for a single nutrient either to the left or to the right in a three-dimensional surface. An additional complexity and concern is the issue of the fourth dimension of time. Time scales on classic nutrient deficiency studies are, by nature, much longer than the shorter time responses that might be the focus of research on nutritional supplements for performance enhancement. A related issue that should be addressed is the importance of time intervals both for the duration of feeding of any supplements and paired control or deficient diets and the intervals between consumption and testing the performance-related responses (Willcutts et al, 1988).

Military nutrition standards are shown in Table 5–1. These standards provided by the Office of the Surgeon General of the Army, published in AR 40–25 (U.S. Department of the Army, 1985), provide a prescription that must be met by ration developers. The military ration is based on a 3,600-kcal daily

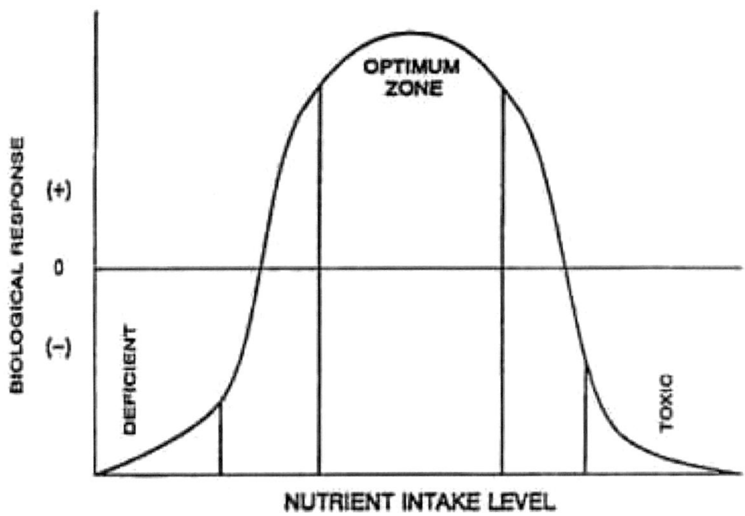

FIGURE 5–1 Optimal nutrition concept. Source: Adapted from Mertz (1981).

TABLE 5–1 Nutritional Standards for Operational Rations

Nutrient	Units	AR 40–25*	RDA M-19–22†
Energy	kcal	3,600	2,900±400
Protein	g	100	56
Carbohydrate	g	440	-
Fat	g	160	-
Vitamin A	µg RE‡	1,000	1,000
Vitamin D	IU	400	300
Vitamin E	mg TE§	10	10
Ascorbic acid	mg	60	60
Thiamin	mg	1.8	1.5
Riboflavin	mg	2.2	1.7
Niacin	mg	24	19
Vitamin B_6	mg	2.2	2.2
Folacin	µg	400	400
Vitamin B_{12}	µg	3	3
Calcium	mg	800	800
Phosphorus	mg	800	800
Magnesium	mg	400	350
Iron	mg	18	10
Zinc	mg	15	15
Sodium¶	g	5–7	1.1–3.3
Potassium¶	g	1.88–5.62	1.88–5.62

*U.S. Department of the Army (1985).

†RDA, Recommended Dietary Allowances for males, ages 19–22 (NRC 1980).

‡RE, retinol equivalents.

§TE, α-tocopherol equivalents.

¶Estimated safe and adequate dietary intakes.

energy requirement, so many of the nutrient requirements have been increased by a calorie multiplier when compared with Recommended Dietary Allowances of the National Research Council (National Research Council, 1980). The Military Recommended Daily Allowances (MRDA) contain a specified minimum value for carbohydrates (440 g or 48.9 percent of calories) because of the established link between carbohydrate intake and optimal performance in high-demand exercise (Costill, 1988). Investigators are now addressing the issue of which specific types of carbohydrates in what mixtures would be best for selected scenarios (Guezennec et al., 1993).

One other difference in recommended macronutrient composition is the high protein requirement of 100 g for the MRDA. It must be recognized that protein is not only used for growth, replacement of injured tissue, and tissue turnover but also as a key source of the precursors of biogenic amines and many of the other secondary metabolites of the protein-derived amino acids.

Additional nutrients that are of concern to ration developers are listed in Table 5–2. One concern is that, since packaged rations may be used for extended periods of time, the nutrients found at trace levels in a normal mixed diet may not be available at appropriate levels. Another concern, which has also been expressed by Irwin Taub (see Chapter 4), is the possible use of some of the nutrients as metabolic enhancers or to meet stress-induced extra metabolic demands. In particular, some combat rations are high in fat, and individuals may be metabolizing fat at high levels. Heinonen et al. (1992) among others have conducted research on carnitine, which is needed to transport the fatty acids into the mitochondria for oxidation. Zeisel et al. (1991) have summarized the recent studies of choline, which point to the possibility that choline is a required nutrient for humans, especially under conditions of stress. Of the trace elements, Anderson (1989) was especially interested in chromium because of its reported links to carbohydrate metabolism.

A key goal is to identify any special nutritional needs that may be created by stressful situations in combat, that include extremes of heat, cold, or altitude, in addition to physical and mental demands. Investigators would then work at engineering foods or special-purpose food supplements to be used in

TABLE 5–2 Other Important Micronutrients

Nutrient	Safe and Adequate Intake*
Biotin	100–200 μg
Choline	400–900 mg
Inositol	–
Carnitine	–
Vitamin K	70–140 μg
Pantothenic acid	4–7 mg
Iodine	150 μg (RDA)†
Chloride	1.7–5.1
Sulfur	?‡
Chromium	50–200 μg
Manganese	2.5–5 mg
Copper	2–3 mg
Molybdenum	150–500 μg
Selenium	50–200 μg
Fluoride	1.5–4.0 mg
Dietary fiber	?

*National Research Council (1980).

†RDA, Recommended Dietary Allowance.

‡A safe and adequate intake of sulfur is assumed if the RDA/MRDA for protein is met.

testing in conjunction with the Military Nutrition Division of the U.S. Army Research Institute of Environmental Medicine (USARIEM).

The current objectives for the ongoing effort to develop performance-enhancing ration supplements are listed below:

- To develop fortified liquid or solid ration components that satisfy the special nutritional needs of troops under stress.
- To provide optimal nutritional support for physiological defense mechanisms against environmental hazards.
- To seek a definition of the special vitamin and mineral requirements of troops.
- To test the net available fortifying micronutrients in formulations after processing, storage, and reconstitution for use.
- To develop a selection procedure for specific protein, peptide, or amino acid supplementation by consideration of precursors of stress-related biogenic amines.

PRACTICAL CONSIDERATIONS FOR RATION DESIGN

In Chapter 4, Irwin Taub provided examples of some of the kinds of structured foods that can be developed and made stable to serve the requirements of military personnel. In any prescription for an optimal nutrient content of rations, it must be recognized that the nutrients must be available after processing, after storage for up to 3 years at 27°C (80°F), to meet military shelf-life requirements, and after any form of reconstitution of the preparation that may be required before use. Some of the technical concerns for ration development are listed in Table 5–3. Certain of those may be of special interest to the Committee on Military Nutrition Research. One key issue is the choice of a carrier for supplemental nutrients. An ideal carrier should maintain the stability of the nutrient, and it should have sensory characteristics that will encourage consumption.

Investigators also need to follow guidelines for fortification that not only match the physical and chemical characteristics of the nutrient with the carrier but also the expectations that a certain food item carries about its nutritional content. For example, it might be best to add caffeine to a cocoa- or coffee-flavored beverage or bar, but not to a fruit bar or drink, where caffeine would not be expected.

The military shelf-life requirements demand that some ration formulations contain food additives as stabilizers or antioxidants. Whenever possible, investigators try to select functional ingredients that would also have a nutritional value. Dunne (1987) developed stable high-fat dairy bars that use a synergistic combination of antioxidants centered on vitamin E (α-tocopherol) and ascorbyl palmitate. Investigators also select food-grade lecithin, which is commonly used as an emulsifier, for the provision of choline. Purified phosphatidylcholine in liposome vesicles is also being explored as a carrier for labile nutrients.

The bottom line regarding the technical concerns listed in Table 5–3 is taste and acceptability; this is also the bottom line for any food item selected for its special nutritional value. If soldiers do not eat the foods, the foods are not nutritious. As a major design consideration, investigators give attention, in addition to nutrient content, to the nutrient-nutrient interactions that may affect sensory properties (color, flavor, and odor). At least three levels of interactions should be considered: (1) chemical interactions that may occur during processing or storage of rations, (2) interactions during digestion and absorption, and (3) metabolic interactions.

Chemical interactions may be either positive or negative. Examples of negative interactions include the interaction of iron, copper or vitamin B_{12} with ascorbate. All three of these reactions require air, and they represent the catalysis of oxidation of ascorbate by redox-active metal ions. In the case of vitamin B_{12} and ascorbate, a mutual destruction has been observed. This destruction is postulated to occur through the formation of active oxygen species [superoxide or hydroxyl radicals] involving the participation of both the CO^{+2} and CO^{+3} states of vitamin B_{12} (Gossamer et al., 1977). Although this destructive interaction caused some concern about negative effects of megadoses of ascorbate supplements, the physiological organometallic coenzyme forms of vitamin B_{12} are quite unlikely to participate in such destructive redox cycles

TABLE 5–3 Technical Concerns for Ration Development

Liquid versus Solids—stability differences, sterilization required
Long-term storage requirements
Minerals and electrolytes—choice of salts
Vitamins—choice of form
Requirements for additives
Stabilizers-antioxidants
pH control buffers and acidulents for liquids
Packaging the product to maximize stability
Taste and acceptability—as a function of temperature

(Dunne, 1971). Another possible destructive interaction is the riboflavin-catalyzed photooxidation of unsaturated lipids. Chemical interactions may also be positive, as in the antioxidant couple, whereby ascorbyl palmitate may serve to regenerate the active form of vitamin E (α-tocopherol) (Cort, 1974).

There are examples of both positive and negative interactions during digestion and absorption that can be used to guide the formulation of nutrient-rich products (Roe, 1991). Negative interactions that retard absorption include the complexing of certain minerals (iron or zinc) with inositol phosphates (phytate), producing insoluble, less available forms or the complexing of calcium or magnesium with the fatty acids produced by digestion of fats, forming insoluble soaps. Examples of positive interactions that may enhance absorption include the interaction of ascorbate with iron and sugars with calcium.

Food technologists may avoid some of the negative chemical interactions by use of encapsulation techniques to shield one or more of the potential reactants. For example, either metal salts of iron or zinc can be purchased as encapsulated forms, and so can ascorbate. The encapsulation agents can be chosen to be released or removed during digestion, so that the positive effects of ascorbate on iron intake can be derived without the risk of loss of nutrient potential during storage. Some of the types of encapsulation are shown in Figure 5–2.

After digestion and absorption there may be continued metabolic interactions involving dietary nutrients that should be considered in the design of supplements (Bodwell and Erdman, 1988). Again, both positive and negative metabolic interactions have been observed. For example, the branched-chain amino acids, being large neutral amino acids, compete with the aromatic amino acids tyrosine, tryptophan, or phenylalanine for the transport system involved in the uptake of these amino acids across the capillaries into the brain. The negative folate-vitamin B_{12} interaction is a subtle and pernicious one, whereby folate masks some of the symptoms of vitamin B_{12} deficiency, but the neurological damage caused by the hidden vitamin B_{12} deficiency is the reason why folate is not allowed as a single nutrient supplement.

This case of vitamin B_{12} and folate may be just one example of the trouble that can be caused by single-nutrient supplements. A single nutrient, especially when given at high doses, does have the potential to perturb metabolic pathways such that the metabolism of other nutrients may be negatively affected. For a brief summary of single-nutrient problems, see the paper by Bendich (1992).

There are positive higher metabolic interactions that should also be considered. Many of these involve product-precursor relationships or the sharing of a common pool of chemical functional groups, such as choline and methionine, which are methyl group donors and part of the key one-carbon

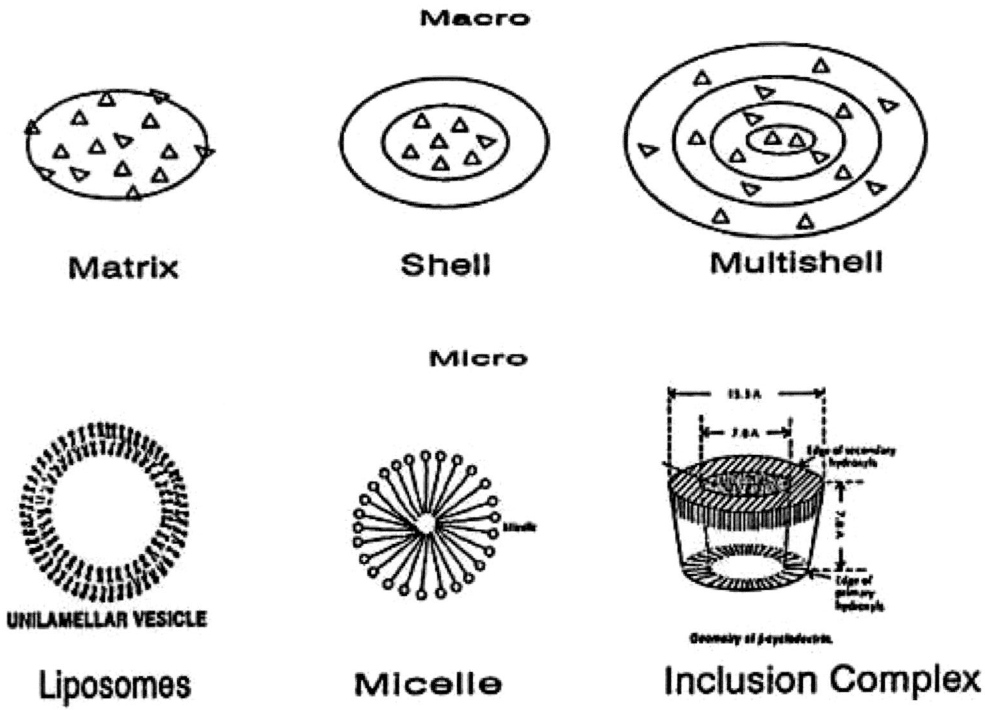

FIGURE 5–2 Encapsulation types. Source: Information on the sizes and structures of macro forms is adapted is from Risch and Reineccius (1988). Information on micro forms is from Brooks and McManus (1990) for liposomes, used with permission; and adapted from Yesair (1989) for micelles; and information for cyclodextrins is from Beesley (1985), used with permission.

metabolism scheme that animal nutritionists, especially those in the poultry industry, have known for some time. These two nutrients are listed among the lipotropic factors in older textbooks. Vitamin E and vitamin A have been shown to interact positively both chemically and metabolically (Machlin and Langseth, 1988). Certain product-precursor relationships are of interest because they involve nutrients that are topics of other chapters in this volume. These nutrients with positive metabolic interactions include phenylalanine and tyrosine, tryptophan and niacin, and lysine and carnitine. A much more complete discussion of nutrient interaction is found in the monograph edited by Bodwell and Erdman (1988). One interesting question is whether all of the aspartame consumed in both commercial and military products can lead to increased phenylalanine- or tyrosine-derived neuroendocrine factors.

BIOCHEMICAL STRATEGIES FOR CONTROLLED DELIVERY OF NUTRIENTS

Investigators at the U.S. Army Natick Research, Development and Engineering Center are exploring some strategies for what can be termed *targeted nutrient delivery*. It is akin to approaches taken by a pharmacokineticist in the design of an oral delivery system for a new drug. Techniques of sustained or controlled release may be explored, but first, one must consider a whole host of barriers or reactants that nutrients and their carriers must traverse on their way through the digestive tract. Figure 5–3 is provided as a guide to the stresses and membrane barriers that exist during enteral nutrition. During normal oral delivery of nutrients, few nutrients may pass directly into the bloodstream through oral cavity membranes. However, the buccal route is exploited for direct delivery of some active water-soluble pharmaceutical agents, including enzymes, which can be absorbed by the body by holding tablets under the tongue, thereby allowing the agents to gain entry to the bloodstream without the delay resulting from the passage of the agent through the digestive tract and thus bypassing a potential first-pass metabolism by the liver through the portal circulation. Some digestion may be initiated in the oral cavity by the action of amylase and a lingual lipase that may continue its action downstream in the digestive tract. In the stomach there is a pH shift plus the addition of the protease pepsin, which is active at acid pH. Again, membrane barriers are significant, so not much leaks out into the bloodstream; one exception, however, is alcohol. As nutrients and carriers enter the small intestine, the medium changes drastically, whereby, along with carbonate to neutralize acid, the pancreatic enzymes and the bile salts enter the system. The bile salts prove to be important at changing the structures of native dietary fats and also of fats or phosphatidylcholine vesicles (liposomes) that might be used as encapsulates for nutrients. In the intestinal mucosal cell there is more or less a division point where the majority of water-soluble nutrients, either by diffusion or facilitated transport, enter the portal circulation system to go to the liver, which is metabolically active in the transformation of many nutrients into final circulating forms. The portal route may take from 1 to 4 h to show evidence of nutrient intake by an increase in the general blood concentration of those nutrients; a commonly studied indicator is the blood glucose level, which peaks about 2 h after the intake of common carbohydrates, including simple sugars. An alternative route is taken by lipids, including long-chain fatty acids. They enter the lymphatic system and are later deposited in the general circulation via the thoracic duct; this pathway is slower, taking 2 to 7 h, but the nutrients are able to avoid first-pass liver metabolism.

One key area of concern is the uptake and subsequent metabolism of amino acids and protein. When considering oral delivery routes for amino acids that

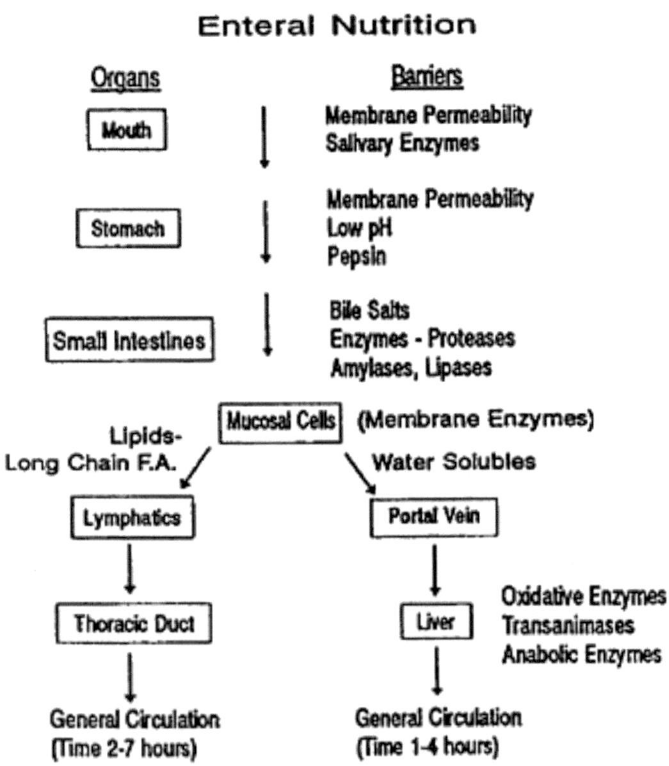

FIGURE 5–3 Diagram indicating the barriers to nutritional delivery where F.A.=fatty acids. SOURCE: Adapted from Briggs and Calloway (1984).

are to serve as biotransmitter precursors, one should consider two sometimes overlooked facts: (1) that certain amino acids, especially the aromatic ones, are classic inducers of catabolic liver enzymes (Ip and Harper, 1973), and (2) that, in some cases, uptake of peptides may be facilitated compared with uptake of single amino acids (Siemensma et al., 1993). A hypothesis can be constructed that, with certain amino acids such as tyrosine and tryptophan, repeated or chronic supplementation of the free amino acids may induce the catabolic liver enzymes, such as tryptophan pyrrolase to such an extent that more precursor amino acid will be oxidized or otherwise changed and less will get to the target tissues, such as the adrenal glands or the brain, to be used for biogenic amine synthetic pathways.

One might then consider alternative strategies that could be used to minimize the effects of diversionary metabolic pathways on those amino acids that are intended to serve as neurotransmitter precursors. One strategy is to restrict the doses to large single bolus forms, such that liver enzyme induction is not a factor, or a candy drop (i.e., pill) that is held under the tongue can be used to enhance buccal uptake. In either of these cases, one may face the issue of deciding whether the delivery is that of a drug or a food; John Vanderveen addresses this issue in Chapter 23. Both of these types of delivery seem limited both by mass and by permeability factors, so they might be best for potential performance-enhancing nutrients that are effective in relatively small quantities (milligrams rather than grams) and that are fairly water soluble.

To provide protection to nutrients either during processing and storage or during the passage through the digestive system, a variety of techniques are available for encapsulating nutrients. The top of Figure 5–2 shows examples of larger microencapsulation products that are found in commercial food, fragrance, or pharmaceutical products (Risch and Reineccius, 1988); these range in size from 2 μm to 1 mm. Only some are true shell-type encapsulated products, such as in the dry powder forms of fat-soluble vitamins. The shell might be made of gelatin or an acacia gum, which can protect fat-soluble vitamin A or D from damage during processing or storage. These shells would resist organic solvents, but they would release their contents in aqueous environments. Mulitshell encapsulants may offer added protection or offer the possibility of a controlled or an extended duration of release of the contents. Many of the commercial encapsulated micronutrients use a spray-drying process to produce matrix "encapsulated" products in which the active nutrient is embedded in a matrix made of starch, for example, but is not truly isolated from the environment.

The bottom of Figure 5–2 shows smaller encapsulated forms, sometimes called nanocapsules, which may range in size from 20 nm to 200 mm. Inclusion complexes of the cyclodextrins are included in Figure 5–2 because of their potential to trap and carry small, volatile molecules (Bender and

Komiyama, 1978), but they are not yet approved for use as a food in the United States. Micelles and derivatives of micelles are starting to receive consideration as carriers to exploit the alternative lymphatic route to the bloodstream (Yesair, 1989); these may be as small as 5 to 10 nm in diameter. The liposome shown in Figure 5–2 is a simple unilamellar vesicle, perhaps 50 to 200 nm in diameter, that can be made from phosphatidylcholine or related polar lipids (Deamer and Uster, 1983). Larger multilamellar liposomes are also commonly used as potential microencapsulants or carriers; these onion-like structures may form spontaneously (Brooks and McManus, 1990). Investigators at the U.S. Army Natick Research, Development and Engineering Center are finding that they can get a stable vesicle by sonicating the mulitilamellar vesicles and waiting for subsequent thermal fusion or curing of the resulting smaller unilamellar vesicles. Whitburn and Dunne (1991) have been able to stabilize the vesicles to some degree against freeze-drying, providing the possibility of creating stable dry dosage nanocapsules.

To date investigators have not found that liposomes are true magic bullets for the oral delivery of high-impact nutrients. The location of the carried cargo nutrient, the amount of cargo that can be carried, and the stability of vesicles depend on the nature of the cargo, the nature of the polar lipids forming the vesicle, and the preparation procedures. Investigators have not had much success encapsulating caffeine, for instance. Investigators have been assessing the effects on loading efficiencies and cargo leakage as a function of (1) the presence of membrane additives (e.g., cholesterol), (2) bilayer phospholipid chain length, and (3) medium additives. There is still much to learn about matching the carried nutrient to the encapsulating agent to achieve a true targeted and controlled nutrient delivery system. The information presented in this volume should help investigators focus their efforts on the most promising nutrients that could be enhanced by a controlled or sustained delivery system.

CONCLUSIONS AND RECOMMENDATIONS

Not all of the strategy described here is a nutritional "Star Wars" concept, in that many of the nutrients or food ingredients considered to have potential performance-enhancing capabilities are available as food-grade materials. Investigators have been using a strategy of the dual-purpose use of such ingredients as shown in Table 5–4, which lists examples of substances with both nutritional function and special functionalities in the food technology sense. The strategy is to emphasize the proper form of the ingredients that will best fill their functional and nutritional roles. A simple example is α-tocopherol acetate, which is present in many multivitamin preparations. When used in this form, the product is not protected by the chemical antioxidant function of free α-tocopherol.

TABLE 5–4 Dual-Function Ingredients for Ration Bars

Ingredient	Function	Nutritional Role
α-tocopherol	Antioxidant	Vitamin E
Ascorbyl palmitate	Antioxidant	Vitamin C
Lecithin	Surfactant and emulsifier	Choline source
Pectin	Binder and texturizer	Soluble dietary fiber
Whey protein	Binder	Essential amino acids
Bran	Matrix Structure	Insoluble dietary fiber

SOURCE: Dunne (1987), used with permission.

Investigators have developed several criteria for the optimal fortification of supplementation that may well be applied to any performance-enhancing supplements. These criteria are listed below:

- The supplementation regimen should be based on knowledge of the nutrient content of an individual's basic diet. This knowledge may be simpler for combat rations than for normal diets, but many advances in analytic techniques may be required.
- Supplements should be in a form that is acceptable and consumable by troops under battlefield conditions. Carriers must be highly preferred items.
- Fortified items should be designed to maximize nutrient retention in the form that they are consumed by users. Both storage stability and nutrient stability when reconstituted for use need to be optimized.
- The interactive effects among different components must be considered and controlled. Reactive micronutrients will be separated by encapsulation or by use of separate carriers.
- The levels and specific forms of individual fortifying nutrients should be chosen to give maximum bioavailability, with little or no chance of negative effects from either under- or oversupplementation.
- Supplementation should be based on knowledge of the metabolic roles of the supplement's components and the basic dietary components.

Finally, four major concerns related to the issues listed above set the stage for later issues. These are:

- Where do certain potential performance-enhancing supplements lie in the gray zone between food and drugs?
- What will be the acceptance by users, and how can it be maximized?
- What real tests of efficacy are available to establish the positive effects of any supplement on mental and/or physical performance?
- How do investigators establish and use proper time frames for both usage and testing of supplements?

A related issue linking the first and last questions is to consider the differences between a bolus dose of a single amino acid, which might well be considered a drug, and graduated regular doses over a longer term of that amino acid in peptide forms, which is more akin to a food.

A bit of history outlined in Table 5–5 may put the task in perspective. In the prime period of Army human nutrition research Consolazio and colleagues established a time course for the onset of nutrient deficiency syndromes (Consolazio, 1983). From the data there seems to be a hierarchy of effects, with fatigue being a major and leading effect. However, one must note that with the exception of water, the time course for the first signs of deficiency is in days.

The present task is to come back 20 years later to determine whether it is possible to observe the effects in hours, not days, by modulating intakes of specific nutrients under stressful conditions in which subtle differences in performance can be detected. There may be improved technology for the delivery of nutrients, but investigators must still deal with the major issues of evaluating the effects of nutrients on performance.

TABLE 5–5 Time Course for Onset of Nutrient Deficiency Effects

Nutrient	Time for Deprivation Effect	Primary Symptom of Deprivation
Water	A few hours	Fatigue, mental confusion
Total energy	2–3 days	Fatigue
Electrolytes ($Na^{+}CL^{-}$)	≥3 days	Fatigue, muscle cramps
Carbohydrate	≥3 days	Fatigue
B Vitamins	1–2 weeks	Fatigue, neurological effects
Vitamin C	Several weeks	Fatigue
Protein	Several weeks	Varies
Vitamin A	Several months	Uncertain
Fats	Many months	Varies; essential fatty acid deficiency
Trace Minerals	Several months	Anemias or blood cell functions

SOURCE: Consolazio (1983), used with permission.

REFERENCES

Anderson, R.A. 1989 Essentiality of chromium in humans. Pp. 75–81 in The Science of the Total Environment. Amsterdam: Elsevier Sciences Publishers.

Army Regulation 40–25 1985 *See* U.S. Departments of the Army, the Navy, and the Air Force.

Beesley, T.E. 1985 Inclusion Complexing: A new Basis for HPLC Selectivity. American Laboratory 17(5):78–87.

Bender, M.L., and M.Komiyama 1978 Cyclodextrin Chemistry. Berlin: Springer-Verlag.

Bendich, A. 1992 Safety Issues Regarding the Use of Vitamin Supplements. Ann. N.Y. Acad. Sci. 669:300–310.

Bodwell, C.E., and J.W.Erdman, Jr. Eds. 1988 P. 389 in Nutrient Interactions. New York: Marcel Dekker, Inc.

Brooks, G.J., and R.C.McManus 1990 Finding new uses for liposomes in cosmetics. INFORM (Am. Oil Chem. Soc.) 1:891–895.

Consolazio, C.F. 1983 Recommended dietary allowances. Prog. Food Nutr. Sci. Nutr. Performance 7:13–27.

Cort, W.M. 1974 Antioxidant activity of tocopherols, ascorbyl palmitate, and ascorbic acid and their mode of action. J. Am. Oil Chem. Soc. 51:321–325.

Costill, D.L. 1988 Carbohydrates for exercise: Dietary demands for optimal performance. Int. J. Sports Med. 9:1–18.

Deamer, D.W., and P.S.Uster 1983 Pp. 27–51 in Liposome Preparation: Methods and Mechanisms, in Liposomes, M.J.Ostro, Ed. New York: Marcel Dekker.

Dunne, C.P. 1971 Reactions of the Carbon-Cobalt Bond of Alkyl Vitamin B_{12} Derivatives. Ph.D. Thesis. Brandeis University, Waltham, Mass.

1987 Fundamental research and engineered caloric dense rations-introduction: Some nutritional perspectives. Activities Report of the R&D Associates 39:145–150.

Gossamer, A., B.Grüning, L.Ernst, W.Becker, and W.S.Sheldrick 1977 Reaction of dicyanocobyrinic heptamethyl ester with ascorbic acid. Angew. Chem. Int. Ed. Engl. 16:481–482.

Guezennec, C.Y., P.Satabin, F.Duforez, J.Koziet, and J.M.Antoine 1993 The role of type and structure of complex carbohydrates response to physical exercise. Int. J. Sports Med. 14:224–231.

Heinonen, O.J., J.Takala, and M.H.Kvist 1992 Effect of carnitine loading on long-chain fatty acid oxidation, maximal exercise capacity and nitrogen balance. Eur. J. Appl. Physiol. 65:13–17.

Ip, C.C.Y., and A.E.Harper 1973 Effects of dietary protein content and glucagon administration on tyrosine metabolism and tyrosine toxicity in the rat. J. Nutr. 103:1594–1607.

Machlin, L.J., and L.Langseth 1988 Pp. 287–311 in Vitamin-Vitamin Interactions in Nutrient Interactions, C.E.Bodwell and J.W.Erdman, Jr., eds. New York: Marcel Dekker.

Mertz, W. 1981 The essential trace elements. Science 213:1332–1338.

National Research Council 1980 Recommended Dietary Allowances, 9th Ed. Washington, D.C.: National Academy of Sciences Press.

Risch, S.J., and G.A.Reineccius 1988 Flavor Encapsulation. ASC Symposium Series 370. Washington, D.C.:American Chemical Society.

Roe, D.A. 1991 Pp. 459–471 in Bioavailability of Nutrients Added to Human Foods in Nutrient Additions to Food—Nutritional Technological and Regulatory Aspects, J.C.Bayernfeind and P.A.Lachance, eds. Trumbell, Conn.: Food and Nutrition Press, Inc.

Siemensma, A.D., W.J.Weijer, and H.J.Bak 1993 The importance of peptide lengths in hypoallergenic infant formulae. Trends Food Sci. Technol. 4:16–21.

U.S. Departments of the Army, the Navy, and the Air Force 1985 Army Regulation 40–25/Naval Command Medical Instruction 10110.1/Air Force Regulation 160–95. Nutrition Allowances, Standards, and Education. May 15. Washington, D.C.

Willcutts, K.F., A.R.Wilcox, and K.K.Grunewald 1988 Energy metabolism during exercise at different time intervals following a meal. Int. J. Sports Med. 9:240–243.

Whitburn, K.D., and C.P.Dunne 1991 Pp. 161–181 in Evaluation of Stabilizers for Synthetic Vesicles and Milk Fat Globules Under Drying Stress in Microemulsions and Emulsions in Foods. M.El-Nokaly and D. Cornell, eds. ACS Symposium Series 448. Washington, D.C.: American Chemical Society.

Yesair, D.W. 1989 Composition for Delivery of Orally Administered Drugs and Other Substances. U.S. Patent No. 4,874,795. October 17, 1989;

Zeisel, S.H., K.A.DaCosta, P.D.Franklin, E.A.Alexander, J.T.Lament, N.F.Sheard, and A.Beiser 1991 Choline, an essential nutrient for humans. FASEB. 5:2093–2098.

DISCUSSION

AUDIENCE MEMBER: Dr. Dunne, you made the distinction between taking a bolus as opposed to taking an encapsulated form and putting it into the food, making the encapsulated form a food. Those of us who work in this field need guidelines as to what the U.S. Food and Drug Administration will accept and how we should proceed in trying to formulate this complex.

PATRICK DUNNE: Our strategy is that if we are going to put any nutrient in rations on a regular basis, it must be an additive approved for use in foods. So levels of use would be set by certain parameters, whether it is generally recognized as safe (GRAS) or as an approved food additive. There is an upper value of how much you would be able to take in on a daily basis if it is a food. So we bring in that regulatory response and we would do it on a regular basis. With the bolus, however, I would say that first, your level of use might be different for a drug dose, and the timing factors would be different.

RICHARD WURTMAN: The trouble is, amino acids are not GRAS. In addition to that, compounds that are GRAS are GRAS for specific functionalities. The effects of amino acids on performance and behavior do not qualify.

PATRICK DUNNE: My own feeling is we would get somewhere into a middle ground if we focused on peptides or protein hydrolysates that happen to have the right enrichment in the amino acids that we are more interested in.

RICHARD WURTMAN: Then, of course, you get into the problem that the efficacy of a compound like tyrosine will be specifically impaired if it is presented along with proteins unless you make a peptide that has tyrosine plus nonessential amino acids, and that gets very expensive.

PATRICK DUNNE: The question of making versus selecting a natural peptide is where we might also have a distinction. We would prefer not to have synthetic peptides, but there are ways with specific receptor technology to enrich for tyrosine, for instance, in a casein hydrolysate.

PART III

Military Issues

PART III INCLUDES THREE CHAPTERS in which the performance and measurement issues of interest to the military are reviewed. The first chapter is a discussion of four categories of physiological factors that are involved in physical task performance: metabolic capacity, neuromotor control, energy substrates, and tissue homeostasis. The second chapter presents a review of recent research on sleep deprivation and its effects on performance during continuous combat operations, and the third chapter provides an overview of the history, methodological approaches, and methodological issues related to research in food intake, contextual factors, and performance enhancement.

6

Evaluation of Physical Performance

James A.Vogel[1]

INTRODUCTION

The performance of physical tasks involves many physiological and psychological factors and processes. Many of these factors or processes are potential targets for performance-enhancing interventions, commonly referred to as *ergogenic aids.* Military personnel are required to perform heavy, physically demanding tasks under stressful conditions, which has stimulated the military's interest in the identification of useful ergogenic aids. Decisions on the potential ergogenic aids that should be used will depend on appropriate evaluations of their physical performance-enhancing capabilities. This chapter discusses the methods and steps that should be taken in carrying out these physical performance evaluations.

The selection of appropriate physical performance tests for evaluating candidate ergogenic aids should start with the identification of the likely target of action. These targets of action are one or more of the components or factors

[1] James A.Vogel, Department of the Army, U.S. Army Research Institute of Environmental Medicine, Natick, MA 01760–5007

Physical performance can be evaluated at several levels, ranging from the performance of isolated in vitro nerve-muscle preparations to the performance of an actual physical task in the field, that determine physical activity. This chapter categorizes these components and then describes how each is assessed.

This chapter is limited to a discussion of the later stages of physical performance evaluation, that is, performance testing in the intact whole body and, more specifically, in controlled laboratory and field task performance testing.

PHYSICAL PERFORMANCE FACTORS AND THEIR EVALUATION

Performance of physically demanding tasks is a function of both psychological and physiological factors (Table 6–1). Psychological factors include those related to willingness and motivation to carry out the task, whereas physiological factors are concerned with the control of and energy generation for muscular contraction. The food components evaluated for their physical performance-enhancing potential could be targeted at both types of factors, but they are most often aimed at the physiological component and therefore will be the focus of this chapter. The reader is referred to Dishman (1989) for a review of the psychological factors in physical performance.

Physiological Factors

The four categories of physiological factors involved in physical task performance are (1) metabolic energy-generating system capacity, (2) neuromotor control, (3) energy substrate supply, and (4) tissue homeostasis. Each physical task may include components of each category, but the extent to which each component is involved varies greatly. The physical task of firing a rifle is predominantly determined by neuromotor control factors, whereas that of running for long distances is predominantly determined by the other three groups of factors. Potential physical performance-enhancing food additives could be targeted at any of the four categories of factors, and therefore, each category is considered below.

TABLE 6–1 Factors That Determine Physical Performance

Psychological factors
Arousal
Concentration
Motivation
Physiological factors
Metabolic capacity
Phosphagen stores
Glycolytic capacity
Aerobic capacity
Neuromotor control
Central nervous system processing
Nerve impulse to muscle
Inhibition and recruitment
Energy substrates
Carbohydrates, fatty acids
Supply, utilization
Tissue homeostasis
Hydrogen ion concentration
Osmolality
Temperature

Metabolic Capacity

The metabolic capacity to generate energy for muscular activity consists of three separate energy sources, with each source predominating in a particular duration and intensity of physical activity. These three types of muscular activity, summarized in Table 6–2, are commonly measured as muscular strength, anaerobic power, and aerobic power. Muscular strength, defined as the maximal force that can be generated in one muscular contraction, derives its energy almost exclusively from stored high-energy phosphagens, ATP, and creatinine phosphate (CP). Anaerobic power, also commonly referred to as *muscular endurance,* is defined as the muscular force generated during brief, intense exercise (repetitive contractions) which derives its energy primarily from phosphagens (ATP and CP) replenished from the anaerobic glycolytic metabolic pathway. Aerobic power is defined as the rate at which energy can be generated from oxygen-requiring phosphorylation of food substrates to replenish ATP and CP. The aerobic metabolic system is used primarily during prolonged physical activity of low- to moderate-level intensity.

TABLE 6–2 Sources of Energy for Muscular Contraction and Their Corresponding Types of Muscular Activity

Energy Source	Type of Activity	Measure
Stored ATP-CP	Single contraction	Muscular strength
Anaerobic glycolysis	Brief high intensity	Anaerobic power
Aerobic metabolism	Low-moderate intensity	Aerobic power

Thus, evaluation of an ergogenic aid predicted to act on energy supply delivery must be tailored to the appropriate energy system and its corresponding type of muscular activity.

Muscular Strength. The supply of stored energy for immediate muscular contractions, such as that required for lifting, pulling, or pushing, can be assessed by measuring muscular strength, or the maximal force that can be generated in a single movement. This supply is determined by both the concentration of phosphagens per unit of muscle and the amount of muscle involved, that is, the total available ATP and CP.

Muscle strength can be assessed in several modes: (1) isoinertial, which is the maximal force generated during the movement of a mass, as in lifting free weights or moving weight stacks on a weight machine (DeLorme, 1962); (2) isokinetic, which is the torque produced during maximal contraction at a constant velocity, as measured by various isokinetic devices such as the Cybex II (Sapega et al., 1983); and (3) isometric, which is the force generated during a static contraction, that is, contraction against an immovable mass (Caldwell et al., 1974). There is no single best choice among these three modes of strength measurement. Although precision and reproducibility of force quantification may be superior with isometric and isokinetic devices, the isoinertial mode more often mimics actual task performance and therefore has greater face validity (validity with actual tasks as opposed to artificial measures). It seems prudent to begin with controlled laboratory measures of isometric and isokinetic forces and then to use the more realistic isoinertial measures. If free weights, machines, or other force-measuring devices are unavailable, the maximal jump-and-reach test (Harman et al., 1991) is an example of a good means of measuring body strength that requires no equipment.

Several reports (Knapik et al., 1980; Sharp and Vogel, 1992; Sharp et al., 1980; Teves et al., 1985) contain normative strength data for U.S. Army populations.

Anaerobic Power. Measurement of anaerobic power is uniquely difficult since it cannot readily be isolated from the power provided by other energy systems. Markers of anaerobiosis, such as oxygen debt and lactic acid formation, have proven to be unsatisfactory. Measurement of anaerobic power, then, has focused on a physical performance test that measures the energy derived predominantly from the anaerobic glycolytic repletion of the high-energy phosphagens. Such performance tests measure very-high-intensity activities performed for 20 to 60 s.

Two currently accepted anaerobic power tests are the 20-s Wingate test (Patton et al., 1985), which uses a modified cycle ergometer, and the 60-s repeated contraction procedure of Thorstensson (1976), which uses an isokinetic dynamometer. The Wingate procedure records power output during a 20-s all-out effort when resistance is suddenly applied to the flywheel of the cycle ergometer. The Thorstensson test measures power output during 50 repeated maximal isokinetic contractions performed for a 60-s period. Normative Wingate data for men and women have been reported by Murphy et al. (1986). An example of Thorstensson endurance data for soldiers can be found in the report by Wright et al. (1983).

When ergometers or dynamometers are unavailable, suitable tests of anaerobic power include sprint runs and stair-climbing tests (Margaria et al. (1966).

Aerobic Power. The body's capacity to generate energy through the metabolic pathway of oxidative phosphorylation of diet-supplied substrates includes a number of components: pulmonary ventilation, oxygen saturation of the blood, pumping action of the heart, blood flow to the muscles, oxygen diffusion into the muscle cells, and action of the oxidative enzymes of the cell mitochondria. Some of these are possible sites for ergogenic aids. Aerobic power is measured as the maximal rate of oxygen consumption during exercise, referred to as maximal oxygen uptake $\dot{V}_{O_2\,max}$. Since oxygen consumption by the muscles depends on oxygen transfer at both the alveolar-capillary and capillary-cell interfaces, measurements of $\dot{V}_{O_2\,max}$ should involve exercise bouts that last long enough for oxygen consumption to reach a steady state for that particular exercise intensity, usually 3 to 5 min. The classical procedure for determining $\dot{V}_{O_2\,max}$ in humans is to employ uphill running on a treadmill using progressive, rest-interrupted exercise loads until a plateau in oxygen uptake with increasing exercise loads is achieved (Mitchell et al., 1958). This procedure generally gives the highest and most reproducible values. Other procedures (such as continuously increasing, uninterrupted loads) and other ergometric devices (cycle, rowing, arm crank ergometers) are commonly used. The primary variable leading to differences between various procedures and devices is the amount of muscle mass involved in the exercise. Stationary-cycle ergometers give values 7 to 10 percent lower than those obtained from running on a treadmill (Hermansen and Saltin, 1969; McArdle et al., 1973), whereas stationary repetitive lifting ergometry provides values approximately 22 percent below those provided by running on a treadmill (Sharp et al., 1988). Population data on the aerobic power of soldiers has been reported by Vogel et al. (1986).

Neuromotor Control

The second physiological determinant of physical performance is neuromotor control of the initiation, coordination, and maintenance of muscular activity. This is composed of central nervous system processing of afferent signals, transmission of efferent signals to the muscle, and the subsequent depolarization of the muscle myofibril to bring about muscle contraction. Neuromotor control is typically assessed by measuring reaction time, agility, and coordination. Even though these measures are more commonly applied to tasks that are not physically demanding, they can be used to assess performance of tasks that are complex and demanding, such as the repeated loading and firing of a howitzer.

Total reaction time, or the time from the recognition of a signal until a motor action takes place, can be fractionated into its components with the use of electromyography (Kroll, 1974), thereby allowing evaluation of the efficiency of each of the subcomponents of neuromotor control. Premotor time corresponds to the central processing component, while motor time represents the muscle contractile component. A typical procedure involves the presentation of a sudden visual signal to which the subject responds by hitting a target. The activity of the involved muscle is measured electromyographically (Clarkson, 1978).

A laboratory test of gross motor agility and coordination has been reported by Fitzgerald et al. (1986). For this test, a subject stands between two sets of shelves. During a 1-min time interval, the subject removes a 7.3-kg sliding drawer from a shelf at a 150-cm height on the left side, rotates 180 degrees and inserts the drawer into a shelf at a 50-cm height on the right side. The subject repeats this pattern by removing a second sliding drawer from the shelf on the upper right side and inserting this into a shelf on the lower left side. The process is then reversed, moving the shelves from the lower positions back to the upper ones. The motion is repeated as many times as possible within the 1-min period.

Examples of fine motor control tests that assess eye-hand coordination and steadiness include the arm-hand steadiness task (Kobrick et al., 1988, p. 6), the cord and cylinder manipulation test (Johnson, 1981, pp. 166–167), and marksmanship. Marksmanship can now be quantified in the laboratory by the use of laser marksmanship systems (Noptel ST-1000, Oulu, Findland) (Tharion et al., 1992).

Substrates and Tissue Homeostasis

The last two groups of physiological factors that determine physical performance are discussed in the context of the capacity to sustain performance at a submaximal level. The previous factors were presented in terms of their influence on maximal power output or control, but in actuality, most military tasks are performed at less than maximal ability so that they can be repeated or sustained over a period of time. For muscular activity to be sustained for a prolonged or indefinite period, energy substrates must be available to the aerobic energy system for oxidation and there must be an environment that favors the action of the oxidative enzymes.

This does not mean that maximal aerobic power is not a determining factor in sustained physical activity. The intensity of a particular physical task or activity is determined by the absolute energy requirement of the task and the aerobic power of the individual; the higher the person's $\dot{V}_{O_2\,max}$, the lower the intensity of the exercise and, therefore, the lower the imposition on substrate requirements and tissue homeostasis.

Energy Substrate Supply. During prolonged muscle activity, the muscles use both carbohydrates and free fatty acids for oxidative metabolism, with the proportions of each dependent on the intensity of exercise; the higher the intensity, the higher the utilization of glycogen. Since muscle carbohydrate stores (glycogen) are limited compared with the ample stores of lipids, potential ergogenic aids may target not only substrate stores but also their relative utilization during submaximal endurance exercise. Muscle glycogen levels during controlled endurance testing can be assessed directly through biopsies or indirectly through endurance times to exhaustion (Bergstrom and Hultman, 1967). The ratio of carbohydrate to fat utilization during such testing can be assessed through measurements of respiratory quotients or isotopic labeling of the substrates.

Tissue Homeostasis. Physical exercise inevitably tends to disrupt the optimal cell environment in terms of its hydrogen ion concentration, osmolality, fluid volume, and temperature. Prevention or attenuation of debilitating changes in these variables is another target for ergogenic aids. A common example is a buffering agent to counteract metabolic acidosis. Such ergogenic aids must be evaluated, as with substrate factors, in the context of submaximal endurance exercise tests, the final topic of this chapter.

Assessment of Submaximal Endurance Capacity

Endurance capacity tests are the most common types of evaluations used to assess potential physical performance enhancing agents. This is because they more realistically mimic real tasks than maximal power tests do. They not only provide a quantifiable endpoint of performance but they also provide a situation in which the actual physiological factors can be measured in a controlled and quantifiable setting.

Endurance capacity testing is probably best conducted in the laboratory, where conditions and exercise intensity can be controlled, usually by treadmill walking/running or stationary-cycle ergometry. Task endurance tests performed in the field are possible and are also discussed here.

Laboratory Tests of Aerobic Endurance

Exercise Mode. Treadmill and cycle ergometry are both commonly used for endurance testing, and each of these has advantages and disadvantages. The advantages of cycle ergometry are the ease of quantifying and controlling the exercise load, its physical safety, and the ease of performing such procedures as drawing blood and obtaining muscle biopsies. Discomfort while on the cycle seat, local muscle fatigue, and boredom tend to be disadvantages of stationary cycling. Treadmill walking or running has greater face validity for military tasks but has the disadvantages of the complications of foot blisters, greater safety concerns and less convenience in making ancillary measurements. Exercise load during treadmill walking can be adjusted by changing the speed and grade as well as the external loads that the subject carries. It is advantageous to conduct endurance testing by using pairs of subjects who are side by side, for motivational purposes.

Exercise Intensity. The absolute or relative exercise load chosen for an endurance test depends on the physiological factor(s) that is being targeted as well as considerations of subject time and cooperation. To be able to elicit a detectable endpoint of physical performance (exhaustion), an intensity relative to maximal aerobic power of between 70 and 90 percent is recommended. Intensities lower than this extend endurance times to the point that motivational and discomfort factors rather than physiological limitation become dominant. Intensities greater than this tend to bring in factors of strength and anaerobic power rather than the factors of substrate and tissue homeostasis that limit aerobic metabolism. Depending on the ergogenic aid being evaluated, greater intensities should be chosen if carbohydrate metabolism is of interest. Exercise intensities of about 75 percent $\dot{V}_{O_2\ max}$ produce endurance times of about 2 h, a convenient testing time for the laboratory setting.

Work-Rest Cycles. Although endurance tests to an exhaustion endpoint can be conducted in a continuous fashion without rest stops, short rest stops can have a motivational benefit as well as practical benefits for the ease of measurements. Gleser and Vogel (1971) demonstrated that rest periods of various lengths and work-rest ratios of 9:1, 18:2, 12:3 and 27:3 or no rest at all had no effect on endurance time during cycle ergometry at 75 percent $\dot{V}_{O_2\ max}$ (Figure 6–1). The work-rest ratio of 18:2 was a popular choice among the volunteers.

Endpoint Criteria. The point of "exhaustion" during treadmill or cycle endurance exercise can be problematic. Cycle ergometry has the advantage of using the inability to maintain a preset pedal rate at the prescribed exercise intensity as a well-defined endpoint. For the treadmill, a subject's judgment of when he or she is unable to continue (e.g., for 1 more min) or when a subject continues to drift back on the treadmill belt or grab the handrails can be used as endpoints of the test. All of these suggestions assume that the subjects' have experience in the test protocol.

An alternative to an exhaustion endpoint is the change in a physiological parameter above some preset threshold indicating that the subject has approached a physiological limit in such parameters as heart rate, core temperature, or blood lactate concentration. Such indicators may not, however, correspond well with actual exercise endurance time.

Test Experience. Gleser and Vogel (1971) also demonstrated that in endurance testing, subjects must be conditioned to or experienced with the test protocol before an asymptote in their performance is reached. They found that this was reached by the third week of weekly testing (Figure 6–2).

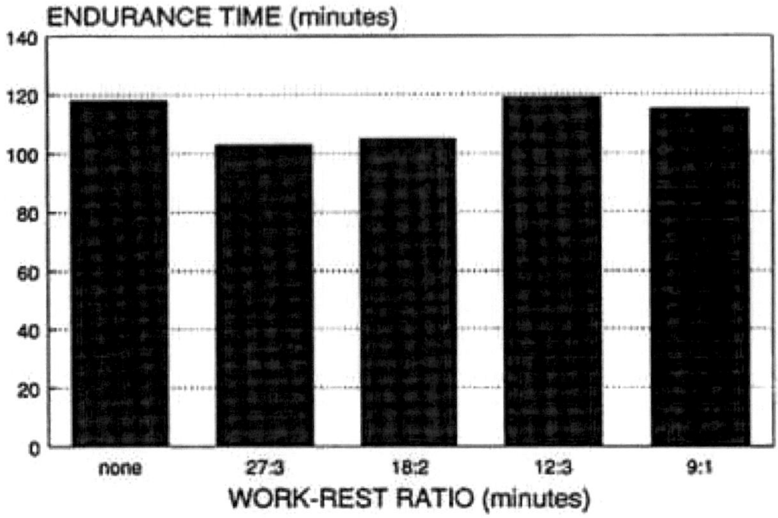

FIGURE 6–1 Influence of various work-rest ratios on endurance time on the cycle ergometer at 75 percent of $\dot{V}_{O_2\ max}$ SOURCE: Adapted from Gleser and Vogel (1971).

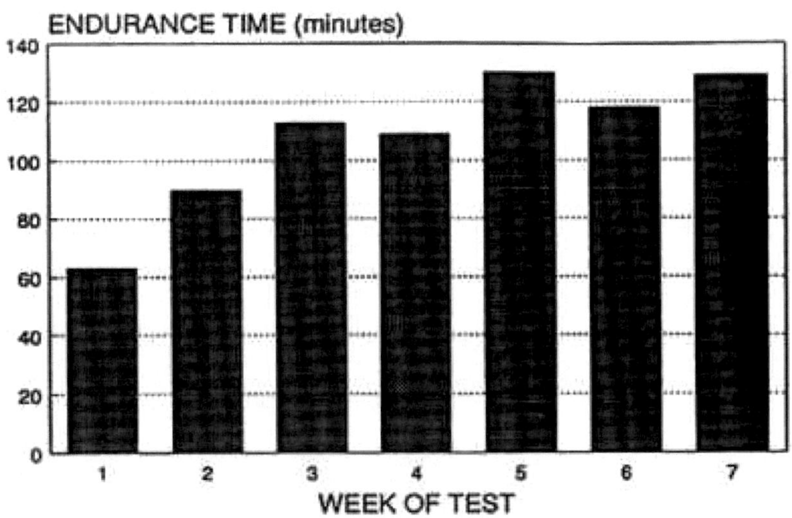

FIGURE 6–2 Effect of repeated weekly test experience on the endurance time of cycle ergometry at 75 percent of $\dot{V}_{O_2\ max}$. SOURCE: Adapted from Gleser and Vogel (1971).

Field Task Tests of Aerobic Endurance

Potential ergogenic aids that show positive effects during laboratory endurance testing should be further evaluated under actual field conditions. Despite the difficulties in conducting such tests because of the lack of control of motivation and external conditions, it is an important step in the evaluation of an ergogenic aid for military use. Potential aids that show a positive benefit in the relatively sterile environment of the laboratory but that lose their effects in the "noise" of the operational environment in the field may not deserve further consideration.

Field task tests should be conducted first in an isolated setting and should then be incorporated into a realistic operational combat scenario. Such field task tests generally differ from the laboratory version in that they utilize an actual military task, are typically self-paced, and most often use an endpoint of best-effort time to completion.

An isolated setting would consist of one in which the test task is performed before and after administration of the ergogenic aid and without other activities or stresses. An example of this type of field endurance test is a road march carrying a load for a given distance, observing the time for completion after asking the subjects for a maximal best effort and with the task performed by itself, not in an operational setting. Such an example is described by Knapik et al. (1990) for a road march over 20 km with a load of 46 kg. The standard deviation of that study's completion time (63 min, for a mean time of 304 min) demonstrates the high variability that is possible in such a test. This suggests the importance of using well-motivated subjects for this type of testing.

The final evaluation performed in a realistic operational setting would consist of a quantifiable task incorporated as part of a total operational scenario, such as a field training exercise or simulated unit combat training exercises. In this case the soldier is performing many tasks and is working under numerous demands, but with a single endurance task being used to evaluate the ergogenic aid.

It could be argued that testing under realistic operational conditions in the field is advantageous since it adds other stresses and demands on the soldier in addition to the exercise load of the task being evaluated, thereby creating a more vulnerable environment in which the potential performance-enhancing agent can exert its effect. This is more likely to be the case with psychoactive agents than with ergogenic agents.

RECOMMENDATIONS

The following steps should be taken in the evaluation of potential physical performance enhancing agents.

- Identify the target of action as a psychological or a physiological factor. Physiological factor targets should be further identified as being related to metabolic energy capacity, neuromotor control, or substrate supply and tissue homeostasis.
- Metabolic capacity targets should be further identified as one of the three energy-generating systems, and an appropriate measure should be selected for that system: strength, anaerobic power, or aerobic power.
- If energy substrate supply or tissue homeostasis is the target of the agent, then an aerobic endurance test should be chosen.
- Aerobic endurance testing should optimally be carried out in three stages: first, in a controlled laboratory setting using treadmill or other ergometric devices; second, in an isolated field setting for the task; and finally, as part of a total operational scenario setting.

REFERENCES

Bergstrom, J., and E.Hultman 1967 A study of the glycogen metabolism during exercise in man. J. Clin. Lab. Invest. 19:218–228.

Caldwell, L.S., D.B.Chaffin, F.N.Dukes-Dobos, K.H.E.Kroemer, L.L.Lauback, S.H.Snook, and D.E.Wasserman 1974 A proposed standard procedure for static muscle strength testing. Am. Ind. Hyg. Assoc. J. 35:201–206.

Clarkson, P.M. 1978 The effect of age and activity level on simple and choice fractionated response time. Eur. J. Appl. Physiol. 40:17–25.

DeLorme, T.L. 1962 Measurement and evaluation of weight training. Pp. 96–105 in Weight Training in Sports and Physical Education, F.D.Sills, L.E.Morehouse, and T.L.DeLorme, eds. Washington D.C.: American Association for Health, Physical Education, and Recreation.

Dishman, R.K. 1989 Psychology of sports competition. Pp. 129–164 in Sports Medicine, A.J.Ryan and F.L. Allman, Jr., eds. New York: Academic Press.

Fitzgerald, P.I., J.J.Knapik, W.L.Daniels, J.A.Vogel, and B.E.Joyce 1986 Influence of Atropine on Physical Performance in the Heat. Technical Report No. 16– 86. Natick, Mass: U.S. Army Research Institute of Environmental Medicine.

Gleser, M.A., and J.A.Vogel 1971 Endurance exercise: Effect of work-rest schedules and repeated testing. J. Appl. Physiol. 31:735–739.

Harman, E.A., M.T.Rosenstein, P.N.Frykman, R.M.Rosenstein, and W.J.Kraemer 1991 Estimation of human power output from vertical jump. J. Appl. Sport. Sci. Res. 5:116–120.

Hermansen, L., and B.Saltin 1969 Oxygen uptake during maximal treadmill and bicycle exercise. J. Appl. Physiol. 26:31–37.

Johnson, R.F. 1981 Effects of Explosive Ordnance Disposal (EOD) Armor on the Gross Body Mobility, Psychomotor Performance, Speech Intelligibility, and Visual Field of Men and Women. Technical Report No. 81/031. Natick, Mass.: U.S. Army Natick Research and Development Laboratories.

Knapik, J.J., J.W.Wright, D.M.Kowal, and J.A.Vogel 1980 The influence of U.S. Army basic initial entry training on the muscular strength of men and women. Aviat. Space Environ. Med. 51:1086–1090.

Knapik, J., M.Bahrke, J.Staab, K.Reynolds, J.Vogel, and J.O'Connor 1990 Frequency of Loaded Road March Training and Performance on a Loaded Road March. Technical Report No. 13–90. Natick, Mass.: U.S. Army Research Institute of Environmental Medicine.

Kobrick, J.L., R.F.Johnson, and D.J.McMenemy 1988 Nerve Agent Antidotes and Heat Exposure: Summary of Effects on Task Performance of Soldiers Wearing BDU and MOPP-IV Clothing Systems. Technical Report No. 1–89. Natick, Mass.: U.S. Army Research Institute of Environmental Medicine.

Kroll, W. 1974 Fractionated reaction and reflex time before and after fatiguing isotonic exercise. Med. Sci. Sports 6:260–266.

Margaria, R., P.Aghemo, and E.Ravelli 1966 Measurement of muscular power (anaerobic) in man. J. Appl. Physiol. 21:1662–1664.

McArdle, W.D., F.I.Katch, and G.S.Pechar 1973 Comparison of continuous and discontinuous treadmill and bicycle test for max Med. Sci. Sports 5:156–160.

Mitchell, J.H., B.J.Sproule, and C.B.Chapman 1958 The physiological meaning of the maximal oxygen intake test J. Clin. Invest. 37:538–547.

Murphy, M.M., J.F.Patton, and F.A.Frederick 1986 Comparative anaerobic power of men and women. Aviat. Space Environ. Med. 57:636–641.

Patton, J.F., M.M.Murphy, and F.A.Frederick 1985 Maximal power outputs during the Wingate anaerobic test. Int. J. Sports Med. 6:82–85.

Sapega, A.A., J.S.Torg, G.Drillings, and J.Vegso 1983 Modifications for enhanced data collection and analysis with the Cybex isokinetic dynamometer. Physician Sports Med. 11:103–110.

Sharp, D.S., J.E.Wright, J.A.Vogel, J.F.Patton, W.L.Daniels, J.Knapik, and D.M.Kowal 1980 Screening for Physical Capacity in the U.S. Army: An Analysis of Measurers Predictive of Strength and Stamina. Technical Report No. 8–80. Natick, Mass.: U.S. Army Research Institute of Environmental Medicine.

Sharp, M.A., and J.A.Vogel 1992 Maximal lifting strength in military personnel. Pp. 1261–1267 in Advances in Industrial Ergonomics and Safety IV, S.Kumar, ed. London: Taylor & Francis.

Sharp, M.A., E.Harman, J.A.Vogel, J.J.Knapik, and S.J.Legg 1988 Maximal aerobic capacity for repetitive lifting: Comparison with three standard exercise testing modes. Eur. J. Appl. Physiol. 57:753–760.

Teves, M.A., J.E.Wright, and J.A.Vogel 1985 Performance on Selected Candidate Screening Test Procedures before and after Army Basic and Advanced Individual Training. Technical Report No. 13–85. Natick, Mass.: U.S. Army Research Institute of Environmental Medicine.

Teves, M.A., J.A.Vogel, D.E.Carlson, and D.D.Schnakenberg 1986 Body Composition and Muscle Performance Aspects of the 1985 CFFS Test. Technical Report No. 12–86. Natick, Mass.: U.S. Army Research Institute of Environmental Medicine.

Tharion, W.J., R.W.Hoyt, B.E.Marlowe, and A.Cymerman 1992 Effects of high altitude and exercise on marksmanship. Aviat. Space Environ. Med. 63:114–117.

Thorstensson, A. 1976 Muscle strength, fibre types and enzyme activities in man. Acta Physiol. Scand. Suppl.: 443:1–45.

Vogel, J.A., J.F.Patton, R.P.Mello, and W.L.Daniels 1986 An analysis of aerobic capacity in a large United States population. J. Appl. Physiol. 60:494–500.

Wright, J.E., J.A.Vogel, J.B.Sampson, J.J.Knapik, J.F.Patton, and W.L.Daniels 1983 Effects of travel across time zones (jet-lag) on exercise capacity and performance. Aviat. Space Environ. Med. 54:132–137.

7

The Effects of Sleep Deprivation on Performance During Continuous Combat Operations

Gregory Belenky[1], *David M.Penetar, David Thorne, Kathryn Popp, John Leu, Maria Thomas, Helen Sing, Thomas Balkin, Nancy Wesensten, and Daniel Redmond*

INTRODUCTION

Good cognitive performance is central to successful combat operations. Command, control, communication, and intelligence are central to successful operations at all levels, from the crew, squad, and platoon levels through the division and corps levels. Battles are won or lost at the small-unit level (company, platoon, squad, and crew) (English, 1984). A single, small group

[1] Gregory Belenky, Walter Reed Army Institute of Research, Department of Behavioral Biology, Washington, DC 20307–5100

delivering modest amounts of fire at the right place and at the right time often determines the outcome of a major engagement (Marshall, 1978).

Sleep deprivation impairs alertness, cognitive performance, and mood. The ability to do useful mental work declines by 25 percent for every successive 24 h that an individual is awake. Thorne et al. (1983) have studied cognitive performance using a variety of computer-based cognitive performance tests during 72 h of total sleep deprivation in normal volunteer subjects. Those data and their analysis are summarized in Figure 7–1. The performance data in Figure 7–1 are expressed as throughput—the product of speed and accuracy. During sleep deprivation, performance declines, but it usually declines in such a way as to preserve the accuracy of response at the expense of speed. The throughput measure captures the combination of speed and accuracy and measures the amount of useful (i.e., accurate) work done per unit of time. Sleep deprivation degrades the most complex mental functions, including the ability to understand, adapt, and plan under rapidly changing circumstances. In contrast, simple psychomotor performance and physical strength and endu

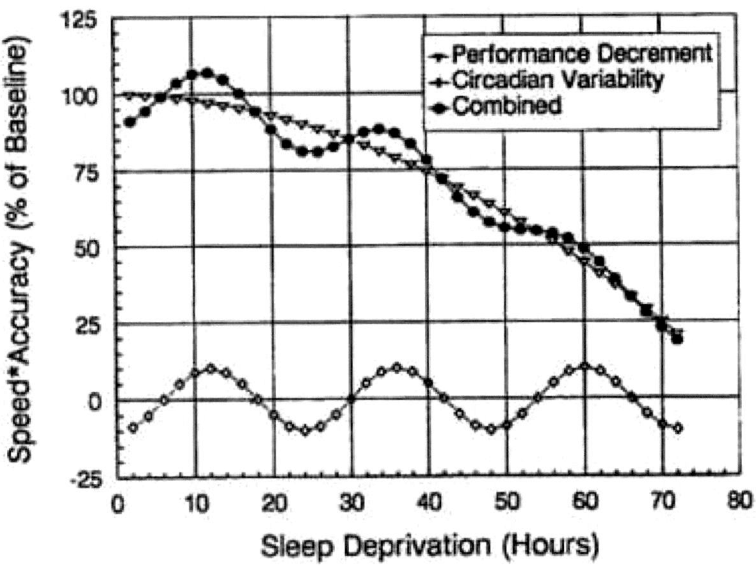

FIGURE 7–1 Effect of 72 h of total sleep deprivation on cognitive performance of normal volunteer subjects. The combined curve is decomposed into circadian variability and a negatively accelerating decrement in performance.

endurance are unaffected. For example, a soldier can shoot as tight a cluster of rounds at a fixed target after 90 h without sleep as he or she can when well rested, but if he or she has to shoot at targets that pop up at random at random locations on a firing range, then his or her performance drops to below 10 percent of baseline (Haslam and Abraham, 1987).

Pilot data from Thomas et al. (1988) suggest that sleep deprivation-induced decrements in performance are accompanied by decreases in brain glucose metabolism, particularly in the frontal areas. This provides a neurobiological correlate for the performance decrements. Whether the brain is less able to use glucose and hence is less able to do work, or is doing less work and hence uses less glucose, remains to be determined by future research.

Brief fragmented sleep has little recuperative value and is similar to total sleep deprivation in its effects on performance. Bonnet (1987) fragmented the sleep of normal volunteers by sounding an increasingly loud tone every 2–3 min until the subjects met the arousal criterion. For one group of subjects, the arousal criterion was a full awakening, as indicated by a movement and a verbal response. For a second group, the arousal criterion was a simple postural adjustment, with no verbal response required. For a third group, the arousal criterion was simply a change in the electroencephalogram (EEG), with no movement or verbal response required. All three arousal criteria destroyed the recuperative value of sleep as measured by the subjects' alertness and performance on the next day. Bonnet's results were not the result of sleep restriction, as subjects in all groups had near normal total sleep times, but rather they were the result of sleep fragmentation. Bonnet's results are of great relevance to performance during continuous combat operations. If fragmentation of sleep, even fragmentation of sleep with no obvious behavioral manifestation (i.e., the change in the EEG only group), destroys the recuperative value of sleep, then not only duration but also continuity of sleep is important. In consultations to U.S. Army combat units, investigators stressed the need for sleep. Often, commanders have taken and applied the advice only to come back with something like: "I took a four-hour nap and awoke feeling no better than when I went to sleep." When asked where they slept, a typical answer was "in the corner of my TOC." (TOC is an acronym for Tactical Operations Center.) During continuous operations, the TOC is a busy, noisy place (people moving around and talking, radios giving off bursts of static) 24 h a day. Behaviorally (as judged by not moving and not talking), these commanders remained asleep for the period of the nap. It is hypothesized that they suffered frequent EEG-only arousals that fragmented their sleep and destroyed its recuperative value.

Continuous combat is characterized by brief fragmented sleep. In anecdotal accounts of actual combat operations and objective studies of simulated combat operations, brief, fragmented sleep is the rule rather than the exception. Pleban et al. (1990) have studied sleep during the 58 days of U.S. Army Ranger School. These 58 days involve simulated light infantry operations against a superior force. In one study of one class, Ranger candidates averaged 3.2 h of sleep each night over the 58 days of the school (Pleban et al., 1990). In a second study of two classes, Ranger candidates averaged 3.6 h of sleep each night (Popp and Redmond, in preparation). This sleep was not accrued in a single sleep period but in a several naps over each 24-h period. Anecdotally, cognitive performance in Ranger candidates was marginal, with frequent episodes of what the Rangers call "droning," in which candidates can put one foot in front of another and respond if challenged but have difficulty grasping their situation or acting on their own initiative.

Investigators in our research group have studied sleep during simulated armored and mechanized infantry operations at the National Training Center (NTC) in the high desert of Southern California. The operations involve battalion-sized task forces, consist of force on force and live fire exercises, and last for 14 days. As in the Ranger School study, sleep is brief and fragmented at NTC. Notable in the NTC study was the fact that there was a clear correlation between sleep and rank and between sleep and echelon of command and control. Whereas the personnel at the squad and crew levels averaged between 7 and 8 h of sleep each night, those at the battalion and brigade levels averaged little more than 4 h of sleep each night. Thus, from the perspective of sleep and its effects on performance, one would expect personnel at lower echelons to be more effective than personnel at higher echelons. This is what was observed, with the more junior people improving their performance over the course of the exercise and the more senior people "droning," to use the Ranger School term, toward the end of the exercise.

McNally and colleagues (1989) have used data from Thorne et al. (1983) on the effects of total sleep deprivation on individual cognitive performance as input to the Army Unit Resiliency Analysis (AURA) model. The AURA model is detailed, modeling the performance of individual soldiers in the unit and, from this, the performance of the unit as a whole. It is this modeling of individual performance that allowed McNally et al. (1989) to use the laboratory data of Thorne et al. (1983) as input data. Specifically, they modeled the effects of sleep deprivation on artillery company performance with 4, 5, 6, or 7 h of sleep each night. They measured artillery company performance in rounds per tube (artillery piece) per day accurately delivered to the target. This is a measure of productivity similar to the throughput measure Thorne et al. (1983) used in their laboratory studies of sleep-deprived normal volunteers. The results of McNally et al. (1983) are depicted in Figure 7–2. What is obvious from Figure 7–2 is that deliberately restricting unit sleep in the hopes of greater output is unproductive. For 2–3 days, the unit that slept less was able, by virtue of having more time in which to work, to put more rounds accurately on target in any 24-h period, but after the third day, their efficiency degraded to the point that even with this extra time to work their output was less. Even though the unit that slept for 4 h each night had 3 h more in each 24-h period in which to work, their overall output for the 24-h period fell below that for the unit that slept for 7 h each night by the third day of operations. In addition, according to the model, the unit's aggregate output continued to fall as the days passed. These modeling results provide a qualitative estimate of the effects of partial sleep deprivation on unit performance over days and weeks of continuous operations.

Data from individual subjects in prolonged sleep deprivation show a gradual, systematic decline in performance (Thorne et al., 1983) (Figure 7–1). Modeling of unit performance during continuous operations when subjects are given 4, 5, 6, or 7 h sleep each night shows the same gradual, systematic decline (McNally et al., 1989). In realistic operational simulations and in actual

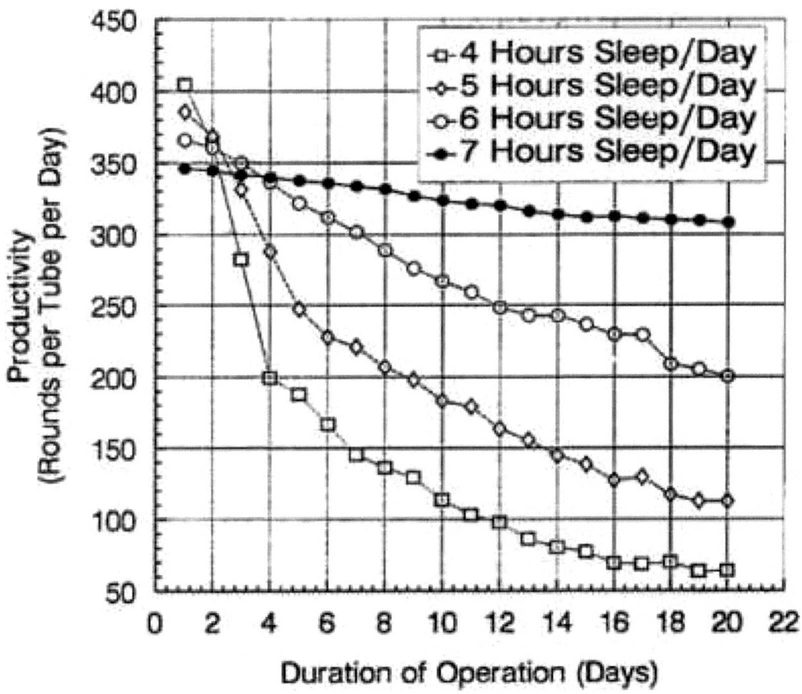

FIGURE 7–2 Effect of 4, 5, 6, or 7 h of sleep each night on artillery company performance during 21 days of continuous operations. These are modeling data derived from the Army Unit Resiliency Analysis model of artillery company performance.

operations, these systematic declines in performance may be of no great consequence for a few days if the task at hand is simple and familiar and if an accurate although slower response is sufficient to complete the task. However, the task may be complex, unfamiliar, and/or intrinsically time-limited, and then sudden, severe, and even catastrophic failure can occur. Examples are illustrative.

Banderet and colleagues (1981) conducted a detailed, realistic simulation of artillery fire direction center (FDC) team operations. FDCs are manned by five-person teams. Their task is to plot the location of a target as given by observers farther forward and to derive range, bearing, angle of gun elevation, and charge. Targets may be called in on the fly with requests for immediate fire (fire missions) or may be called in advance for firing upon at a later time (preplanned targets). In either case, the FDC should derive range, bearing, etc., upon receipt of the target location, and in the case of a fire mission, the FDC should send this information directly to the guns or, in the case of a preplanned target, hold the information until a call for fire on that target is received. In the process of plotting target location, the FDC updates its situation map and clears the target to be sure that the location plotted is not that of a hospital, school, church, etc. At the time that Banderet et al. did their study, FDC teams were able to process two fire missions concurrently. In that study, FDC teams from the 82nd Airborne Division were run through simulated operations for 36 h. Throughout the 36 h, their ability to accurately derive range, bearing, elevation, and charge was unimpaired. However, after about 24 h they stopped keeping up their situation map and stopped computing their preplanned targets immediately upon receipt. They lost their grasp of their place in the operation. They no longer knew where they were located relative to friendly and enemy units. They no longer knew what they were firing at. Early in the simulation, when the investigators called for fire on, for example, a hospital, they would check their situation map, appreciate the nature of the target, and question the request. Later, without a current situation map, they would fire without hesitation, regardless of the nature of the target. Early in the simulation, when the investigators called in two concurrent fire missions and called for fire on a preplanned target, they would, having already plotted and derived information for the preplanned target, fire on all three quickly and accurately. Later, when the investigators called in two concurrent fire missions and called for fire on a preplanned target, the team, having neglected to plot and derive information for the preplanned target, would try to plot and derive information for three targets concurrently, and the targets, if fired on at all, were fired on only after long delays.

One of the authors of this chapter (G.Belenky) conducted after-action debriefings with personnel involved in friendly-fire incidents in the 100-h ground war during Operation Desert Storm. At dusk, after 48-plus h of continuous operations (i.e., operations with brief, fragmented sleep), a platoon of six Bradley fighting vehicles was ordered to cease forward advance and to set up a screen line. No further movement was planned until the next morning. The platoon was flanked to the right and left by other Bradley fighting vehicle platoons. Supporting each platoon of Bradley fighting vehicles was a platoon of four M-1 tanks. These tanks took up positions some distance to the rear of the Bradleys. This was the position at last light. At about 0100 h, hot spots were observed in the thermal imaging sights moving toward the screen line. For reasons that remain obscure, even though the debriefing occurred soon after the event, these hot spots were simply observed until they ran into the screen line, at which point they resolved themselves into six Iraqi armored personnel carriers. This was not an attack; the Iraqis were still in column and were presumably just as surprised as the Americans. A firefight ensued in which all the Iraqi vehicles were destroyed. In the process, two Bradley fighting vehicles were destroyed. Fortunately, there were no American casualties. Conversely, there were no Iraqi survivors. Later, it was established that the Bradley fighting vehicles were destroyed by friendly fire. From the debriefings, here is apparently what happened. The two Bradleys that were destroyed were on the left of the platoon's screen line. The one or two Bradleys that destroyed them were on the right of the platoon's screen line. The advancing Iraqi column coming from the front and right encountered the screen line at an angle in proximity to the two Bradleys on the far left. The advancing Iraqi column was destroyed in a formation that was still in a column and trailing off at an angle to the right. The two Bradleys on the left were maneuvering in and around the first two Iraqi vehicles that were, by then, destroyed and burning. The Bradleys on the right, believing the Bradleys on the left to be Iraqis, engaged and destroyed them. Thanks to the crew protection built into the Bradleys, the five-men crews in both vehicles escaped unhurt. On debriefing, it was apparent that the two Bradleys on the right believed that they were firing forward and were unaware that they were enfilading their own line. Although no objective measures of sleep duration and continuity were made in this platoon, by self-report sleep for the prior 48-plus h had been brief and fragmented. This friendly fire incident is consistent with the known effects of sleep deprivation on performance. The ability to lay cross hairs on a target and accurately squeeze off rounds remained intact. What was lost was orientation and grasp of the tactical situation. The crews of the Bradley fighting vehicles that fired on their own comrades held to the sound tactical idea that "if it's in front of us it dies." However, they were no longer clear as to where front was.

CONCLUSIONS AND RECOMMENDATIONS

In conclusion, soldiers can fight for extended periods of time with only brief, fragmented sleep, but they become progressively less productive as the days pass and are increasingly prone to abrupt and serious failures in command and control. Commanders at all echelons should encourage sleep. Deliberately restricting sleep at any echelon in the hope of getting more out of soldiers and units is unproductive. In contrast, an adequate duration and continuity of sleep will sustain individual and unit performance indefinitely. To paraphrase General George Patton, the idea is not to give up sleep for your country but to make the other poor bastard give up sleep for his.

REFERENCES

Banderet, L.E., J.W.Stokes, R.Francesconi, D.M.Kowal, and P.Naitoh 1981 Artillery teams in simulated sustained combat: Performance and other measures. Pp. 581–604 in DHHS (Department of Health and Human Services) NIOSH (National Institute for Occupational Safety and Health) Report 81–127: The Twenty-Four Hour Workday: Proceedings of a Symposium on Variations in Work-Sleep Schedules, L.C. Johnson, D.I.Tepas, W.P.Colquhon, and M.J.Colligan, eds. Washington, D.C.: U.S. Government Printing Office .

Bonnet, M.H. 1987 Sleep restoration as a function of periodic awakening, movement, or electroencephalographic change. Sleep 10:364–373.

English, J.A. 1984 On Infantry. Pp. 145–147 New York: Praeger.

Haslam, D.R., and P.Abraham 1987 Sleep loss and military performance. Pp. 167–184 in Contemporary Studies in Combat Psychiatry, G.Belenky, ed. Westport, Conn.: Greenwood Press.

Marshall, S.L.A. 1978 Men Against Fire. Pp. 138–156. Gloucester, Mass.: Peter Smith. McNally, R.E., A.M. Machovec, D.T.Ellzy, and S.R.Hursh

1989 Evaluation of Sleep Discipline in Sustaining Unit Performance. SAIC Contract No. MDA903–88-D-1000: McClean, Va: Science Applications International Corporation.

Pleban, R.J., P.J.Valentine, D.M.Penetar, D.P.Redmond, and G.Belenky 1990 Characterization of sleep and body composition changes during ranger training. Milit. Psychol. 2:145–156.

Thomas, M., H.Sing, G.Belenky, D.Thorne, T.Balkin, D.Penetar, D.Redmond, J.Norcross, P. Newhouse, H.Mayberg, H.Holcomb, B.Sadzot, R.Dannals, J.Links, and H. Wagner 1988 Positron emission tomography measurement of human regional cerebral glucose utilization following 48 hours of sleep deprivation. Soc. Neurosci. Abstr. 14:48.

Thorne, D.R., S.G.Genser, H.C.Sing, F.W.Hegge 1983 Plumbing human performance limits during 72 hours of high task load. Pp. 17–40 in Proceedings of the 24th DRG Seminar on the Human as a Limiting Element in Military Systems. Toronto: Defence and Civil Institute of Environmental Medicine.

8

The Role of Context in Behavioral Effects of Foods

Herbert L.Meiselman and F.Matthew Kramer[1]

INTRODUCTION

The situation in which we eat, the eating context, is receiving increasing attention as a major factor in the control of eating habits. Traditionally, more attention was placed on the food itself and the personality characteristics and physiology of the eater. Placing food in its context has led to research and discussion of a number of situational or contextual variables such as the effort needed to obtain food (Collier, 1989; Meiselman et al., 1988), the time of day food is eaten (Birch et al., 1984; Kramer et al., 1992), the presence of other food, and social dynamics (de Castro and Brewer, 1991). Schutz (1988) sought to capture the overall impact of eating contexts in his measurement of "appropriateness," which indicates how well a food fits into a particular situation.

The emerging role of context has been reflected in its inclusion in recent international meetings. At the First International Conference on Food Choice,

[1] Herbert L.Meiselman and F.Matthew Kramer, U.S. Army Natick, ATTN: SATNC-Y, Natick, MA 01760–5020

a multidisciplinary meeting held in Brussels, Belgium, in July 1992, a number of sessions were devoted to the cultural and social context of eating, and papers throughout the meeting addressed context as well. At the meeting on Advances in Sensory Science, held in Helsinki, Finland, in August 1992 in memory of Professor Rose Marie Pangborn, an entire session was devoted to context.

The U.S. Army's interest in context began with large field studies of the military ration, the Meal Ready to Eat, in the early 1980s. The traditional approach was to research and evaluate food product development and improvement. In the early 1980s, however, researchers began to realize that without attention to the eating situation they could never fully understand what controls eating and what should be done to maximize soldiers' intakes of needed nutrients. Some of that research is presented in articles by Meiselman et al. (1988) and Hirsch and Kramer (1993).

Not only was it necessary to rethink what controls eating, but it was also necessary to rethink how to conduct research. Researchers began to doubt the adequacy of short-term laboratory tests, and so they focused more on longer-term field tests that better covered the situational variables that are now viewed as critical. The questioning of how human food research is conducted led to a recent critical review of methodology in the journal *Appetite* (Meiselman, 1992).

The role of context has long been realized in the experimental design literature (Campbell and Stanley, 1966). The difference now may be that while context was traditionally seen as a source of confounding to be controlled, more effort is currently being put into defining and studying the impact of context. The change in research is not only in how research is conducted but also in the focus.

A useful example might be derived from the growing body of research on noncaloric substances such as sugar and fat substitutes as human foods. The initial studies were simple, looking at the impact of a sweet drink (e.g., aspartame-containing beverages) on the subsequent intake of a test meal. In principle, to the subjects the drinks or other vehicles were made to seem equivalent, so that any differences in response to the drinks could be attributed to the fact that one contained calories and the other did not. Among these early studies of aspartame were reports (Blundell and Hill, 1986) suggesting that consumption of such items enhanced hunger and possibly intake as well, implying that diet drinks would not only fail to produce useful reductions in caloric intake but might actually be associated with increases. Early studies also indicated that typical two-group comparisons could not readily separate out the role of calories versus the role of sweetness (Blundell et al., 1988). Given the nature of these findings, aspartame and other noncaloric sweeteners have been the subject of many recent studies (see Rolls [1991] for a review), but those studies have not yet clarified their impacts on food habits. What those studies have made clear is that the results and conclusions reflect the context of the study. Depending on the investigation, aspartame is associated with an increase, decrease, or no change in eating or other outcome measures (Rolls, 1991). The context of the studies has varied across the means of administration (flavored or unflavored beverages, food and meal ingredients, chewing gum, capsule form), timing of administration (preload before a measurement period, during a meal or meals, at multiple times during the day), outcome measures (consumption, palatability, hunger or other subjective ratings, thermic effect of ingestion), length of study (single meals, 24-h impact, 1 to 2 weeks), and participant expectations (whether subjects were informed that they were taking aspartame, use of aspartame as a diet aid).

The role of context in studying the effects of foods on performance and mood and then applying those effects covers a wide area. One could discuss the context of the research situation, its physical and social environment, and the food and its immediate context. One could discuss the nonresearch eating situation in which, ultimately, foods of interest are consumed. One could also discuss the military context, which investigators are trying to address using performance- and mood-altering foods. Not all aspects of the topic can be covered because of the current state of the art, but this chapter should remind the reader of context and perhaps raise the reader's assessment of its role in the effects of food on performance and mood. Context can be covered by looking at foods, the people who eat them, and the environment in which researchers test and try to predict peoples responses.

DETERMINING A BASELINE

Studies of the effects of foods on performance or mood generally need a baseline condition against which treatment effects can be measured. Kruesi and Rapaport (1986) point out that baseline data can be used to estimate variance and help to control problems of individual differences, a key problem in these tests. However, Kruesi and Rapaport also note the potential problems of treatment order effects whenever a baseline precedes a treatment.

Christensen (1991) discussed several alternatives for controlling the immediate previous nutritional states of test subjects. For a diet that is to be consumed the next day, for example, the experimenter can request abstinence from eating following the evening meal or can administer a standard meal before the test. Both conditions might require that subjects receive instructions about what else they can or cannot eat or drink. The subjects' "normal" eating is being changed, which sets up potential changes in, for example, eating habit patterns and concern about what is being done to them.

In some cases, Christensen (1991) recommends an elimination or washout phase for 2 to 3 weeks, such as those used in allergy research. They point out that the elimination phase allows for baseline assessment of behavior and permits the full range of the response to manifest itself after reintroduction of the food. A washout phase can clearly show the benefits of avoiding the food and the detriments or advantages of adding the food to the diet. However, this method or approach is likely to influence subjects' expectations. Washout phases must be done with the subjects' permission and cooperation. The subjects must think, for example, that they are doing something to help themselves, something aversive, or something difficult. A washout condition is not like a neutral baseline where one measures "normal" behavior before the introduction of the treatments. The washout condition is a treatment itself that can produce, for instance, withdrawal effects (for caffeine, see Griffiths and Woodson [1988]), varying widely in incidence, severity, and duration. Therefore, subjects must be warned of potential adverse effects, perhaps exacerbates their expectancies. Christensen and colleagues (1991) farther point out that the treatment does not always result in prewashout levels.

In addition to attending to dietary baselines, one must also consider the subjects' overall baseline condition. Their prior psychological state could be significant if mood changes are a possible or likely outcome of the dietary treatment. Psychological state could also affect performance on some tasks (e.g., demanding cognitive tasks).

Researchers need to decide whether to consider baseline behavior and mood under conditions of nutrition similar to those that occur in field or nonfield situations. It has been well documented that soldiers in the field, on average, do not eat all of their food. Many eat so little that they lose weight. This issue of underconsumption is dealt with below; the issue here is to highlight the problem of specifying the nutrient status under which the baseline is determined.

Thus, before one even begins a test with a food stimulus, there is a context problem. In what way does one determine baseline performance, and in what way does one examine behavior or mood without any treatment? Many ways of establishing baselines might be as potent as treatments in changing food habits.

EXPECTANCY

Studies in both humans and animals have repeatedly shown that subjects' expectancies and attributions regarding an "intervention" can dramatically change cognitive, emotional, and behavioral responses. Placebo effects are of critical importance in drug-behavior research. The risk of such attitudinal effects has led investigators to use, for example, double-blind crossover designs with or without washout phases to be able to conclude that any effects that they find are due to the drug or nutrient under study.

Although studies designed to control for the cognitive effects of expectancies, for example, are an important and necessary step in the evaluation of potential performance-enhancing substances for the practitioner or, for the purpose of this volume, the U.S. military, the issue is whether these interventions will be potent in both the expected and unexpected real-life scenarios soldiers face. One cannot approach these questions from a purely physiological point of view. For instance, Siegel (1988) in rat models and Marlatt and Rohsenow (1980) in a study of humans have shown that in situations in which pharmacologically active doses of potent, addictive drugs are administered with the organism either expecting or not expecting the substance, the consequences of ingestion are determined more by the organism's expectancy than by whether or not the substance is consumed.

Caffeine is a good example because it is commonly used in an effort to maintain alertness and performance by both civilian and military personnel. Caffeine has been shown to be effective at maintaining alertness and to function as a potent reinforcer (Griffiths and Woodson, 1988). A recent double-blind trial found that withdrawal symptoms can occur in chronic caffeine users even when that use is modest (i.e., about 0.59 1 [2.5 cups] of coffee per day). These findings indicate the potency of caffeine. Nonetheless, studies of caffeine (Fillmore and Vogel-Sprott, 1992; Kirsch and Weixel, 1988) have found clear effects of expectancies on measures as diverse as mood, blood pressure, and motor performance. Parallel studies on placebos, alcohol, and eating likewise indicate that expectancies improve behavioral outcomes (Lick and Bootzin, 1975; Marlatt and Rohsenow, 1980; Polivy, 1976).

Given the potential importance of these cognitive mediators, research is needed not just on controlling them to determine the utility of various substances but also on understanding and applying these influences in relevant situations. For example, Cardello and Sawyer (1992) have shown that one's expectation of a food determines its acceptability and is related to how much is consumed. A number of studies have shown that military food and food in a military package are perceived unfavorably, which may explain, in part, the typical underconsumption of rations by soldiers. Studies of expectancies and attributions would help not only in determining the ultimate usefulness of agents but also in developing guidelines for administering the substances (e.g., nutrient supplements within food items versus in pill form) and educating soldiers to obtain the best match of cognitive and physiological forces.

CONTROLLING THE FOOD, STIMULUS, AND TREATMENT

A number of reviews have highlighted the need for carefully controlled treatment conditions. Kruesi and Rapaport (1986) call for double-blind treatment conditions in which neither the subject nor the experimenter can identify treatment conditions. Blind conditions are essential when the subject or experimenter is likely to have beliefs or expectations about the treatment in particular or the behavioral effects of foods in general. Christensen (1991) even suggests that expectancy can produce behavior that mimics treatment effects under the placebo condition and that one must use continuation of an effect to determine a real treatment effect. Many people claim sensitivity to monosodium glutamate, but very few people actually show an allergic reaction under blind conditions (Meiselman, 1987).

To utilize blind conditions, there must be a treatment substitute (placebo) that is indistinguishable from the treatment. Substituting decaffeinated coffee for caffeinated coffee, for example, appears possible in the short term; but making large dietary changes, like substituting aspartame for sugar in all foods and over an extended period of time, is often not possible (Christensen 1991).

Neither the treatment nor the placebo condition should require the subject to expend more effort. Studies have shown that increased effort affects food choices and intake in both laboratory and natural eating environments (Engell and Hirsch, 1991; Meiselman, et al., 1994). When the effort to obtain a food is increased, selection and, as a result, intake of that food decrease. Moreover, the depressed intake does not necessarily appear to recover quickly or fully when the need for increased effort to obtain a food is removed.

Controlling the treatment often requires placement of the treatment at a certain frequency within the 24-h cycle. The experimenter must decide how often and at what times to deliver the treatment. These times and cycles might not coincide with the subject's normal daily patterns of eating or activity. The issue is whether to allow the subject to control the timing of treatment, or permit the experimenter to test all subjects at the same treatment time.

PEOPLE

Individual Differences

It is a truism to say that the effects of a given nutrient or other form of intervention vary from person to person. In broad terms, individual differences in response can be either continuum based (i.e., the dose-response relationship varies across individuals) or category based (i.e., a subset of individuals does not respond to the intervention or some individuals might respond in a paradoxical manner). One needs to determine not only the average response but also who responds and to what degree, and one must attempt to determine whether the differences between people are due to their intrinsic characteristics or to other outside influences. In part, this speaks to determining the dosage method that best captures the population of interest. Another assumption that may need to be addressed is person-situation consistency. In other words, if one can reliably describe how a given set of people will respond to the intervention in a particular situation, can one generalize across situations; or is it the case that exposure to physical or psychological stress will change who does and who does not respond? The ultimate goal is to derive a situation- and person-specific dosing system.

Individual differences also can play a mediating role. For example, caffeine may function fairly successfully as an alertness enhancer in most people, or tyrosine might aid in the reduction of stress-based decrements in performance. However, as noted previously, if the relevant source items are not consumed—a real risk with military rations—then the effectiveness or lack thereof is moot. A well-known fact in dietetic studies is that intraindividual variation for most nutrients is as large or larger than interindividual variation (Beaton et al., 1979). Thus, if the agent of interest has a relatively narrow range of effectiveness or is otherwise inflexible regarding its daily required dose, a substantial chance of ineffectiveness arises solely because of soldiers' inconsistencies in consuming source rations or items.

Also of relevance here is that to determine the true daily intake of nutrients in the face of large intraindividual variations, repeated assessment of intake over a number of representative days is required (about 7–14 days depending on the nutrient of interest) (Basiotis et al., 1987; Beaton et al., 1979; Nelson et al., 1989). Similarly, inter- and intravariations in subjects' responses to nutrients could be determined and used to guide the length of evaluations as well as to help investigators understand better the individual variation. Beaton and colleagues (Beaton et al., 1979; Tarasuk and Beaton, 1992a,b) discuss at length the nature and implications of within-subject variability in nutrient intake. A study by Caputo and Mattes (1992) is typical. Subjects were overfed or underfed with carbohydrate or fat. The authors concluded that, although as a group, subjects compensated better for dilutions than for supplementations of energy intake, individual patterns of compensations were highly variable. Likewise, Epstein (1980, 1983) has championed this focus on extended assessment over time as the best approach to obtaining stable behavioral measures. In general, studies on the role of nutrition on behavior might have to be longer than is currently the norm.

Clinical Disorders

One aspect of individual differences may be represented by individuals with clinical deficiencies or excesses. For example, food and mood (Herman et al., 1987; Leathwood and Pollet, 1982–1983; Morley et al., 1986) are frequently linked, as are mood and performance. Both anxiety and depression have been linked to changes in behavioral activation and food intake. Although the "typical" response to such negative moods—especially at high levels—is a decrement in food intake as well as performance, there are subgroups that tend to show enhanced eating in the face of such stressors. Although clinical disorders per se may not be of central importance to examining the nutrition-performance relationship in the military, such studies do provide a basis for examining the potential role of underlying physiological or psychological states on the relationship.

For example, although both fear and hunger alone can potentiate behavior, when both are present the combination of an aversive and appetitive stimulus can lead to different experimental conclusions, depending on the assessment methodology. As reported by Gray (1987), fear reduces the probability of eating in a hungry subject, but if eating does occur it is more vigorous than that in a nonfearful subject. It is not unreasonable to expect that different mood states will influence the probability of behavioral choices and, in turn, also influence the strength of that behavior once it is chosen.

A more apt example of pathology relates to the impact of jet lag or shift work on performance. This topic has received considerable attention from U.S. Army Research Institute of Environmental Medicine (USARIEM) as well as many other military and civilian research centers (Moline et al., 1990; Tepas, 1990). Circadian rhythms appear to be intimately linked to metabolism, mood, and behavior, and as has been shown repeatedly, disruptions of these rhythms are also disruptive to performance (Armstrong, 1980; Boulos and Terman, 1980; Halberg, 1989). Given the nature of military operations, challenges to circadian rhythms are to be expected, and in instances of rapid deployment, they pose a potentially serious risk. Circadian rhythms may also have a mediating role on food and performance relationships (Mistlberger, 1990). Metabolic research suggests that physiological responses to nutrients vary depending on the time of day when the nutrients are ingested. In addition, the timing of a meal appears to influence some, although not all, biological rhythms. The appropriate type of dietary component and the appropriate dose and schedule of ingestion depend, among other factors, on the schedule in force prior to the disruption, the specifics of the actual disruption, and the feeding and sleep schedule that is possible following the disruption.

Social Influence

Although social sources of influence are pervasive, much remains to be learned about how social factors influence performance and behavior. Social influences are difficult to assess, in part because such influences can be manifested in several ways. Social influences may be categorized in terms of time of occurrence (e.g., influences that occur at the time of measurement versus influences that reflect past experience) and by pathway (e.g., behavioral or verbal modeling and social context) and whether the influences have a direct or indirect impact on what is being measured. Social influences can enhance or detract from concurrent physiological factors (Goldman et al., 1991). Furthermore, social influences can be evaluated in terms of individuals or groups. The majority of food intake research focuses on individuals, as in studies of how much a subject consumes when a confederate eats a relatively large or small meal. The military, however, has a long-standing interest in issues such as unit morale and cohesion and how these group-oriented variables affect unit performance.

A growing body of work (de Castro and Brewer, 1991; Redd and de Castro, 1992) indicates that consumption increases for individuals as the number of people with whom they are eating increases. This social facilitation has been seen with other behaviors (Latane, 1981). The findings of de Castro and colleagues appear to be at least partially explained by the fact that meal length increases as well, while the rate of eating remains nearly the same. However, the data to date do not clearly indicate that increased meal length is the sole determinant of this social facilitation of eating.

Studies have also found that the behaviors or actions of others (e.g., a sergeant and the soldiers under his or her command) can have substantial direct effects on consumption and acceptability. For example, research at Fort Devens found that soldiers ate significantly more rations at a meal and rated foods as more acceptable when their sergeant made a moderate positive comment and ate most of their meal than when he made a moderate negative comment and ate approximately two-thirds of his meal (Engell et al., 1990). Similarly, following a 2-week ration field test, soldiers who reported that they typically ate their meals in a social setting (i.e., with a small group of friends or colleagues) consumed approximately 5 percent more calories than soldiers who reported that they typically ate either alone or in the midst of a large, undifferentiated group of fellow soldiers (F.M.Kramer, U.S. Army Natick, unpublished data, 1991).

Studies with military and civilian personnel have also shown that social influences such as modeling and persuasion can influence attitudes and behaviors toward food (Edelman et al., 1986; Polivy et al., 1979; Smith, 1961). An interesting aspect of that research was that changes in behavior (e.g., consumption) and attitudes (e.g., hedonic ratings) were not always consistent with one another (Meiselman et al., 1988). For example, Smith (1961) found that after an experienced U.S. Army sergeant explained to his men the importance of eating unusual foods such as grasshoppers in order to survive and concluded his talk by actually eating a grasshopper, 90 percent of subjects ate one or more grasshoppers; in contrast, hedonic ratings gave no indication of an attitude change. On the other hand, following a cognitive dissonance approach, after soldiers heard a talk by an aloof professional who offered 50 cents to each person who would eat a grasshopper, only 50 percent of subjects actually chose to do so, although hedonic ratings indicated a significant, positive change in attitude. As in other types of research, different measurement methods or different aspects of a phenomenon may yield varying results and conclusions. To be sure of their findings, investigators need to be cognizant of a multitrait-multimethod approach (Campbell and Fiske, 1959).

CHEMICALS, FOODS, AND MEALS

In a number of human eating research areas, the relevance of stimuli has been discussed (Meiselman, 1992; Spitzer and Rodin, 1981). Studies of nutrition and behavior probably run the range from pure chemical stimuli to entire complex, long-term diets. Different levels of treatment complexity are listed in Table 8–1. Each level of complexity brings with it a set of advantages and a set of disadvantages. Moreover, within each level there can be further distinctions; pure chemical substances can be given in subphysiological doses, physiological doses, or superphysiological doses. Complex meals can be three or more components all on one plate, or they can be multiple courses. Complex diets can involve three meals per day, or they can involve ad libitum consumption of a wide range of foods.

Within the wide range of possible stimuli in food behavior studies, many variables influence food intake habits. For example, Engell (1992) has recently shown that in a meal setting, increased beverage variety leads to increased beverage consumption and increased food consumption. How one constructs laboratory meals and diets in many ways determines the outcomes of studies.

Ultimately, researchers need to know what to serve as an entire diet since that is what all people eat. Although pure substances and simple foods and meals might need to be researched to get the building blocks for diets, can one safely assume that the effects seen in isolation will remain when added to the overall diet? Or, conversely, will dietary components, produce behavioral or mood effects only when added to other dietary components, as Kruesi and Rapaport (1986) suggest?

TABLE 8–1 Levels of Treatment Complexity

Treatment Category	Examples
Pure substances	Subphysiological dosage
	Physiological dosage (Griffiths and Woodson, 1988)
	Greater than physiological dosage—better enhancement of behavioral effect (Spring et al., 1986)
Simple foods	Pure protein (turkey salad) or pure carbohydrate (bread-like wheat starch) (Spring et al., 1986)
	Breakfast drink or no food for breakfast (Benton and Sargent, 1992)
Complex foods	Ham casserole as a meal (van Amelsvoort and Weststrate, 1992)
Simple meals	Different breads with cheese, margarine, and coffee or tea (Holm and Bjorck, 1992)
Complex meals	Buffet lunch on 3 alternate days with preload and taste trays (Rolls et al., 1992)
Simple diets	Liquid diet for space travel, 19 weeks, prisoners (Winitz et al., 1965)
	Two basic meals high and low in energy for 5 days (Caputo and Mattes, 1992)
Complex diets	21-day diet (oat bran, wheat bran intake) in metabolic ward (Anderson et al., 1991)
	Vending machine diet of entrees, desserts, snacks, and beverages for 7 days (Rising et al., 1992)

All investigators should be clear about the current situation and the challenge ahead. The written military requirement for performance-enhancing ration components (dated July 30, 1992) states that the performance enhancing rations "would be sufficiently stable to withstand long-term storage; they would be sufficiently appealing to ensure consumption; and they would be packaged to withstand standard ration abuses and to promote ration acceptance." This requirement expects more from a performance-enhancing ration than was obtained from the current ration, the Meal Ready to Eat (MRE) (Hirsch and Kramer, 1993; Lester et al., in press; Meiselman et al., 1988). At present, the long-term storage requirements for rations lead to difficult demands for both the developer and the consumer, but these are outside the topic of this chapter. However, although the Army provides the soldier 3,900 kcal/day for moderate activity in a temperate climate, at present a soldier eats well under 3,000 kcal/day on average and occasionally eats under 2,000 kcal/day, on average.

Many data have been collected from both short-term (Table 8–2) and long-term (Table 8–3) studies of acceptance and consumption of the MREs. Although earlier studies suggested a gradual increase in MRE consumption, this trend has not continued. It is clear that MRE consumption is far more complicated than simply how acceptable the foods are rated.

Since the goal is to enhance performance in combat, one must also question whether a soldier in actual combat would eat more or less than what field training exercise studies have shown. Questionnaire data collected from U.S. Marines who had been in combat indicated that they ate as little as 58 per

TABLE 8–2 Prototype Testing (Short-Term Study) of Meal Ready to Eat Rations

				Acceptance	
Reference	Specific Ration[*]	Test Duration (days)[‡]	Intake (kcal/day)	Overall	Main Dish
Askew et al. (1987)	MRE IV	12 (3 MREs/ day)	2,282		NA[†]
Popper et al. (1987)	MRE IV	11 (3 MREs/ day)	2,517		5.7
	MRE VII		2,517		6.8
	IMP MRE		2,842	7.86	7.6
Engell et al. (1987)	MRE V	10 (4 MREs/ day)	2,733		6.2
Morgan et al. (1988)	MRE VIII	11 (4 MREs/ day)	3,217		
Lester et. al. (1990)	MRE VIII	3 (4 MREs/ day)	2,550		7.03
			2,289		7.39
			2,206		6.56
Edwards et al. (1989)	MRE VI	10 (4 MREs/ day)	2,009		6.34
	MRE VIII		2,802		7.33
Lester et al. (1993)	MRE VIII	7 (3 MREs/ day)	1,956	5.6	6.8

* Starting in 1980 the Roman numeral indicates the year of production; for example, MRE IV was produced in 1984.

† NA=not available.

‡ IMP MRE was improved MRE.

cent of their normal amount (Popper et al., 1989). Only 3 percent reported eating more than usual on the first combat day, and 29 percent reported eating the same as usual on the first combat day. Therefore, it is highly likely that underconsumption of rations in a real combat situation would be the same or worse than the underconsumption observed in training exercises.

TABLE 8–3 Extended Testing of Meal Ready to Eat Rations

Reference	Specific Ration*	Test Duration (days)	Intake (kcal/day)	Acceptance	
				Overall	Main Dish
Hirsh et al. (1985)	MRE IV	34	2,189	7.05	7.05
Hirsch and Kramer (1993)†	MRE IV	45	3,149	6.05	
Askew et al.	MRE VI	30	2,782	6.53‡	6.99
Thomas et al.§	MRE XII	30	2,441		

* Starting in 1980 the Roman numeral indicates the year of production; for example, MRE IV was produced in 1984.

† Student volunteers.

‡ Final questionnaire.

§ Technical Report in preparation.

At this point, the ability to predict the food intake of soldiers depends on both the food (e.g., its packaging, palatability, and form [e.g., liquid]) and the situation (e.g., effort required, timing of the meal, and social factors). By the time one can actually use a performance-enhancing ration in the field, one might be able to control and predict its acceptance and consumption by soldiers, but there is much work in this area that has yet to be done.

PERFORMANCE AND MOOD OUTCOMES

What is the military looking for with regard to performance-enhancing foods? Researchers are interested in what controls human food consumption habits. The military, however, does not have a special need to study what academia can do just as well. Performance-enhancing foods are a subject of interest and investment for the military because it is believed they can enhance militarily relevant behavior. However, the science of soldier performance is not yet mature. At present it is safe to say that researchers do not know what to measure or how to measure it. The measures of physical performance have not changed much over the years, but there is no way to integrate some of those into an overall physical effectiveness score. Measures of cognitive performance have changed, although integrated measurement of cognitive effectiveness is still far off. Combining physical and cognitive scores has probably never been attempted. Variables such as personality and mood must be factored in as well.

A broader issue in performance enhancement measurement is also one of context. Military thinkers involved with soldiers are necessarily thinking in terms of what capabilities soldiers bring to the battlefield. Recently, a newly proposed Army thrust called the Warrior's Edge focuses on enhancement of a soldier's performance in five capabilities: lethality, mobility, command and control, survivability, and sustainment.

Researchers need to begin to think of how to measure these militarily relevant factors and to demonstrate performance enhancement (or decrements) with these measures. A number of measures of lethality pertaining to firing a rifle exist. Similarly, measures of mobility on foot, either marching or on a treadmill, also exist. Command and control deals with the largely cognitive area of communication and information transfer. The greatest problems are survivability and sustainment. For neither of these is there an established measure.

Perhaps most importantly, researchers need to find ways to combine these measures (and perhaps others) to yield measures of overall soldier effectiveness. The USARIEM has begun some modeling work in this area. The ultimate context for performance-enhancing foods for the military will be the field, and measurement of enhanced soldier performance in the field must be the goal.

Assessment of enhanced soldier performance in the field requires that the enhancements provided by nutrient engineering be of sufficient magnitude to be observable and to make a real difference on the battlefield. The literature in this field is filled with caveats about the sizes of effects. Christensen (1991) distinguish chronic nutritional effects that can produce behavioral changes from acute diet manipulations that produce subtle, nonclinical behavioral changes. He suggests that acute manipulations must be done chronically to observe less subtle behavioral effects. They further warn that the psychological context interacts with chronic effects to produce behavioral changes. This means that short-term tests could produce incorrect estimates of behavioral changes—and might even miss them—and that the psychological context might be a necessary component of such demonstrations.

CONCLUSIONS

Consideration of context when planning or interpreting the effects of foods on the behaviors or moods of soldiers will require the following changes:

- Questions will need to be phrased contextually, and investigators will need to plan and conduct their research contextually. This might involve consideration of foods and meals, people issues (individual differences, social influences), environmental issues (both physical and social) and measures of mood and performance.
- In order to consider context, investigators will need to shift their questions in the following direction: Does carbohydrate (when present in *x* form in *y* foods in *z* diets) affect the behavior (e.g., mobility) or mood (e.g., stress) of people (e.g., young males or soldiers of particular selection criteria) over a 3-, 6-, or 12-month period, as compared with a control condition when tested in *x* environment. Then investigators will need to translate those contextual variables into specific test conditions.
- Investigators will need to limit their generalizations of results with the understanding that the phenomena might not extend to other contexts.

REFERENCES

Anderson, J.W., N.H.Gilinsky, D.A.Deakins, S.F.Smith, D.S.O'Neal, D.W.Dillon, and P.R.Oeltgen 1991 Lipid responses of hypercholesterolemic men to oat bran and wheat bran. Am. J. Clin. Nutr. 54:678–683.

Armstrong, S. 1980 A chronometric approach to the study of feeding behavior. Neurosci. Biobehav. Rev. 4:27–53.

Askew, E.W., I.Munro, M.A.Sharp, S.Siegel, R.Popper, M.S.Rose, R.W.Hoyt, J.W. Martin, K.Reynolds, H.R.Lieberman, D.B.Engell, and C.P.Shaw 1987 Nutritional status and physical and mental performance of special operations soldiers consuming the Ration, Lightweight or the Meal, Ready-to-Eat military field ration during a 30-day field training exercise. Technical Report T7–87. Natick, Mass.: Army Research Institute of Environmental Medicine.

Askew, E.W., J.R.Claybaugh, S.A.Cucinell, A.J.Young, and E.G.Szeto 1987 Nutrient intakes and work performance of soldiers during seven days of excise at 7,200 ft. altitude consuming the meal, Ready-to-Eat ration. Technical Report T3–87. Natick, Mass.: U.S. Army Research Institute of Environmental Medicine.

Askew, E.W., J.R.Claybaugh, S.A.Cucinell, A.J.Young, and E.G.Szeto 1991 Nutrient intakes and work performance of soldiers during seven days of exercise at 7,200 ft. altitude consuming the Meal, Ready-to-Eat ration. Technical Report T3–87. Natick, Mass.: U.S. Army Research Institute of Environmental Medicine.

Basiotis, P.P., S.O.Welsh, F.J.Cronin, J.L.Kelsay, and W.Mertz 1987 Number of days of food intake records required to estimate individual and group nutrient intakes with defined confidence. J. Nutr. 117:1638–1641.

Beaton, G.H., J.Milner, P.Corey, V.M.McGuire, M.Cousins, E.Stewart, M.de Ramos, D. Hewitt, P.V.Grambich, N.Kassim, and J.A.Little 1979 Sources of variance in 24-hour dietary recall data: Implications for nutrition study design and interpretation. Am. J. Clin. Nutr. 32:2546–2559.

Benton, D., and J.Sargent 1992 Breakfast, blood glucose and memory. Biol. Psych. 33:207–210.

Birch, L.L., J.Billman, and S.S.Richards 1984 Time of day influences food acceptability. Appetite 5:109–116.

Blundell, J.E., and A.J.Hill 1986 Paradoxical aspects of an intense sweetener (aspartame) on appetite. Lancet 1:1092–1093 (letter).

Blundell, J.E., P.J.Rogers, and A.J.Hill 1988 Uncoupling sweetness and calories: Methodological aspects of laboratory studies on appetite control. Appetite 11(Suppl):54–61.

Boulos, Z., and M.Terman 1980 Food availability and daily biological rhythms. Neurosci. Biobehav. Rev. 4:119–131.

Campbell, D.T., and D.Fiske 1959 Convergent and discriminant validation by the multitrait-multimethod matrix. Psychological Bull. 56:81–105.

Campbell, D.T., and J.C.Stanley 1966 Experimental and Quasi-Experimental Designs for Research. Skokie, III.: Rand McNally.

Caputo, F.A., and R.D.Mattes 1992 Human dietary responses to covert manipulations of energy, fat, and carbohydrate in a midday meal . Am. J. Clin. Nutr. 56:36–43.

Cardello, A.V., and F.M.Sawyer 1992 Effects of disconfirmed consumer expectations on food acceptability. J. Sensory Studies 7:253–277.

Christensen, L., J.Miller, and D.Johnson 1991 Issues in the design of studies investigating the behavioral concomitants of foods. J. Consult, and Clin. Psych. 6:874–882.

Collier, G. 1989 The Economics of Hunger. Thirst, Satiety and Regulation. Ann. N.Y. Acad. Science., 575:136–154.

de Castro, J.M., and E.M.Brewer 1991 The amount eaten in meals by humans is a power function of the number of people present. Physiol. Behav. 51:121–125.

Edelman, B., D.Engell, P.Bronstein, and E.Hirsch 1986 Environmental effects on the intake of overweight and normal-weight men. Appetite 7:71–83.

Edwards, J.S.A., D.E.Roberts, T.E.Morgan, and L.S.Lester 1989 An evaluation of the nutritional intake and acceptability of the Meal, Ready-to-Eat consumed with and without a Supplemental pack in a cold environment. Technical Report T18–89. Natick, Mass.: U.S. Army Research Institute of Environmental Medicine.

Engell, D. 1992 Sensory influences on meal consumption. Rose Marie Pangborn Memorial Symposium. August 2–6, Jarvenpaa, Finland.

Engell, D.B., D.E.Roberts, E.W.Askew, M.S.Rose, J.Buchbinder, and M.A.Sharpe 1987 Evaluation of the Ration Cold Weather during a 10-day cold weather field training exercise. NATICK Technical Report TR-87/030. Natick, Mass.: U.S. Army Natick Research, Development and Engineering Center.

Engell, D., F.M.Kramer, S.Luther, and S.Adams 1990 The effect of social influences on food intake. Paper presented at the Society for Nutrition Education 1990 Annual Meeting, Anaheim, Calif.

Epstein, S. 1980 The stability of behavior. II. Implications for psychological research. Am. Psychologist 35:790–806.

1983 Aggregation and beyond: Some basic issues on the prediction of behavior. J. Personality 51:360–392.

Fillmore, M., and M.Vogel-Sprott 1992 Expected effect of caffeine on motor performance predicts the type of response to placebo. Psychopharmacology 106:209–214.

Goldman, S.J., C.P.Herman, and J.Polivy 1991 Is the effect of a social model on eating attenuated by hunger? Appetite 17:129–140.

Gray, J.A. 1987 The Psychology of Fear and Stress. Cambridge: Cambridge University Press.

Griffiths, R.R., and P.P.Woodson 1988 Reinforcing effects of caffeine in humans. J. Pharmacol. Exp. Ther. 246:21–29.

Halberg, F. 1989 Some aspects of the chronobiology of nutrition: More work is needed on "when to eat." J. Nutr. 119:333–343.

Herman, C.P., J.Polivy, C.N.Lank, and T.F.Heatherton 1987 Anxiety, hunger, and eating behavior. J. Abnormal Psychol. 96:264–269.

Hirsch, E., and F.M.Kramer 1993 Situational influences on food intake. In Nutrition for Work in Hot Environments. Report of the Committee on Military Nutrition Research, B.M.Marriott, ed., Food and Nutrition Board, Institute of Medicine. Washington, D.C.: National Academy Press.

Hirsch, E., H.L.Meiselman, R.D.Popper, G.Smits, B.Jezior, I.Lichton, N.Wenkam, J.Burt, M.Fox, S.McNutt, T.N.Thiele, and O.Direge 1985 The effects of prolonged feeding Meal, Ready-to-Eat (MRE) operational rations. Technical Report Natick TR-85/035. Natick, Mass.: U.S. Army Natick Research, Development and Engineering Center.

Holm, J., and I.Bjorck 1992 Bioavailability of starch in various wheat-based bread products: Evaluation of metabolic responses in healthy subjects and rate and extent of in vitro starch digestion. Am. J. Clin. Nutr. 55:420–429.

Kirsch, I., and L.J.Weixel 1988 Double-blind versus deceptive administration of a placebo. Behav. Neurosci. 102:319–323.

Kramer, F.M., K.Rock, and D.Engell 1992 Effects of time of day and appropriateness on food intake and hedonic ratings at morning and mid-day. Appetite 18:1–13.

Kruesi, M.J., and J.L.Rapaport 1986 Diet and human behavior: How much do they affect each other? Pp. 113–130 in Annual Review of Nutrition, R.E.Olson, E.Beutler, and H.P.Broquist, eds. Palo Alto, Calif: Annual Reviews Inc.

Latane, B. 1981 The psychology of social impact. Am. Psychologist 36:343–355.

Leathwood, P.D., and P.Pollet 1982- Diet-induced mood changes in normal populations. J. Psychiat. Res. 1983 17:147–154.

Lester, L.S., F.M.Kramer, J.Edinberg, S.Mutter, and D.B.Engell 1990 Evaluation of the Canteen cup stand and ration heater pad: effects on acceptability and consumption of the Meal, Ready-to-Eat in a cold weather environment. Technical Report TR-90/008L. Natick, Mass.: U.S. Army Natick Research, Development and Engineering Center.

Lester, L.S., L.L.Lesher, M.Salomon, D.B.Engell, S.L.Dewey, J.Ward, C.Thomas, and J. Kalick 1993 Nutritional and hedonic consequences of consuming the MRE VIII or the SEP MRE. Technical Report Natick TR-93/015. Natick, Mass.: U.S. Army Natick Research Development and Engineering Center.

Lick, J., and R.Bootzin 1975 Expectancy factors in the treatment of fear: Methodological and theoretical issues. Psychological Bull. 82:917–931.

Marlatt, G.A., and D.J.Rohsenow 1980 Cognitive processes in alcohol use: Expectancy and the balanced placebo design. Pp. 159–199 in Advances in Substance Abuse, Vol. 1, N.K.Mello, ed. Greenwich, Conn.: JAI Press.

Meiselman, H.L. 1987 Use of sensory evaluation and food habits data in product development. Pp. 307–326 In Umami: A Basic Taste Y.Kawamura and M.Kare, eds. New York: Marcel Decker.

1992 Methodology and theory in human eating research. Appetite 19:49–55.

1994 Identifying and demonstrating consumer acceptance variables in a natural eating environment. In Proceedings of Food Preservation 2000, I.Taub and R.Bell, eds. Washington, D.C.: National Academy Press.

Meiselman, H.L., E.S.Hirsch, and R.D.Popper 1988 Sensory, hedonic and situational factors in food acceptance and consumption. Pp. 77–87 in Food Acceptability, D.M.H.Thomson, ed. London: Elsevier Applied Science.

Mistlberger, R. 1990 Circadian pitfalls in experimental designs employing food restrictions. Psychobiology 18:23–29.

Moline, M.L., C.P.Pollack, S.Zendell, L.S.Lester, C.A.Salter, and E.Hirsch 1990 A Laboratory Study of the Effects of Diet and Bright Light Countermeasures to Jet Lag. Technical Report Natick TR-90/024. Natick, Mass.: U.S. Army Natick Research, Development and Engineering Center.

Morgan, T.E., L.A.Hodges, D.Schillig, R.W.Hoyt, E.J.Iwanyk, G.McAnich, T.C.Wells, and E.W.Askew 1988 A comparison of the Meal, Ready-to-Eat, Ration Cold Weather and Ration, Lightweight nutrient intakes during moderate altitude cold weather field training operations. Technical Report T5–89. Natick, Mass: U.S. Army Research Institute of Environmental Medicine.

Morley, J.E., A.S.Levine, and M.L.Willenbring 1986 Stress-induced feeding disorders. Pp. 71–99 in Pharmacology of Eating Disorders: Theoretical and Clinical Developments, M.O.Carruba and J.E.Blundell, eds. New York: Raven Press.

Nelson, M., A.E.Black, J.A.Morris, and T.J.Cole 1989 Between- and within-subject variations in nutrient intake from infancy to old age: Estimating the number of days required to rank dietary intakes with desired precision. Am. J. Clin. Nutr. 50:155–167.

Polivy, J. 1976 Perception of calories and regulation of intake in restrained and unrestrained subjects. Addict. Beh. 1:237–243.

Polivy, J., C.P.Herman, J.C.Younger, and B.Erskine 1979 Effects of a model on eating behavior: The induction of a restrained eating style. J. Personality. 47:100–117.

Popper, R., E.Hirsch, L.Lesher, D.Engell, B.Jezior, B.Bell, and W.T.Matthew 1987 Field Evaluation of Improved MRE, MRE VII, and MRE IV. NATICK Technical Report TR-87/027. Natick, Mass.: U.S. Army Natick Research, Development and Engineering Center.

Popper, R., G.Smits, H.L.Meiselman, and E.Hirsch 1989 Eating in combat: A survey of U.S. Marines. Milit Med. 154:619–623.

Redd, M., and J.M.de Castro 1992 Social facilitation of eating: Effects of social instruction on food intake. Physiol. Behav. 52:749–754.

Rising, R., S.Alger, V.Boyce, H.Seagle, R.Ferraro, A.M.Fontvieille, and E.Ravussin 1992 Food intake measured by an automated food-selection system: Relationship to energy expenditure. Am. J. Clin. Nutr. 55:343–349.

Rolls, B.J. 1991 Effects of intense sweeteners on hunger, food intake, and body weight: A review. Am. J. Clin. Nutr. 53:872–878.

Rolls, B.J., A.E.Andersen, T.H.Moran, A.L.McNelis, H.C.Baier, and I.C.Fedoroff 1992 Food intake, hunger, and satiety after preloads in women with eating disorders. Am. J. Clin. Nutr. 55:1093–1103.

Rose, M.S. and D.E.Carlson 1987 Effect of A-ration meals on body weight during sustained field operations. Technical Report T2–87. Natick, Mass.: U.S. Army Research Institute of Environmental Medicine.

Schutz, H.G. 1988 Beyound preference: Appropriateness as a measure of contextual acceptance of food. Pp. 115–134 in Food Acceptability, D.M.H.Thomson, ed. London: Elsevier Applied Science.

Siegel, S. 1988 State-dependent learning and morphine tolerance. Behav. Neurosci. 102:228–232.

Smith, E.E. 1961 The power of dissonance techniques to change attitudes. Public Opinion Q. 25:626–639.

Spitzer, L., and J.Rodin 1981 Human eating behavior: A critical review of studies in normal weight and overweight individuals. Appetite 2:293–329.

Spring, B J., H.R.Lieberman, G.Swope, and G.S.Griffiths 1986 Effects of carbohydrates on mood and behavior. Pp. 51–60 in Nutrition Reviews, R.E. Olson , ed. Washington, D.C.: Nutrition Foundation.

Tarasuk, V., and G.H.Beaton 1992a Day-to-day variation in energy and nutrient intake: Evidence of individuality in eating behaviors? Appetite 18:43–54.

1992b Statistical estimation of dietary parameters: Implications of patterns in within-subject variation—a case study of sampling strategies. Am. J. Clin. Nutr. 55:22–27.

Tepas, D.I. 1990 Do eating and drinking schedules interact with work schedule variables? Work Stress 4:203–211.

van Amelsvoort, J.M.M., and J.A.Weststrate 1992 Amylose-amylopectin ratio in a meal affects postprandial variables in male volunteers. Am. J. Clin. Nutr. 55:712–718.

Winitz, M., J.Graff, N.Gallagher, A.Narkin, and D.A.Seedman 1965 Evaluation of chemical diets as nutrition for man-in-space. Nature 205:742–743.

DISCUSSION

DAVID D.SCHNAKENBERG: Herb, I want to compliment you on your thought-provoking paper. You have brought out issues that you and I used to talk about.

I would like to add one point to one study that you cited to me, but I feel it was done by Rose and Carlson (1987) on sustained artillery operations. It was serendipity, the study that was done—7 days of continuous artillery operations with very little sleep to see how the performance of these artillerymen would be degraded. The plan was to feed them MREs [Meals Ready to Eat] three times a day. However, the bugs crawled out of some plant in San Antonio, and the Secretary of the Army put a total moratorium throughout the world that "thou shalt not" eat any more MREs until we find the problem in the production plant.

That happened 2 days before the planned study. There was a question: Should they cancel the study or do something else? They could not feed them MRES. So they took hot meals from the dining hall and carried them out to the field, and the cooks prepared and laid out the food for them. They had to stop the action briefly and let the people sit down and eat the meals and then continue on.

That was the study in which soldiers in the field ate 3,700 calories per day over a 7-day period; they lost no water and did not become dehydrated. Much to the frustration I think of Dr. (James) Vogel, they had no performance decrements.

DAVID D.SCHNAKENBERG: So I think that is one example: If there is nothing physiologically or psychologically wrong with a soldier when he goes outside, if you give him something that he likes to eat and in a situation which gives him time to eat it, he will eat to maintain energy balance. However, these factors are often not all in place in the other field studies that have been undertaken.

ROBERT O.NESHEIM: In every one of the MRE tests that we have evaluated as a committee, we have always had that issue that the troops do not eat enough to maintain their weight. The question is, why don't they? I think the context of the situation is a big part of it.

G.RICHARD JANSEN: That gap you mentioned at the end between, say, the real-world situation and experimental protocols, is a real issue.

HERBERT MEISELMAN: I think the focus groups which Natick has conducted might show you some of the things to look at, but you are going to have to develop something very quantitative after that in order to aid the ration developers, logisticians, and nutritionists..

ROBERT O.NESHEIM: I was reminded, as you were talking, about the problems that I dealt with in a food lab at the Quaker Oats Corporation many, many years ago. We would have very good tests on products that had high degrees of acceptability. They compared very favorably against competitive products, but sometimes you would put them out in a test marketplace and they would fall flat on their face.

It is my understanding that more and more of the food research labs are doing less and less of a detailed product evaluation within the labs, but are doing more and more of it out in the field, simply because they are trying to overcome some of that situation.

JOHANNA DWYER: I just wanted to compliment everybody who made presentations this morning because I thought they were fascinating. I want to revisit this issue of continuity. It seems from David Schnakenberg's statement just now about that experiment where they put the hot foods out, and then from some of the sleep data we heard earlier, this continuity issue seems to be very important.

The question I have is, is it possible to sleep in a tank; is there a way to do it? Similarly, does the context of the combat situation simply preclude this, or are there things that we can consider? What are our constraints as we work the next 2 days with respect to this issue?

JOEL GRINKER: That has been documented by behavioral tests by Dr. Smith in England, and there is no question that there is a decline in intake.

It certainly is important, and it gets complicated in terms of circadian rhythms because the circadian rhythm also has a 12-hour cycle, so that sort of confuses things. That may be part of the cause of that 12-hour cycle.

Also, I think Dr. Bonnie Spring will have some things to say later about the effects of different food on the amount of behavioral change.

I have another comment. I was reminded by the sergeants explaining the importance of eating grasshoppers, about the studies during World War II that addressed food acceptance, in order to get the American public to eat organ meats, they did experiments in which they suggested that if, in fact, they had somebody who posed as an expert—the tests showed—that they got a greater acceptance than if they just told people that this is good for them.

EDWARD HORTON: I am fascinated, as I have listened to this morning's presentation, at the parallelism between sleep deprivation and food deprivation and the importance of the context. If you put a person in a context where he cannot get sleep for very long or you put him in a context where he cannot sit down and enjoy a good hot meal, you end up with these deprivation syndromes. There seems to be a lot of parallelism.

I was wondering if people have looked at the recovery from these. After you have been through a sleep deprivation, do you sleep like a babe after a while? After you have been through a period of food deprivation, do you go back and chow down and make up your energy losses and so forth? Looking at periodic recovery, are there ways to enhance recovery after the fact?

HERBERT MEISELMAN: I think part of our problem is that the more we study this, the more we realize that our tests should be longer and longer in the field. There is a real problem with keeping troops in the field in a training exercise for 4, 6, or 8 weeks and with the associated costs. I think we have thought of what you are suggesting, but it is very difficult to do; it is very long-term testing.

EDWARD HORTON: There are two questions. One is adaptation; adaptations occur over time. The other is recovery and thinking of something like the exercise physiology test where you basically give little rest periods between tests.

HERBERT MEISELMAN: In our first test in 1982, we were positive that the troops would find the diet very monotonous. We predicted that their food acceptance ratings would go down over time, an example of classic monotony.

In fact, what happened is that the troop ratings of the foods stayed absolutely flat for 35 days. But over time they ate less and less and less, so that by the end of the test they were eating considerably less than at the beginning but were not aware of it.

So our simple model of this—that the diet would be monotonous and they would not eat it—did not fit. The diet, in effect, was monotonous if you view it from an intake measure but not from a rating measure.

PART IV

Stress and Nutrient Interactions: Metabolic Consequences

IN PART IV THE EXPERT PAPERS that formed the basis for the development of the basic science summary and recommendations in Part I begin. Speakers were selected who were well known for their research in specific areas. Each speaker was asked to review carefully the literature in his or her field of expertise as it related to the six questions posed to the committee and to provide copies of scientific articles as background papers to the CMNR before the workshop. In their presentations and chapters, the invited experts were asked to make critical comments on the relevant research and conclude with their recommendations. When time allowed, there was a recorded question and answer period at the end of each presentation. These discussions are included at the end of the chapters.

Reviewed in this section are the biochemical basis underlying L-tyrosine administration to counter stress; a broad overview of endocrine system responses to military-type stresses; and the nutritional, endocrinological, and physiological aspects of metabolism needed to sustain physical and mental performance under a variety of stressful conditions.

9

Stress and Monoamine Neurons in the Brain

John D.Fernstrom[1]

INTRODUCTION

Stress is a common behavioral and physiologic phenomenon that occurs in combat and other military operations and is believed to contribute to decrements in performance (Owasoyo et al., 1992). Thus, the identification of methods for counteracting stress is highly desirable. One pharmacologic countermeasure for stress currently under evaluation is the administration of an amino acid, L-tyrosine (TYR). The grounds for evaluating this amino acid follow from the fact that it is the precursor for the catecholamine neurotransmitters dopamine (DA) and norepinephrine (NE). These transmitters are found in brain neurons that are involved in the central nervous system's response to stress; indeed, some data indicate that TYR administration can enhance DA and NE synthesis in the brain and, as a result, reverse deficient performance in both rats and humans (Banderet and Lieberman, 1989; Lehnert et al., 1984).

This chapter focuses on the biochemical basis for the assertion that TYR administration might be useful as a pharmacologic countermeasure to stress.

[1] John D.Fernstrom, Department of Psychiatry, University of Pittsburgh School of Medicine, 3811 O'Hara Street, Pittsburgh, PA 15213

The conclusions are that the available evidence suggests that DA and NE synthesis in the brains of stressed individuals should respond to TYR administration by increasing neurotransmitter synthesis and release and that such alterations should affect brain functions. However, given the diversity of effects of stress on the functional states of the various DA and NE receptor subtypes, the exact responses to TYR may not always be simple. Indeed, because of the incomplete body of data regarding the effects of stress on brain catecholamine receptors, their further study in this context would appear essential to an eventual understanding of the utility of TYR and other pharmacologic agents that stimulate DA and/or NE release as stress countermeasures.

TYR administration can also influence the synthesis and release of serotonin (5-hydroxytryptamine; 5HT) in the brain, because of its role as a large neutral amino acid (LNAA). A discussion of the effects of stress on 5HT synthesis and release is thus also warranted, and can be used to evaluate whether an action of TYR on 5HT release might be a desirable consequence of TYR administration.

SYNTHESIS OF MONOAMINES IN THE BRAIN

Dopamine and Norepinephrine

The catecholamine neurotransmitters DA and NE are synthesized from the nonessential amino acid TYR. The initial step is a ring hydroxylation that is mediated by the enzyme tyrosine hydroxylase, forming dihydroxyphenylalanine (DOPA). Tyrosine hydroxylase can also hydroxylate phenylalanine to DOPA; indeed, this amino acid has been shown to be an important substrate for catecholamine biosynthesis (Karobath and Baldessarini, 1972). DOPA is converted to DA by the enzyme aromatic-L-amino acid decarboxylase (AAAD). An additional enzyme, dopamine-ß-hydroxylase, is found in neurons that synthesize and use NE as their transmitter. This enzyme mediates the beta-hydroxylation of DA to NE.

DA undergoes oxidative deamination (mediated by monoamine oxidase; MAO) to dihydroxyphenylacetic acid. A further reaction, O-methylation (mediated by catechol-O-methyltransferase; COMT), produces a second DA metabolite, homovanillic acid. The principal NE metabolite in the brain is methoxyhydroxyphenylethylglycol, which is produced in reactions mediated by MAO and COMT (Cooper et al., 1991).

The rates at which DA and NE are synthesized are controlled at the initial enzymatic step, TYR hydroxylation. Although many phenomena influence TYR hydroxylase activity, and thus DA and NE synthesis, two are especially relevant to the present discussion. First, the activity of TYR hydroxylase is quite sensitive to neuronal activity, increasing and decreasing rapidly in parallel with the rate at which the neurons that produce DA and NE are firing (Cooper et al., 1991). Under stressful conditions, as discussed below, the firing rates of neurons that contain DA and NE increase and probably account for the observed increases in DA and NE synthesis. Second, the TYR hydroxylation rate changes rapidly in response to the TYR concentration within the neuron (Fernstrom et al., 1986). Hence, increasing brain TYR levels can stimulate DA and NE synthesis. However, TYR administration increases catecholamine synthesis only under conditions in which the neurons are active. When they are inactive, increments in the TYR level do not affect DA or NE synthesis (Fernstrom, 1990). As indicated below, stress is associated with increases in the activity of neurons that produce both DA and NE, and indeed, the synthesis of both transmitters is increased. Accordingly, in this context, the supply of additional amounts of TYR should further stimulate the production of each transmitter.

Serotonin

Serotonin (5-hydroxytryptamine; 5HT) is synthesized from the essential amino acid tryptophan (TRP). Like the catecholamines, the initial step in the pathway is hydroxylation, which is mediated by the enzyme tryptophan hydroxylase. The product, 5-hydroxytryptophan, is then decarboxylated to 5HT in a reaction mediated by AAAD (the same enzyme that converts DOPA to DA). Serotonin is metabolized to 5-hydroxyindoleacetic acid in a reaction initiated by MAO (Cooper et al., 1991).

Control of the 5HT synthesis rate is focused on the initial hydroxylation step. Like TYR hydroxylase, TRP hydroxylase activity is sensitive to changes in neuronal activity (Boadle-Biber et al., 1986), rising and falling with the depolarization rate. In addition, TRP hydroxylation and 5HT synthesis rates respond to the local concentration of TRP (Fernstrom, 1990). This relationship is tied to neuronal activity, however, because an increase in the brain TRP level produces a much larger stimulation of 5HT synthesis and release when the 5HT neuron is active than when it is quiescent (Fernstrom et al., 1990; Sharp et al., 1992). As discussed below, stress does not influence the activity of 5HT-producing neurons, but it does increase brain TRP levels. Hence, the increases in 5HT synthesis and turnover that occur with stress may follow from increased substrate levels.

STRESS AND BRAIN NOREPINEPHRINE

Acute Stress

Several types of evidence suggest that stressful stimuli increase the activity of norepinephrine (NE)-producing neurons in the brain. The most direct demonstration has been provided by measurement of the firing rate of NE-producing neurons in the locus ceruleus (a nucleus in the brain stem). Levine et al. (1990) recorded the electrical activities of locus ceruleus neurons in awake, freely moving cats by means of chronically implanted electrodes. They observed that when the animals were exposed to an environmentally meaningful stress (e.g., auditory and visual, but not physical exposure to a dog or an enraged cat), the neuronal firing rate increased substantially. Biochemical methods have also revealed stress-induced increases in the firing rate of NE-producing neurons. In early studies, the turnover rate of NE in the brains of rats exposed to foot shock was estimated by prelabeling the brain NE pool with tritiated NE. The rate of loss of radioactivity was used as an index of transmitter turnover rate and neuronal activity. Using this method, Thierry et al. (1968) observed an increase in NE turnover in many regions of the rat brain (including the brain stem, cerebral cortex, and hypothalamus). A similar result was obtained by a different biochemical method, which also provided a good estimate of NE turnover: the decline in endogenous NE levels following injection of a drug that blocks NE synthesis (α-methyl-*p*-tyrosine). By this method, NE turnover has been found to be increased above normal rates in whole brain and in a variety of brain regions (Bliss et al., 1968; Korf et al., 1973). Finally, brain NE levels have often been observed to fall in parallel with increments in the levels of NE metabolites in stressed rats, an indication that transmitter turnover has accelerated (Nakagawa et al., 1981; Sauter et al., 1978). Indeed, in such cases, the results suggest that synthesis cannot keep up with transmitter utilization.

The influence of acute stressors has also been examined on NE receptors in the brain, primarily the ß and α_2 subtypes. The most consistent finding has been that single episodes of stress do not influence ß-receptor number or affinity in the cerebral cortex or brain stem (Cohen et al., 1986; Nomura et al., 1981; Stone and Platt, 1982; U'Prichard and Kvetňanský, 1980). Inconsistent changes have been reported for the hypothalamus (Cohen et al., 1986; Stone and Platt, 1982) and other brain regions (e.g., the cerebellum and hippocampus [Nomura et al., 1981; U'Prichard and Kvetňanský, 1980]). The α_2-receptor number and affinity have also been examined in a variety of rat brain regions following exposure to acute stressors and have been found to yield no simple effect. In different regions, acute stress is reported to reduce receptor number but not change affinity (hippocampus), reduce receptor number but increase affinity (amygdala), increase receptor number but reduce affinity (midbrain), or have no affect on receptor number or affinity (hypothalamus and brain— stem) (Cohen et al., 1986; Nukima et al., 1987). For some regions, results differ across laboratories (e.g., for the cerebral cortex [Cohen et al., 1986; Nukima et al., 1987]).

On the basis of the available evidence, it appears that an appropriate conclusion for the influence of acute stress on NE receptors in the brain is that they may not be remarkably altered. As a consequence, the clear increases in NE release from nerve terminals may have sustained postsynaptic effects during a single stressful event. In such situations, where NE neurons are firing rapidly, one would certainly expect an increase in neuronal TYR levels, such as can be induced following the oral ingestion of free TYR, to stimulate NE synthesis (Lehnert et al., 1984), and thus provide a continuing source of amine for release.

Chronic Stress

Chronic stress, like single episodes of stress, is associated with increased NE synthesis and turnover (Stanford et al., 1984; Thierry et al., 1968). Such findings are consistent with the notion that NE-producing neurons are synthesizing and releasing above-normal amounts of neurotransmitter. However, unlike the acute stress context, in which NE receptors appear to show little change in their properties, some NE receptor subtypes show sizable changes with chronic stress. In particular, ß-receptor number is reported most consistently to be below normal in the cortex, brain stem, and hypothalamus (whereas the agonist affinity is normal) (Stone and Platt, 1982; Stanford et al., 1984; Torda et al., 1981, 1985). Less consistent changes have been reported for α_2 receptors: increased α_2 receptor populations have been reported in the hypothalamus and brain stem (Torda et al., 1981, 1985), but reduced numbers have been reported in the cerebral cortex (Lynch et al., 1983; Stanford et al., 1984). α_1 receptor properties have been measured in the cortex following chronic stress and have been found to be normal (Lynch et al., 1983).

Norepinephrine receptors are coupled to second messenger systems (e.g., cyclic AMP generation and phospholipase activity), and attempts have been made to link chronic stress-induced alterations in NE receptors to effects on second messenger systems. For example, Torda et al. (1981) reported that pretreatment of rats with a drug that inhibits phospholipase activity, and ultimately cyclic AMP generation, blocks the reduction in ß-receptor number in the hypothalamus and brain stem that follows chronic stress in rats. This finding suggests that the stress-induced increase in NE release by brain neurons, via stimulation of ß-receptors on target neurons and the production of second messenger-mediated effects, initiates events leading to ß-receptor down-regulation. As another example, Stone et al. (1985) observed that in association with the reduction in ß-receptor number in the hypothalamus and brain stem following repeated stress in rats, NE-induced cyclic AMP generation in slices from these regions incubated in vitro was also diminished. It should be noted, however, that cyclic AMP generation in response to isoproterenol, a selective ß-agonist, was not diminished in that study, suggesting that the reduction in second messenger responsiveness may not be the result of ß-receptor down-regulation. The same group of investigators (Stone et al., 1986) later reported that the diminished cyclic AMP response to NE (which stimulates all adrenergic receptors) may be mediated via a reduction in the NE effects on α-receptors.

Whatever the ultimate outcome of this line of investigation, the available evidence clearly indicates that (1) the NE receptor responsiveness changes following repeated exposure to stressful stimuli, (2) these changes are dissimilar from the effects that occur after a single exposure to stress, and (3) NE receptors and their subtypes are not affected uniformly by chronic stress, nor are the changes of a particular receptor subtype the same in different brain regions. Thus, the effects of agents that enhance NE synthesis and release (such as TYR) and that, as a result, produce particular functional effects following single stressful events, may not provide a reliable foundation for predicting functional changes under conditions of continued or repeated stress. Such effects must be sought in the context of chronic stress.

STRESS AND BRAIN DOPAMINE

Acute Stress

Dopamine (DA) neurons are stimulated by stress. This effect has been demonstrated by using biochemical indices similar to those used to study norepinephrine (NE). Thus, stress increases the rate of decline in brain DA levels following administration of an inhibitor of DA synthesis (Thierry et al., 1976), indicating that DA turnover has increased. A similar conclusion has been drawn from results showing that stress increases the brain levels of the major DA metabolite, dihydroxyphenylacetic acid (Dunn, 1988a, Roth et al., 1988). Stress also increases the activity of tyrosine hydroxylase, measured both in vivo (Reinhard et al., 1982) and in vitro (luvone and Dunn, 1986). The direct release of DA from the neuron, as assessed by in vivo dialysis, is also stimulated by stress (Abercrombie et al., 1989). Although the results of some studies suggest that only one or two subgroups of DA-producing neurons are affected by stress (particularly those projecting to the prefrontal cortex [Roth et al., 1988; Thierry et al., 1976]), other data indicate that essentially all DA-producing neurons in the brain can be activated by stressful stimuli (Abercrombie et al., 1989; Dunn, 1988a) (those projecting from the midbrain to the limbic system [nucleus accumbens, amygdala], the cerebral cortex, and the corpus striatum). Almost no data appear to exist regarding DA receptor responses to acute stress. In a single study, the number of D_2 receptors in the prefrontal cortex and striatum were reported to be unchanged soon after a single stressful event (MacLennan et al., 1989).

From such data, it can be predicted that the administration of TYR to animals undergoing acute stress should stimulate DA synthesis and probably DA release in most brain DA-producing neurons. Functional changes might result from such biochemical effects, if the properties of DA receptors are indeed unchanged.

Chronic Stress

Relatively few data have evaluated the response of brain DA-producing neurons in animals repeatedly exposed to stressful stimuli. Available data suggest that DA-producing neurons (like NE-producing neurons) continue to be activated by repeated, stressful events. For example, Dunn (1988a) observed that daily episodes of foot shock for 10 days continued to raise dihydroxyphenylacetic acid levels in the prefrontal cortex, corpus striatum, and brain stem. Similar findings were reported by MacLennan et al. (1989).

At present, it is unclear whether DA receptor sensitivity is influenced by chronic stress. The D_1 class of receptors appears largely to be unaffected (Friedhof et al., 1986; Puglisi-Allegra et al., 1991). Although changes in the D_2 receptor are observed in response to chronic stress, consistent effects have not been obtained. For example, D_2 receptor number is reputed by some to be increased by chronic stress in the caudate, nucleus accumbens, and prefrontal cortex (Friedhoff et al., 1986); others, however, report a reduction in D_2 receptor number following restraint stress (Puglisi-Allegra et al., 1991). Some investigators have also failed to detect stress-induced changes in D_2 receptors (Anderson et al., 1986) or have obtained results suggestive of a lack of effect of chronic stress on the D_2 receptor (MacLennan et al., 1989).

At present, therefore, it appears that recurrent episodes of stress activate DA-producing neurons and probably lead to enhanced DA release. It also appears that the properties of DA receptors are not remarkably altered as a result. However, too few data are presently available to draw firm conclusions regarding DA receptor effects; additional work is clearly indicated. Nevertheless, the available data suggest that the administration of TYR should stimulate DA synthesis and release in animals exposed to chronic stress. As a result, physiologic and behavioral effects may occur, taking into account the functional state of the DA receptor onto which the transmitter is released (i.e., if the DA receptor on a particular neuron is normal or up-regulated, a functional effect would be expected; if it is down-regulated, a diminished response would be anticipated).

STRESS AND BRAIN SEROTONIN

Acute Stress

Acute stress stimulates serotonin (5-hydroxytryptamine; 5HT) synthesis and turnover in the rat brain. Acute stressors (e.g., immobilization or foot shock) rapidly increase the brain level of 5-hydroxyindoleacetic acid (5HIAA), the principal 5HT metabolite (Bliss et al., 1968; Curzon and Green, 1969). Brain 5HT levels are unaffected, suggesting that stress increases both the rate of synthesis and the rate of turnover of 5HT. Other studies support this conclusion. Morgan et al. (1975) observed that restraint stress increased the accumulation of 5HIAA in stressed rats pretreated with probenecid, a drug that blocks 5HIAA removal from the brain. Mueller et al. (1976) showed that stress increased 5HT accumulation in stressed rats pretreated with pargyline, a drug that blocks 5HT metabolism. These results provide convincing evidence that stress increases both 5HT synthesis and turnover. Similar observations have also been made in mice (Soblosky and Thurmond, 1986).

The mechanism responsible for the stress-induced increase in 5HT synthesis and turnover differs from that thought to account for the increases in dopamine (DA) and norepinephrine (NE) synthesis and turnover. First, unlike DA- and NE-producing neurons in the brain, the depolarization rate of 5HT-producing neurons is unaffected by stressful events. Using cats, Wilkinson and Jacobs (1988) observed that when animals are exposed to highly relevant environmental stressors (e.g., giving them visual and auditory but not physical exposure to an agitated dog or to an enraged cat, which causes clear sympathetic activation), the firing rate of 5HT-producing neurons is unaltered. Neuronal activation with stress therefore cannot be the source of increased transmitter synthesis in 5HT-producing neurons, as it probably is in DA- and NE-producing neurons. Second, stress elevates the brain levels of the 5HT precursor tryptophan (TRP) (Curzon et al., 1972; Dunn, 1988b), an effect that has not been observed for L-tyrosine (TYR), the precursor of DA and NE (Kennett et al., 1986). Since 5HT synthesis is known to be sensitive to small, physiologic changes in brain TRP concentrations (Fernstrom, 1990), the stress-induced rise in brain TRP levels may cause the stimulation of 5HT synthesis.

The mechanism by which stress raises brain TRP levels may center on the blood-brain barrier carrier for transporting TRP and the other large neutral amino acids (LNAAs) into the brain. Immobilization has been reported to increase the brain levels of most LNAAs (including TRP), suggesting that stress may stimulate the shared LNAA transporter (Kennett et al., 1986). This effect may derive from the stress-induced release of epinephrine into the circulation; epinephrine is known to increase brain levels of the LNAA (Eriksson and Carlsson, 1988). Further support for an LNAA transport-mediated effect of stress comes from the work of Kennett and Joseph (1981), who reported that the administration of a large dose of valine (an LNAA) blocks the stress-induced rise in brain TRP levels. Valine or TYR treatment also eliminated the stress-induced rise in neuronal 5-hydroxyindole release (Joseph and Kennett, 1983).

To summarize, the above evidence suggests that a single stressful event raises the amount of TRP taken up by the brain, possibly via the release of epinephrine into the circulation, causing brain TRP levels to rise and thus 5HT synthesis to increase. The increase in 5HT synthesis may lead to an increase in 5HT release, since stress appears to enhance 5HT-mediated brain functions (Kennett and Joseph, 1981). The administration of LNAAs, like valine or TYR, can attenuate the stress-induced increase in brain 5HT levels, with unknown consequences to brain function.

Chronic Stress

Few data with which to evaluate the effects of chronic stress on 5HT neurons appear to be available. Soblosky and Thurmond (1986) reported increases in mouse brain 5HIAA levels (with no change in 5HT) after the repeated administration of stressors for several days, suggesting that 5HT turnover (and synthesis) might be increased. However, it is unknown at present whether such changes are induced by alterations in brain TRP levels or in the activity of 5HT neurons. Chronic stress also reportedly increases postsynaptic sensitivity to 5HT, since many 5HT-mediated behaviors appear to be more responsive to 5HT agents when administered to chronically stressed rats (Kennett et al., 1985). However, the basis for this effect is presently unexplained, since in the only available report (Ohi et al., 1989), 5HT receptor kinetics have been found to be unaffected by chronic stress. These findings are not totally convincing, however, since ß-receptor properties were also found to be normal in that study. This result stands in contrast to the bulk of published data showing ß-receptor function to be increased (see above).

At present, because of the disparate nature of the small pool of available data, it is not possible to state with certainty how chronic stress affects 5HT neuronal function.

CONCLUSIONS AND RECOMMENDATIONS

- Single and repeated episodes of stress cause the synthesis, turnover, and, probably, release in the brain of both dopamine (DA) and norepinephrine (NE) to increase. These effects probably derive from the stress-induced increases in the firing rate of DA- and NE-containing neurons. Under such conditions, in which DA and NE utilization is substantially increased, the administration of tyrosine should stimulate DA and NE synthesis and probably release.
- With acute stress, no clear changes in the properties of NE receptors are apparent, although data are often conflicting. Almost no data regarding the effects of acute stress on DA receptors appear to be available. With chronic stress, ß-adrenergic receptors are down-regulated, suggesting that postsynaptic responses in brain circuits employing ß-receptors may be attenuated (although the functional effects of such changes do not appear to have been evaluated). α_1-Adrenergic receptors are unaffected by chronic stress, but both increases and decreases have been reported for α_2-receptor numbers in different brain regions. For DA receptors, chronic stress does not appear to change D_1 receptors; data on the D_2 receptor are few and conflicting. It is thus difficult to conclude with any confidence whether and how D_2 receptors change following repeated stress.
- Overall, given this diversity of catecholamine receptor responses to chronic stress and the relatively small number of studies that have defined them, it is presently impossible to conclude how brain circuits with catecholamine-producing neurons and postsynaptic receptors should respond to repeated stressful events. Additional studies should be encouraged, to define with more certainty the effects of stress on catecholamine receptors in particular brain regions and then to attempt to correlate such changes with functions specific to the affected regions. Without such information, the pharmacologic development and application of agents like L-tyrosine (TYR) or drugs that selectively target particular catecholamine receptors cannot be attempted with any hope of obtaining highly selective and useful effects on performance.
- Single episodes of stress cause the synthesis, turnover, and possibly release ofserotonin (5-hydroxytryptamine; 5HT) in the brain to increase. These effects do not derive from stress-induced increases in the firing rate of 5HT neurons but, rather, derive from increases in brain tryptophan (TRP) levels,

possibly induced by an effect of stress on the transport of TRP into the brain. Under such conditions, in which the increase in 5HT synthesis is probably dependent on an increased supply of TRP to the brain, the administration of TYR to stimulate catecholamine production could block the stress-related increase in 5HT synthesis (by antagonizing TRP transport into the brain). The impact of such an effect on performance is unknown, but clearly, it should be examined. Potential effects could be imagined on sleep and sensitivity to painful and other environmental stimuli, phenomena that have previously been connected to 5HT neuronal function.

- Finally, too few data are presently available to conclude how repeated or chronic stress influences 5HT synthesis and release. Additional information is therefore required before any notion can be formulated regarding how the administration of TYR might have an impact on serotonergic function under conditions of repeated stress.

Overall, given the impact of stress on performance, and on health in general, it is surprising that the influence of stress on the monoamine-producing neurons in the brain (probably the most examined group of transmitter-specific neurons in the past quarter century) is so incompletely studied or understood. A greater body of fundamental information on this relationship should be collected to better approach the applied question of how amino acids and drugs can be utilized effectively to combat the decrements in performance that accompany stress.

REFERENCES

Abercrombie, E.D., K.A.Keefe, D.S.DiFrischia, and M.J.Zigmond 1989 Differential effect of stress on in vivo dopamine release in striatum, nucleus accumbens, and medial frontal cortex. J. Neurochem. 52:1655–1658.

Anderson, S.M., J.R.Leu, T.Eggleston, G.F.Davis, and G.J.Kant 1986 Effects of chronic stress on dopamine D_2 receptors measured by [^{3}H]spiperone binding to rat brain membranes. Soc. Neurosci. Abstr. 12:417 (abstract).

Banderet, L., and H.Lieberman 1989 Treatment with tyrosine, a neurotransmitter precursor, reduces environmental stress in humans. Brain Res. Bull. 22:759–762.

Bliss, E.L., J.Ailion, and J.Zwanziger 1968 Metabolism of norepinephrine, serotonin and dopamine in rat brain with stress. J. Pharmacol. Exp. Ther. 164:122–134.

Boadle-Biber, M.C., J.N.Johannessen, N.Narasimhachari, and T.H.Phan 1986 Tryptophan hydroxylase: Increase in activity by electrical stimulation of serotonergic neurons. Neurochem. Int. 8:83–92.

Cohen, R.M., M.R.Cohen, and C.A.McLellan 1986 Foot shock induces time and region specific adrenergic receptor changes in rat brain. Pharmacol. Biochem. Behav. 24:1587–1592.

Cooper, J.R., F.E.Bloom, and R.H.Roth 1991 The Biochemical Basis of Neuropharmacology, 6th ed. New York: Oxford University Press.

Curzon, G., and A.R.Green 1969 Effects of immobilization on rat liver tryptophan pyrrolase and brain 5-hydroxytryptamine metabolism. Br. J. Pharmacol. 37:689–697.

Curzon, G., M.H.Joseph, and P.J.Knott 1972 Effects of immobilization and food deprivation on rat brain tryptophan metabolism. J. Neurochem. 19:1967–1974.

Dunn, A.J. 1988a Changes in plasma and brain tryptophan and brain serotonin and 5-hydroxyindoleacetic acid after footshock stress. Life Sci. 42:1847–1853.

1988 Stress-related activation of cerebral dopaminergic systems. Ann. N.Y. Acad. Sci. 537:188–205.

Eriksson, T., and A.Carlsson 1988 ß-Adrenergic control of brain uptake of large neutral amino acids. Life Sci. 42:1583–1589.

Fernstrom, J.D. 1990 Aromatic amino acids and monoamine synthesis in the central nervous system: Influence of the diet J. Nutr. Biochem. 1:508–517.

Fernstrom, M.H., E.A.Volk, J.D.Fernstrom, and P.M.Iuvone 1986 Effect of tyrosine administration on dopa accumulation in light- and dark-adapted retinas from normal and diabetic rats. Life Sci. 39:2049–2057.

Fernstrom, M.H., M.S.Massoudi, and J.D.Fernstrom 1990 Effect of 8-hydroxy-2-(di-n-propylamino)-tetralin on the tryptophan-induced increase in 5-hydroxytryptophan accumulation in rat brain. Life Sci. 47:283–289.

Friedhoff, A.J., H.Rosengarten, and E.A.Stone 1986 Increase in D_2 receptor density in rat brain after repeated stress. Soc. Neurosci. Abstr. 12:192 (abstract),

Iuvone, P.M., and A.J.Dunn 1986 Tyrosine hydroxylase activation in mesocortical 3,4-dihydroxyphenylethylamine neurons following footshock. J. Neurochem. 47:837–844.

Joseph, M.H., and G.A.Kennett 1983 Stress-induced release of 5-HT in the hippocampus and its dependence on increased tryptophan availability: An in vivo electrochemical study. Brain Res. 270:251–257.

Karobath, M., and R.J.Baldessarini 1972 Formation of catechol compounds from phenylalanine and tyrosine with isolated nerve endings. Nature New Biol. 236:206–208.

Kennett, G.A., and M.H.Joseph 1981 The functional importance of increased brain tryptophan in the serotonergic response to restraint stress. Neuropharmacology 20:39–43.

Kennett, G.A., S.L.Dickinson, and G.Curzon 1985 Enhancement of some 5-HT-dependent behavioral responses following repeated immobilization in rats. Brain Res. 330:253–263.

Kennett, G.A., G.Curzon, A.Hunt, and A.J.Patel 1986 Immobilization decreases amino acid concentrations in plasma but maintains or increases them in brain. J. Neurochem. 46:208–212.

Korf, J., G.K.Aghajanian, and R.H.Roth 1973 Increased turnover of norepinephrine in the rat cerebral cortex during stress: Role of the locus coeruleus. Neuropharmacology 12:933–938.

Lehnert, H., D.K.Reinstein, B.W.Strowbridge, and R.J.Wurtman 1984 Neurochemical and behavioral consequences of acute, uncontrollable stress: effects of dietary tyrosine. Brain Res. 303:215–223.

Levine, E.S., W.J.Litto, and B.L.Jacobs 1990 Activity of cat locus coeruleus noradrenergic neurons during the defense reaction. Brain Res. 531:189–195.

Lynch, M, J.Littleton, R.M.McKernan, M.J.Durcan, T.McMillan, and I.C.Campbell 1983 α-Adrenoceptor number and function in rat cortex after ethanol and immobilization stress. Brain Res. 288:145–149.

MacLennan, A.J., M.A.Pelleymounter, S.Atmadja, A.Jakubovic, S.F.Maier, and H.C.Fibiger 1989 D_2 dopamine receptors in the rat prefrontal cortex: Characterization and alteration by stress. Brain Res. 477:300–307.

Morgan, W.W., P.K.Rudeen, and K.A.Pfeil 1975 Effect of immobilization stress on serotonin content and turnover in regions of the rat brain. Life Sci. 17:143–150.

Mueller, G P., C.P.Twohy, H.T.Chen, J.P.Advis, and J.Meites 1976 Effects of L-tryptophan and restraint stress on hypothalamic and brain serotonin turnover, and pituitary TSH and prolactin release in rats. Life Sci. 18:715–724.

Nakagawa, R., M.Tanaka, Y.Kohno, Y.Noda, and N.Nagasaki 1981 Regional responses of rat brain noradrenergic neurones to acute intense stress. Pharmacol. Biochem. Behav. 14:729–732.

Nomura, S., M.Watanabe, N.Ukei, and T.Nakazawa 1981 Stress and ß-adrenergic receptor binding in the rat's brain. Brain Res. 224:199–203.

Nukima, I., G.B.Glavin, and F.S.LaBella 1987 Acute cold-restraint stress affects α_2-adrenoceptors in specific brain regions of the rat. Brain Res. 401:30–33.

Ohi, K., M.Mikuni, and K.Takahashi 1989 Stress adaptation and hypersensitivity in 5-HT neuronal systems after repeated foot shock . Pharmacol. Biochem. Behav. 34:603–608.

Owasoyo, J.O., D.F.Neri, and J.G.Lamberth 1992 Tyrosine and its potential use as a countermeasure to performance decrement in military sustained operations. Aviat. Space Environ. Med. 63:364–369.

Puglisi-Allegra, S., E.Kempf, C.Schleef, and S.Cabib 1991 Repeated stressful experiences differently affect brain dopamine receptor subtypes. Life Sci. 48:1263–1268.

Reinhard, J.F., M.J.Bannon, and R.H.Roth 1982 Acceleration by stress of dopamine synthesis and metabolism in prefrontal cortex: Antagonism by diazepam. Naunyn-Schmiedeberg's Arch. Pharmacol. 318:374–377.

Roth, R.H., S.Y.Tam, Y.Ida, J.X.Yang, and A.Y.Deutch 1988 Stress and the mesocorticolimbic dopamine systems. Ann. N.Y. Acad. Sci. 537:138–147.

Sauter, A.M., Y.Baba, E.A.Stone, and M.Goldstein 1978 Effect of stress and of phenylethanolamine-N-methyltransferase inhibition on central norepinephrine and epinephrine levels. Brain Res. 144:415–419.

Sharp, T., S.R.Bramwell, and D.G.Grahame-Smith 1992 Effect of acute administration of L-tryptophan on the release of 5-HT in rat hippocampus in relation to serotoninergic neuronal activity: An in vivo microdialysis study. Life Sci. 50:1215–1223.

Soblosky, J.S., and J.B.Thurmond 1986 Biochemical and behavioral correlates of chronic stress: Effects of tricyclic antidepressants. Pharmacol. Biochem. Behav. 24:1361–1368.

Stanford, C., M.Fillenz, and E.Ryan 1984 The effect of repeated mild stress on cerebral cortical adrenoceptors and noradrenaline synthesis in the rat Neurosci. Lett. 45:163–167.

Stone, E.A., and J.E.Platt 1982 Brain adrenergic receptors and resistance to stress. Brain Res. 237:405–14.

Stone, E.A., A.V.Slucky, J.E.Platt, and R.Trullas 1985 Reduction of the cyclic adenosine 3',5'-monophosphate response to catecholamines in rat brain slices after repeated restraint stress. J. Pharmacol. Exp. Ther. 233:382–388.

Stone, E.A., J.E.Platt, A.S.Herrera, and K.E.Kirk 1986 Effect of repeated restraint stress, desmethylimipramine or adrenocorticotropin on the alpha and beta adrenergic components of the cyclic AMP response to norepinephrine in rat brain slices. J. Pharmacol. Exp. Ther. 237:702–707.

Thierry, A.M., F.Javoy, J.Glowinski, and S.S.Kety 1968 Effects of stress on the metabolism of norepinephrine, dopamine and serotonin in the central nervous system of the rat. I. Modifications of norepinephrine turnover. J. Pharmacol. Exp. Ther. 163:163–171.

Thierry, A.M., J.P.Tassin, G.Blanc, and J.Glowinski 1976 Selective activation of the mesocortical dopamine system by stress. Nature 263:242–244.

Torda, T., I.Yamaguchi, F.Hirata, I.J.Kopin, and J.Axelrod 1981 Mepacrine treatment prevents immobilization-induced desensitization of beta-adrenergic receptors in rat hypothalamus and brain stem. Brain Res. 205:441–444.

Torda, T., R.Kvetn`anský, and M.Petríková 1985 Effect of repeated immobilization stress on central and peripheral adrenoceptors in rats. Endocrin. Exp. 19:157–163.

U'Prichard, D.C., and R.Kvetn`anský 1980 Central and peripheral adrenergic receptors in acute and repeated immobilization stress. Pp. 299–308 in Catecholamines and Stress: Recent Advances, E.Usdin, R. Kvetn`anský, and I.J.Kopin, eds. New York: Elsevier/North Holland.

Wilkinson, L.O., and B.L.Jacobs 1988 Lack of response of serotonergic neurons in the dorsal raphe nucleus of freely moving cats to stressful stimuli. Exp. Neurol. 101:445–457.

DISCUSSION

CHANDON PRASAD: I would like to make a comment with regard to receptor binding, particularly dopamine receptor binding. When one looks at the earlier binding studies, and even the new ones, one must be very careful in interpreting their results.

JOHN FERNSTROM: I agree with you 100 percent. Most investigators worry to some extent about that problem. I think your point is well taken. I think the conclusion would be that more studies are needed in this area; they are not there now.

GEORGE BRAY: At the end of each of your sections, you state what tyrosine might do to monoamine synthsis and receptors. Does that tell us that we are going to hear about tyrosine later or that no one has done the experiments?

JOHN FERNSTROM: I was originally thinking, when I was invited to give this talk, that I would be responsible for that. But then when the workshop program was finally sent to me, I saw that there were several people who investigate tyrosine effects on the list of participants. So I assumed they would be discussing this information, and did not spend much time myself dealing with it.

RICHARD WURTMAN: I think you set it up beautifully, too. There were several people in my laboratory who did some studies on the effect of giving tyrosine to stress-immobilized animals. They found that the stress per se depleted hypothalamic locus ceruleus. Norepinephrine modified behavior; that is, there was less spontaneous activity, less poking their nose in the hole in the ground, which I guess means something to a rat (I am not sure what). But also, of course, stress caused striatocortical activation of corticosterone release. Then they found that giving tyrosine blocked all of these effects.

I have been waiting to see some other laboratories confirm or not confirm —I would hope confirm—these findings because they are from our lab, and I believe them; but if they are really powerful, it means that physicians might have an available strategy for diminishing cortisone responses, for example, in somebody who has broken their leg and has diabetes.

I am not aware of any studies. Do you know of any other studies?

JOHN FERNSTROM: No. In fact, your study with Lehnert was more interesting than you have stated, because tyrosine was put in the diet. So the animals were actually eating increased amounts of tyrosine supplied chronically in their diets. Then an acute stress was provided, and the effect of the tyrosine was to prevent the stress-induced depletion of brain NE. It would be very interesting to do a chronic stress study, too, to see if tyrosine supplementation would continue to be beneficial.

10

Endocrine and Immune System Responses to Stress

William R.Beisel[1]

INTRODUCTION

The interacting responses of the endocrine and immune systems characterize various forms of stress. Although only partially defined, these responses evolve in combination with stress-induced responses of the central nervous system (CNS).

To encompass the complexities of this neuroendocrine-immune axis, equally complex titles for the field are now emerging, as typified by the term *psychoneuroendocrineimmunology*. Recent reviews of this subject include a book edited by Chrousos et al. (1988), two conferences of the New York Academy of Sciences (see Bomberger and Haar [1988] and Goetzl et al. [1990]), and a review by Chrousos and Gold (1992).

Molecular participants in these responses to stress include traditional hormones, neuropeptides, immunologically generated cytokines, and the secondary and tertiary messengers formed within responding cells. These

[1] William R.Beisel, John Hopkins School of Public Health, 615 N. Wolfe Street, Baltimore, MD 21205

participants in stress responses can act as autocrines, paracrines, or circulating endocrines (or endogenous mediators) with far-ranging effects.

Neuroendocrine-immune system responses to stress are characterized by multiple checks and balances and interacting feedback loops. Other prominent features include redundancy, which is most evident with cytokines, many of which have overlapping activities, plus the ability to enlist related cytokines. Many cytokines also exhibit pleiotropy, with multiple functions (Dantzer and Kelley, 1989).

Neural cells and lymphocytes are capable of producing some of the peptide hormones, and many have receptors that allow them to respond to hormonal stimuli.

Responses of the neuroendocrine-immune axis vary with the form, duration, and severity of the inciting stress. Different patterns of response may also evolve longitudinally, over time, if stress is protracted.

Because the molecular mediators involved in responses to stress show differences in the timing and magnitude of their endogenous production, it is not surprising that their physiologic, metabolic, and nutritional consequences are not consistent. Furthermore, the immunological consequences of stress may impair host defense mechanisms against infectious diseases and malignancies. Host defense mechanisms against infectious diseases are of special concern when military populations are under consideration.

Valuable insights have been obtained by studying responses to stress in laboratory animals. However, because of differences between species, such models may not accurately reflect the stress-induced responses that occur in humans.

HISTORICAL PERSPECTIVES

The first hormone to be discovered, just prior to the turn of the century, was adrenalin (epinephrine), a major contributor to immediate cardiovascular responses to stress. Several decades elapsed, however, before William Cannon, in 1929, summarized his theories of homeostasis and his easily understood concept of "fight or flight" (Kopin et al., 1988).

Contributions of Hans Selye

Two additional decades elapsed before Hans Selye divided stress reactions into three stages: an initial sympathoadrenomedullary "alarm reaction," a subsequent "stage of resistance" with activation of the hypothalamic-pituitary-adrenocortical axis, and a final stage of exhaustion and death (Kopin et al., 1988).

Selye's resistance stage included his general adaptation syndrome. This was characterized by adrenocortical secretion and hypertrophy, gastrointestinal ulceration, and thymic and lymphoid shrinkage. These concepts of Selye gained widespread acceptance, in part because they immediately preceded the clinical availability and use of cortisone and adrenocorticotropic hormone (ACTH).

Selye taught his students that "to measure is to know." This dictum is reflected in the subsequent logarithmic growth in knowledge during the 1950s, 1960s, and 1970s about each hormone or hormone group. These knowledge bursts depended on advances in steroid and protein chemistry, which allowed hormones and their metabolic products to be assayed in body fluids. Use of radioisotopic iodine was also a major factor in allowing thyroid physiology to be deciphered.

Studies of Endogenous Pyrogen

Following Paul Beeson's observation (1948) that endotoxin-free substances obtained from neutrophils were capable of inducing fever, many studies of endogenous pyrogen (EP) were initiated. This research consumed much of the professional lifetimes of individuals such as W.Barry Wood, Jr., Elisha Adkins, Phyllis Bodel, and Patrick A.Murphy.

Studies of Infectious Stress

In the early 1960s, Beisel (1991) initiated comprehensive prospective longitudinal studies of the endocrine, metabolic, physiological, and nutritional responses to the stress of infectious disease in research volunteers. These studies were superimposed on ongoing tests of new, experimental vaccines conducted at the U.S. Army Medical Research Institute for Infectious Diseases (USAMRIID).

The USAMRIID group measured day-to-day changes in glucocorticoids and was the first to report increases in aldosterone, growth hormone, insulin, and glucagon during the stress of infectious illnesses and the depression of thyroid function. Similar changes have subsequently been found in individuals with other forms of stress.

However, hormonal changes failed to account for the metabolic and nutritional changes detected in plasma glycoproteins, amino acids, and trace elements or for other components of acute-phase reactions in volunteers (Beisel, 1991). The dilemma was solved, however, by USAMRIID's discovery of leukocyte products that induced acute-phase reactions and that stimulated endocrine responses as well. These hormone-like substances were originally named leukocytic endogenous mediator(s) (LEMs) (Pekarek and Beisel, 1971);

they are now called interleukin-1, interleukin-6, and/or tumor necrosis factor, the three "proinflammatory" cytokines.

Studies in Ranger Trainees

Beginning in the late 1970s, a Norwegian group led by Aakvaag and coworkers (1978), Opstad and colleagues (1980, 1981, 1982, 1983, 1984, 1985, 1991, 1992), and Øektedalen (1982, 1983a,b,c) initiated a comprehensive (still ongoing) study of the endocrinological responses of Ranger trainees during 5-day exercises, which included the stresses of food and sleep deprivation as well as severe physical demands. Similar studies have recently been conducted in U.S. Army Rangers. U.S. Army Rangers, who also underwent comprehensive physiological and nutritional measurements as well as immunological studies (Moore et al., 1992)[1]

Immunological Progress

Logarithmic growth in immunological knowledge also accompanied new research techniques. Identification of populations and subpopulations of T and B lymphocytes in 1968 led to current concepts of the humoral and cell-mediated arms of the immune system and their interrelationships.

Another direction of immunological growth focused on the cytokines. The mutual identity of lymphocyte-activating factor, EP, and LEM was recognized, and in 1979, the three were renamed interleukin-1 (IL-1). The interleukin designation was then used for numerous other cytokines (Beisel, 1991). A few new cytokines may still be identified, but cytokine research still has other major objectives; that is, questions remain about how cytokine genes are regulated, how cytokine gene regulation relates to immune system functions and clinical disease, and how their effects are modulated by circulating cytokine receptors and receptor antagonists.

ENDOCRINE RESPONSES TO STRESS

Most traditional hormones have been implicated in responses to stress, although data on their concentrations in body fluids are relatively scarce and

[1] Additional data on U.S. Army Ranger trainees were presented at a meeting of the Committee on Military Nutrition Research, Food and Nutrition Board, Institute of Medicine, National Academy of Sciences, in March, 1993 and are referred to here as unpublished data.

data on production rates are scarcer still. Despite these shortcomings, major hormonal responses to military stresses are now fairly well defined. Hormonal responses to stress are not simply "all out" but are modulated and carefully controlled by feedback loops. Furthermore, CNS peptide mediators that normally function as neurotransmitters may reach concentrations in plasma that allow them to function as hormones (Geelhoed, 1987).

Catecholamines

Acute responses to stress, that is, Cannon's "fight or flight" and Selye's "alarm reaction," focus on catecholamines. These are products of the CNS's locus ceruleus and the sympathetic nervous system. A dense network of CNS neurons produces norepinephrine, and epinephrine is released from the adrenal medulla and sympathetic nerve terminals (Chrousos and Gold, 1992). These and other neurotransmitters initiate immediate responses to stress (Kopin et al., 1988), including tachycardia, hyperventilation, sweating, piloerection, dilation of pupils and bronchi, vasomotor changes, and altered gut motility.

Increased concentrations of epinephrine and norepinephrine occur during Ranger training (Opstad, 1991; Opstad et al., 1980), as an early component of trauma or surgical stress (Geelhoed, 1887), during intense physical exercise (Landmann et al., 1984), and in patients who suffer strokes (O'Neill et al., 1991) or severe lobar pneumonia (Feldman et al., 1989). Food restriction stress in mice induces gastric ulcers and increases plasma catecholamine values (Nakamura et al., 1990).

Catecholamine responses to infectious disease stress vary with the severity of illness. Although no changes may be detected in subjects with mild, brief infections, increased plasma epinephrine and norepinephrine concentrations urqwoccur in subjects with septic shock (Beisel, 1991) and critically severe infections (Feldman et al., 1989). It should also be noted that vitamin C is required for the production of these catecholamines. The highest concentrations of vitamin C found in the human body are in the catecholamine-producing areas of both the CNS and adrenal glands.

Adrenocortical Responses

Secretion of increased levels of adrenocortical hormones, central to Selye's general adaptation syndrome, is initiated by corticotropin-releasing factor (CRF) from hypothalamic neurons; this is followed by the release of ACTH from the anterior pituitary gland. Thus, the central hormonal role in stress is now often ascribed to CRF (Audhya et al., 1988; Koob et al., 1988; McEwen et al., 1988).

CRF and ACTH

In addition to its role in stimulating greater adrenocorticoid secretion, CRF appears to act in mediating the release of oxytocin, vasopressin, and vasoactive intestinal peptide (Koob et al., 1988; McEwen et al., 1988) and by initiating visceral and paracrine responses to stress (Audhya et al., 1988; Lenz, 1990; Murison and Badde, 1990).

CRF is produced by many CNS neurons in addition to those in the hypothalamus. Its production in the brain's locus ceruleus gives it a role in stimulating norepinephrine production (Valentino, 1988). Because of its presence in the thymus and spleen, CRF can play a role in neuroimmunomodulation (Audhya et al., 1988; Irwin et al., 1990; Jain et al., 1991). Like CNS opioids, CRF may also have analgesic functions (Bianchi et al., 1991).

Neuronal production of CRF can be stimulated by IL-1 (Rothwell and Grimble, 1992) and platelet-activating factor (PAF) (Rougeot et al., 1990). In contrast, CRF is not stimulated by some stimuli that induce ACTH release, including epinephrine, norepinephrine, angiotensin II, oxytocin, arginine vasopressin, tumor necrosis factor (TNF), IL-2, and IL-6 (Plotsky, 1988; Rothwell and Grimble, 1992). ACTH concentrations in plasma are increased during stress (Chakraborti, 1989; Plotsky, 1988). The responsiveness of adrenocortical cells to ACTH is heightened by immune system activation (Torres-Aleman et al., 1988).

Adrenal Glucocorticoids

The principal glucocorticoids, cortisol in humans and corticosterone in rodents, show relatively modest responses to most stresses. Beisel and coworkers (1967, 1969) found that the normal circadian periodicity of plasma cortisol concentrations was lost during early febrile stages of infections induced in volunteers. Although morning cortisol concentrations were not elevated, the normal circadian decline in cortisol concentrations in the afternoon failed to occur. This combination resulted in a modest increase in 24-h urinary 17-hydroxy-corticosteroids (17-OHCS) excretion (Beisel, 1991).

Increased plasma cortisol concentrations may occur in patients with infections of great severity or terminally ill patients; in such instances, the increased cortisol concentrations can usually be explained by impairment of the hepatic enzymes that convert plasma cortisol to water-soluble metabolites (Beisel, 1991).

Some of the largest adrenocortical responses occur after trauma or surgical stress (Geelhoed, 1987). However, only modest elevations of plasma cortisol and urinary 17-OHCS have been reported with various other stresses such as heat (Armstrong et al., 1989), high-altitude and cold (Chakraborti, 1989), and in patients with strokes (Mulley et al., 1989; O'Neill et al., 1991).

The stress of Ranger training also is accompanied by a modest adrenocorticoid response (Opstad, 1991, 1992; Opstad and Aakvaag, 1983; Opstad et al., 1980) and a loss of circadian rhythm (Opstad and Aakvaag, 1981). Similar small increases in plasma cortisol concentrations were seen in U.S. Rangers (Moore et al., 1992). Elevations of plasma corticosterone concentrations occur during various forms of experimental stress in rodents (Flores et al., 1990; Kandil and Borysenko, 1988; Kant et al., 1987).

The cortisol response to stress in humans is always proportionally greater than the responses of any other, less potent adrenal glucocorticoids or the adrenal androgens (Beisel, 1991). In fact, adrenal androgen concentrations were found to decrease during Ranger training (Opstad, 1992).

Increased body temperatures caused by the stress of a hot, humid environment produced an adreno-cortical response, along with sizable losses of body nitrogen, electrolytes, and minerals (Beisel et al., 1968).

The physiologic effects (and side effects) of these combined glucocorticoid responses to stress are quite small when compared with those of highly potent synthetic adrenocortical steroids. Furthermore, production of adrenocortical steroids may fall below normal concentrations if disease or surgical stress is protracted (Beisel, 1991; Geelhoed, 1987).

ADRENAL MINERALOCORTICOIDS

The increases in aldosterone concentrations produced during the stress of febrile infections and surgical procedures explains the renal retention of sodium (Beisel, 1991). The increase in aldosterone concentrations may be accompanied by a seemingly inappropriate secretion of antidiuretic hormone, which occurs in some infections, especially those localized within the skull (Beisel, 1991). This combination may lead to retention of dangerous amounts of salt and water.

An increase in the amount of secreted aldosterone and renin has been noted during heat stress (Armstrong et al., 1989) and Ranger training (Opstad et al., 1985).

Growth Hormone

A stress-induced increase in plasma immunoreactive growth hormone (GH) concentrations was first reported during the stress of infectious disease (Beisel, 1991). Similar increases have been shown to occur in patients with severe pneumonia (Feldman et al., 1989) and have been reported in Norwegian Rangers (Aakvaag et al., 1978; Opstad, 1991; Opstad and Aakvaag, 1981, 1983; Opstad et al., 1980). Six- to 10-fold increases were found in U.S. Army Rangers by MAJ K.Friedl and colleagues (Moore et al., 1992).

Increased GH secretion by the pituitary could be due to growth hormone-releasing factor stimulation (Dieguez et al., 1988) or stress-induced increases in pituitary dopamine values (Aakvaag et al., 1978). It is also possible that lymphocyte secretion of GH could contribute to increased concentrations of GH in plasma (Kelley, 1990).

Thyroidal Responses

Stress-induced activation of the hypothalamic-pituitary-adrenal axis produces secondary suppression of thyroidal responses (Chrousos and Gold, 1992). The concentrations of plasma protein-bound iodine, thyroxine (T4), triiodothyronine (T3), and thyroid-stimulating hormone (TSH) fall during infectious illnesses (Beisel, 1991). The decrease in T3 concentrations can be explained, in part, by an increase in "reverse" T3. These altered values all rebound to normal concentrations during convalescence.

An identical pattern of thyroidal suppression was observed repeatedly during the stress of Ranger training (Opstad and Aakvaag, 1981, 1983; Aakvaag et al., 1978; Opstad et al., 1980, 1984). These Ranger data were compatible with an almost complete halt in thyroidal T4 release (Aakvaag et al., 1978).

Analogous thyroidal suppression occurs in older or poorly conditioned long-distance runners (Hesse et al., 1989). Low thyroid hormone concentrations also characterize traumatic or surgical stress (Geelhoed, 1987).

Other Pituitary Hormones

Like the thyroidal hormone responses, the reproductive hormone axis is inhibited at all levels by components of the hypothalamic-pituitary-adrenal axis (Chrousos and Gold, 1992). Initially, prolactin (PRL) concentrations were thought to be increased by acute stress (Aakvaag et al., 1978), and small increases in PRL concentrations have been found in patients with severe pneumonia (Feldman et al., 1989). In contrast, a decline in plasma PRL concentrations was noted in each Ranger group studied (Aakvaag et al., 1978; Opstad and Aakvaag, 1982; Opstad et al., 1980, 1991). These declines in PRL concentrations were minimized by allowing extra sleep time, but not by increasing the daily food intake of the Rangers.

Luteinizing hormone concentrations have shown variable changes in Rangers, with increases and decreases being noted in different groups (Aakvaag et al., 1978; Opstad, 1992; Opstad and Aakvaag, 1983). Another pituitary gonadotropin, follicle-stimulating hormone, showed consistent declines in the plasma of Rangers (Aakvaag et al., 1978; Opstad, 1992).

Testosterone

Testosterone and other androgens share similar fates. Sharp and sustained declines in the concentrations of testosterone and other gonadal androgens occurred in the serum of all Ranger groups tested (Aakvaag et al., 1978; Opstad, 1992; Opstad and Aakvaag, 1983). Declines of 25 and 33 percent were also detected in U.S. Rangers (Moore et al., 1992). It is not known whether testosterone concentration declines were secondary to declines in PRL and the gonadotropin concentrations or whether they were due to some direct testicular effect of heavy exercise.

Pancreatic Hormones

Within 12 h after the onset of fever in infected volunteers, baseline concentrations of both insulin and glucagon in plasma became elevated; glucose tolerance curves and insulin responses also became abnormal, resembling those of adult-onset diabetics (Beisel, 1991). Simultaneous elevations of both insulin and glucagon are most unusual, because these hormones usually act reciprocally. These changes, plus the appearance of cellular insulin resistance, have been attributed to the effects of interleukin-1 (IL-1) (Beisel, 1991).

Increased plasma glucagon values were found in patients with recent strokes (O'Neill et al., 1991). An increase in the insulin concentrations in the plasma of fully fed Rangers was reversed when food restriction stress was added to their training (Opstad and Aakvaag, 1981).

Intestinal Hormones

Øektedalen et al. (1982, 1983a,b,c) reported three- to sixfold increases in plasma secretin values in fasting Ranger trainees and athletes who participated in long cross-country ski races. These high values rapidly returned to normal after a meal or oral glucose feeding.

Plasma vasoactive intestinal peptive and pancreatic peptide values were also elevated in these ski racers, whose gastric acid secretions showed a threefold increase.

Other Hormones and Neuroendocrines

Nussey et al. (1988) found increases in plasma oxytocin and arginine vasopressin concentrations during surgical stress in elderly patients.

Opioid peptides (endorphins, enkephalins, and dynorphin) are produced by lymphocytes and phagocytic cells as well as by the central nervous system (CNS) (Teschemacher et al., 1990). The stresses of severe exercise, surgery, hyperthermia, and severe pain all trigger the release of beta-endorphin but not methionine-enkephalin (Vescovi etal., 1990). Similar beta-endorphin increases are seen in critically ill children (Dindar et al., 1990).

A depression in the concentrations of insulin-like growth factor (somatomedin C) to 30–50 percent of the baseline concentrations in plasma was measured during all four phases of U.S. Army Ranger training (Moore et al., 1992), despite the concomitant rise in plasma growth hormone values.

IMMUNE SYSTEM RESPONSES TO STRESS

Stress and a variety of psychiatric illnesses, notably the affective disorders, may be associated with immunosuppression (Khansari et al., 1990). However, studies attempting to link various forms of stress to an increased susceptibility to infectious diseases or malignancies seldom include direct measurements of immune system competence.

Sophisticated tests of immune functions have generally not been available in clinical laboratories (although the Acquired Immunodeficiency Syndrome (AIDS) epidemic may be changing that, especially for the important task of counting of helper T-lymphocyte [CD4] numbers). Furthermore, interpretation of delayed dermal hypersensitivity skin tests as a measure of cell-mediated immunity (CMI) requires a competent, well-trained observer.

Nevertheless, the available data suggest that stress may reduce functional immune system competence, especially CMI. Emotional stresses such as the death of a family member, divorce, and major depressions all have immunological links, that is, depressed lymphocyte counts and decreased responsiveness of lymphocytes to mitogens (Bonneau et al., 1990).

Changes in Lymphoid Cells and Tissues

Thymic involution, a component of Selye's general adaptation syndrome, was first recognized in the early 1800s as a component of severe cachexia; it remains a major problem in malnourished children and in adults with disease-induced cachexia. Involution is most prominent in T-cell areas of the thymus and other lymphoid tissues. In contrast, B-cells and plasma cells are usually spared (Beisel, 1991). Stresses that induce cachexia or deficiencies in levels of body zinc can also induce a reversible state of thymic involution. Other stresses can also influence thymic cells; for example, auditory stress in mice inhibits migration of prethymic stem cells into the thymus (Bomberger and Haar, 1988).

Thymic involution is accompanied by reduced production of zinc-containing hormones by thymic epithelial cells. These peptides (thymosin, thymopoietin, thymopentin) have essential roles in the continued maintenance of T-cell functions throughout the body (Beisel, 1991). These thymic peptides can also increase the production of adrenocorticotropic hormone (ACTH) (Khansari et al., 1990) and may play a role in stressful situations.

Lymphocyte Counts in Stress

Reductions in lymphocyte counts, T-cell counts, and CD4/CD8 cell ratios are seen during some stresses (reduced CD4 cell counts in patients with AIDS are attributed to direct viral invasion of those cells). Lymphopenia caused by corticosteroid-induced lympholysis is a phenomenon of rodents but not of humans.

Simultaneous intravenous injections ofcortisol and epinephrine in healthy adult volunteers caused an initial increase in lymphocyte numbers (particularly suppressor CD8 cells and natural killer [NK] cells); these responses were followed by a decline in lymphocyte numbers and then a normalization within 24 h (Brohee et al., 1990).

Humoral Immunity and Stress

Paradoxically, concentrations of total serum immunoglobulins (IgM, IgG, and IgA) all tend to be increased in children with severe malnutrition. In contrast, secretory IgA is diminished. Antibody responses to a new vaccine also tend to be reduced, but not eliminated, in these children (Beisel, 1991).

U.S. Army Rangers showed diminished antibody responses to two standard vaccines when they were inoculated 2 weeks after beginning their stressful training (Bernton, 1992). Similarly, subjects experiencing major stresses tended to have lower baseline serum IgG values and a poorer 3-week response to immunization with a novel test antigen, keyhole limpet hemocyanin (KLH), than did a control population (Snyder et al, 1990).

Neonatal mice subjected to immobilization stress had diminished antibody responses to test antigens (Taylor and Ross, 1991). Rats subjected to electrical shocks had reduced IgG antibody responses to KLH immunization (Laudenslager et al., 1988). However, Korneva and Shkhinek (1990) found that the nature, intensity, and duration of a stress altered the humoral immune responses to standardized antigens: poor responses were seen after cold or traumatic stresses, average responses were seen after rotation or immobilization stresses, and enhanced responses were seen after repeated swimming stresses.

Peak antibody titers after immunization may coincide with a rise in circulating glucocorticoids in mice (Blalock, 1988).

Cell-Mediated Immunity and Stress

Cell-mediated immune responses to stress include poor responses of lymphocytes to mitogens, diminished delayed dermal hypersensitivity (DDH) responses, and decreased NK cell activity. Although DDH responses have widely been used to study immunological dysfunctions in patients with trauma-or disease-induced cachexia or other forms of malnutrition (Beisel, 1991), DDH has rarely been measured in humans with other types of stresses.

U.S. Army Rangers showed significant declines in DDH responses after 4 weeks of training, with a slight rebound in the sixth week, in a study conducted by LTC E.Bernton (Bernton, 1992). In another Ranger group, however, DDH responses were quite variable; an increase that coincided with a rebound in lymphocyte responsiveness to mitogens was noted during the last phase of training (Moore et al., 1992).

Lymphocyte Responses to Mitogens

In U.S. Army Rangers, lymphocytes showed diminished in vitro responses to mitogens during the second and third phases of training, with a rebound in the fourth and final phase (Moore et al., 1992). Walter Reed Army Institute of Research investigators found slight but progressive declines in lymphocyte numbers during a 6-week period in other trainees (Bernton, 1992). Stresses of avoidable electric shock or loud noise in volunteers each led to poor in vitro lymphocyte responses to mitogens (Weisse et al., 1990).

Sheep exposed to heat stress showed diminished in vitro lymphocyte mitogenesis, and their sera caused reduced mitogenesis of lymphocytes from unstressed sheep (Niwano et al., 1990). In contrast, the lymphocytes of rats subjected to involuntary treadmill running exercise periods (45 minutes per day, for 8 weeks) showed significant increases in mitogen responsiveness (Tharp and Pruess, 1991). This apparent difference may be explained by the study of Hoffman-Goetz et al. (1988), who subjected mice to treadmill running stress. Well-trained mice showed improved lymphocyte mitogenesis, whereas lymphocytes from untrained novice mice showed decreased mitogenic activity.

Natural Killer Cell Activity

Both lymphocyte mitogenesis and NK cell numbers were found to be decreased in medical students taking final examinations (Bonneau et al., 1990). NK cell activity as well as NK cell surface markers were reduced in individuals categorized as "noncopers" in comparison with the findings for "copers" (Schlesinger and Yodfat, 1988).

Studies in animals showed a reduction in NK cell activity in mice subjected to rotation-induced stress (Kandil and Borysenko, 1988), but an increase in mice stressed by food restriction (Nakamura et al., 1990). A decrease in NK cell activity and NK cell recycling capacity occurred in rats subjected to surgical stress (Pollock et al., 1989). This impaired role of NK cells was shown most dramatically by Zoller et al. (1989), who observed survival in all rats subjected to leg amputation 7 days after footpad implants of adenocarcinoma cells; in contrast, 80 percent of rats died of metastases if a simple laparotomy was done 2 days before the leg amputation.

Cytokine Responses to Stress

The cytokines include interleukins, tumor necrosis factor (TNF; cachectin), interferons, lymphotoxin, colony-stimulating factors, and cell growth factors.

The number of identifiable cytokines continues to grow, and many are important participants in body responses to stress. In many types of stress, cytokines play a major role in triggering and modulating acute-phase reactions, which include hormonal responses and immune system activation.

Many cytokines have now been isolated and produced by recombinant DNA technology. Preclinical and clinical studies have employed several of the cytokines in immunocompromised hosts (Roilides and Pizzo, 1992). These studies have shown dangers as well as benefits from cytokines such as interleukins 1 and 2 (IL-1 and IL-2), TNF, and gamma interferon.

In studies in animals and trials in humans, high doses of these cytokines cause hypotensive shock, capillary leak syndrome, and multiorgan failure. This form of shock is due to the vasodilatory effects of nitric oxide (NO), which is formed when these cytokines activate NO synthase in vascular endothelial cells (Kilbourn and Belloni, 1990).

NO has thus been identified as the "vascular relaxing factor" of septic shock (Hibbs et al., 1992). NO-induced hypotension is not always reversible, even with the most potent pressor agents.

Microbicidal and Tumoricidal Effects of NO

Although the cytokine-induced generation of NO may have lethal consequences, it can also provide an alternative mechanism for the microbicidal and tumoricidal activities of macrophages and other body cells, a mechanism that is totally independent of the well-studied actions of free oxygen radicals generated during the respiratory burst of phagocytic cells.

Following its intracellular induction by cytokine actions, NO synthase produces NO from the terminal guanidino nitrogen atoms of arginine, an amino acid that might be a candidate for use as a nutritional supplement. NO aids in killing tumor cells and some infectious agents by functioning in arginine-dependent cell-mediated immune responses, and by interfering with DNA replication and iron-containing mitochondrial enzymes in tumor cells and microbes (Hibbs et al., 1992). In the process, NO is metabolized to nitrites and then to nitrates, the form in which it is excreted in urine.

During mild infections in humans or induced nonlethal experimental endotoxemia in rats, urinary nitrate excretion can jump 10-fold (Wagner and Tannenbaum, 1982). This newly defined, cytokine-induced microbicidal mechanism is totally dependent on the presence of arginine. Arginine is the only substrate for this NO- and citrulline-generating pathway in endothelial cells and certain phagocytes. Of note, as part of the "urea cycle" in hepatocytes, an analogous pathway proceeds in the opposite direction, that is citrulline is processed into arginine, which, in turn, is converted to urea and ornithine.

The Immunological Role of Arginine

In addition to its immunological role as the precursor for NO production in body cells, there is growing evidence that arginine supplementation may have immunostimulatory activity, and that arginine becomes an indispensable amino acid after trauma or severe sepsis (Jeevanandam et al., 1993; Kirk and Barbul, 1992; Nirgiotis et al., 1991). Following trauma in rodents, arginine supplements enhance thymic size, prevent thymic involution, and stimulate lymphocyte functions, including the synthesis of IL-2 and the production of natural killer cells. In this latter role, arginine also promotes host antitumor responses in a number of tumor models (Kirk and Barbul, 1992).

The formation of NO and citrulline from arginine in various body cells is totally dependent on the action on intracellular NO synthase. Recent evidence shows that, unlike rodents, human mononuclear phagocytes (monocytes and macrophages) do not possess the enzyme, NO synthase, and under tightly controlled conditions, cannot be induced to produce NO following cellular activation by endotoxin or various cytokines (Schneemann et al., 1993). No reports have yet been forthcoming about similar studies in human granulocytes. Additional studies are also needed to evaluate the potential role of alanine supplements in severely stressed humans.

The Acute Phase Reaction

The triad of IL-1, TNF, and IL-6 initiates and sustains acute-phase reactions, with their attendant fever, myalgia, cephalalgia, somnolence, anorexia, hypermetabolism, immune system activation, hepatic production of acute-phase proteins, muscle protein catabolism, amino acid fluxes from muscle to liver, and the sequestration of iron and zinc (Beisel, 1991).

These responses are accompanied by activation of the pituitary-adrenal axis; release of other hormones such as growth hormone, aldosterone, insulin, and glucagon; alterations in lipid and carbohydrate metabolism; as well as losses of body weight, muscle mass, and body nutrient stores (Beisel, 1991; Parker, 1991).

The acute-phase reaction can be triggered by infectious microorganisms, trauma, or any stress that activates macrophages, thereby initiating the release of IL-1. This can include strenuous exercise. The magnitude and duration of acute-phase reactions depend on the production and release of IL-1, TNF, and IL-6.

Although acute-phase reactions may have some beneficial aspects, an excess production of IL-1 or TNF can be quite detrimental (Moldawer and Lowry, 1992), in part because of increased cellular release of phospholipase A_2, leukotrienes, and prostaglandins (Larson and Henson, 1983; Vadas, 1984). Acute-phase reactions during very severe illnesses or bacterial endotoxemias can be complicated by hypotensive shock attributed to the previously described cytokine-induced formation of nitric oxide (Kilbourn and Belloni, 1990).

Interleukin-1

IL-1 peptides have alpha or beta forms with dissimilar amino acid sequences but with apparently identical actions. These forms can have similar or dissimilar receptors with varying affinities for the many cell types that respond to IL-1 (Scarborough, 1990). Cytokine receptors can become soluble and circulate in plasma, where they may serve to modulate cytokine activities (Kern et al., 1992).

As illustrated in Figure 10–1, IL-1 or TNF, as prototype cytokines, initiate cellular responses when they contact cell receptors. This activates cell wall phospholipase A_2 (in a process accompanied by calcium influx), causing the release of arachidonic acid, eicosapentanoic acid, or platelet-activating factor from cell wall phospholipids. Release of these lipids is blocked by glucocorticoid hormones (Claman, 1988).

The fatty acid composition of cell wall phospholipids, as influenced by dietary intake of unsaturated fatty acids of the omega-3 or omega-6 varieties, determines which second messenger acids will be released into the cell (Rothwell and Grimble, 1992). A dietary supplement of linoleic acid in healthy volunteers was shown to increase neutrophil phagocytosis, arachidonic acid release, and leukotriene B_4 generation (Jannace et al., 1992).

Cellular responses to these second messenger acids are then governed by the specific enzymes that are contained in individual responding cells. These enzymes convert second messenger acids to third messenger leukotrienes (LTs) or prostaglandins (PGs). Cells that possess lipooxygenase enzymes convert arachidonic or eicosapentanoic acids to LTs, whereas cells that possess cyclooxygenase enzymes convert these acids to PGs (Beisel, 1991; Kinsella et al., 1990).

Arachidonic acid is converted to LTs of the 4 series or PGs of the 2 series. A diet rich in omega-3 fish oils increases eicosapentanoic acid levels in cell walls and leads to less active LTs of the 5 series and PGs of the 3 series (Rothwell and Grimble, 1992).

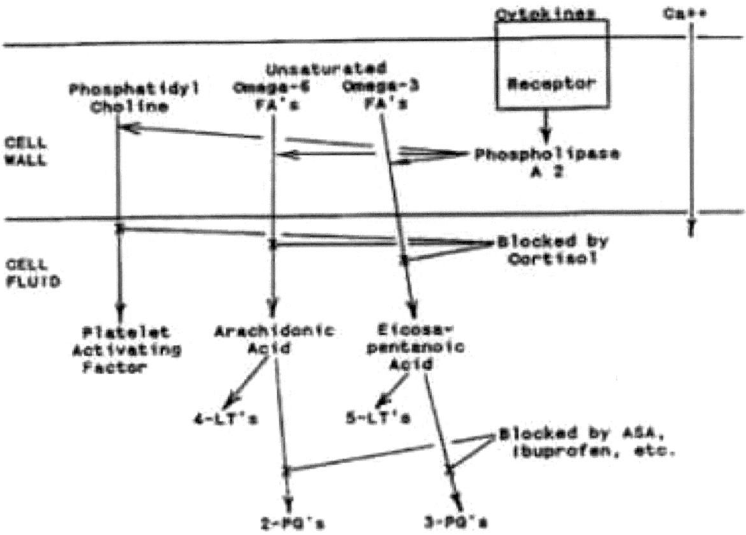

FIGURE 10–1 Cellular actions of prototype cytokines. Following the attachment of cytokines such as interleukin-1 (IL-1) or tumor necrosis factor (TNF) to cell wall receptors, phospholipase A_2 is activated; this is accompanied by an influx of calcium. This enzymatic action on cell wall phospholipids creates platelet-activating factor from phosphatidylcholine, arachidonic acid from omega-6 fatty acids (FAs), and eicosapentanoic acid from omega-3 fatty acids. These effects are blocked by cortisol and other potent glucocorticoids. Arachidonic acid is converted to 4-series leukotrienes (LTs) or 2-series prostaglandins (PGs). Eicosapentanoic acid is converted to 5-series LTs or 3-series PGs. PG production is blocked by drugs such as ibuprofen or aspirin (ASA).

Importantly, drugs such as aspirin or ibuprofen can block IL-1-induced production of PGs in the hypothalamus, skeletal muscle, and other cells (Beisel, 1991). Such symptomatic therapy could be of importance for military personnel with minor infections, inflammation, trauma, or other common military stresses by minimizing decrements in the physical and mental performances of soldiers as well as by reducing losses of their body nutrients and muscle mass.

For example, in studies of groups of U.S. Army Medical Research Institute for Infectious Diseases (USAMRIID) volunteers working 8 h/day on computer-generated problems, large performance decrements were shown to accompany illness produced by infectious diseases (Alluisi et al., 1973). However, symptomatic therapy with aspirin and propoxyphene hydrochloride (Darvon) markedly reduced fever and the symptoms of illness. At the same time, this symptomatic therapy totally eliminated performance decrements (Beisel et al., 1974). Also, when the hypermetabolic effects of fever are minimized, losses of body nutrients are reduced, and skeletal muscle protein is preserved (Beisel, 1991).

Tumor Necrosis Factor

Like IL-1, TNF can be produced by many of the body's cells. However, TNF is produced in greatest amounts by macrophages, which are stimulated by endotoxin from gram-negative bacteria. TNF is less potent than IL-1 in initiating fever and may even have antipyretic effects, as shown in rats subjected to stress (Long et al., 1990). Unlike IL-1, TNF inhibits cellular lipoproteinase enzymes, allowing triglycerides to accumulate in plasma (Beisel, 1991). TNF helps mediate the development of hypotensive septic shock, and TNF can lead to the development of chronic cachexia (Moldawer and Lowry, 1992; Tracey, 1992).

Concentrations of solable TNF receptors in serum were found to correlate with both malarial counts and severity of disease in African patients (Kern et al., 1988).

Interleukin-6

IL-6, the third member of the acute-phase reaction triad, is mainly responsible for stimulating hepatic production of acute-phase proteins. IL-6 also has antiviral properties, stimulates T cells, and augments antibody secretion by plasma cells (Rothwell and Grimble, 1992).

Epinephrine administration in rats causes marked increases in IL-6 concentrations in plasma (van Gool et al., 1990). Although little is known about IL-6 values in subjects under stress, Kramer and colleagues (Moore et al., 1992) detected an initial increase in IL-6 concentrations in plasma during Ranger training (National Academy of Sciences, 1993); this was followed by a progressive decrease to only 35 percent of the baseline level; IL-6 concenstrations in supernatants of whole blood cultures also fell to 40–80 percent of baseline concentrations during all four phases of Ranger training.

Potential Importance of Stress Proteins

Bacteria subjected to high temperatures or other stresses have long been known to manufacture unique new heat shock proteins that provide survival value. However, stressed cells from higher species, including humans, produce a family of similar proteins now termed *stress proteins* (Lindquist, 1986).

Stress proteins from invading microorganisms are important immunologically because they can serve as antigens recognized by host T cells (Lamb and Young, 1990).

Stress proteins in humans have value in traumatized or glucose-starved cells because they can bind to damaged, partially unfolded, or denatured cellular proteins and assist in restoring them to their normal, prestress configuration. Stress proteins also help protect damaged cells from the free radicals generated by inflammatory reactions, and they protect cells against TNF and NK cells (Sugawara et al., 1990). Stress proteins also exist in healthy cells and may play a role in normal protein assembly (e.g., immunoglobulin heavy chain formation in lymphocytes).

The stress proteins formed in cells traumatized during the rigors of military training have potential importance in the hormonal and immunological responses to stress. Their presence in lymphocytes is stimulated by IL-2. Stress proteins can bind to and temporarily inactivate intracellular glucocorticoid receptors (Lamb and Young, 1990). Stress proteins and other cellular proteins released from damaged cells may also serve as antigens that can initiate harmful autoantibody reactions (Lamb and Young, 1990; Leclere and Weryha, 1989).

Military Aspects of the Acute-Phase Reaction

The major knowledge gap in considering endocrine and immune system responses to military stresses is a deficiency of specific data concerning the possible occurrence of acute-phase reactions in soldiers. This reaction occurs with major wounds or infections as generalized nonspecific host responses that help to activate the immune system.

On the other hand, acute-phase reactions contribute to (or cause) the malaise, myalgia, headaches, somnolence, losses of body weight and muscle mass, and decrements in physical and mental performance that accompany military stresses in soldiers who do not have major wounds or infections. Indirect evidence suggests the occurrence of acute-phase reactions.

Data are needed to confirm or reject the possibility that acute-phase reactions are frequent companions of severe military stress. The data that are needed include those that can be obtained from assays of acute-phase reaction components such as acute-phase reactant glycoproteins, triad cytokines (IL-1, IL-6, and TNF) and their receptors, phospholipase A_2, leukotrienes, and prostaglandins in plasma. The acute-phase glycoproteins include haptoglobin,

C-reactive protein, amyloid A, alpha-1 antitrypsin, ceruloplasmin, and alpha-1 acid globulin (orosomucoid).

Malnutrition and Immune System Dysfunctions

The immunological dysfunctions associated with malnutrition have been studied in some detail. Protein energy malnutrition (PEM) produces severe immunological problems. These include lymphoid tissue atrophy, depression of thymic hormone production, dysfunction of all aspects of cell-mediated immunity, and to a lesser extent, an impaired humoral response to new antigens (Beisel, 1991).

Individuals with cachexia caused by protracted semistarvation experience the disappearance of allergic and hypersensitivity reactions, and eosinophils are rarely found in their blood (Winick, 1979). The effects of other stresses on allergic illnesses, IgE values, eosinophils, basophils, mast cells, and histamine release have not been studied, however (Parker, 1991).

Many individual micronutrients are also important for proper immune system function, each in its own manner (Beisel, 1991). Important vitamins include A, beta carotene (as distinct from vitamin A), vitamin C, vitamin E, pyridoxine, folic acid, vitamin B_{12}, and to a lesser extent, the other B vitamin group members, vitamin D, and vitamin K. Important trace element deficiencies (or excesses) include those of zinc, iron, copper, and selenium (Beisel, 1982, 1991).

Immune system dysfunctions associated with severe PEM and/or single-nutrient malnutrition have been termed *nutritionally acquired immunodeficiency syndrome* (NAIDS); unlike AIDS, NAIDS is potentially curable (Beisel, 1991).

U.S. Ranger trainees experienced a significant decline in serum retinol and smaller declines in erythrocyte indicators for several of the B vitamins (Moore et al., 1992).

Nutritional Support for the Immune System

Attempts to improve immune system functions in cachectic patients have included supplementation of diets with vitamins, minerals, unsaturated fatty acids, single amino acids (especially arginine, glutamine, and alanine), precursors of nucleotides, purines (adenine and guanine), pyrimidines (uracil, cytosine, and thymine), and yeast RNA (Balch, 1990).

Supplementation of military diets with single (or combinations) of nutrients such as these could have immunological consequences. Too little information is available, however, to determine whether the immunological consequences would be helpful or harmful in healthy subjects subjected to severe military stresses.

For instance, polyunsaturated fatty acid supplements increase the fluidity of cell walls in lymphocytes, phagocytes, and other body cells (Kinsella et al., 1990); the omega-3 versus omega-6 composition of these fatty acid supplements helps determine the activities of the leukotrienes and protaglandins produced in response to cytokines (Rothwell and Grimble, 1992). Would such changes be helpful or harmful to the multiply stressed soldier?

On the other hand, infectious stress is known to accelerate the metabolic degradation or loss of body vitamins, but the administration of multivitamin supplement at the Recommended Dietary Allowance maintained virtually normal vitamin concentrations in the plasma of USAMRIID volunteers experiencing an experimental viral infection (Beisel et al., 1972).

HORMONAL AND IMMUNOLOGICAL INTERACTIONS DURING STRESS

Responses of both the immune and endocrine systems differ according to the nature of the stress, its intensity, and its duration (Korneva and Shkhineks, 1990; Landmann et al., 1984), with many interactions becoming apparent (Weigent et al., 1990).

Perhaps the most important response with regard to military personnel, is the complex interaction between cytokines and the central nervous system-pituitary-adrenal axis. IL-1, IL-2, and TNF can stimulate this axis to cause increased cortisol secretion, and at the same time, they activate the immune system. Cytokines and glucocorticoids stimulate gluconeogenesis. The cytokine-induced stimulation of new protein synthesis in hepatocytes requires the permissive presence of cortisol (Beisel, 1985).

Along with these synergistic relationships, however, are antagonistic ones. Cortisol blunts fever, inflammatory reactions, the formation of arachidonic acid, leukotrienes (LTs) and prostaglandins (PGs); and cortisol is immunosuppressive (Beisel, 1985).

Activated lymphocytes are capable of secreting small quantities of a number of hormones, including adrenocorticotropic hormone (ACTH), growth hormone (GH), somatostatin, vasoactive intestinal peptide (VIP), thyroid-stimulating hormone (TSH), prolactin (PRL), and many pain-reducing opioids. Lymphocytes also have cell surface receptors for ACTH, VIP, PRL, GH, catecholamines, and endorphins (Khansari et al., 1990). Releasing factors and cytokines of lymphocytic origin can increase the concentrations of many hormones in plasma and help to mediate pituitary-adrenal axis activation (Blalock, 1988).

Conversely, lymphocytes have receptors for many hormones, including ACTH, GH, PRL, VIP, steroids, opioids, catecholamines, and releasing factors and can be influenced by these hormones (Khansari et al., 1990). Thymic involution follows hypophysectomy in rats (Kelley, 1990).

Hormonal Effects on Immune System Functions

Corticotropin-releasing factor (CRF) mediates the decrease in natural killer (NK) cell activity caused by stress (Irwin et al., 1990; Jain et al., 1991). CRF also leads to a 75 percent reduction in T-cell mitogenesis in rats stressed by electric shocks; this reduction can be blunted by CRF antagonists or antibodies (Jain et al., 1991). The glucocorticoids suppress NK cell activity and reduce the amounts of cytokines and antibodies produced by lymphocytes (Khansari et al., 1990). These steroids also block the intracellular production of arachidonic acid following interleukin-1 (IL-1) stimulation (Claman, 1988).

Catecholamines suppress lymphocyte mitogenesis (Khansari et al., 1990), stimulate the production of IL-6 in rats (van Gool et al., 1990), and participate in immunoregulatory functions (Besedovsky et al., 1979).

GH enhances the activities of NK and T cells; aids in the production of antibodies, TNF, and thymulin; modulates the effects of IL-2; and enhances macrophage activation (Khansari et al., 1990). GH also helps prime macrophages for superoxide anion production (Edwards et al., 1988) and thus augments the actions of gamma interferon (Kelley, 1990).

PRL stimulates T-cell gene transcription and mitogenesis, T-cell-dependent macrophage tumoricidal activity, and the production of gamma interferon and IL-2 (Bernton et al., 1988; Khansari et al., 1990; Yu-Lee et al., 1990).

The neuropeptide VIP has numerous immunological functions. It influences the homing and recycling of lymphocytes, NK cell activity, and production of antibodies and cytokines. VIP also functions in hypersensitivity reactions by conveying signals from mast cells, basophils, and eosinophils to lymphocytes (Goetzl et al., 1990; Wenger et al., 1990). A 5- to 10-fold increase in high-affinity VIP receptors occurs during stress (Wiik, 1990).

The endorphin opioids enhance NK cell, T-cell, B-cell, and macrophage activities; lymphocyte mitogenesis; and antibody production (Bonneau et al., 1990; Khansari et al., 1990).

Gonadal hormones, ACTH, melatonin, somatostatin, thyroxine, vasopressin, and oxytocin are other hormones that have immunomodulatory properties (Khansari et al., 1990).

CONCLUSIONS

Stress initiates many interacting endocrine, immune system, and central nervous system (CNS) responses. Responses to stress vary widely, depending on the nature, severity, and duration of the stress. Excellent physical conditioning may minimize the magnitude of stress responses.

Endocrine responses to stress have been studied in some detail. Many hormonal changes during stress are components of the acute-phase reaction and tend to be relatively stereotyped.

Acute emotional and physical stresses may evoke immediate CNS-catecholamine responses. Physical and disease-related stresses are generally accompanied by activation of the CNS-pituitary-adrenal axis and increased levels of secretion of aldosterone, growth hormone, and sometimes, insulin and glucagon. In contrast, thyroid hormones, gonadatropins, and androgens show decreased outputs.

More information is needed about stress-induced changes in intestinal hormones and neuroendocrine hormones.

Impairments in both cell-mediated and humoral immunities have been noted during stress, but little is known about the effects of stress on allergic and hypersensitivity reactions. Additional data are needed to define changes in cell-mediated and humoral immunities and lymphocyte subsets (especially natural killer cells and CD4 and CD8 cells) during military stresses.

The major immune system response to stress is the activation of cells that release cytokines, including the triad of interleukins 1 and 6 and tumor necrosis factor, which combine to initiate acute-phase reactions. Military stresses that include strenuous and prolonged physical exercise, numerous cuts and bruises, dermal inflammations, and nagging minor infections are likely to trigger acute-phase reactions, but definitive laboratory data to document the occurrence of such reactions have not yet been obtained. This is an important knowledge gap.

Cytokine-induced acute-phase reactions during stress contribute to deterioration of cognitive and psychomotor performance. Additional studies are needed to determine whether the drugs that block the prostaglandin-releasing actions of the cytokines would prevent or minimize stress-induced (1) decrements of military performance, (2) catabolism of skeletal muscle protein, and (3) catabolic losses of essential micronutrients.

Immune system dysfunctions are caused by protein energy malnutrition and/or inadequacies of certain essential vitamins and minerals. Nutritional rehabilitation with vitamins, minerals, certain amino and fatty acids, and nucleotide precursors appears to hasten immune system recovery.

Similar supplements may have a role in military stresses that generate losses of body weight, muscle mass, and essential micronutrients. There is little to suggest, however, that nutritional supplementation of healthy individuals can induce a state of supernormal immunity. Rather, some nutrient excesses can suppress immunological functions.

Studies in animals are needed to evaluate the possible immunological importance of stress proteins in military-type stresses.

RECOMMENDATIONS

- First of all, do no harm.
- Gather additional data during military stress situations to document the possible occurrence of acute-phase reactions, cell-mediated immune system and humoral immune system dysfunctions, changes in lymphocyte subsets, changes in essential micronutrients, and changes in intestinal hormones and hormonal neurotransmitters.
- Conduct studies in animals to explore the possible role of stress proteins in military-type stresses.
- If warranted by additional data, protect the immune system during military stress with a daily multivitamin, multimineral preparation. This should include all vitamins in the amounts specified in the Recommended Dietary Allowance (RDAs)plus beta carotene; and the minerals iron, zinc, copper, and selenium, also in RDA amounts.
- If new data confirm the occurrence of acute-phase reactions during military stress, the value of drug prophylaxis with ibuprofen (or aspirin) should be tested in an attempt to reduce decrements in performance and the loss of body weight and skeletal muscle mass. The doses of these drugs should be sufficient to minimize the prostaglandin-related effects of acute-phase reactions without masking the symptoms of major infections.
- Carefully consider the possible adverse immunological consequences of any nutritional supplement given to enhance military performance.
- Remember that the value of nutritional supplements or pharmaceutical agents in preventing performance decrements may equal or exceed their potential value as performance enhancers.

REFERENCES

Aakvaag, A., T.Sand, P.K.Opstad, and F.Fonnum 1978 Hormonal changes in serum in young men during prolonged physical strain. Eur. J. Appl. Physiol. 39:283–291.

Alluisi, E.A., W.R.Beisel, P.J.Bartelloni, and G.D.Coates 1973 Behavioral effects of tularemia and sandfly fever in man. J. Infect. Dis. 128:710–717.

Armstrong, L.E., R.P.Francesconi, W.J.Kraemer, N.Leva, J.P.Deluca, and R.W.Hubbard 1989 Plasma cortisol, renin, and aldosterone during an intense heat acclimation program. J. Sports Med. 10:38–42.

Audhya, T., D.Zwickler, B.Hutchinson, C.Brown, and C.S.Hollander 1988 Stress-inducing changes in corticotropin-releasing factor (CRF) in immune tissues and hypothalamus: Studies toward defining a role for CRF in neuroimmunomodulation. Trans. Assoc. Am. Physicians 101:62–69.

Balch, F.H. 1990 Symposium proceedings: Update on immunonutrition. Nutrition 6:1–106.

Beeson, P.B. 1948 Temperature elevating effects of a substance obtained from polymorphonuclear leukocytes. J. Clin. Invest. 27:548.

Beisel, W.R. 1982 Single nutrients and immunity. Am. J. Clin. Nutr. 35(Feb. Suppl.):417–68.

1985 Evolving concepts of the roles of interleukin-1 (IL-1) and cortisol in stress: Similarities and differences. Pp. 3–12 in The Physiologic, Metabolic, and Immunologic Actions of Interleukin-1, M.J.Kluger, J.J.Oppenheim, and M.C.Powanda, eds. New York: Alan R.Liss, Inc.

1991 Nutrition and infection. Pp. 507–542 in Nutritional Biochemistry and Metabolism, 2nd ed., M.C.Linder, ed. New York: Elsevier.

Beisel, W.R., J.Bruton, K.D.Anderson, and W.D.Sawyer 1967 Adrenocortical responses during tularemia in human subjects. J. Clin. Endocrinol. Metab. 27:61–69.

Beisel, W.R., and M.I.Rapoport 1969 Interrelations between adrenocortical functions and infections illnesses. N. Engl. J. Med. 280:541–546, 594–604.

Beisel, W.R., R.F.Goldman, and R.J.T.Joy 1968 Metabolic balance studies during induced hyperthermia in man. J. Appl. Physiol. 24:1–10.

Beisel, W.R., B.B.Morgan, Jr., P.J.Bartelloni, G.D.Coates, F.R.DeRubertis, and E.A.Alluisi 1974 Symptomatic therapy in viral illness. A controlled study of effects on work performance. J. Am. Med. Assoc. 228:581–587.

Beisel, W.R., Y.F.Herman, H.E.Sauberlich, R.H.Herman, P.J.Bartelloni, and J.E.Canham 1972 Experimentally induced sandfly fever and vitamin metabolism in man. Am. J. Clin. Nutr. 25:1165–1173.

Bernton, E.W. 1992 Immunological aspects of the Walter Reed Army Institute of Research Study of Class 11–91. Unpublished paper presented at a Meeting of the Food and Nutrition Board Committee on Military Nutrition Research, Review of a Nutritional Assessment of Ranger Training Class 11–91, National Academy of Sciences, February 5, 1992 , Washington, D.C.

Bernton, E.W., M.S.Meltzer, and J.W.Holaday 1988 Suppression of macrophage activation and T-lymphocyte function in hypoprolactinemic mice. Science 239:401–403.

Besedovsky, H.O., A.del Rey, E.Sorkin, M.DaPrada, and H.H.Keller 1979 Immunoregulation mediated by the sympathetic nervous system. Cell. Immunol. 48:346–355.

Bianchi, M., P.Sacerdote, L.Locatelli, P.Mantegazza, and A.E.Panerai 1991 Corticotropin releasing hormone, interleukin-1, and tumor necorsis factor share characteristics of stress mediators. Brain Res. 546:139–142.

Blalock, E.J. 1988 Immunologically-mediated pituitary-adrenal activation. Adv. Exp. Med. Biol. 2–45:217–223.

Bomberger, C.L., and J.L.Haar 1988 Effect of sound stress on the migration of prethymic stem cells. Ann. N.Y. Acad. Sci. 540:700–701.

Bonneau, R.H., J.K.Kiecolt-Glaser, and R.Glaser 1990 Stress-induced modulation of the immune response. Ann. N.Y. Acad. Sci. 594:253–269.

Brohee, D., M.Vanhaeverbeek, B.Kennes, and P.Neve 1990 Leukocyte and lymphocyte subsets after a short pharmacological stress by intravenous epinephrine and hydrocortisone in healthy humans. Int. J. Neurosci. 53:53–62.

Chakraborti, S. 1989 Adrenocortical activity and plasma camp levels of humans under high altitude stress. Clin. Chim. Acta 184:329–332.

Chrousos, G.P., and P.W.Gold 1992 The concepts of stress and stress system disorders. Overview of physical and behavioral homeostasis. J. Am. Med. Assoc. 267:1244–1252.

Chrousos, G.P., D.L.Loraiux, and P.W.Gold 1988 Mechanisms of physical and emotional stress. Adv. Exp. Med. Biol. 245:1–530.

Claman, H.N. 1988 Corticosteroids and the immune response. Adv. Exp. Med. Biol. 245:203–208.

Dantzer, R., and K.W.Kelley 1989 Stress and immunity: An integrated view of relationships between the brain and the immune system. Life Sci. 44:1995–2008.

Dieguez, C., M.D.Page, and M.F.Scanlon 1988 Growth hormone neuroregulation and its alterations in disease states. Clin. Endocrinol. 28:109–143.

Dindar, A., H.Gunoz, and O.Neyzi 1990 ß-Endorphin levels of children in acute stress. Diabetes Res. Clin. Pract. 9:245–249.

Edwards, III, C.K., S.M.Ghiasuddin, J.M.Schepper, L.M.Unger, and K.W.Kelly 1988 A newly defined property of somatotropin: Priming of macrophages for production of superoxide anion. Science 239:769–770.

Feldman, C., B.Joffe, V.P.Panz, H.Levy, L.Walker, J.M.Kallenbach, and H.C.Stefel 1989 Initial hormonal and metabolic profile in critically ill patients with community-acquired lobar pneumonia. S. Afr. Med. J. 76:593–596.

Flores, C.M., M.C.Hernandez, K.M.Hargreaves, and B.M.Bayer 1990 Restraint stress-induced elevations in plasma corticosterone and ß-endorphin are not accompanied by alterations in immune functions. J. Neuroimmunol. 28:219–225.

Geelhoed, G.W. 1987 Endocrine emergencies in critical illness. Pp. 773–800 in Trauma: Emergency Surgery and Critical Care, J.H.Siegl, ed. New York: Churchill Livingstone.

Goetzl, E.J., T.Grotmol, R.W.Van Dyke, C.W.Turck, B.Wershil, S.J.Galli, and S.P. Sreedharan 1990 Generation and recognition of vasoactive intestinal peptide by cells of the immune system. Ann. N.Y. Acad. Sci. 594:34–44.

Hesse, V., C.Vilser, J.Scheibe, G.Jahreis, and T.Foley 1989 Thyroid hormone metabolism under extreme body exercises. Exp. Clin. Endocrinol. 94:82–88.

Hibbs, Jr., J.B., C.Westenfelder, R.Taintor, Z.Vavrin, C.Kabliz, R.L.Baranowski, J.H.Ward, R.L.Menlove, M.P.McMurry, J.P.Kushner, and W.E.Samlowski 1992 Evidence for cytokine-inducible nitric oxide synthesis from L-arginine in patients receiving interleukin-2 therapy. J. Clin. Invest. 89:867–877.

Hoffman-Goetz, L., R.J.Thorne, and M.E.Houston 1988 Splenic immune responses following treadmill exercise in mice. Can. J. Physiol. Pharmacol. 66:1415–419.

Irwin, M., W.Vale, and C.Rivier 1990 Central corticotropin-releasing factor mediates the suppressive effect of stress on natural killer cytotoxicity. Endocrinology 126:2837–2844.

Jain, R., D.Zwickler, C.S.Hollander, H.Brand, A.Saperstein, B.Hutchinson, B.Brown, and T.Audhya 1991 Corticotropin-releasing factor modulates the immune response to stress in the rat. Endocrinology 128:1329–1336.

Jannace, P.W., R.H.Lerman, J.I.Santos, and J.J.Vitale 1992 Effects of oral soy phosphatidylcholine on phagocytosis, arachidonate concentrations, and killing by human polymorphonuclear leukocytes. Am. J. Clin. Nutr. 56:599–603.

Jeevanandam, M., M.R.Ali, N.J.Holaday, and J.K.Weis 1993 Relative nutritional efficacy of arginine and ornithine salts of alpha-ketoisocaproic acid in traumatized rats. Am. J. Clin. Nutr. 57:889–896.

Kandil, O., and M.Borysenko 1988 Stress-induced decline in immune responsiveness in C3H/HeJ mice: Relation to endocrine alterations and tumor growth. Brain Behavior Immun. 2:32–49.

Kant, G.J., J.R.Leu, S.M.Anderson, and E.H.Mougey 1887 Effects of chronic stress of plasma corticosterone, ACTH, and prolactin. Physiol. Behavior 40:775–779.

Kelley, K.W. 1990 The role of growth hormone in modulation of the immune response. Ann. N.Y. Acad. Sci. 594:95–103.

Kern, P., C.J.Hemmer, H.Gallati, S.Neifer, P.Kremsner, M.Dietrich, and F.Porzsolt 1992 Soluble tumor necrosis factor receptors correlate with parasitemia and disease severity in human malaria. J. Infect. Dis. 166:930–934.

Khan, N.A., and V.Karla 1988 Urinary 5HIAA and VMA and their relationship with immunoregulatory cells in stress administered subjects. Arch. Immunol. Ther. Exp. 36:717–721.

Khansari, D.N., A.J.Murgo, and R.E.Faith 1990 Effects of stress on the immune system. Immunol. Today 11:170–175.

Kilbourn, R.G., and P.Belloni 1990 Endothelial cell production of nitrogen oxide in response to interferon gamma in combination with tumor necrosis factor, IL-1, or endotoxin. J. Natl. Cancer Inst. 82:772–776.

Kinsella, J.E., B.Lokesh, S.Broughton, and J.Whelan 1990 Dietary polyunsaturated fatty acids and eicosanoids: Potential effects on the modulation of inflammatory and immune cells: An overview. Nutrition 6:24–44.

Kirk, S.J., and A.Barbul 1992 Arginine and Immunity. Pp. 160–161 in Encyclopedia of Immunology, I.M.Roitt and P.J.Delves, eds. London: Academic Press.

Koob, G.F., K.Thatcher-Briton, A.Tazi, and M.LeMoal 1988 Behavioral pharmacology of stress: Focus on CNS corticotropin-releasing factor. Adv. Exp. Med. Biol. 245:25–34.

Kopin, I.J., G.Eisenhofer, and D.Goldstein 1988 Sympathoadrenal medullary system and stress. Adv. Exp. Med. Biol. 245:11–23.

Korneva, E.A., and E.K.Shkhinek 1990 Neuroendocrine mechanisms underlying stress-induced changes in immune reactions. Int. J. Neurosci. 51:225–226.

Lamb, J.R., and D.B.Young 1990 T cell recognition of stress proteins. A link between infectious and autoimmune disease. Mol. Biol. Med., 7:311–321.

Landmann, R.M.A., F.B.Muller, C.H.Perini, M.Wesp, P.Erne, and F.R.Buhler 1984 Changes of immunoregulatory cells induced by psychological and physical stress: Relationship to plasma catecholamines. Clin. Exp. Immunol. 58:127–135.

Larson, G.L., and P.M.Henson 1983 Mediators of inflammation. Annu. Rev. Immunol. 1:335–359.

Laudenslager, M.L., M.Fleshner, P.Hofstadter, P.E.Held, L.Simons, and S.F.Maier 1988 Suppression of specific antibody production by inescapable shock: Stability under varying conditions. Brain Behavior Immun. 2:92–101.

Leclere, J., and G.Weryha 1989 Stress and auto-immune endocrine diseases. Horm. Res. 31:90–93.

Lenz, H.J. 1990 Mediation of gastrointestinal stress responses by corticotropin-releasing factor. Ann. N.Y. Acad. Sci. 597:81–91.

Lindquist, S. 1986 The heat-shock response. Annu. Rev. Biochem. 55:1151–1191.

Long, N.C., A.J.Vander, S.L.Kunkel, and M.J.Kluger 1990 Antiserum against tumor necrosis factor increases stress hyperthermia in rats. Am. J. Physiol. 258:R591-R595.

McEwen, B.S., R.E.Brinton, and R.M.Sapolsky 1988 Glucocorticoid receptors and behavior: Implications for the stress response. Adv. Exp. Med. Biol. 245:35–45.

Moldawer, L.L., and S.F.Lowry 1992 Interactions between cytokine production and inflammation: Implications for therapies modulating the host defense to infection. Pp. 511–523 in Nutrient Modulation of the Immune Response, S.Cunningham-Rundles, ed., New York: Marcel Deckker, Inc.

Moore, R.J., K.E.Friedl, T.R.Kramer, L.E.Martinez-Lopez, R.W.Hoyt, R.T.Tulley, J.P. Delany, E.W.Askew and J.A.Vogel

1992 Technical Report 13–92, U.S. Army Research Institute of Environmental Medicine, Natick, Mass.

Mulley, G.P., R.C.Wilcox, and M.J.G.Harrison 1989 Plasma cortisol as a measure of stress response in acute stroke. Stroke 20:1593.

Murison, R., and H.K.Badde 1990 The role of corticotropin-releasing factor in rat gastric ulcerogenesis. Ann. N.Y. Acad. Sci. 597:71–80.

Nakamura, K., A.Aoike, T.Hosokaws, K.Rokutan, K.Koyana, Y.Nishi, A.Yoshida, and D.Kawai 1990 Effect of food-restriction stress on immune response in mice. J. Neuroimmunol. 30:23–29.

National Academy of Sciences 1992 A Nutritional Assessment of U.S. Ranger Training Class 11–91. A Brief Report of the Committee on Military Nutrition Research. B.M.Marriott, ed. Washington, D.C.: National Academy Press.

1993 Review of the Results of Nutritional Intervention, Ranger Training Class 11–92 (Ranger II). A Brief Report of the Committee on Military Nutrition Research. B.M.Marriott, ed. Washington, D.C.: National Academy Press.

Nirgiotis, J.G., P.J.Hennessey, and R.J.Andrassy 1991 The effects of an arginine-free enteral diet on wound healing and immune function in the post-surgical rat. J. Pediat Surg. 26:936–941.

Niwano, Y., B.A.Becker, R.Mitra, C.W.Caldwell, E.B.Abdalla, and H.D.Johnson 1990 Suppressed peripheral lymphocyte blastogenesis in pre- and postpartal sheep by chronic heat-stress, and suppressive property of heat-stressed sheep serum on lymphocytes. Dev. Comp. Immunol. 14:139–149.

Nussey, S.S., S.R.Page, V.T.Y.Ang, and J.S.Jenkins 1988 The response of plasma oxytocin to surgical stress. Clin. Endocrinol. 28:277–282.

Øektedalen, O., P.K.Opstad, and O.B.Schaffalitzky de Muckadell 1982 Secretin—a new stress hormone? Regulatory Peptides 4:213–219.

Øektedalen, O., P.K.Opstad, and O.B.Schaffalitzky de Mukadell 1983a The plasma concentrations of secretin and vasoactive intestinal polypeptide (VIP) after long-term strenuous exercise. Eur. J. Appl. Physiol. 52:5–8.

Øektedalen, O., P.K.Opstad, O.B.Schaffalitzky de Mukadell, O.Fausa, and O.Flaten 1983b Basal hyperchlorhydria and its relation to the plasma concentrations of secretin, vasoactive intestinal polypeptide (VIP) and gastrin during prolonged strain. Regulatory Peptides 5:235–244.

Øektedalen, O., P.K.Opstad, H.Waldum, and R.Jorde 1983c The fasting levels and the post-prandial response of gastroenteropancreatic hormones before and after prolonged fasting. Scand. J. Gastroenterol. 18:555–560.

O'Neill, P.A., I.Davies, K.J.Fullerton, and D.Bennett 1991 Stress hormone and blood glucose response following acute stress in the elderly. Stroke 22:842–847.

Opstad, P.K. 1991 Alterations in the morning plasma levels of hormones and the endocrine responses to bicycle exercise during prolonged strain. The significance of energy and sleep deprivation. Acta Endocrinol. (Copenhagen) 125:14–22.

1992 Androgenic hormones during prolonged physical stress, sleep, and energy deprivation. J. Clin. Endocrinol. 74:1176–1183.

Opstad, P.K., and A.Aakvaag 1981 The effect of a high calorie diet on hormonal changes in young men during prolonged physical strain and sleep deprivation. Eur. J. Appl. Physiol. 46:31–39.

1982 Decreased serum levels of oestradiol, testosterone, and prolactin during prolonged physical strain and sleep deprivation, and the influence of a high calorie diet. Eur. J. Appl. Physiol. 49:343–348.

1983 The effect of sleep deprivation on the plasma levels of hormones during prolonged physical strain and calorie deficiency. Eur. J. Appl. Physiol. 51:97–107.

Opstad, P.K., A.Aakvaag, and T.O.Rognum 1980 Altered hormonal response to short-term bicycle exercise in young men after prolonged physical strain, caloric deficit, and sleep deprivation. Eur. J. Appl. Physiol. 45:51–62.

Opstad, P.K., D.Falch, O.Øktedalen, F.Fonnum, and R.Wergeland 1984 The thyroid function in young men during prolonged exercise and the effect of energy and sleep deprivation. Clin. Endocrinol. 20:657–669.

Opstad, P.K., O.Øktedalen, A.Aarvaag, F.Fonnum, and P.K.Lund 1985 Plasma renin activity and serum aldosterone during prolonged physical strain. Eur. J. Appl. Physiol. 54:1–6.

Parker, C.W. 1991 Environmental stress and immunity: Possible implications for IgE-mediated allergy. Perspect. Biol. Med., 34:197–212.

Parker, L.N., E.R.Levin, and E.T.Lifrak 1985 Evidence for adrenocortical adaptation to severe illness. J. Clin. Endocrinol. Metab. 60:947–952.

Pekarek, R.S., and W.R.Beisel 1971 Characterization of the endogenous mediator(s) of serum zinc and iron depression during infection and other stresses. Proc. Soc. Exp. Biol. Med. 138:728–732.

Plotsky, P.M. 1988 Hypophysiotropic regulation of stress-induced ACTH secretion. Adv. Exp. Med. Biol. 245:65–81.

Pollock, R.E., E.Lotzova, and S.D.Stanford 1989 Surgical stress impairment of murine natural killer cell cytotoxicity involves pre- and postbinding events. J. Immunol. 143:3396–3403.

Roilides, E., and P.A.Pizzo 1992 Modulation of host defenses by cytokines: Evolving adjuncts in prevention and treatment of serious infection in immunocompromised hosts. Clin. Infect. Dis. 15:508–524.

Rothwell, N.J., and R.F.Grimble 1992 Metabolic and nutritional effects of TNF. Pp. 237–253 in Tumor Necrosis Factors: The Molecules and Their Emerging Role in Medicine, B.Beutler, ed. New York: Raven Press.

Rougeot, C, M.P.Junier, J.Weidenfeld, P.Praquet, and F.Dray 1990 Intracerebroventricular injection of platelet-activating factor induces secretion of adrenocorticotropin, beta-endorphin and corticosterone in conscious rats: A possible link between the immune and nervous systems. Neuroendocrinology 51:267–275.

Scarborough, D.E. 1990 Cytokine modulation of pituitary hormone secretion. Ann. N.Y. Acad. Sci. 594:169–187.

Schneemann M., G.Schoedon, S.Hofer, N.Blau, L.Guerrero, and A.Schaffner 1993 Nitric oxide synthase is not a constituent of the antimicrobial armature of human mononuclear phagocytes. J. Infect. Dis. 167:1358–1363.

Schlesinger, M., and Y.Yodfat 1988 Effect of psychosocial stress on natural killer cell activity. Cancer Detect. Prevent. 12:9–14.

Snyder, B.K., K.J.Roghmann, and L.H.Sigal 1990 Effect of stress and other biopsychosocial factors on primary antibody response. J. Adolesc. Health Care. 11:472–479.

Sugawara, S., M.Nowicki, S.Zie, H.J.Song, and G.Dennert 1990 Effects of stress on lysability of tumor targets by cytotoxic T cells and tumor necrosis factor. J. Immunol. 145:1991–1998.

Taylor, C.E., and L.L.Ross 1991 Alteration of antibody response to pneumococcal polysaccharide type III in rats by neonatal immobilization stress. Brain Behav. Immunol. 3:160–170.

Teschemacher, H., G.Koch, H.Scheffler, A.Hildebrand, and V.Brantl 1990 Opioid peptides immunological significance? Ann. N.Y. Acad. Sci. 594:66–88.

Tharp, G.D., and T.L.Pruess 1991 Mitogenic response of T-lymphocytes to exercise and stress. J. Appl. Physiol. 70:2535–2538.

Torres-Aleman, I., I.Barasoain, J.Borrell, and C.Guaza 1988 Immune activation and psychoneurogenic stress modulate corticosterone-releasing effects of lymphokines and ACTH. Am. J. Physiol. 255:R839-R845.

Tracey, K.J. 1992 The acute and chronic pathophysiologic effects of TNF: Mediation of septic shock and wasting (cachexia). Pp. 255–273 in Tumor Necrosis Factors: The Molecules and Their Emerging Role in Medicine, B.Beutler, ed. New York: Raven Press.

Vadas, P. 1984 Plasma phospholipase A2 levels correlate with the hemodynamic and pulmonary changes in Gram negative septic shock in man. J. Lab. Clin. Med. 104:873–881.

Valentino, R.J. 1988 CRH effects on central noradrenergic neurons: Relationship to stress. Adv. Exp. Med. Biol. 245:47–64.

van Gool, J., H.van Vugt, M.Helle, and L.A.Aarden 1990 The relation among stress, adrenalin, interleukin 6 and acute-phase proteins in the rat. Clin. Immunol. Immunopathol. 57:200–210.

Vescovi, P.P., G.Gerra, G.Pioli, M.Medrazzoni, L.Manninette, and M.Passeri 1990 Circulating opioid peptides during thermal stress. Horm. Metab. Res. 22:44–46.

Wagner, D.A., and S.R.Tannenbaum 1982 Enhancement of nitrate biosynthesis by *Escherichia coli* lipopolysaccharide. Pp. 437–441 in Nitrosamines and Human Cancer, P.N.MaGee, ed. Cold Spring Harbor, N.Y.: Cold Spring Harbor Laboratory.

Weigent, D.A., D.J.J.Caar, and J.E.Blalock 1990 Bidirectional communication between the neuroendocrine and immune systems. Ann. N.Y. Acad. Sci. 579:17–27.

Weisse, C.S., C.N.Pato, C.G.McAlister, R.Littman, A.Brier, S.M.Paul, and A.Baum 1990 Differential effects of controllable and uncontrollable acute stress on lymphocyte proliferation and leukocyte percentages in humans. Brain Behavior Immunol. 4:339–351.

Wenger, G.D., M.S.O'Dorisio, and E.J.Goetzl 1990 Vasoactive intestinal peptide. Messenger in a neuroimmune axis. Ann. N.Y. Acad. Sci. 594:140–119.

Wiik, P. 1990 VIP inhibition of monocyte respiratory burst ex vivo during prolonged strain and energy deficiency. Int. J. Neurosci. 51:195–196.

Winick, M., ed. 1979 Hunger Disease. Studies by the Jewish Physicians in the Warsaw Ghetto. New York: John Wiley & Sons.

Yu-Lee, L.-Y., A.M.Stevens, J.A.Hrachovy, and L.A.Schwarz 1990 Prolactin-mediated regulation of gene transcription in lymphocytes. Ann. N.Y. Acad. Sci. 594:146–155.

Zoller, M., U.Heumann, M.Betzler, H.Stimmel, and S.Matzka 1989 Depression of nonadaptive immunity after surgical stress: Influence on metastatic spread. Invasion Metastasis 9:46–68.

11

The Metabolic Responses to Stress and Physical Activity

Edward S.Horton[1] and William R.Beisel[2]

INTRODUCTION

Metabolic responses to stress and physical activity are extremely complex, involving many interacting variables. These multiple factors include endocrinological, physiological (cardiovascular and neuromuscular), biochemical, nutritional, and central nervous system (CNS) components, at a minimum. This chapter will attempt to focus upon several of these interacting factors (i.e., nutrient substrates, endocrine/CNS controls, and physiologic responses during exercise) that seem most important and that also have the support of reliable current data.

[1] Edward S.Horton, Joslin Diabetes Center, Boston, MA 02215

[2] William R.Beisel, Johns Hopkins School of Hygiene and Public Health, Baltimore, MD 21205

UNDERLYING CONCEPTS

Initially, some basic concepts must be made clear. First, there are many different kinds of stress to consider: physical exercise, sleep deprivation, psychological stress, environmental stresses (e.g., heat, cold, high altitude, depth, etc.), trauma, and infection, to name a few. In animal models, there are also standardized stresses, such as immobilization or electrical shock.

Second, the human body responses to the military stresses under discussion are obviously very complex and as noted earlier, involve many systems throughout the body. Despite differences in the kinds of stress, body responses may have some broad or generalized commonalities, or in other situations, body responses to a given form of stress may be very specific. For example, acute-phase responses associated with various infections or trauma are rather stereotyped, whereas metabolic responses to exercise may be far less specific.

Third, it must be remembered that these adaptations by the body to the military stresses under discussion, both acute and chronic, are really designed to help in survival. Yet, some of these adaptations may, at times, actually become deleterious.

Thus, researchers must separate out the positive and the negative responses, and in the words of an old song, "Accentuate the Positive, Eliminate the Negative." Researchers must identify the adaptations that are beneficial to the organism and attempt to determine how they can be enhanced, but at the same time, no harm must be done, as noted earlier (see Chapter 10). Certainly a recommended nutritional "enhancement" should not interfere with potentially beneficial aspects of the stress response.

THE FOCUS ON FUEL METABOLISM

Because of the complexities of the metabolic responses to military stresses, researchers must focus on the most important response factors that they are trying to enhance. When evaluating stress situations in a military environment, the goal is to enhance the chances for survival of soldiers. For survival, soldiers must be able to think and to act—sometimes quite strenuously. Errors in thinking have occurred because of sleep deprivation, and maintaining physical performance has been a problem under the circumstances of military stress.

A focus on body fuel metabolism is important, because humans must have fuel available for both the CNS (primarily glucose) and for skeletal muscle (a mixture of glucose and fatty acids) in order to do two things: to think properly and then to act physically on the decisions made.

Metabolic Fuel Homeostasis During Physical Exercise

The metabolic fuel homeostasis that occurs during physical exercise, a militarily important form of stress, involves multiple levels of integration. These multiple levels of metabolic integration will be reviewed in this chapter and compared with experimental models of stress, for (or because) there are many similarities between physical exercise in human subjects and CNS models of stress in laboratory animals. Such animal models may reveal strategies that might help to "accentuate the positive." John Ivy's discussion of ergogenic aids (see Chapter 12) provides some of the possible strategies.

Fuel Homeostasis Under Baseline Conditions

In the normal, nonstressed individual, after an overnight fast and in the resting state, about two-thirds to three-quarters of glucose uptake from blood occurs in non-insulin-dependent pathways. As much as 50 percent is taken up by the brain and CNS in general, and about 15–25 percent by blood cells and kidneys. Only about one-fourth to one-third of glucose uptake goes to insulin-dependent pathways, with about 15–20 percent going into skeletal muscle.

At rest, skeletal muscle derives about 85 percent of its energy from fatty acid oxidation, only about 10 percent from glucose oxidation, and maybe 1–2 percent from oxidation of branched chain amino acids.

The blood glucose concentration stays very constant in these circumstances, because glucose is being taken up by all of these tissues, and at the same time an equivalent amount is being produced, primarily by the liver. Hepatic glycogenolysis accounts for most (about 75 percent) of liver glucose production, with only about 25 percent coming from gluconeogenesis.

At the same time, lipolysis in fat cells is releasing free fatty acids and glycerol. Lipolysis provides free fatty acids for direct oxidation in muscle, liver, and other tissues. Meanwhile, pyruvate, lactate, and amino acids are being released from the intestine and muscle. All of these nutrients provide substrates that feed gluconeogenic pathways in the liver.

Fuel Homeostasis During Exercise

With the onset of exercise, dramatic changes occur in the body because of the rapid increase in energy demands. Initially, rapidly increases, sympathetic CNS activity (Shimazu, 1992), which stimulates glycogenolysis within the muscle itself. As an immediate result, there is a breakdown of muscle glycogen stores, with the production of glucose for anaerobic glycolysis and then, ultimately, for oxidative metabolism in muscle.

At the same time, there is also an activation of lipolysis and a release of free fatty acids and glycerol in and around muscle tissue as well as in adipose tissue. Initially the breakdown of muscle glycogen is more important. In these early moments, before oxidative metabolism begins, lactate may actually be released from muscle, and sometimes a little glucose is also released.

Soon after the onset of exercise, blood flow to the muscle is increased. This allows more substrates to be delivered to muscle. Glucose transport mechanisms in the cell wall are activated also, allowing for an increased uptake of glucose by muscle (Goodyear et al., 1992). However, the blood glucose concentration is maintained at quite a constant level during exercise by a very tightly matched production of glucose by the liver.

Levels of Metabolic Integration During Exercise

The dramatic changes in fuel supply and utilization during exercise are under a very tightly regulated control system that operates at least at five different levels. As previously noted, activation of the sympathetic nervous system is the initial, first-level, response to the onset of exercise (Shimazu, 1992). The very rapid stimulation of sympathetic outflow is measurable by the increase in circulating norepinephrine, and its spillover from the nerve terminals. There is also an activation of a whole cascade of counterregulatory hormone responses over time during exercise, with increases epinephrine, glucagon, cortisol, and growth hormone (Shimazu, 1992). The pattern of hormone responses constitutes the second level of integration. Interactions among insulin, glucagon, and the catecholamines are of major importance in substrate mobilization during exercise.

A third level of integration is the availability of substrates, particularly free fatty acids, lactate, pyruvate, glycerol for gluconeogenesis, and glucose itself. The fourth level of integration is the regulation of blood flow, which controls the delivery rate of substrates to exercising muscle. Fifth, there are local cellular factors that regulate glucose uptake and its intracellular metabolism.

FACTORS THAT INFLUENCE FUEL UTILIZATION DURING EXERCISE

A number of factors influence the pattern of fuel utilization during exercise. These include the intensity of exercise; the duration of exercise; and the effects of prior physical conditioning, of prior dietary intake, and of the existing hormonal milieu.

The first highly important factor is the intensity of exercise. As noted earlier, an oxidation primarily of free fatty acids for energy (with only about 10 percent coming from glucose oxidation) typifies the resting state in skeletal muscle. Exercising at about half the maximum aerobic capacity (i.e., 50 percent of $\dot{V}_{O_2\ max}$) requires a 50/50 mixture of glucose and free fatty acids, with amino acid oxidation still supplying only 1–2 percent of the energy.

When exercise intensity increases to higher levels, that is 75 percent of $\dot{V}_{O_2\ max}$ or greater, muscles become progressively more dependent on glucose oxidation rather than on fatty acid oxidation.

The duration of exercise also influences the metabolic fuel mixture. The uptake of glucose from blood increases progressively during exercise, peaking after 60–90 min. Then, as exercise persists, free fatty acid concentrations in blood increase, and the muscle gradually shifts over to burning more fatty acids and less glucose.

The effects of physical training tend to cause a more effective adaptation of skeletal muscle, allowing them to oxidize fatty acids more effectively, and thus to spare both muscle and liver glycogen.

The antecedent diet can influence this fuel mixture rather acutely, as can changes in the hormonal milieu, particularly the concentrations of insulin, glucagon, or the catecholamines.

BICYCLE ERGOMETER STUDIES

Classical data produced by John Wahren and his group in Stockholm (Wahren et al., 1971) demonstrated the increase in glucose uptake by leg muscles when exercising on a cycle ergometer. Coincident with an increase in oxygen uptake at the onset of exercise was a striking increase in muscle glucose uptake. Glucose uptake was then heightened by increases in the intensity of exercise due to the combination of increased blood flow to the legs and to activation of glucose transport in muscle cells.

This adaptation takes some time to be fully present. The increase in glucose uptake continues for at least 40 min. at moderate intensity exercise, that is about 50 percent of $\dot{V}_{O_2\ max}$. This observation would suggest an increasing extraction of glucose by the muscles over that period of time. With an increasing duration of exercise, glucose uptake by muscle begins to decline, and there is an increased dependency on free fatty acids for energy metabolism. Free fatty acid uptake becomes progressively greater, so that after 3–4 h of moderate exercise, free fatty acids are the predominant fuel being utilized.

A key to this adaptation is that the liver increases hepatic glucose output to match exactly the peripheral needs, with few exceptions. After 40 min of exercise, the increase in hepatic glucose production is almost entirely due to an increase in glycogenolysis. However, with increasing duration of exercise as hepatic glycogen stores begin to fall, glycogenolysis becomes less significant and gluconeogenesis increases, becoming an important part of hepatic glucose production.

There are two circumstances where blood glucose concentrations are not maintained within a very narrow range. These situations are during brief, high-intensity exercise and during very prolonged, exhaustive, marathon-type endurance exercise.

During an 8–12 min maximum stress test, blood glucose values of a cyclist will overshoot baseline values for a brief time. This is the result of intense sympathetic nervous system stimulation, with an activation of hepatic glucose production that transiently exceeds peripheral glucose utilization.

During prolonged, exhaustive exercise, the liver is simply not able to keep up with the glucose demands. When glycogen stores become depleted in both muscle and liver, the marathon runner must slow down, become hypoglycemic, or ingest glucose.

ENDOCRINE INTERACTIONS

Sympathetic nervous system activation, which stimulates glycogenolysis within muscle and lipolysis within fatty tissues, is the initial endocrine response to exercise stress. This response is accompanied by an activation of both the adrenocortical axis and the adrenomedullary axis, with rises in both plasma cortisol and epinephrine values. Epinephrine, in turn, stimulates an increase in glucagon secretion and a suppression of insulin secretion.

With exercise above 50 percent of $\dot{V}_{O_2\,max}$ both norepinephrine and epinephrine concentrations in plasma rise quite linearly in proportion to the intensity of exercise. Epinephrine, as a counterregulatory hormone, also responds to low blood glucose concentrations. Both of these catecholamines stimulate lipolysis, but epinephrine is also a major factor in mobilizing hepatic glucose production.

Plasma insulin concentrations actually fall during exercise, due to stimulation of alpha adrenergic receptors that suppress insulin secretion. When exercise stops, there is a rebound release of insulin and then a gradual return to baseline values.

Glucagon responds more slowly as a function of both the intensity and duration of exercise. Rising catecholamine values are believed to stimulate glucagon release. Glucagon is the primary hormone responsible for stimulating hepatic glucose output, although catecholamines from plasma and/or from direct sympathetic innervation of the liver may also contribute.

As noted, glucagon stimulates hepatic glucose production, while insulin suppresses it. The declining insulin glucagon ratio during exercise is a contributing factor in stimulating hepatic glucose output. On the other hand, the insulin norepinephrine ratio is the key regulator of the lipolytic response, with a decline in the ratio-stimulating lipolysis, as seen during exercise.

INFORMATION DERIVED USING THE PANCREATIC CLAMP TECHNIQUE

To sort out effects of individual counterregulatory hormones on hepatic glucose production, Alan Cherrington and his colleagues at Vanderbilt University (Cherrington et al., 1993; McGuinness et al., 1993) have used the pancreatic clamp technique in the conscious dog model, with implanted hepatic vein and peripheral vascular catheters. By measuring artery-vein concentration differences and by using tracer infusions, rates of glycogenolysis and gluconeogenesis can be estimated. Then, in addition, a pancreatic clamp can be established by infusing sufficient somatostatin to maintain basal insulin and glucagon values. With this technique, effects of each individual counterregulatory hormone can be measured.

When an excess of glucagon is infused (Cherrington et al., 1993; McGuinness et al., 1993), a prompt and sustained increase of arterial glucose concentration is seen, followed by a more gradual increase in peripheral vein glucose. About 70–75 percent of this glucogenic response is due to glycogenolysis; a very small increase in hepatic gluconeogenesis is more delayed.

When epinephrine is infused and all other hormones held constant, an increase in arterial blood glucose values is also seen. This increase is smaller than the one caused by glucagon, but it is also due to an increase in hepatic glucose production. To accomplish this, epinephrine also increases glycogen breakdown and initiates a slow increase in gluconeogenesis (Cherrington et al., 1993; McGuinness et al., 1993). However, epinephrine has a far greater effect on gluconeogenesis than does glucagon. This can be explained by the lack of peripheral effects of glucagon, whereas epinephrine stimulates peripheral lipolysis and increases the delivery of gluconeogenic substrates to the liver, for example glycerol, lactate, and alanine (Cherrington et al., 1993; McGuinness et al., 1993).

Norepinephrine also causes a rise in plasma glucose concentrations, with a gradual slight increase in hepatic gluconeogenesis and a gradual slight decline in glycogenolysis. The effects of norepinephrine are primarily on non-hepatic tissues, where, like epinephrine, norepinephrine increases the production of gluconeogenic substrates for delivery to the liver (Cherrington et al., 1993; McGuinness et al., 1993).

Cortisol alone has little short-term effect on hepatic glucose production or on peripheral utilization (Cherrington et al., 1993; McGuinness et al., 1993).

With an insulin-glucose infusion, there is an increase in peripheral glucose utilization and a suppression of hepatic glucose production (Cherrington et al., 1993; McGuinness et al., 1993).

Combinations of counterregulatory hormones can also be studied, and over longer intervals of time. In an attempt to study the more chronic effects of these hormones, Cherrington's group (Cherrington et al., 1993; McGuinness et al., 1993) infused a combination of epinephrine, norepinephrine, glucagon, and cortisol over a 3-d period. Arterial glucose and insulin concentrations increased, as did the concentrations of all infused hormones. There was also an increase in glucose turnover during this 3-d period, with increased rates in both the production and utilization of glucose.

Such an increase in glucose turnover rates is part of the normal stress response, which appears to be driven by increased hepatic glucose production. There is also an increase in glucose utilization in the periphery, despite some possible degree of insulin resistance.

In other studies of chronic responses, Horton's group infused norepinephrine into rats for 10-d (Lupien et al., 1990). They also found an increased glucose turnover under basal conditions. This increase in glucose turnover persisted even under conditions of insulin stimulation, with no evidence of insulin resistance. The chronic norepinephrine infusion had apparently changed the glucose transport system by increasing blood flow to skeletal muscle as well as to brown fat (Lupien et al., 1990).

Some of the mechanisms by which exercise stress increases glucose turnover thus include changes in hepatic metabolism, changes in blood flow to skeletal muscle, and changes in the glucose transport system itself.

INFORMATION FROM OTHER ANIMAL MODELS

Another model of stress (stress caused by intracerebro-ventricular carbachol infusions) resembles the stress caused by exercise. In experiments done by Mladen Vranic and his group in Toronto (Miles et al., 1991), carbohydrate metabolism was studied after an injection (via a small catheter) of carbachol (an analogue of acetylcholine) into the third cerebral ventricle of dogs, thus stimulating paraventricular nucleus neurons and other nearby brain areas.

This simple injection produced a mild stress response, with activation of the adrenocortical axis, the adrenomedullary axis, and the sympathetic nervous system (Miles et al., 1991; Yamatani et al., 1992). Increases in cortisol, epinephrine, norepinephrine, and glucagon occurred, but insulin values remained unchanged (possibly because of a balanced alpha-, and beta-adrenergic stimulation of pancreatic beta cells). These hormonal changes were accompanied by a very large increase in hepatic glucose production rates, a surprising, matching increase in peripheral glucose uptake and only a small increase in blood glucose (Miles et al., 1991).

The surprising increase in peripheral glucose uptake, in the absence of an increase in plasma insulin, may have resulted from an increased blood flow to muscles and/or possibly to an activation of the glucose transport system in muscle cells.

To determine if the increase in glucose clearance was insulin-dependent or not, Vranic's group did other studies before and after the production of partial alloxan diabetes in the dogs (Miles et al., 1991; Yamatani et al., 1992). A submaximal insulin infusion was used to stabilize both insulin and glucose values in the normal baseline range. In these stabilized diabetic dogs, the carbachol infusion produced marked hyperglycemia, far in excess of the slight rise in blood glucose seen in nondiabetic dogs. The diabetic dogs showed a similar increase in hepatic glucose production, but they lacked the increase in peripheral glucose clearance seen in normal dogs. These findings suggest that at least a permissive amount of insulin (i.e., an amount sufficient to trigger some cellular uptake of glucose) must be present in order to see an increase in muscle glucose uptake in response to this mild model of stress (Miles et al., 1991; Yamatani et al., 1992).

INTERPRETATIONS OF THE METABOLIC DATA

Data on glucose homeostasis during exercise stress reveal a combination of stimulated hepatic glucose production and activated peripheral glucose uptake. This combination is obviously useful, because it provides the glucose energy needed for muscular contractions.

The animal stress model with CNS simulation-activation leads to an increase in glucose turnover, which could provide additional glucose for CNS function and also initiate a stimulated muscle cell uptake of glucose in case muscular exercise would also ensue. However, in the absence of physical activity, little benefit would result from creating severe hyperglycemia. There must be, then, a mechanism for increasing peripheral glucose clearance in stress situations that is independent of the increase in peripheral glucose uptake stimulated by physical exercise.

The skeletal muscle's uptake of glucose is an important area for study, because glucose transport in skeletal muscle is the major rate-limiting step in glucose utilization. Since skeletal muscle is the largest organ system in the body responsible for using glucose, it becomes important to understand how glucose is transported across the plasma membrane and is utilized for energy production in muscle tissue.

Glucose transport occurs primarily by a carrier-mediated pathway involving a whole family of glucose transporter protein isoforms, named Glut 1 through Glut 5. The key transporter isoform in skeletal muscle appears to be Glut 4. The glucose transport system responds to mediators that include insulin, muscle fiber contraction (in skeletal muscle), growth hormone, and glucose itself.

But the main point, in terms of exercise stress, is that insulin and exercise *independently* stimulate glucose transport in skeletal muscle. Contractions of skeletal muscle, in in vitro systems, can activate the glucose transport system in a total absence of insulin.

Thus there are two major (and apparently independent) stimuli. One is insulin, which normally activates the glucose transport system in a rested, fed state, and during recovery from exercise. And the second, the contraction stimulus, which is responsible for increasing muscle uptake of glucose during exercise and which can act in the absence of insulin.

With this dual system, plasma insulin values fall during exercise. This decrease allows for an increased hepatic glucose production, and at the same time, the contraction stimulus is enough to activate glucose uptake in skeletal muscle. This beautifully coordinated system thereby allows for both the increase in hepatic gluconeogenesis and the increase in skeletal muscle uptake of glucose.

SUMMARY AND RECOMMENDATIONS

- Glucose homeostasis is an important factor in attempting to preserve or enhance function during the stress response.
- It is very important to maintain blood glucose concentrations and the hepatic output of glucose during prolonged stress. However, any attempt to change either hepatic glucose output or peripheral glucose uptake by manipulating the CNS with current levels of knowledge may induce deleterious effects.

- Recommendations about ergogenic aids and the enhancement of performance during endurance exercise are contained in Chapter 12.
- Additional research is needed to understand fully the role of the sympathetic nervous system, centrally mediated hormone responses, and direct neuronal effects on both hepatic glucose production and peripheral glucose utilization. The central role of the CNS, and how it might be enhanced, remains unclear.
- Additional research is also needed on the effects of various neurotransmitters, beta-blockers, and beta-receptors on metabolic homeostasis during stress.

REFERENCES

Cherrington, A.D., R.W.Stevenson, K.E.Steiner, C.C.Connolly, M.Wada, and R.E. Goldstein 1993 Acute hormonal regulation of gluconeogenesis in the conscious dog. Pp. 199–208 in New Concepts in the Pathogenesis of NIDDM, S.Efendie, C.J.Ostensen, and M. Vranic, eds. New York: Plenum Publishers.

Goodyear, L.J., M.F.Hirshman, and E.S.Horton 1992 The glucose transport system in skeletal muscle: Effects of exercise and insulin. Pp. 201–215 in Integration of Medical and Sports Sciences. Y.Sato, J.Poormans, I. Hashimoto, and Y.Oshida, eds. Basel, Switzerland: Karger.

Lupien, J.R., M.F.Hirshman, and E.S.Horton 1990 Effects of norepinephrine infusion on in vivo insulin sensitivity and responsiveness. Am. J. Physiol. 259(2 Pt1):E210-E215.

McGuinness, O.P., T.Fugiwara, S.Murrell, D.Bracy, D.Neal, D.O'Connor, and A.D. Cherrington 1993 Impact of chronic stress hormone infusion on hepatic carbohydrate metabolism in the conscious dog. Am. J. Physiol. 265(2 Pt1):E314–E322.

Miles, P.D.G., K.Yamatani, H.L.A.Lickley, and M.Vranic 1991 Mechanism of glucoregulatory responses to stress and their deficiency in diabetes. Proc. Natl. Acad. Sci. 88:1296–1300.

Shimazu, T. 1992 The hypothalamus and neural feed-forward regulation of exercise metabolism Pp. 20–32 in Integration of Medical and Sports Sciences, Y.Sato, J.Poormans, I. Hashimoto, and Y.Oshida, eds. Basel, Switzerland: Karger.

Wahren, J., P.Felig, G.Ahlborg, and L.Jorfeldt 1971 Glucose metabolism during leg exercise in man. J. Clin. Invest. 50:2715–2725.

Yamatani, K., Z.Q.Shi, A.Giacca, R.Gupta, S.Fisher, H.L.A.Lickley, and M.Vranic 1992 Role of FFA-glucose cycle in glucoregulation in total absence of insulin. Am. J. Physiol. 263(4Pt 1):E646–53.

PART V

Potential Performance-Enhancing Food Components

IN PART V, the performance-enhancing capacities of several food components are reviewed. Prior to the workshop the Army identified a number of food components that they specifically requested the Committee on Military Nutrition Research to evaluate. In response to this request the committee invited ten well known scientists to provide reviews of these food components and make their own recommendations regarding the potential of these food components to enhance performance. The first chapter presents an overview of ergogenic aids. This is followed by a discussion of issues relating nutrients and neurotransmitter release and behavioral consequences. Discussed next are the performance-enhancing effects of protein and amino acids, followed by a description of the results of human and animal studies evaluating the effects of tyrosine supplements on mental performance under stressful conditions, and the effects of tyrosine in reducing cognitive deficits resulting from cold stress. Treated next in this section are, the role of carbohydrate in fatigue and the effects of carbohydrate on cognitive performance. Reviews of the effects of choline on human performance; the effects of caffeine on cognitive performance, mood, and alertness; and the effects of carnitine on enhancing physical performance, close this section.

12

Food Components That May Optimize Physical Performance: An Overview

John L.Ivy[1]

INTRODUCTION

For years people have routinely searched for ways to optimize physical performance, increase the amount of work that can be accomplished under various environmental extremes, and enhance recovery from a physically exhausting task. Aids that are used to increase physical performance or enhance recovery from physical exertion are referred to as *ergogenic aids.* The word *ergogenic* is derived from the Greek word *ergon* meaning "work" and the suffix *-genic* meaning "producing." Therefore, the word ergogenic literally means "work producing" or "tending to increase work."

Ergogenic aids are generally classified into five categories: (1) mechanical, (2) psychological, (3) physiological, (4) pharmacological, and (5) nutritional. An example of a mechanical ergogenic aid is the fiberglass pole for pole vaulting or the lightweight frame on a racing bike. A psychological ergogenic aid might be hypnosis or mental rehearsal. Blood doping or erythropoietin injections are considered powerful physiological ergogenic aids by virtue of their ability to increase red blood cell mass and increase maximum aerobic capacity. Pharmacological ergogenic aids might be the xanthines such as caffeine or the amphetamines. Carbohydrate and protein supplements are

[1] John L.Ivy, Belmont Hall 222, University of Texas, Austin, TX 78712

examples of nutritional ergogenic aids. It should be noted that many ergogenic aids can be classified into more than one category. For example, caffeine can be classified as a nutritional or a pharmacological ergogenic aid. Likewise, bicarbonate could be classified as a physiological or pharmacological ergogenic aid.

Of the various aids known to have ergogenic effects, many are natural foods or derivatives of food products. This chapter identifies some of the more effective food components that have been found to enhance physical performance and describes their methods of action. Some potential yet unproved ergogenic aids are also discussed.

Food components or food derivatives that might have ergogenic effects are generally classified as either a nutritional or a pharmacological ergogenic aid. Such aids enhance performance by:

1. acting as a central or peripheral nervous system stimulant,
2. increasing the stored amount or availability of a limiting substrate,
3. acting as a supplemental fuel source or reducing reliance on a limiting substrate during prolonged physical exertion,
4. reducing or neutralizing metabolic by-products that interfere with energy-producing reactions or muscle contraction, and
5. enhancing recovery.

ACTIONS OF SPECIFIC FOODS AND DERIVATIVES OF FOOD PRODUCTS

Ergogenic Aids That Act as Central or Peripheral Nervous System Stimulants

Several food components or substances derived from plant extracts have been used to stimulate the brain, ward off feelings of fatigue, and renew vigor and enthusiasm. These substances may stimulate the brain directly, may increase the production or release of neurotransmitters that activate certain stimulatory regions of the brain, or prevent the release of inhibitor neurotransmitters. Examples of these neurostimulating aids are caffeine, which is found in a variety of foods, and norpseudoephedrine, which is found in the leaves of the African plant *Catha edulis.*

Recently, it was suggested that branched-chain amino acid (BCAA) supplementation may prevent central nervous system fatigue (Blomstrand et al., 1988, 1991). One of the hypotheses proposed to explain central nervous system fatigue is related to an increase in the concentration of 5-hydroxytryptamine (serotonin) in one or more specific areas of the brain. An increase in serotonin levels in the brain can theoretically arise from two peripheral effects of endurance exercise. First, an increase in BCAA utilization by muscle may cause a decrease in plasma BCAA levels, which would raise the plasma tryptophan/BCAA ratio. Since BCAAs compete with free tryptophan for amino acid transporters in the brain (Pardridge and Oldendorf, 1975), an increase in the tryptophan/BCAA ratio should favor the entry of tryptophan into the brain. Tryptophan is a precursor of serotonin, and therefore, as the levels of tryptophan increase in the brain, there is a proportional increase in serotonin levels (Newsholme and Leech, 1983). Second, an increase in the plasma free fatty acid concentration could compete with tryptophan for binding sites on albumin and increase the plasma free tryptophan concentration. An increase in plasma free fatty acid levels generally occurs with prolonged aerobic exercise. Whatever the circumstances, it has been suggested that BCAA supplementation may be beneficial in that it may prevent a rise in the tryptophan/BCAA ratio, thereby reducing the uptake of tryptophan by the brain and blunting or preventing a rise in brain serotonin levels. However, there has been little definitive research that supports this idea.

Another possible mechanism of action of food components is the facilitation of excitation-contraction-coupling. This facilitating effect could occur at the neuromuscular junction by increasing the release of the neurotransmitter acetylcholine or, possibly, by preventing the depletion of this neurotransmitter by providing choline supplements (R.T.Wurtman, Massachusetts Institute of Technology, personal communication, 1992). As with BCAA supplementation, however, there has been no definitive research that supports this idea.

Ergogenic Aids That Increase the Stored Amount or Availability of a Limiting Substrate

Carbohydrate is an essential fuel source for prolonged exercise of moderate intensity. At intensities ranging between 60 and 80 percent of maximum aerobic power (maximum oxygen uptake [$\dot{V}_{O_2\ max}$], the major source of carbohydrate is muscle glycogen. Numerous studies have demonstrated that the capacity to exercise at exercise intensities ranging from 60 to 80 percent $\dot{V}_{O_2\ max}$ is directly related to the preexercise muscle glycogen level (Ahlborg et al., 1967; Bergström and Hultman, 1967; Bergström et al., 1967). Because of the paramount importance of muscle glycogen during prolonged, moderate-intensity exercise, the regulation of muscle glycogen synthesis and mechanisms for increasing the muscle glycogen stores have been studied extensively. For years it has been known that the consumption of a high-carbohydrate diet will elevate glycogen stores above normal levels. To maximize muscle glycogen stores, however, a specific regimen of exercise and diet must be followed. Although several regimens have been developed, the 7-day protocol developed by Sherman et al. (1981) is the most practical. First, the muscle glycogen level is depleted by exercise. During the next 3 days, exercise should be of moderate intensity and duration and a well-balanced mixed diet composed of about 45 percent carbohydrate should be consumed. During the last 3 days, the exercise duration is tapered and the carbohydrate content of the diet is increased to 70 percent. This protocol has been found to double the normal muscle glycogen concentration.

Oxygen availability is also an important determinant of aerobic endurance. Increasing oxygen delivery or availability to the working muscles has been found to increase maximum aerobic power and aerobic endurance. The increase in aerobic endurance is thought to be due to a reduced reliance on carbohydrate stores and/or reduced lactate production during submaximal exercise. Blood doping and erythropoietin injections have been used to increase the oxygen-carrying capacity of the blood and to increase $\dot{V}_{O_2\ max}$ by increasing the red blood cell mass (Spriet, 1991). These procedures, however, are potentially dangerous because of the possibility of infection and increased blood viscosity, which can place undue stress on the exercising heart.

Phosphate loading, which has been found to increase $\dot{V}_{O_2\ max}$ is an alternative to blood doping and other procedures that increase red blood cell mass (Cade et al., 1984; Kreider et al., 1990; Stewart et al., 1990). Typically, this procedure consists of consuming between 600 and 1,000 mg of sodium phosphate three to four times per day for 3 to 6 days. It has been reported that this procedure will increase $\dot{V}_{O_2\ max}$ by 6 to 12 percent, increase the anaerobic threshold, and increase the run time to exhaustion during a continuous ramp protocol on the treadmill (Cade et al., 1984; Kreider et al., 1990; Stewart et al., 1990). It is believed that the increased phosphate consumption elevates the 2,3-diphosphoglycerate concentration of the blood and that this improves tissue oxygen extraction from blood by reducing the affinity of oxygen for hemoglobin (Bredle et al., 1988; Cade et al., 1984; Stewart et al., 1990). It should be mentioned, however, that other possibilities for the ergogenic effects of phosphate loading have been suggested (Bredle et al., 1988; Kreider et al., 1990) and that positive effects have not always been found (Bredle et al., 1988; Duffy and Conlee, 1986).

Ergogenic Aids That Act as a Supplemental Fuel Source or Reduce Reliance on a Limiting Fuel Store

Several nutritional supplements have been used as a supplemental fuel source. The most popular and probably the most effective is simple carbohy drates. Generally, these supplements are composed of glucose or a combination of maltodextrins, glucose, and fructose. The mechanism by which carbohydrate supplements improve aerobic endurance performance may be determined by the intensity of the exercise. During the onset of moderate-intensity aerobic exercise (60–75 percent $\dot{V}_{O_2\ max}$), muscle glycogen is a primary fuel source (Ahlborg et al., 1967; Bergström and Hultman, 1967; Bergström et al., 1967). As exercise continues and the muscle glycogen stores decline, the muscle becomes increasingly more dependent on blood glucose for its carbohydrate needs (Gollnick et al., 1981). This, however, does not appear to be a problem as long as the liver is able to maintain an adequate blood glucose concentration of approximately 3.5 mM (Coyle et al., 1986). However, when the muscle glycogen stores have been depleted and the blood glucose concentration falls below 3.5 mM, muscle glucose uptake cannot meet the carbohydrate requirements of the active muscle. Once the carbohydrate requirement cannot be met, muscle fatigue rapidly ensues. Carbohydrate supplements taken during the activity are able to maintain the blood glucose concentration above a critical level and prolong the time to fatigue during exercise of moderate intensity (Coyle et al., 1983, 1986).

Carbohydrate supplementation has also been found to be beneficial during low-intensity exercise (40–50 percent $\dot{V}_{O_2\ max}$) (Ivy et al., 1983; Yaspelkis and Ivy, 1991). However, the mechanism of action of the carbohydrate supplementation during low-intensity exercise appears to differ from that during moderate-intensity exercise. During low-intensity exercise, the rate of muscle glycogen utilization is significantly reduced by carbohydrate supplementation (Yaspelkis and Ivy, 1991). The difference in the muscle glycogen response elicited by a carbohydrate supplement during moderate- and low-intensity steady-state exercise is likely due to the differences in the plasma glucose and insulin responses. Ingestion of carbohydrate supplements during low-intensity exercise increases insulin and plasma glucose concentrations and maintains these variables at elevated levels throughout the exercise bout (Ivy et al., 1983; Yaspelkis and Ivy, 1991). In contrast, carbohydrate supplementation during moderate-intensity exercise aids only in the maintenance of plasma glucose and insulin concentrations (Coyle et al., 1983, 1986; Ivy et al., 1979). Recently, Yaspelkis et al., 1993) observed that carbohydrate supplementation elevated plasma glucose and insulin levels during prolonged, continuous variable-intensity exercise (45–75 percent $\dot{V}_{O_2\ max}$) and enhanced aerobic endurance. The increase in plasma insulin levels was the highest that those investigators had observed during exercise. Associated with the increase in endurance was a sparing of muscle glycogen (Yaspelkis et al., 1993). Therefore, it appears that when exercise intensity is fluctuating between low and moderate intensity, carbohydrate supplementation may enhance aerobic endurance by reducing dependency on muscle glycogen as a fuel source.

Another approach to increasing aerobic endurance is to increase the blood free fatty acid concentration prior to the onset of aerobic exercise. Raising the blood free fatty acid concentration increases the amount of fatty acid uptake by the muscle and reduces reliance on muscle glycogen and blood glucose for energy production. This process has been found to be effective in both rats and humans (Costill et al., 1977; Hickson et al., 1977). The most effective procedure for the elevation of plasma free fatty acid is to ingest a high-fat meal several hours prior to exercise. This elevates the plasma triglyceride level. Once plasma triglycerides are elevated, heparin is injected intravenously to activate lipoprotein lipase, which hydrolyzes the triglycerides to glycerol and free fatty acids. This can effectively raise the free fatty acid concentration in the blood to more than 1 mM. However, this mechanism is impractical and potentially dangerous because of the anticlotting effect of the heparin.

Because of the lipolytic effect of caffeine, the use of this xanthine to elevate plasma free fatty acid levels prior to exercise has also been investigated. Several studies have found that ingestion of caffeine approximately 1 h prior to exercise increased the plasma free fatty acid concentration (Costill et al., 1978; Essig et al., 1980). This was accompanied by a decrease in the exercising respiratory exchange ratio and an increase in aerobic endurance. However, other studies have found an increase in aerobic performance following caffeine ingestion without an increase in plasma free fatty acid concentrations (Graham and Spriet, 1991; Ivy et al., 1979; Spriet et al., 1992). For example, Ivy et al. (1979) used nine trained cyclists to study the effects of caffeine on work production during 2 h of isokinetic cycling exercise. Ingestion of 250 mg of caffeine 60 min before the ride and ingestion of an additional 250 mg of caffeine at 15-min intervals over the first 90 min of exercise increased work production by 7.4 percent without increasing the subjects' perception of exertion. Of interest was the observation that the subjects started exercising at a higher work rate from the start of exercise and maintained a higher work rate than the controls during the course of the 2-h ride. Plasma free fatty acid levels in the test subjects were not significantly different from those in the controls although fat oxidation, based on the respiratory exchange ratio, in the test subjects became significantly greater than those in the controls after 60 min of exercise. It was concluded that the ergogenic effect of caffeine was both neurological and metabolic in nature and independent of an increase in plasma free fatty acid levels.

Recently, Spriet et al. (1991, 1992) performed a series of studies investigating the mechanism of caffeine's ergogenic effects on running and cycling performance at a relatively high aerobic exercise intensity (80–85 percent $\dot{V}_{O_2\ max}$). It was found that high concentrations of caffeine ingested prior to exercise resulted in an elevation in plasma epinephrine levels and a sparing of muscle glycogen early in exercise. This spared glycogen was available late in exercise and coincided with a prolonged time to exhaustion. It was further suggested that increased utilization of intramuscular triglyceride and/or extramuscular free fatty acids after caffeine ingestion may have inhibited carbohydrate oxidation early in exercise via elevations in muscle citrate and the acetyl-coenzyme A to coenzyme A ratio (acetyl CoA/CoA-SH) ratio. Plasma free fatty acid levels, however, were not significantly different during the caffeine and control treatments.

The combination of pyruvate and dihydroxyacetone (PD) is another food component that has potential as an ergogenic aid. Stanko et al. (1990a) found that consumption of pyruvate and dihydroxyacetone as part of a standard diet improved submaximal arm endurance by 20 percent. The experimental paradigm called for substituting 100 g of PD (1:3) for an isocaloric amount of carbohydrate in the diet over 7 consecutive days. Both arteriovenous glucose difference and blood fractional glucose extraction were higher after dietary consumption of the PD than after consumption of the control diet, suggesting an enhanced muscle glucose uptake. In addition, the muscle glycogen concentration was higher for the PD treatment compared with that for the control treatment before exercise but did not differ between the two groups at exhaustion. It was suggested that the greater muscle glycogen stores and the increased muscle glucose uptake delayed the onset of fatigue and extended the submaximal endurance capacity during the PD trial.

In a subsequent study by the same group, the ergogenic effects of PD were investigated during cycling at an exercise intensity of 70 percent $\dot{V}_{O_2\ max}$(Stanko et al., 1990b). The experimental paradigm used was similar to that of their first study, except that the PD and the placebo were provided separately from the meals. This resulted in similar muscle glycogen concentrations for the two treatment groups at the onset of exercise. Time to fatigue was 20 percent longer for the PD treatment group compared with that for the placebo group. The whole-leg arteriovenous glucose difference was greater for the PD treatment group than for the placebo group at rest and during the first 30 min of exercise, but there was no difference in the respiratory exchange ratio between the two groups. There was also no difference in muscle glycogen levels at the time of exhaustion between the treatment groups. It was suggested that the greater glucose extraction may have spared muscle glycogen and that the spared muscle glycogen and/or the increased glucose extraction provided the necessary fuel for prolongation of exercise endurance capacity. A potential problem with this supplement, however, is that pyruvate is available only as a sodium or a calcium salt. Therefore, the high concentrations of pyruvate required for the ergogenic effect may produce a mineral overload.

Medium-chain triglycerides (MCTs) have also been experimented with as a substitute fuel source during prolonged moderate-intensity exercise. MCTs have been described as a food fat that can be more rapidly hydrolyzed, absorbed, and metabolized than ordinary long-chain triglycerides (Greenberger et al., 1966; Schwabe et al., 1964). Since MCTs are absorbed into the blood as medium-chain fatty acids (Greenberger et al., 1966) and metabolized as quickly as glucose (Schwabe et al., 1964), it has been speculated that they might provide an alternate carbon source for muscle metabolism during prolonged exercise. To date, however, there have been no studies that have demonstrated an advantage to ingesting large amounts of MCTs before or during prolonged aerobic exercise. In addition, there is a significant problem with the oral administration of MCTs. By themselves, MCTs are highly unpalatable and produce stomach discomfort and diarrhea when taken in high concentrations (Ivy et al., 1980). Therefore, even if they appeared to enhance aerobic endurance, their use is questionable.

Ergogenic Aids That Reduce or Neutralize Metabolic By-Products

During intense exercise, in which glycolysis is primarily responsible for resynthesis of ATP, lactic acid is formed and accumulates in the muscle and blood. The decrease in muscle pH because of lactic acid accumulation is assumed to be one of the major factors limiting exercise performance. The inhibitory effect of an increase in the intramuscular hydrogen ion concentration (H^+) has been related to impairment of glycolytic enzyme activity (Chasiotis et al., 1983; Trivedi and Danforth, 1966), direct interference with excitation-contraction-coupling (Fuchs et al., 1970; Nakamura and Schwartz, 1972), and alterations in the plasma membrane potential because of excessive potassium ion (K^+) efflux (Heigenhauser and Jones, 1991). The magnitude of the decrease in muscle pH is determined by the amount of lactic acid accumulation, the muscle buffering capacity, and the flux rate of lactic acid from muscle to blood.

Early studies by Dennig and colleagues (1931) suggested that administration of buffering substances such as sodium bicarbonate ($NaHCO_3$) could improve high-intensity exercise performance, whereas substances that compromised the buffering capacity of the blood would worsen intense exercise performance. Those early studies, however, were conducted on only one subject, and several subsequent studies from other laboratories found no effect of $NaHCO_3$ on exercise performance (Asmussen et al., 1948; Johnson and Black, 1953). It was not until 1976 that a well-controlled study on the ergogenic effects of $NaHCO_3$ was conducted. Sutton et al. (1976) found that, in comparison with a control condition, the ingestion of $NaHCO_3$ increased by approximately 65 percent the duration of time subjects could cycle at 90 percent $\dot{V}_{O_2\ max}$. In a second study, the same group evaluated the effects of metabolic acidosis and metabolic alkalosis on high-intensity exercise performance (Jones et al., 1977). Subjects were provided calcium carbonate ($CaCO_3$) as a control (placebo), ammonium chloride (NH_4Cl) to induce acidosis, and $NaHCO_3$ to induce alkalosis. Compared with the control, acidosis reduced exercise duration by 70 percent while alkalosis increased exercise duration by 63 percent. Of interest was the observation that the blood pH and plasma lactate concentration were highest during the $NaHCO_3$ trial and lowest during the NH_4Cl trial. It was suggested that the endurance performances associated with NH_4Cl and $NaHCO_3$ treatments were due, in part, to their effect on the efflux rate of lactate from muscle. That is, NH_4Cl impaired muscle lactate efflux and increased the rate of muscle lactate accumulation, and $NaHCO_3$ facilitated muscle lactate efflux and decreased the rate of muscle lactate accumulation. It has been demonstrated in various animal models that a low blood pH impairs and that a high blood pH facilitates lactate efflux from muscle to blood (Hirche et al., 1975).

Another approach to increasing high-intensity exercise performance is to reduce the rate of muscle lactate production. Pangamic acid, which is also referred to as vitamin B_{15}, is a naturally occurring substance with vitamin-like properties. The active agent in pangamic acid is thought to be dichloroacetate (DCA). DCA stimulates pyruvate dehydrogenase indirectly by inhibiting pyruvate dehydrogenase kinase (Whitehouse et al., 1974). Pyruvate dehydrogenase catalyzes the rate-limiting step in the aerobic oxidation of pyruvate and lactate. Maximal stimulation of pyruvate dehydrogenase activity by DCA has been shown to lower blood lactate concentrations during exercise in animals and during postexercise recovery in humans (Carraro et al., 1989; Schneider et al., 1981). Schneider et al. (1981) found that DCA-treated rats were able to swim approximately 40 percent longer than controls when the exercise intensity was near the maximal work load. This increase in performance was associated with lower levels of blood and muscle lactate at rest and during the swim. At exhaustion, blood lactate was the same in the two groups, even though the DCA-treated rats had worked for a significantly longer period of time.

Heat is another metabolic by-product of exercise that can also impair physical performance and endurance. If environmental conditions are extreme and the exercise period is prolonged, the increased metabolic rate that occurs during exercise can result in dehydration and hyperthermia unless adequate water is consumed. The amount of water lost during exercise is determined by the need to regulate body heat. During exercise in the heat, evaporation is the principal means of body heat loss. As sweat comes into contact with the skin, a cooling effect occurs as the sweat evaporates. For each liter of water that vaporizes, 580 kcal of heat is dissipated from the body and transferred to the environment. In a few hours of hard exercise in the heat, water loss from sweating can reach 3 to 4 liters. A water loss equivalent to 2 percent of body weight will impair cardiovascular function and the thermal regulatory mechanisms of the body (Bijlani and Sharma, 1980; Drinkwater, 1976; Gisolfi and Copping, 1974). Water loss of 4 percent of body weight will reduce muscle endurance and work capacity (Buskirk et al., 1958; Saltin, 1964). Water loss that exceeds 6 percent of body weight will drastically hamper physical performance and possibly lead to severe heat injury. Therefore, water becomes a very important ergogenic aid during prolonged exercise in a hot environment.

Ergogenic Aids That Enhance Recovery

Because of the importance of muscle glycogen for prolonged moderate-intensity exercise, replenishment of the muscle glycogen stores is essential for high levels of daily physical activity and training. Following the depletion of muscle glycogen levels by a prolonged exercise bout, normal glycogen stores can be replenished within a 24-h period if sufficient carbohydrate is ingested. This generally requires consumption of 500 to 550 g of carbohydrate daily (Costill et al., 1981). If the carbohydrate concentration of the diet is inadequate, successive days of intense, prolonged exercise may result in a gradual reduction in the muscle glycogen stores and a deterioration in performance (Costill et al., 1971).

To optimize the rate of muscle glycogen replenishment, a carbohydrate supplement of approximately 1.0 g/kg of body weight should be consumed immediately after the cessation of exercise (Ivy et al., 1988a,b) Continuation of supplementation every 2 h will maintain a rapid rate of storage for up to 6 h after exercise (Blom et al., 1987). Increasing the amount of carbohydrate consumption above 1.0 g/kg of body weight per supplement appears to provide no additional benefit (Ivy et al., 1988b). Supplements composed of glucose or glucose polymers are more effective for the replenishment of muscle glycogen stores after exercise than supplements predominantly composed of fructose (Blom et al., 1987). However, some fructose is recommended because it is more effective than glucose in replenishing liver glycogen stores (Nilsson and Hultman, 1974). It has also been found that theaddition of protein (~ 0.3 to 0.4 g/kg of body weight) to a carbohydrate supplement will increase the rate of muscle glycogen storage (Zawadzki et al., 1992). This is due to the synergistic insulin response produced from the combination of carbohydrate and protein. Finally, carbohydrates in solid or liquid form can be consumed immediately after exercise with similar results (Reed et al., 1989). However, liquid supplements are recommended because they are easy to digest and are less filling, and therefore do not tend to adversely affect an individual's normal appetite. They also provide a source of fluid for rapid rehydration.

Because of the adverse effects of dehydration on physical performance, it is also important to rehydrate prior to any subsequent physical exertion. Although water has generally been recommended as the fluid of choice for rehydration, recent studies have suggested that electrolyte or glucose-electrolyte solutions actually may be superior to water (Morimoto et al., 1981; Nose et al., 1988). Following exercise dehydration there is a prolonged period of delayed rehydration. This is due in part to a decreased dipsogenic drive that occurs with large amounts of water consumption. This reduced drive to consume fluid appears to be related to a disproportionate recovery of plasma volume with respect to total body water (Nose et al., 1988). Apparently, a reduced plasma osmolality or a low sodium chloride (NaCl) concentration inhibits the dipsogenic response. When carbohydrate-electrolyte solutions rather than water are ingested, this prevents the rapid decline in plasma osmolality and NaCl concentration, thus prolonging the dipsogenic response of dehydration, and increases voluntary fluid consumption. It has also been reported that plasma volume and osmolality are significantly greater after 4 h of recovery from exercise-dehydration when a carbohydrate-electrolyte solution is ingested than when an equal volume of water is ingested (González-Alonso et al., 1992). This results in reduced urine loss and significantly greater water retention. These findings strongly suggest that a carbohydrate-electrolyte solution is more effective than water for the rapid replenishment of body fluids following exercise-dehydration.

CONCLUSIONS

Many natural foods or derivatives of food products have ergogenic effects. Their mechanisms of action as well as the types of physical performance they enhance are quite varied. Some have been found to be beneficial during prolonged moderate-intensity exercise, whereas others enhance anaerobic performance. For maximum effectiveness, it is important to understand their limitations and the proper way in which they should be used.

- Carbohydrates may be beneficial in extending the time to fatigue when taken before and during prolonged moderate-intensity aerobic exercise. In combination with protein, they stimulate the rapid recovery of muscle glycogen stores following exercise. In combination with electrolytes and water, they are effective in rehydration postexercise.
- Caffeine appears to be a strong enhancer of aerobic endurance. This may be due to its ability to spare muscle glycogen and facilitate neural processes.

- The chronic feeding of pyruvate-dihydroxyacetone may increase aerobic endurance, but a major disadvantage of this supplement is that the concentrations shown to be effective may result in a mineral overload.
- Although it has been suggested that medium-chain triglycerides may enhance aerobic endurance, this has not been substantiated, nor have there been any definitive results demonstrating a positive effect of choline supplementation on physical performance.
- Branched-chain amino acids may enhance aerobic endurance by reducing the rate of brain serotonin accumulation during prolonged exercise. However, more research is needed to substantiate this hypothesis.
- For maximum performance during prolonged physical exertion in a hot and humid environment, water or fluid supplementation is essential.
- For high-intensity aerobic and anaerobic performance, phosphate loading may be beneficial because of the ability of phosphate to increase the blood 2,3-diphosphoglycerate concentration and reduce the affinity of oxygen for hemoglobin.
- Anaerobic capacity may be enhanced by preexercise ingestion of sodium bicarbonate or dichloroacetate. Sodium bicarbonate increases blood pH, which helps with the buffering of lactate and its efflux from the exercising muscle. Dichloroacetate increases the activity of pyruvate dehydrogenase and thus reduces the rate of lactate accumulation.

REFERENCES

Ahlborg, B., J.Berström, L.G.Ekelund, and E.Hultman 1967 Muscle glycogen and muscle electrolytes during prolonged physical exercise. Acta Physiol. Scand. 70:129–142.

Asmussen, E., W.Van Dobelin, and M.Nielson 1948 Blood lactate and oxygen debt after exhaustive work at different oxygen tensions. Acta Physiol. Scand. 15:57–62.

Bergström, J., and E.Hultman 1967 A study of the glycogen metabolism during exercise in man. Scand. J. Clin. Lab. Invest. 19:218–226.

Bergström, J., L.Hermansen, E.Hultman, and B.Saltin 1967 Diet, muscle glycogen and physical performance. Acta Physiol. Scand. 71:140–150.

Bijlani, R.L., and K.N.Sharma 1980 Effect of dehydration and a few regimes of rehydration on human performance. Ind. J. Physiol. Pharm. 24:255–266.

Blom, P.C.S., A.T.Høstmark, O.Vaage, K.R.Kardel, and S.Maehlum 1987 Effect of different post-exercise sugar diets on the rate of muscle glycogen synthesis. Med. Sci. Sports Exerc. 19:491–496.

Blomstrand, E., F.Celsing, and E.A.Newsholme 1988 Changes in plasma concentrations of aromatic and branched-chain amino acids during sustained exercise in man and their possible role in fatigue. Acta Physiol. Scand. 133:115–121.

Blomstrand, E., P.Hassmén, B.Ekblom, and E.A.Newsholme 1991 Administration of branched-chain amino acids during sustained exercise—effects on performance and on plasma concentration of some amino acids. Eur. J. Appl. Physiol. 63:83–88.

Bredle, D.L., J.M.Stager, W.F.Brechue, and M.O.Farber 1988 Phosphate supplementation, cardiovascular function, and exercise performance in humans. J. Appl. Physiol. 65:1821–1826.

Buskirk, E.R., P.P.Lampietto, and D.E.Bass 1958 Work performance after dehydration: Effects of physical conditioning and heat acclimatization. J. Appl. Physiol. 12:189–197.

Cade, R., M.Conte, C.Zauner, D.Mars, J.Peterson, D.Lunne, N.Hommen, and D.Parker 1984 Effects of phosphate loading on 2,3-diphosphoglycerate and maximal oxygen uptake. Med. Sci. Sports Exerc. 16:263–268.

Carraro, F., K.Samuel, J.I.Rosenblatt, and R.R.Wolfe 1989 Effect of dichloroacetate on lactate concentration in exercising humans. J. Appl. Physiol. 66:591–597.

Chasiotis, D., E.Hultman, and K.Sahlin 1983 Acidotic depression of cyclic AMP accumulation and phosphorylase b to a transformation in skeletal muscle of men. J. Physiol. (London) 335:197–204.

Costill, D.L., R.Bowers, G.Branam, and K.Sparks 1971 Muscle glycogen utilization during prolonged exercise on successive days. J. Appl. Physiol. 31:834–838.

Costill, D.L., E.F.Coyle, G.Dalsky, W.Evans, W.Fink, and D.Hoopes 1977 Effects of elevated plasma FFA and insulin in muscle glycogen usage during exercise. J. Appl. Physiol. 43:695–699.

Costill, D.L., G.Dalsky, and W.Fink 1978 Effects of caffeine ingestion on metabolism and exercise performance. Med. Sci. Sports 10:155–158.

Costill, D.L., W.M.Sherman, W.J.Fink, C.Maresh, and M.Witten 1981 The role of dietary carbohydrate in muscle glycogen resynthesis after strenuous running. Am. J. Clin. Nutr. 34:1831–836.

Coyle, E.F., J.M.Hagberg, B.R.Hurley, W.H.Martin, A.A.Ehsani, and J.O.Holloszy 1983 Carbohydrate feeding during prolonged strenuous exercise can delay fatigue. J. Appl. Physiol. 55:230–235.

Coyle, E.F., A.R.Coggan, M.K.Hemmert, and J.L.Ivy 1986 Muscle glycogen utilization during prolonged strenuous exercise when fed carbohydrate. J. Appl. Physiol. 61:165–172.

Dennig, H., J.H.Talbott, H.T.Edwards, and D.B.Dill 1931 Effect of acidosis and alkalosis upon capacity for work. J. Clin. Invest. 9:601–613.

Drinkwater, B.L. 1976 Thermoregulatory responses of women to intermittent work in the heat. J. Appl. Physiol. 41:57–62.

Duffy, D.J., and R.K.Conlee 1986 Effects of phosphate loading on leg power and high intensity treadmill exercise. Med. Sci. Sports Exerc. 18:674–677.

Essig, D., D.L.Costill, and P.J.van Handel 1980 Effects of caffeine ingestion on utilization of muscle glycogen and lipid during leg ergometer cycling. Int. J. Sports Med. 1:86–90.

Fuchs, F., Y.Reddy, and F.N.Briggs 1970 The interaction of cations with the calcium-binding site of troponin. Biochim. Biophys. Acta 221:407–409.

Gisolfi, C.V., and J.R.Copping 1974 Thermal effects of prolonged treadmill exercise in the heat. Med. Sci. Sports 6:108–113.

Gollnick, P.D., B.Pernow, B.Essén, E.Jannson, and B.Saltin 1981 Availability of glycogen and plasma FFA for substrate utilization in leg muscle of man during exercise. Clin. Physiol. 1:27–42.

González-Alonso, J., C.L.Heaps, and E.F.Coyle 1992 Rehydration after exercise with common beverages and water. Int. J. Sports Med. 13:399–406.

Graham, T.E., and L.L.Spriet 1991 Performance and metabolic responses to a high caffeine dose during prolonged exercise. J. Appl. Physiol. 71:2292–2298.

Greenberger, N.J., J.B.Rodgers, and K.J.Isselbacher 1966 Absorption of medium and long-chain triglycerides: Factors influencing their hydrolysis and transport. J. Clin. Invest. 45:217–222.

Heigenhauser, G.J.F., and N.L.Jones 1991 Bicarbonate loading. Pp. 183–212 in Ergogenics, Enhancement of Performance in Exercise and Sport, D.R.Lamb and M.H.Williams, eds. Ann Arbor, Mich.: William C.Brown.

Hickson, R.C., M.J.Rennie, R.K.Conlee, W.W.Winder, and J.O.Holloszy 1977 Effects of increased plasma fatty acids on glycogen utilization and endurance. J. Appl. Physiol. 43:829–833.

Hirche, H., V.Hombach, H.D.Langohr, U.Wacher, and J.Busse 1975 Lactic acid permeation rate in working gastrocnemii of dogs during metabolic alkalosis and acidosis. Pflüegers Arch. 356:209–222.

Ivy, J.L., D.L.Costill, W.J.Fink, and R.W.Lower 1979 Influence of caffeine and carbohydrate feedings on endurance performance. Med. Sci. Sports 11:6–11.

Ivy, J.L., D.L.Costill, W.J.Fink, and E.Maglischo 1980 Contribution of medium and long chain triglyceride intake to energy metabolism during prolonged exercise. Int. J. Sports Med. 1:15–20.

Ivy, J.L., W.Miller, V.Dover, L.G.Goodyear, W.H.Sherman, S.Farrell, and H.Williams 1983 Endurance improved by ingestion of a glucose polymer supplement. Med. Sci. Sports Exerc. 15:466–471.

Ivy, J.L., A.L.Katz, C.L.Cuttler, W.M.Sherman, and E.F.Coyle 1988a Muscle glycogen synthesis after exercise: Effect of time of carbohydrate ingestion. J. Appl. Physiol. 64:1480–1485.

Ivy, J.L., M.C.Lee, J.T.Brozinick, and M.J.Reed 1988b Muscle glycogen storage after different amounts of carbohydrate ingestion. J. Appl. Physiol. 65:2018–2023.

Johnson, W.R., and D.H.Black 1953 Comparison of effects of certain blood alkalinizers and glucose upon competitive endurance performance. J. Appl. Physiol. 5:577–78.

Jones, N.L., J.R.Sutton, R.Taylor, and C.J.Toews 1977 Effect of pH on cardiorespiratory and metabolic responses to exercise. J. Appl. Physiol. 43:959–964.

Kreider, R.B., G.W.Miller, M.H.Williams, C.T.Samma, and T.A.Nasser 1990 Effects of phosphate loading on oxygen uptake, ventilatory anaerobic threshold, and run performance. Med. Sci. Sports Exerc. 22:250–256.

Morimoto, T., K.Miki, H.Nose, S.Yamada, K.Hirakawa, and C.Matsubara 1981 Changes in body fluid and its composition during heavy sweating and effect of fluid and electrolyte replacement. Jpn. J. Physiol. 18:31–39.

Nakamura, Y., and A.Schwartz 1972 The influence of hydrogen ion concentration on calcium binding and release by skeletal muscle sarcoplasmic reticulum. J. Gen. Physiol. 59:22–32.

Newsholme, E.A., and A.R.Leech 1983 Pp. 784–787 in Biochemistry for the Medical Sciences. Chicester, United Kingdom: Wiley.

Nilsson, L.H., and E.Hultman 1974 Liver and muscle glycogen in man after glucose and fructose infusion. Scand. J. Clin. Lab. Invest. 33:5–10.

Nose, H., G.W.Mack, X.Shi, and E.R.Nadel 1988 Role of osmolality and plasma volume during rehydration in humans. J. Appl. Physiol. 65:325–331.

Pardridge, W.M., and W.M.Oldendorf 1975 Kinetic analysis of blood-brain barrier transport of amino acids. Biochim. Biophys. Acta 401:128–136.

Reed, M.J., J.T.Brozinick, M.C.Lee, and J.L.Ivy 1989 Muscle glycogen storage postexercise: Effect of mode of carbohydrate administration. J. Appl. Physiol. 66:720–726.

Saltin, B. 1964 Circulatory response to submaximal and maximal exercise after thermal dehydration. J. Appl. Physiol. 19:1125–1132.

Schneider, S.H., P.M.Komanicky, M.N.Goodman, and N.B.Ruderman 1981 Dichloroacetate: Effects on exercise endurance in untrained rats. Metabolism 30:590–595.

Schwabe, A.D., L.R.Bennett, and L.P.Bowman 1964 Octanoic acid absorption and oxidation in humans. J. Appl. Physiol. 19:335–337.

Sherman, W.M., D.L.Costill, W.J.Fink, and J.M.Miller 1981 The effect of exercise and diet manipulation on muscle glycogen and its subsequent utilization during performance. Int. J. Sports Med. 2:114–118.

Spriet, L.L. 1991 Blood doping and oxygen transport. Pp. 213–284 in Ergogenics, Enhancement of Performance in Exercise and Sport, D.R.Lamb and M.H.Williams, eds. Ann Arbor, Mich.: William C.Brown.

Spriet, L.L., D.A.MacLean, D.J.Dyck, E.Hultman, G.Cederblad, and T.E.Graham 1992 Caffeine ingestion and muscle metabolism during prolonged exercise in humans. Am. J. Physiol. 262:E891-E898.

Stanko, R.T., R.J.Robertson, R.J.Spina, J.J.Reilly, Jr., K.D.Greenawalt, and F.L.Goss 1990a Enhancement of arm exercise endurance capacity with dihydroxyacetone and pyruvate. J. Appl. Physiol. 68:119–124.

Stanko, R.T., R.J.Robertson, R.W.Galbreath, J.J.Reilly, Jr., K.D.Greenawalt, and F.L.Goss 1990b Enhanced leg exercise endurance with a high-carbohydrate diet and HRT dihydroxyacetone and pyruvate. J. Appl. Physiol. 69:1651–1656.2

Stewart, I., L.McNaughton, P.Davies, and S.Tristram 1990 Phosphate loading and the effects on in trained cyclists. Res. Q. Exerc. Sport 61:80–84.

Sutton, J.R., N.L.Jones, and C.J.Toews 1976 Growth hormone secretion in acid-base alterations at rest and during exercise. Clin. Sci. 50:241–247.

Trivedi, B., and W.H.Danforth 1966 Effect of pH on the kinetics of frog muscle phosphofructokinase. J. Biol. Chem. 241:4110–4112.

Whitehouse, S., R.H.Casper, and P.J.Randle 1974 Mechanism of activation of PDH by DCA and other halogenated carboxylic acids. Biochem. J. 141:761–774.

Yaspelkis, III, B.B., and J.L.Ivy 1991 Effect of carbohydrate supplements and water on exercise metabolism in the heat. J. Appl. Physiol. 71:680–687.

Yaspelkis, III, B.B., J.G.Patterson, P.A.Anderla, A.Ding, and J.L.Ivy 1993 Carbohydrate supplementation spares muscle glycogen press during variable intensity exercise. J. Appl. Physiol. 75:1477–1485.

Zawadzki, K.M., B.B.Yaspelkis III, and J.L.Ivy 1992 Carbohydrate-protein complex increases the rate of muscle glycogen storage after exercise. J. Appl. Physiol. 72:1854–1859.

13

Effects of Nutrients on Neurotransmitter Release1

Richard J.Wurtman[2]

INTRODUCTION

Contrary to earlier expectations, it has now become well established that the amounts of neurotransmitter released when certain neurons fire normally vary over a broad range. One process that generates such variations involves receptors on the neurons' own presynaptic terminals: when activated by the neurotransmitter molecules that the neuron has released into the synapse, by concurrently released neuromodulators such as adenosine, or by other transmitters (e.g., the enkephalins) released at axoaxonal synapses, these receptors initiate intracellular events that diminish the number of neurotransmitter molecules released subsequently.

Another type of process that particularly affects the release of amine neurotransmitters depends on changes in the composition of the blood plasma induced by eating or by prolonged physical activity. Changes in plasma levels of choline or of certain amino acids lead to changes in brain levels of the

[1] Portions of this manuscript have been adapted from Wurtman (1988).

[2] Richard J.Wurtman, Massachusetts Institute of Technology, E25–604, Cambridge, MA 02139

precursors for these neurotransmitters—choline for acetylcholine, tryptophan for serotonin, and tyrosine for the catecholamines. These, in turn, regulate the *rates* at which the transmitters are synthesized, their *concentrations* within nerve terminals, and ultimately, the *quantities released* each time the neurons fire. For one transmitter—serotonin—the relevant variations in plasma composition probably affect most, if not all, of the neurons that release it. For other transmitters (e.g., the catecholamines), individual nerve cells can become more or less precursor dependent at any time, depending on the rates at which they happen to be firing.

Unlike the receptor-mediated presynaptic modulation of transmitter release, precursor-dependent modulation depends primarily on metabolic events occurring outside the brain and arising from a particular type of voluntary behavior, such as eating or exercise. Indeed, the primary physiological role of this dependency may be sensory (i.e., to provide the omnivore's brain with information about what has been eaten or about important changes in macronutrient requirements, so that the individual can better decide what to eat next). However, because precursor-dependent neurotransmitters are involved in a wide variety of normal (and pathological) brain mechanisms besides those controlling food intake, this relationship may have broad physiological and medical implications. It also provides benign ways of influencing neurotransmission, and thus mental and physical performance.

FOOD CONSUMPTION, TRYPTOPHAN AVAILABILITY, AND BRAIN SEROTONIN SYNTHESIS

The initial observation that physiological changes in precursor availability (i.e., after food consumption) could affect neurotransmitter synthesis was made in studies on rats performed in 1971 (Fernstrom and Wurtman, 1971). Animals were allowed to eat a test diet that contained carbohydrates and fat but that lacked protein. Soon after the start of the meal, brain levels of the essential (and scarce) amino acid tryptophan were found to have risen, thus increasing the substrate saturation of the enzyme that controls serotonin synthesis, tryptophan hydroxylase. The resulting increase in brain serotonin levels was associated with an increase in brain levels of serotonin's metabolite, 5-hydroxyindole acetic acid, thus suggesting that serotonin release had also been enhanced. (Direct evidence that physiological variations in brain tryptophan concentrations affect serotonin release was not obtained until 1987 [Schaechter and Wurtman, 1989].)

The rise in brain tryptophan levels after consumption of this test diet was accompanied by either a small increase (rats) or no change (humans) in plasma tryptophan levels. Both of these changes had been unanticipated, since the insulin secretion elicited by dietary carbohydrates was known to lower plasma levels of most of the other amino acids. However, the unusual response of plasma tryptophan to insulin was soon recognized as resulting from the amino acid's unusual propensity to bind loosely to circulating albumin. Insulin causes nonesterified fatty acid molecules to dissociate from albumin and to enter adipocytes. This dissociation increases the protein's capacity to bind circulating tryptophan; hence, whatever reduction insulin causes in free plasma tryptophan levels is compensated for by a rise in the tryptophan bound to albumin, yielding no net change in total plasma tryptophan levels in humans (Madras et al., 1974). Because this binding is of low affinity, the albumin-bound tryptophan is almost as able as free tryptophan to be taken up into the brain.

Considerably more difficult to explain were the data then obtained on what happens to brain tryptophan and serotonin levels after rats consume a meal rich in protein. Although plasma tryptophan levels were found to rise, reflecting the contribution of some of the tryptophan molecules in the protein, brain tryptophan and serotonin levels either failed to rise or, if the meal contained sufficient protein, actually fell (Fernstrom and Wurtman, 1972). The explanation for this paradox was found to lie in the transport systems that carry tryptophan across the blood-brain barrier (Pardridge, 1977) and into neurons. The endothelial cells that line central nervous system capillaries contain various macromolecules that shuttle specific nutrients or their metabolites between the blood and the brain's extracellular space. One such macromolecule mediates the transcapillary flux (by facilitated diffusion) of tryptophan and other large neutral amino acids (LNAAs) such as tyrosine; others move choline, basic or acidic amino acids, hexoses, monocarboxylic acids, adenosine, adenine, and various vitamins. The amount of any LNAA transported by the macromolecule depends on its ability to compete with the other circulating LNAAs for binding sites. Thus, the ability of circulating tryptophan molecules to enter the brain is increased when plasma levels of the other LNAAs fall (as occurs after insulin is secreted) and is diminished when the plasma levels of the other LNAAs rise, even if plasma tryptophan levels remain unchanged. Since all dietary proteins are considerably richer in the other LNAAs than in tryptophan (only 1.0–1.5 percent of most proteins), consumption of a protein-rich meal decreases the plasma/tryptophan ratio (the ratio of the plasma tryptophan concentration to the summed concentrations of its major circulating competitors for brain uptake, principally, tyrosine; phenylalanine; the branched-chain amino acids leucine, isoleucine, and valine; and methionine). This, in turn, decreases tryptophan's transport into the brain and slows its conversion to serotonin. (Similar plasma ratios predict brain levels of each of the other LNAAs —including drugs such as levodopa (L-dopa)—following meals or other treatments that modify plasma amino acid patterns (Wurtman et al., 1980). This is why a high-protein meal interferes with levodopa's therapeutic effect, whereas a high-carbohydrate, protein-free meal can lead to abnormal movements caused by too much levodopa suddenly entering the brain (Wurtman et al., 1988).

The fact that administration of pure tryptophan could increase brain serotonin synthesis, thereby affecting various serotonin-dependent brain functions (e.g., sleepiness and mood), has been known since at least 1968. What was novel and perhaps surprising about the above findings was their demonstration that brain tryptophan levels—and serotonin synthesis—normally undergo important variations in response, for example, to the decision to eat a carbohydrate-rich (as opposed to a protein-rich) breakfast or in response to the administration of a very low dose of tryptophan (Fernstrom and Wurtman, 1971).

It remained possible, however, that mechanisms external to the serotonin-releasing neuron might exist. These mechanisms kept such food-induced increases in serotonin's synthesis from causing parallel changes in the amounts released into synapses. Indeed, it was known that if rats were given very large doses of tryptophan that were sufficient to raise brain tryptophan levels well beyond their normal range, the firing frequencies of their serotonin-releasing raphe neurons decreased markedly; this was interpreted as reflecting the operation of a feedback system designed to keep serotonin release within a physiological range. Similar decreases in raphe firing had also been observed in animals given drugs, such as monoamine oxidase (MAO) inhibitors or serotonin-reuptake blockers, which cause persistent increases in intrasynaptic serotonin levels. Indeed, the administration of serotonin uptake inhibitors such as fluoxetine can cause the prolonged inhibition of serotonin release (Gardier and Wurtman, 1991). However, when rats were given small doses of tryptophan that were sufficient to raise brain tryptophan levels but not beyond their normal peaks or when they consumed a carbohydrate-rich meal, which raised brain tryptophan levels physiologically, no decreases in raphe firing occurred. Hence, food-induced changes in serotonin synthesis were found to affect the amounts of serotonin released per firing without slowing the neuron's firing frequencies, thus "allowing" modulation of the net output of information from serotonergic neurons.

BRAIN SEROTONIN, NUTRIENT CHOICE, AND CARBOHYDRATE CRAVING

If rats are allowed to pick from foods in two pans presented concurrently and containing differing proportions of protein and carbohydrate, they choose among the two so as to obtain fairly constant (for each animal) amounts of these macronutrients. However, if before "dinner" they receive either a carbohydrate-based snack or a drug that facilitates serotonergic neurotransmission, they quickly modify their food choice, selectively diminishing their intake of carbohydrates (Wurtman and Wurtman, 1979). These observations support the hypothesis that the responses of serotonergic neurons to food-induced changes in the relative concentrations of plasma amino acids allow these neurons to serve a special function as sensors in the brain's mechanisms governing nutrient choice (Wurtman, 1983, 1988). Perhaps these neurons participate in a feedback loop through which the composition of breakfast (i.e., its proportions of protein and carbohydrate) can, by increasing or decreasing brain serotonin levels, influence the choice of lunch. The ability of serotonin-containing neurons to distinguish between two foods (or the net compositions of two meals or snacks) depends upon the extent to which the foods produce significantly different plasma tryptophan/LNAA ratios. Thus, a food (e.g., berries for rats or popcorn for people) which contains carbohydrates but little or no protein is easily distinguished from one (e.g., meat or eggs) that is rich in protein. Less easily distinguished would be one containing, say, 10 percent protein from one containing 15 percent protein, unless one of the foods happens to lack carbohydrates entirely (Yokogoshi and Wurtman, 1986). Perhaps the food-plasma-serotonin connection evolved because certain carbohydrates taste *too* good; to maintain its muscle mass, the bear must eventually stop eating honey and go catch a fish.

A similar mechanism may operate in humans and may underlie the tendency of people in all known cultures to eat about 13 percent of their total calories as protein and about four to five times as much carbohydrate as protein. Subjects housed in a research hospital were allowed to choose from six different isocaloric foods (containing varying proportions of protein and carbohydrate but constant amounts of fat) at each meal, taking as many small portions as they liked; they also had continuous access to a computer-driven vending machine stocked with mixed carbohydrate-rich and protein-rich isocaloric snacks. It was observed (Wurtman and Wurtman, 1989) that the basic parameters of each person's food intake (total number of calories, grams of carbohydrate and protein, and number and composition of snacks) tended to vary only within a narrow range on a day-to-day basis and to be unaffected by placebo administration.

To assay the involvement of brain serotonin in maintaining this constancy of nutrient intake, pharmacological studies were undertaken in individuals in whom the feedback mechanism might be impaired. These were obese people who claimed to suffer from carbohydrate craving, manifested as their tendency to consume large quantities of carbohydrate-rich snacks, usually at a characteristic time of day or evening (Wurtman et al, 1985). (Too few protein-rich snacks were consumed by the subjects to allow assessment of drug effects on this source of calories.) Administration of dexfenfluramine, an antiobesity drug that increases intrasynaptic serotonin levels by releasing the transmitter and then blocking its reuptake, suppressed this carbohydrate craving. Other drugs thought to enhance serotonin-mediated neurotransmission selectively (e.g., the antidepressants zymelidine, fluvoxamine, and fluoxetine) have also been found to cause weight loss over the short term and may also selectively suppress carbohydrate intake. This contrasts with the weight gain (and carbohydrate craving) often associated with less chemically specific antidepressants such as amitriptyline.

Severe carbohydrate craving is also characteristic of patients suffering from seasonal affective disorder syndrome (SADS), a variant of bipolar clinical depression associated with a fall onset, a higher frequency in populations living far from the equator, and concurrent hypersomnia and weight gain (O'Rourke et al., 1989). A reciprocal tendency of many obese people to suffer from affective disorders (usually depression) has also been noted. Since serotonergic neurons apparently are involved in the actions of both appetite-reducing and antidepressant drugs, they might constitute the link between a patient's appetitive and affective symptoms. Some patients with disturbed serotonergic neurotransmission might present themselves to their physicians with problems of obesity, reflecting their overuse of dietary carbohydrates to treat their dysphoria. (The carbohydrates, by increasing intrasynaptic serotonin, would mimic the neurochemical actions of bona fide antidepressant drugs, such as the MAO inhibitors and tricyclic compounds [Wurtman, 1983].) Other patients might complain of depression, and their carbohydrate craving and weight gain would be perceived as secondary problems. Another group might include women suffering from premenstrual syndrome (PMS) who experience late-luteal-phase mood disturbances, weight gain, carbohydrate craving (Brzezinski et al., 1990), and sometimes bloating and fluid retention. Yet another group includes people attempting to withdraw from nicotine (Spring et al., 1991), a drug that releases serotonin (Ribeiro et al., submitted for publication). The participation of serotonergic neurons in a large number of brain functions besides nutrient choice regulation might have the effect of making such functions hostages to eating (seen in the sleepiness that can, for example, follow carbohydrate intake), just as it could cause mood-disturbed individuals to consume large amounts of carbohydrates for reasons related to neither the nutritional value nor the taste of these foods. In support of this view, it was observed that the serotonergic drug dexfenfluramine can be an effective treatment for both the affective and the appetitive symptoms of SADS (O'Rourke et al., 1989), PMS (Brzezinski et al., 1990), and smoking withdrawal (Spring et al., 1991).

UNDER WHAT CIRCUMSTANCES WILL NUTRIENT INTAKE AFFECT NEUROTRANSMISSION?

On the basis of the tryptophan-serotonin relationship, one can formulate a sequence of biochemical processes that would have to occur in order for any nutrient precursor to affect the synthesis and release of its neurotransmitter product.

First, plasma levels of the precursor (and of other circulating compounds, such as the LNAAs, that affect tryptophan's availability to the brain) must be allowed to increase after its administration (or after its consumption as a constituent of foods). In other words, plasma levels of tryptophan, the other LNAAs, or choline cannot be under tight homeostatic control comparable to, for example, that of plasma calcium or osmolarity. In actuality, plasma levels of tryptophan, tyrosine, and choline do vary severalfold after the consumption of normal foods, and those of the branched-chain amino acids may vary by as much as five- or sixfold.

Second, the brain level of the precursor must be dependent on its plasma level (i.e., there must not be an absolute blood-brain barrier for circulating tryptophan, tyrosine, or choline). In fact, such absolute barriers do not exist for these nutrients; rather, facilitated diffusion mechanisms that allow these compounds to enter the brain at rates that depend on the plasma levels of these ligands are in operation.

Third, the rate-limiting enzyme within presynaptic nerve terminals that initiates the conversion of the precursor to its neurotransmitter product must, similarly, be unsaturated with this substrate so that when presented with more tryptophan, tyrosine, or choline it can accelerate synthesis of the neurotransmitter. (Tryptophan hydroxylase and choline acetyltransferase [CAT] do indeed have very poor affinities for their substrates tryptophan and choline.) As discussed below, tyrosine hydroxylase activity becomes tyrosine-limited when neurons containing the enzyme have been activated and the enzyme has been phosphorylated (Wurtman, 1988; Wurtman et al., 1980).

Available evidence suggests that only some of the neurotransmitters present in the human brain are subject to such precursor control, principally, the monoamines mentioned above (serotonin; the catecholamines dopamine, norepinephrine, and epinephrine; and acetylcholine) and, possibly, histidine and glycine. Pharmacological doses of the amino acid histidine do elevate histamine levels within nerve terminals, and the administration of threonine, a substrate for the enzyme that normally forms glycine from serine, can elevate glycine levels within spinal cord neurons (and, probably, thereby ameliorate some of the clinical manifestations of spasticity [Growdon et al., 1991]). One large family of neurotransmitters, the peptides, is almost certainly not subject to precursor control. Brain levels of these compounds have never been shown to change with variations in brain amino acid levels; moreover, there are sound theoretical reasons why it is unlikely that brain peptide synthesis would respond. The immediate precursor for a brain protein or peptide is not an amino acid per se, as is the case for some of the monoamine neurotransmitters, but the amino acid molecule attached to its particular species of transfer RNA (tRNA). In brain tissue, the known enzymes that catalyze the coupling of an amino acid to its tRNA have very high affinities for their amino acid substrates, such that their ability to operate at full capacity in vivo is probably unaffected by amino acid levels (except possibly in pathological states that are associated with major disruptions in brain amino acid patterns, such as phenylketonuria).

Little information is available concerning the possible precursor control of the nonessential amino acids, such as glutamate, aspartate, and γ-aminobutyric acid (GABA), even though these are probably the most abundant neurotransmitters in the brain. It is difficult to do experiments on these relationships; the precise biochemical pathways that synthesize glutamate and aspartate within nerve terminals are not well established, and for GABA, although it is well established that its precursor is glutamate, brain levels of that amino acid cannot be raised experimentally without sorely disrupting normal brain functions. The macromolecule that transports acidic amino acids such as glutamate and aspartate across the blood-brain barrier is unidirectional and secretes these compounds from the brain into the blood by an active transport mechanism (Pardridge, 1977). Hence, administration of even an enormous dose of monosodium glutamate will not affect brain glutamate levels unless it elevates plasma osmolarity to the point of disrupting the blood-brain barrier.

TYROSINE EFFECT ON DOPAMINE AND NOREPINEPHRINE SYNTHESIS

Because tyrosine administration had not been shown to increase brain dopamine or norepinephrine levels in otherwise untreated animals, it was initially assumed that the catecholamine neurotransmitters were not under precursor control, even though (1) plasma tyrosine levels do increase severalfold after protein intake or tyrosine administration; (2) the LNAA transport system does ferry tyrosine, like tryptophan, across the blood-brain barrier; and (3) tyrosine hydroxylase, which catalyzes the rate-limiting step in catecholamine synthesis, is unsaturated in vivo (Wurtman et al., 1980). It did seem possible, however, that a pool of neuronal dopamine or norepinephrine might exist for which synthesis did depend on tyrosine levels, but which was of too small a size in relation to the total catecholamine mass to be detected.

Hence, studies were performed to determine whether catecholamine synthesis or release could be affected by changes in brain tyrosine concentrations. At first, catecholamine synthesis was estimated by following the rate at which dopa, the product of tyrosine's hydroxylation, accumulated in the brains of rats treated acutely with a drug that blocks the next enzyme in catecholamine formation (aromatic L-amino acid decarboxylase). Tyrosine administration did increase dopa accumulation, whereas other LNAAs decreased both dopa accumulation and brain tyrosine levels. Catecholamine release was then estimated by measuring the brain levels of metabolites of dopamine (homovanillic acid [HVA], dihydroxyphenylacetic acid [DOPAC]) or norepinephrine (methoxyhydroxyphenylglycol sulfate [MHPH-SO_4]). Administration of even large doses of tyrosine had no consistent effect on these metabolites. However, if the experimental animals were given an additional treatment designed to accelerate the firing of dopaminergic or noradrenergic tracts (e.g., dopamine receptor blockers, cold exposure, partial lesions of dopaminergic tracts, and reserpine), the supplemental tyrosine caused a marked augmentation of catecholamine release (Wurtman, 1988; Wurtman et al., 1980). These initial observations formed the basis for the hypothesis that catecholaminergic neurons become tyrosine sensitive when they are physiologically active and lose this capacity when they are quiescent.

The biochemical mechanism that couples a neuron's firing frequency to its ability to respond to supplemental tyrosine involves phosphorylation of the tyrosine hydroxylase enzyme protein, a process that occurs when the neurons fire. This phosphorylation, which is short-lived, enhances the enzyme's affinity for its cofactor (tetrahydrobiopterin) and makes the enzyme insensitive to end product inhibition by catechols; these changes allow its net activity to depend on the extent to which it is saturated with tyrosine. An additional mechanism underlying this coupling may be an actual depletion of tyrosine within nerve terminals as a consequence of its accelerated conversion to catecholamines (Milner et al., 1987). If slices of rat caudate nucleus are superfused with a standard Krebs-Ringer solution (which lacks amino acids) and are depolarized repeatedly, they are unable to sustain their release of dopamine; concurrently, their contents of tyrosine, but not of other LNAAs, decline markedly. The addition of tyrosine to the superfusion solution enables the tissue to continue releasing dopamine at initial rates and also protects it against depletion of its tyrosine. The concentrations of tyrosine needed for these effects are proportional to the number of times the neurons are depolarized. (Of course, the intact brain is continuously perfused with tyrosine-containing blood, making it highly unlikely that tyrosine levels fall to a similar extent, even in continuously active brain neurons. However, they might decline somewhat, since tyrosine is poorly soluble in aqueous media and diffuses relatively slowly.)

More recently, in vivo dialysis techniques have been used to assess tyrosine's effects on brain dopamine release. When otherwise untreated animals receive the amino acid systemically, there is, after 20–40 min, a substantial increase in dopamine output from nigrostriatal neurons unaccompanied by detectable increases in dopamine's metabolites DOPAC or HVA. However, this effect is short-lived, and dopamine release returns to basal levels after 20–30 min. This latter response probably reflects receptor-mediated decreases in the firing frequencies of the striatal neurons (to compensate for the increase in dopamine release that occurs with each firing) and, perhaps, local presynaptic inhibition. If animals are given haloperidol, a dopamine receptor-blocking agent, before—or along with—the tyrosine, the supplemental tyrosine continues to amplify dopamine output for prolonged periods (During et al., 1989).

Tyrosine has now been shown to enhance the production and release of dopamine or norepinephrine in a variety of circumstances. This amino acid may ultimately have considerable utility in treating catecholamine-related diseases or conditions; it may also prove useful in promoting performance— particularly in high-stress situations.

EFFECTS OF CHOLINE ON SYNTHESIS OF ACETYLCHOLINE AND PHOSPHATIDYLCHOLINE

The amounts of acetylcholine released by physiologically active cholinergic neurons depend on the concentrations of choline available. In the absence of supplemental free choline, the neurons will continue to release constant quantities of the transmitter, especially when stimulated (Maire and Wurtman, 1985). However, when choline is available (in concentrations bracketing the physiological range), a clear dose relationship is observed between its concentration and acetylcholine release (Blusztajn and Wurtman, 1983; Marie and Wurtman, 1985). When no free choline is available, the source of the choline used for acetylcholine synthesis is the cells' own membranes (Blusztajn et al., 1987). Membranes are very rich in endogenous phosphatidylcholine (PC), and this phospholipid serves as a reservoir of free choline, much as bone and albumin serve as reservoirs for calcium and essential amino acids. It has been suggested that a prolonged imbalance between the amounts of free choline available to a cholinergic neuron and the amounts needed for acetylcholine synthesis might alter the dynamics of membrane phospholipids to the point of interfering with normal neuronal functioning ("autocannibalism") (Blusztajn and Wurtman, 1983; Nitsch et al., 1992a), for example, in patients with Alzheimer's disease. In that event, providing the brain with supplemental choline would serve two purposes: it would enhance acetylcholine release from physiologically active neurons and it would replenish the choline-containing phospholipids in their membranes (Wurtman, 1985).

Neurons can draw on three sources of free choline for acetylcholine synthesis: that stored as PC in their own membranes, that formed intrasynaptically from the hydrolysis of acetylcholine (and taken back up into the presynaptic terminal by a high-affinity process estimated to be 30–50 percent efficient in the brain), and that present in the bloodstream (and taken into the brain by a specific blood-brain barrier transport system). The PC in foods (e.g., liver and eggs) is rapidly hydrolyzed to free choline in the intestinal mucosa (or is broken down more slowly after passage into the lymphatic circulation). Consumption of adequate quantities of PC can lead to severalfold elevations in plasma choline levels, thereby increasing brain choline levels and the substrate saturation of CAT.

The PC molecules consumed in the diet, as well as those formed endogenously in neuronal membranes, are very heterogeneous with respect to their fatty acid compositions. Some PCs (e.g., those in soybeans and nerve terminals) are relatively rich in polyunsaturated fatty acids; others (e.g., those in eggs) are highly saturated. PCs are also heterogeneous with reference to their mode of synthesis. Brain neurons produce PC by three distinct biochemical pathways: the sequential methylation of phosphatidylethanolamine (PE), the incorporation of preexisting free choline via the CDP-choline cycle, or the incorporation of free choline via the base exchange pathway (in which a choline molecule substitutes for the ethanolamine in PE or the serine in phosphatidylserine [PS]). Quite possibly, the different varieties of PC may subserve distinct functions; for example, one type of PC, distinguished by its fatty acid composition or its mode of synthesis, could be preferentially utilized to provide a choline source for acetylcholine synthesis or could be formed preferentially during the processes of cell division or synaptic remodeling. Similarly, one particular species might be especially involved in the pathogenesis of particular degenerative diseases afflicting cholinergic neurons (e.g., Alzheimer's disease).

Supplemental choline or PC has been used with some success in the treatment of tardive dyskinesia. A summary of related publications (Nasrallah et al., 1984) concluded that choline and the cholinesterase inhibitor physostigmine were about equally efficacious and that choline was less toxic. Most patients exhibited some reduction in the frequency of abnormal movement, but in only a few cases was there complete cessation of the movements. Choline sources have also been tried in the treatment of Alzheimer's disease. Most well-controlled studies have treated subjects for relatively short intervals (6–8 weeks) and have focused on younger subjects, with little or no success. A single double-blind study administered the PC for 6 months (Little et al.,

1985). Improvement was noted in about one-third of the subjects; the average age of the responders was 83 years and that of nonresponders was 73 years, a relationship thought to be compatible with evidence that Alzheimer's disease may be more restricted to cholinergic neurons in subjects who become symptomatic at a later age. Occasional reports have also described the useful effects of choline or PC in treating mania, ataxia, myasthenic syndromes, and Tourette's syndrome. Very recently it has been observed (Nitsch et al., 1992a) that the brains of people dying of Alzheimer's disease (but not Down's Syndrome) contain reduced levels of PC and free choline (and PE and free ethanolamine) but major increases in those of the PC metabolite glycerophosphocholine and the PE metabolite glycerophosphoethanolamine. These changes were not restricted to regions containing plaques, tangles, or amyloid. Since low brain choline levels both impair acetylcholine synthesis and accelerate the breakdown of membrane PC and since adequate acetylcholine may be needed to prevent the formation of the amyloid protein of Alzheimer's disease (Nitsch et al., 1992b), supplemental choline and ethanolamine could have a role in the prevention of this disease.

CONCLUSIONS AND RECOMMENDATIONS

- The design of experiments to display the potentially useful effects of foods and nutrients on the ability to perform well, particularly under stressful circumstances, will require considerable sophistication. These chemicals are not nearly as potent as drugs and, in fact, lack intrinsic potency, having first to be converted to a neurotransmitter within a nerve terminal and then to be released from that terminal. (Of course, they are also likely to be significantly less toxic than drugs; this is perhaps their major advantage.) Such experimental design should be entrusted to people who are well trained in studying human behavior and who also fully understand the ground rules that determine when the food or nutrient is most likely to be effective (e.g., for tyrosine, when particular catecholamine-releasing neurons are firing frequently for long periods).
- At this point, too few adequate experiments have been done with human subjects to begin to assess the utilities of neurotransmitter precursors such as tyrosine or choline in increasing or sustaining performance; in fact, a number of poorly designed studies muddy the waters. Tyrosine's effect on performance must be examined in situations in which subjects are under real stress. Choline's effects on memory must be studied in experiments in which the nutrient is given for a sufficiently long period of time (i.e., one compatible with what is known about the dynamics of the choline-phosphatidylcholine interaction).

- The peripheral actions of the neurotransmitter precursors may turn out to be very useful (e.g., tyrosine's ability to normalize blood pressure when it is both too high and too low [Wurtman et al., 1980] and choline's ability to sustain exercise tolerance in subjects whose plasma choline levels have been reduced by, for example, long-distance running [Conlay et al., 1986; Sandage et al., 1992]).
- The development of foods or nutrients used to sustain performance—or otherwise to improve normal behaviors—requires guidance by the U.S. Food and Drug Administration, and perhaps other agencies as well, regarding how these compounds will be regulated. It is absolutely mandatory that all such preparations be safe and of adequate purity; it is also essential that they be adequately labeled, providing the user with full information about their indications, dosages, contraindications, and side effects. However, if and when it can be shown that their use is largely nutritional (i.e., to meet the body's needs for more of the particular nutrient because environmental circumstances have increased those needs), then perhaps they can be designated as *foods.*
- Considerable additional research should be done to identify special populations with unusual responses to foods or nutrients that affect neurotransmitters (e.g., the carbohydrate cravers who overconsume carbohydrate-rich snacks in order to relieve depressive symptoms). Heterogeneity of response will doubtless also exist among people in the military (e.g., those with mild seasonal depression or premenstrual syndrome and those giving up smoking).

ACKNOWLEDGMENTS

Some of these studies were supported by National Institute of Mental Health grant MH-28783, U.S. Air Force grant AFOSR-830366, National Aeronautics and Space Administration grant NAG-2–210, and National Institutes of Health grant RR00088–24 to the Clinical Research Center, Massachusetts Institute of Technology.

REFERENCES

Blusztajn, J.K., and R.J.Wurtman 1983 Choline and cholinergic neurons. Science 221:614–620.

Blusztajn, J.K., M.Liscovitch, U.I.Richardson, and R.J.Wurtman 1987 Phosphatidylcholine as a precursor of choline for acetylcholine synthesis. Pp. 341–346 in Cellular and Molecular Basis of Cholinergic Function. M.J.Dowdall and J.N. Hawthorne, eds. Chichester (Sussex), U.K.: Ellis Harwood.

Brzezinski, A.A., J.J.Wurtman, R.J.Wurtman, R.Gleason, T.Nader, and B.Laferrere 1990 D-fenfluramine suppresses the increased calorie and carbohydrate intakes and improves the mood of women with premenstrual syndrome. Obstet. Gynecol. 76:296–301.

Conlay, L., R.J.Wurtman, J.K.Blusztajn, G.Lopez-Coviella, T.J.Maher, and G.E.Evoniuk 1986 Decreased plasma choline concentrations in marathon runners. N. Eng. J. Med. 315:892.

During, M.J., I.N.Acworth, and R.J.Wurtman 1989 Dopamine release in rat striatum: Physiological coupling to tyrosine supply. J. Neurochem. 52:1449–1454.

Fernstrom, J.D., and R.J.Wurtman 1971 Brain serotonin content: Physiological dependence on plasma tryptophan levels. Science 173:149–152.

1972 Brain serotonin content: Physiological regulation by plasma neutral amino acids. Science 178:414–416.

Gardier, A., and R.J.Wurtman 1991 Persistent blockade of potassium-evoked serotonin release from rat frontocortical terminals after fluoxetine administration. Brain Res. 540:325–330.

Growdon, J.H., T.M.A.Nader, D.Schoenfeld, and R.J.Wurtman 1991 L-Threonine in the treatment of spasticity. Clin. Neuropharm. 14(5):403–412.

Little, A., R.Levy, P.Chaqui-Kidd, and D.Hand 1985 A double-blind placebo controlled trial of high-dose lecithin in Alzheimer's disease. J Neurol. Neurosurg. Psychiatry 48:736–742.

Madras, B.K., E.L.Cohen, R.Messing, H.N.Munro, and R.J.Wurtman 1974 Relevance of serum-free tryptophan to tissue tryptophan concentrations. Metabolism 23:1107–1116.

Maire, J.-C., and R.J.Wurtman 1985 Effects of electrical stimulation and choline availability on release and contents of acetylcholine and choline in superfused slices from rat striatum. J. Physiol. (Paris) 80:189–195.

Milner, J.D., D.K.Reinstein, and R.J.Wurtman 1987 Dopamine synthesis in rat striatum: Mobilization of tyrosine from non-dopaminergic cells. Experientia 43(10):1109.

Nasrallah, H.A., F.L.Dunner, R.E.Smith, M.McCalley-Whitters, and A.D.Sherman 1984 Variable clinical response to choline in tardive dyskinesia. Psychol. Med. 14:697–700.

Nitsch, R., J.K.Blusztajn, A.Pittas, B.E.Slack, J.H.Growdon, and R.J.Wurtman 1992a Evidence for a membrane defect in Alzheimer's disease brain. Proc. Natl. Acad. Sci. USA 89:1671–1675.

Nitsch, R., B.Slack, R.Wurtman, and J.Growdon 1992b Processing of Alzheimer amyloid precursor stimulated by activation of muscarinic acetylcholine receptors. Science 258(9):304–307.

O'Rourke, D., J.Wurtman, R.Wurtman, R.Chebli, and R.Gleason 1989 Treatment of seasonal depression with D-fenfluramine. J. Clin. Psychiatry 50:343–347.

Ribeiro, E., R.Bettiker, M.Bogdanov, and R.J.Wurtman 1993 Effects of systemic nicotine on serotonin release in rat brain. Brain Res. 621:311–318.

Pardridge, W.M. 1977 Regulation of amino acid availability to the brain. Pp. 141–204 in Nutrition and the Brain, vol. 7, R.J.Wurtman and J.J.Wurtman, eds. New York: Raven Press.

Sandage, B.W., Jr., L.Sabounjian, R.White, and R.J.Wurtman 1992 Choline citrate may enhance athletic performance. Abstract. Fall meeting of the American Physiological Society.

Schaechter, J., and R.J.Wurtman 1989 Tryptophan availability modulates serotonin release from rat hypothalamic slices. J Neurochem. 53:1925–1933.

Spring B., J.Wurtman, R.Gleason, R.Kessler, and R.J.Wurtman 1991 Weight gain and withdrawal symptoms after smoking cessation: A preventive intervention using D-fenfluramine. Health Psy. 10(3):216–223.

Wurtman, J.J., and R.J.Wurtman 1979 Drugs that enhance central serotonergic transmission diminish elective carbohydrate consumption by rats. Life Sci. 24:895–904.

Wurtman, J.J., R.J.Wurtman, S.Mark, R.Tsay, W.Gilbert, and J.Growdon 1985 D-fenfluramine selectively suppresses carbohydrate snacking by obese subjects. Int. J. Eating Disord. 4:89–99.

Wurtman, R.J. 1983 Behavioral effects of nutrients. Lancet 1:145–147.

1985 Alzheimer's disease. Sci. Am. 252:62–75.

1988 Presynaptic control of release of amine neurotransmitters by precursor levels. NIPS (Am. Physiol. Soc.) 3:158–163.

Wurtman, R.J., and J.J.Wurtman 1989 Carbohydrates and depression. Sci. Ame. :68–75.

Wurtman, R.J., F.Hefti, and E.Melamed 1980 Precursor control of neurotransmitter synthesis. Pharmacol. Rev. 32:315.

Wurtman, R.J., B.Caballero, and E.Salzman 1988 Facilitation of levodopa-induced dyskinesias by dietary carbohydrates. N. Engl. J. Med. 319:1288–1289.

Yokogoshi, H., and R.J.Wurtman 1986 Meal composition and plasma amino acid ratios: Effects of various proteins or carbohydrates, and of various protein concentrations. Metabolism 35:837–842.

DISCUSSION

WILLIAM WATERS: It occurred to me during various presentations that there is a difference between what happens to a nutrient when it is taken in a pure form and when it is taken in a natural food form. Does anybody have any information that they might share with us?

RICHARD WURTMAN: Take tryptophan ortyrosine as an example. If these are taken as constituents of dietary protein, much of what is taken in is just converted by the body to its own protein; very little of it enters the brain because of competition with other large neutral amino acids.

On the other hand, if tryptophan or tyrosine are taken alone, the body converts little or none of it to its own protein and much of it goes into the brain because of the lack of competition. That is the good news if you are looking for a drug effect; but not if you're not looking for a drug effect.

WILLIAM WATERS: The qualitative difference is: does that translate into behavior?

RICHARD WURTMAN: In the case of tryptophan versus carbohydrate, for instance, I think Harris Lieberman or Bonnie Spring would be better able to answer whether or not the effects of tryptophan are qualitative.

BONNIE SPRING: My comment was just that, qualitatively, they are very similar, but tryptophan is much more powerful.

WILLIAM WATERS: My comment was to agree with Bonnie Spring and to emphasize the fact that tryptophan produces clear effects that are quite easy to observe.

WILLIAM BEISEL: Should there be any concern for high-dose tryptophan, for the possibility that it may go to oxidative metabolism?

RICHARD WURTMAN: Timothy Maher was on the committee that reviewed that.

TIMOTHY MAHER: We have concerns that I will discuss tomorrow regarding the use of any amino acid in its pure form apart from protein. There were many concerns about the conversion of amino acids into other products that have never been studied. Therefore, your concern is one that is shared because the answer is not known.

ELDON ASKEW: This is directed to John Ivy: It seems like the provision of sugars during exercise elicits insulin responses to exercise, but the provision of simple sugar seems to be what would be provided during exercise. In the recovery phase you want something that stimulates insulin production to stimulate glycogen synthesis. Is it not appropriate to use polymers, glucose polymers, in the recovery phase? Should we be using a simpler sugar in the recovery phase?

JOHN IVY: Actually, some of the polymers that are used in drinks have a glycemic index—not much difference—so I do not think it is much of a problem.

IRWIN TAUB: For John Ivy also: You show that the fats were not very good as an additional energy source during exercise. That is, of course, short term. But what about high fat on a longer-term basis? Would that ultimately lead to some sparing with a glycogen, for example?

JOHN IVY: Let me back up. I think if you can get the fat in and get it converted out of the free fatty acids or somehow get large amounts of medium-chain triglycerides in, which seems to be difficult—I do not know all the ins and outs about possibilities for that—it may be beneficial. Taking a high-fat meal and then injecting heparin so that the triglycerides are broken down into free fatty acids does seem to be beneficial in sparing carbohydrate and enhancing endurance performance.

If you are talking about taking high-fat meals over a long period of time, we can go back a long ways. I think back during World War II they were looking at that with the Canadian Army, giving something called pemmican. That did not improve performance at all. In fact, it caused deterioration.

ROBERT NESHEIM: I think Ed Horton had a comment relative to that.

EDWARD HORTON: I think the pemmican studies were faulty because there was no adaptation. But a lot of people have looked at adaptation of high-fat, low-carbohydrate diets both in terms of intensity and duration of exercise.

I think the bottom line of that is that you can adapt: you lower your RQ [respiratory quotient], and you burn more fatty acid and less carbohydrate at moderate-intensity exercise. But everybody has shown that once you have to put out high-intensity exercise you still have an absolute requirement for carbohydrate oxidation. So they have not really panned out in terms of being able to enhance performance at high intensities.

IRWIN TAUB: But, as was pointed out, marching is equivalent to 40 percent $\dot{V}_{O_2\ max}$ [maximum oxygen uptake]. So the question is, would it be useful in that context?

EDWARD HORTON: I think that the answer is maybe, when you are interested in trying to get high-caloric-density foods so that you can get more calories in with less weight. In fact, we reviewed this a couple of years ago in quite some detail. I think that the feeling was that you are okay at moderate-intensity exercise, but everybody has to put out a high-intensity exercise at some point. Under those circumstances, the high-fat diets do not stack up to having carbohydrates.

JOHN MILNER: I was really trying to understand what was going on. You presented information that the carbohydrate loading would improve performance. Then you turned right around and said that increasing free fatty acids would also do that.

I think that, mechanistically, when one is up, the other is down; so it should not work that way. Can you tell me mechanistically why you would think that an elevation in free fatty acids would be the same as ....

EDWARD HORTON: They function differently.

JOHN MILNER: So is it energy supply that really is a principal factor more than anything else?

EDWARD HORTON: If you have a substantial amount of free fatty acids in the blood, the rate of uptake of muscle free fatty acids is somewhat proportional to the amount available. You increase beta-oxidation. The high free fatty acid levels in the blood seem to block glucose transport as well as increase citrate levels in the muscle, which blocks lipolysis.

So you convert your reliance—you increase your reliance—on fats and spare carbohydrate, and therefore, you are able to work longer.

Typically, when you start exercising, you are not burning optimally the carbohydrates that are required for the exercise. You are actually burning more than what is required because there are plenty available. But if you can block that use initially above and beyond what is necessary, you can spare the carbohydrate and work longer. That is what the fats seem to be doing.

JOHN MILNER: So it is just this sparing, short-term effect in essence?

EDWARD HORTON: Short term from the standpoint that you can work 4 hours rather than 3 hours at 70 percent of maximum $\dot{V}_{O_2\ max}$.

PEGGY BORUM: My question has to do with the different fuel sources that are available. This afternoon we heard that it makes a difference, depending upon what is eaten and also on the intensity and duration of exercise.

My assumption is that these studies like Alan Sherrington's in dogs, were with dogs that were well fed. What we heard this morning is that many individuals in the field are actually not maintaining their energy requirements and are actually not taking in enough fuel on a chronic basis, that is, they are losing weight. When you superimpose these experiments that did not have that element, how does that affect the fuel that is actually available to the muscles of these individuals when we give them stress such as sleep deprivation and then ask them to exercise at a fairly high intensity for an extended period of time?

EDWARD HORTON: That is a good point because you are right; most of the studies that have been done on dietary manipulation have been done on people who are on good caloric intakes.

PEGGY BORUM: Or dogs.

EDWARD HORTON: We have not really talked at all about protein turnover in these people out in the field in terms of what is happening to protein synthesis and protein degradation and the protein turnover rates that are going on when they are hypocaloric (losing weight). We know that they have a negative caloric balance and are losing weight. That certainly has to have an impact on muscle strength and for its immobilization of amino acids for gluconeogenesis, for example.

I think there is some real need for studies in that area that look at the effect of the stress hormone response, for example, on gluconeogenesis and glucose output in the liver when you may have a limitation of substrate in the form of amino acid substrates.

STEVEN ZEISEL: A number of people have described insulin growth factor [IGF] 1 and IGF 2 and shown that IGF 1, for instance, dropped very markedly during early malnutrition, very modest malnutrition.

Now they are using IGF 1 to increase anabolic metabolism and appetite in patients who have cachexia. Have any of you studied changes in IGF 1 at the same time you are studying the other parameters during exercise and starvation in these marching soldiers?

KARL FRIEDL: We looked at it in Rangers last year. It went down to about 50 percent of the normal level. I guess that is an adaptation of the semistarvation, the intense exercise, and the weight loss and sleep deprivation. It is a multistress environment.

DAVID SCHNAKENBERG: It is a cross between people who are doing nutrition work and people who are doing sleep work. Most people are engaged in doing sleep research. Do you know of any studies where they have tried to monitor what people are eating during the course of these 72 hours? Is there any change in terms of what they are eating during that period of time as to how much and when; or do you force people to eat?

GREGORY BELENKY: We keep track pretty much; we limit them. In our PET studies, which we are doing in collaboration with John Hopkins at the Gerontological Research Center, we are actually letting them ad lib it and we are keeping track of exactly what they eat and what they do not so we will have a much better notion of what their caloric intake is.

What we have done up to this time is simply state that this is the meal, this is what you get, here it is. During the sleep deprivation period, we provide snacks at around 2:00 in the morning. Of course, we see the nice regular decline in body temperature across the sleep deprivation period superimposed on the circadian cycle.

RICHARD WURTMAN: How many different foods can they choose from? Do they have a range of carbohydrate, protein, et cetera?

HARRIS LIEBERMAN: Yes, basically they have TV dinners, Healthy Choice, for example.

RICHARD WURTMAN: So they cannot decide they want to eat just the carbohydrates; they have to go with the whole thing?

HARRIS LIEBERMAN: No.

RICHARD WURTMAN: That is a shame because it does not really answer your question to see whether or not these people become carbohydrate cravers in the middle of the night, for instance. I would predict that they would.

DAVID SCHNAKENBERG: They are just looking at the possibility that there may be some opportunities for using diet as an augmentation to maintaining awareness.

HARRIS LIEBERMAN: First, I wanted to say that there is some evidence in the literature on both animals and humans that sleep deprivation produces hyperphagia. I do not know of anyone who actually studied whether that hyperphagia is specific or related to carbohydrate; one would certainly guess that it might be.

The other thing I wanted to mention was undernutrition. The Ranger study is really an extreme of undernutrition. There was a very important study that Eldon Askew did—the RLW30 study—where soldiers were deprived of a portion of their nutrition for a period of a month. They got about 2,000 calories per day but were burning something like 3,200 calories.

As part of that study, we measured both their physical and mental performances. There were only the subtlest changes in both as a function of a full month of undernutrition.

ROBERT NESHEIM: I remember that those studies were done for a month.

ELDON ASKEW: And they had plenty of sleep.

ROBERT NESHEIM: Yes, plenty of sleep.

MELVIN MATHIAS: John Ivy, you were alluding to this branched-chain amino acid cocktail and exercise enhancement. You were only using a neurotransmitter mechanism. Maybe Wayne Askew or Ed Horton can expand on the glucose-alanine cycle and the status of it. I do appreciate that there is not much energy in that cycle, but I think it still has some interest. I do not know how important that might be in the branched chain or if they used that in a hypothesis.

JOHN IVY: They did not use it in a hypothesis. I brought it up just because I saw that people were going to talk about it. I do not know much about the study.

ROBERT NESHEIM: There will be some more discussion of amino acids tomorrow.

JOHN MILNER: There are other studies also showing increases in protein synthesis or retention—the increase in protein degradation especially in the diaphragm. So I assume that some of that relates to that as well as anything else.

WILLIAM BEISEL: You have to remember there is a profound metabolic adaptation to the difference between simple starvation and the cachexia that results from the acute-phase reaction which causes hypermetabolism and gets most of the energy from muscle breakdown. So we have a profound difference here, and we have to determine what the soldiers are facing.

PATRICK DUNNE: As more of a follow-up on the pathways that we are looking at in muscle, in the branched-chain, I hear one strategy is to recognize that muscle will use branched-chain amino acids for energy much better than other tissues will. So, indeed, you might be sparing some of your other energy requirements and maybe feeding your alanine cycle. That is one of the strategies.

EDWARD HORTON: If you look at it quantitatively, the branched-chain amino acids oxidized by exercising muscle never contribute more than 1 or 2 percent of the total energy. It is true that the amino groups are basically converting to alanine with pyruvate, so you can feed that way.

Quantitatively, it is just a very small thing. I cannot believe that it has any major effect on exercise performance in the same way that giving a carbohydrate supplement would or from trying to get the body to use more fatty acids and spare carbohydrates. It is just quantitatively too small.

PATRICK DUNNE: With regard to the related issue of all proteins not being the same, which protein were you using in your supplement?

JOHN IVY: We were using milk isolate and whey.

PATRICK DUNNE: So it is basically a whey protein. Richard Wurtman showed that different proteins give some spectrum of ratio of the large neutral amino acids to the others. So one could be very leery when you say a universal response to protein. A casein may have one response.

PEGGY BORUM: I think part of the theory is that in exercise and in other conditions where free fatty acid levels increase in the plasma, the free fatty acid competes with the tryptophan, at least theoretically, and that you wind up getting more free tryptophan instead of it being bound to albumin because the free fatty acids and the tryptophan are competing.

Theoretically, that is very interesting, but I do not know whether anyone has any data to show that really takes place, where, if you increase the free fatty acid concentration in the plasma, you actually increase the tryptophan concentration in the plasma enough to increase serotonin production in the brain.

RICHARD WURTMAN: We spent about 2 years figuring it out. It does not matter because albumin-bound tryptophan is transported into the brain about 79 percent as effectively as free tryptophan. There is a slight retardation associated with binding of the tryptophan molecule to albumin, but it is so slight that unless you have a mega increase in free fatty acid levels, it is not going to matter or have much of an effect on brain tryptophan levels.

There used to be a great debate 15 or 18 years ago about the determinant of tryptophan's uptake into the brain: is it competition with large neutral amino acids, or is it the proportion that is bound to albumin?

Then definitive studies were done by Pardriole's and other people showing just what I have said.

PEGGY BORUM: But if you add free fatty acids into the mix, does the presence of free fatty acids have some effect?

RICHARD WURTMAN: Yes, it will increase free tryptophan in plasma, but it will not have much of an effect on the passage of plasma tryptophan into the brain.

PEGGY BORUM: That is the only effect?

RICHARD WURTMAN: That is the only effect.

EDWARD HORTON: I wanted to come back to the question that Peggy Borum asked earlier, and what Bill Beisel just said kind of triggered my thinking about this. If you look at people in negative caloric balance—simple starvation, with, say, anorexia nervosa, or people who have been starving or who are hypocaloric—hepatic glucose production actually decreases to very low baseline levels. Go back to the classic George Cahill-type studies. They decrease their gluconeogenic amino acids, they slow down hepatic glucose production to about half of normal, and basically reach an adapted state.

It is just the opposite of what is happening in these stress situations, and that is what I was trying to point out. With stress, it is very similar to exercise, where you increase peripheral utilization, and hepatic glucose production increases to match the peripheral utilization. In a stress situation, you are driving hepatic glucose production it seems, and it is very catabolic.

So if you take somebody out in the field and you are not giving them enough calories to meet their demands and they are under a lot of stress, they are going to be very, very catabolic under that circumstance.

ROBERT NESHEIM: I think that is true. Studies of moderate undernutrition in people show how they adapt. They cut down on their activities. If you are in a situation where you cannot cut down your activities—and as a matter of fact, you are forced to be active—then the picture is totally different.

JOHN IVY: Edward Horton, do you think that individuals under stress and exercise, for example, in a situation of combat where they are actually physically active and under stress, would require more carbohydrates?

EDWARD HORTON: I cannot tell you what the experimental data would show, but I would predict that they would. The real question to me is whether by giving them more carbohydrate in their diet can you affect hepatic glucose production and slow it down. You might be able to to some extent, but I think that some of the earlier studies looking at endotoxin responses show that you cannot shut it off. Also, some of the trauma studies from John Penny show that you cannot shut off hepatic glucose production even when giving glucose.

14

Performance-Enhancing Effects of Protein and Amino Acids

Carol E.Greenwood[1]

INTRODUCTION

The objective of this chapter is to consider whether manipulations of dietary amino acids (AAs) can be used to enhance the performance of military personnel in combat situations. The ultimate concern is whether the combined physiologic and psychologic stresses associated with combat situations, which can lead to negative effects on the performance of the individual, can be overcome or minimized through the provision of specialized diets or AA supplements. Time frames involving both acute and chronic administration will be considered, and the following questions will be asked. First, can the performance of an individual be influenced over the short term (several hours) by provision of specialized meals or AAs? Second, since military personnel may find themselves in combat situations for prolonged periods of time, can the overall diet be modified to help individuals overcome the continuing stress associated with combat situations?

This chapter specifically deals with the potential performance-enhancing effects of AAs. AAs can be provided to the individual either as intact proteins

[1] Carol E.Greenwood, Department of Nutritional Sciences, Faculty of Medicine, University of Toronto, Toronto, Ontario, Canada M5S 1A8 and Baycrest Centre for Geriatric Care, North York, Ontario, Canada M6A 2E1

or in the free form. Furthermore, free AAs either can be administered as single supplements or can be incorporated into existing foods. Therefore, provision of AAs in all these forms will be considered.

EFFECT OF DIETARY PROTEIN: LONG-TERM CONSIDERATIONS

Under normal circumstances, the adequacy of protein in the typical North American diet is not a concern. The Recommended Nutrient Intake (RNI) (Health and Welfare, Canada, 1990a) for protein for Canadians meets or exceeds the needs of almost all individuals in the population. Furthermore, chronic levels of protein intake are well above the RNI (Food and Agriculture Organization of the United Nations/World Health Organization/United Nations University), 1985; Health and Welfare Canada, 1990a; National Research Council, 1980, 1985).

The relevant issue here is whether the chronic high levels of stress under combat situations influence the protein requirements of the individual. Unfortunately, direct experimental evidence is not available; however, there is evidence that the chronic physiologic stress associated with endurance training in athletes may raise protein requirements. The protein requirements needed to maintain the nitrogen (N) balance of bodybuilders and endurance athletes were 12 and 88 percent higher, respectively, in comparison with those of sedentary individuals (Tarnopolsky et al., 1988). If it is assumed that the physical demands of combat are analogous to those experienced by endurance athletes, then these data would suggest that protein requirements are indeed increased under combat situations. The 88 percent increase in protein requirements would raise the RNI for protein from 0.86 g/kg/day in adult males to 1.61 g/kg/day (Table 14–1). Under normal circumstances, the potential increase in protein requirements would be more than offset by the increased energy intake associated with high activity levels. For example, changes in nutrient intake were examined in Navy servicemen during a 5-day period known as Hell Week (Smoak et al., 1988), during which subjects are subjected to conditions similar to those anticipated under combat situations. During Hell Week, average energy intake increased from 18.7 to 24.4 MJ/day. This was accompanied by an increase in protein intake from 189 to 260 g/day (approximately 2.6 and 3.4 mg/kg/day, respectively, on the basis of reported average body weights of 72.9 and 75.6 kg, respectively, at the beginning and end of the experimental period), which could be accounted for entirely on the basis of increased energy intake. Clearly, even if protein requirements were increased during the simulation of combat conditions, the diet provided more than sufficient protein to meet these additional requirements.

TABLE 14–1 Effect of Exercise on Protein Requirements of Athletes

Training Status	Protein Intake to Maintain N Balance (g/kg/day)*	Increase in Protein Needs to Maintain N Balance (percent)	Predicted Safe Levels of Protein Intake (g/kg/day)
Sedentary individuals	0.73	—	0.86†
Bodybuilders	0.82	12	0.96
Endurance athletes	1.37	88	1.61

*Values taken from Tarnopolsky et al. (1988).

†The recommended safe level of protein intake for male adults (Health and Welfare Canada, 1990a) was used as the baseline for sedentary individuals. Predicted safe levels of protein intake for bodybuilders and endurance athletes were calculated on the basis of the percent increase in protein needs to maintain N balance.

Unfortunately, however, despite its intent, Hell Week is unable to simulate all situations associated with real combat. Under these conditions, actual food intake would be expected to decrease (see chapters 7 and 8), and the decrease may be severe enough that the individual is in both negative energy balance and negative N balance. Thus, perhaps of more relevance is the degree to which food shortage, in and of itself, has a negative impact on performance. The impact of energy deficit, in combination with food supplementation, on work performance was examined in Gambian subsistence farmers during a period of natural food shortage (Diaz et al., 1991). No benefit of food supplementation on work productivity could be detected. Thus, it would appear that, at least over the short term, food shortages or energy deficits do not impair an individual's ability to perform physically demanding tasks. What was not addressed in that study, however, was whether higher forms of performance, such as cognitive performance including decision making, were influenced by the energy deficit. Obviously, it will be important to determine whether cognitive skills are sensitive to energy deficits and whether they can be improved with food supplements.

EFFECT OF DIETARY PROTEIN: SHORT-TERM CONSIDERATIONS

The degree to which short-term (meal-to-meal) changes in protein and carbohydrate (CHO) ingestion have an impact on mood and performance has received considerable attention over the past several years (see chapters 17 and 15 for a more extensive review). These studies were a natural extension of research demonstrating that acute administration of specific AAs and/or ingestion of relatively pure CHO and protein sources could alter neuronal synthesis and perhaps the release of certain monoaminergic neurotransmitters (Wurtman et al., 1981). Given this area of research focus, it is therefore appropriate to ask whether controlled manipulations of the protein or CHO content of individual meals can produce desired performance outcomes.

Probably the most extensively examined aspect of protein ingestion is its influence on appetite regulation (Anderson and Li, 1987). Ingestion of high-protein meals is associated with satiety in both experimental animals (Li and Anderson, 1982) and humans (Barkeling et al., 1990). In comparison with high-CHO meals, intake of high-protein meals selectively reduces protein intake as well as total food intake in the subsequent meal. Whether these satiating effects of protein would continue to be observed under stressful conditions is unknown. Indeed, physiologic and psychologic changes associated with highly stressful circumstances could easily be hypothesized to override the normal signals that regulate appetite. Nevertheless, these research data open the possibility that high-protein meals may prolong satiety in the individual, and there may be certain circumstances in which this effect of protein ingestion could be used to advantage.

The mood or performance of the individual may also be influenced by the protein or CHO content of individual meals (see Chapter 17 for a more extensive review). That is, consumption of high-CHO meals in comparison with consumption of either mixed meals or high-protein meals may be associated with fatigue (Deijen et al., 1989; Spring et al., 1989). However, the response to CHO ingestion is variable and differs depending on the age and gender of the individual (Spring et al., 1982–83). Unfortunately, the degree to which behavioral effects of CHO consumption would be observed under combat situations is unknown at present because prior studies have been conducted under nonstressful circumstances.

ROLE OF INDIVIDUAL AAS OR MIXTURES OF AAS

Space limitations preclude an extensive examination of all AAs with regard to their potential performance-enhancing effects, and detailed reports on the impact of single-AA supplementation can be found elsewhere (Health and Welfare Canada, 1990b; (Federation of the American Societies for Experimental Biology, Life Sciences Research Office, 1992). At present, the most promising effect of AA supplementation appears to be with tyrosine (TYR).

The benefit of TYR supplementation probably relates to the fact that it is a precursor to the neurotransmitter norepinephrine and can increase norepinephrine synthesis under conditions in which the neuron is actively firing, such as stress (Wurtman et al., 1981). Provision of TYR under stressful conditions simulating certain combat situations may be associated with a reversal of the observed neurochemical changes and behavioral improvement (see Chapters 15 and 16 for an overview of the impact of TYR supplementation). Clearly, this area warrants further investigation.

There is little evidence at present that provision of other AAs will be of benefit (reviewed in Health and Welfare Canada, 1990b; Life Sciences Research Office, 1992). Indeed, most other AAs appear to have little or no behavioral effects in humans. The one exception may be tryptophan (TRP), which, at high doses, may be an effective hypnotic and useful in the treatment of certain forms of insomnia as well as a useful adjunct to monoamine oxidase inhibitors in the treatment of affective disorders (reviewed in Health and Welfare Canada, 1990b); however, this effect of TRP is unlikely to have application in combat situations.

Consideration should be given, however, to the provision of the branched-chain amino acids (BCAAs), isoleucine, leucine, and valine, as a mixed AA supplement. Early interest in this area related to observations that BCAA catabolism may be increased during prolonged exercise (Henriksson, 1991; Wagenmakers et al., 1989), and the question arose as to whether these AAs should be provided to replenish those presumably used by the exercising muscle. The degree of activation of BCAA catabolism after prolonged, intense exercise is small, however (Wagenmakers et al., 1989), and is not observed in all studies (Tarnopolsky et al., 1991). Furthermore, evidence suggests that proteins or AAs do not contribute substantially as an energy source during exercise (Henriksson, 1991; Wagenmakers et al., 1989). Thus, there appears to be little justification for BCAA supplementation on the basis of replenishing the BCAAs oxidized during exercise.

Nevertheless, there is a report of improved mental performance, measured as the performance in the Stroop Color and Word Test, in subjects given BCAAs during a 30-km cross-country race (Blomstrand et al., 1991). The authors suggest that this effect of the BCAAs may relate to changes in the plasma AA profile and uptake of other AAs, such as TRP, into the brain. Clearly, this area warrants replication and perhaps further experimentation.

ROLE OF DIET IN MODULATING RESPONSE TO AA SUPPLEMENTATION

The background diet fed to an individual, the form in which supplementation is accomplished, and the frequency of AA supplementation may all have an impact on an individual's response to AAs. Careful consideration of these factors must be taken to determine the most effective means of providing AA supplements.

Clearly, if the intent of AA supplementation, for example, TYR, is to raise brain AA levels, the least effective way to accomplish this is to incorporate the AA into prepared meals, especially those containing protein. This is simply due to the fact that plasma levels of other AAs that compete for the same brain uptake carrier will also rise following protein ingestion (Wurtman et al., 1981) . This is particularly important for the large neutral amino acids (LNAAs), including TYR and TRP, since relatively large increases in plasma levels of the competing LNAAs would be anticipated. The overall impact would be to minimize TYR's or TRP's ability to enter the central nervous system (CNS). Rather, the more effective way to increase brain TYR or TRP levels would be to administer it in the absence of other foods during a postprandial period when the plasma levels of the other competing AAs would be at their lowest.

In addition to this acute effect of meal ingestion, the protein level in the chronic background diet may also have an impact on responsiveness to AA supplementation. Plasma AA levels are not only reflective of recent meal ingestion but are also sensitive to the chronic level of protein intake (Glanville and Anderson, 1985; Peters and Harper, 1985). For example, when rats are fed diets that vary in protein concentration from 15 to 50 percent (w/w), and plasma AA levels are measured in the fasting state, a dose-dependent increase in indispensable AAs is observed (Peters and Harper, 1985), with the greatest changes being observed in the BCAAs. Because the BCAAs compete with other LNAAs for entry into the brain, it was postulated that the chronic background diet fed to an animal would influence the ability of the administered TRP to enter the CNS even when the TRP was given to fasting animals. Indeed, brain TRP levels were significantly lower in animals fed a 40 percent protein diet in comparison with those consuming a 12 percent protein diet (Table 14–2). Thus, it would appear that the lower the protein concentration of the chronic diet, the greater the likelihood that individual LNAAs will enter the CNS, even when they are administered in the fasting state.

Finally, consideration should be given to the frequency of AA administration. Sustained high plasma levels of a supplemented AA may result in hepatic induction of AA catabolic enzymes (Harper et al., 1970), thereby minimizing the impact of supplementation. Intermittent dosing schedules may have to be developed to circumvent an increase in AA catabolism.

TABLE 14–2 Effect of Chronic Dietary Protein Level on the Response of Brain Tryptophan Levels to Tryptophan Administration*

Dietary Protein Level (percent)	Brain Tryptophan Levels (μg/g)† after the Administration of the Following Dose of Tryptophan (mg/kg of body weight)				
	0	25	50	75	100
12	5.4±0.5‡	18.8±0.7§	35.2±2.0″	64.1±4.3#	59.0±5.4#
40	5.9±0.6‡	14.2±0.7‡§	18.2±1.1§	33.9±3.2″	44.9±4.3#

* Rats were fed either 12 or 40 percent casein diets for 15–16 days and received intraperitoneal injections of tryptophan 8 h after ingestion of the last meal. Brain tryptophan levels were measured 60 min after peripheral tryptophan administration.

†Data are means±standard errors of the means (*n*=6/dose). Values in the same row not sharing the same superscripts are significantly different (*P*<0.05). Data adapted from Shwery (1989).

SUMMARY AND CONCLUSIONS

There is evidence that the protein requirements of endurance athletes may be increased, thereby suggesting that the chronic physical demands of combat situations may increase the protein requirements of military personnel. However, if energy needs are met in the individual, the increase in protein consumption associated with increased food intake will more than meet the protein requirements of the individual. More realistic, however, is a situation in which food intake is decreased under combat situations because of a number of adverse physical and psychologic conditions. Although an energy deficit may not be associated with diminished performance of physically demanding tasks, the impact of an energy deficit on other indices of performance, including cognitive performance, is not well understood.

Provision of meals high in either protein or CHO may influence satiety and certain aspects of mood and performance. However, this effect of meal composition is variable and can be influenced by the age and gender of the individual. Furthermore, the impact of altering meal composition on mood and behavior has not been examined under stressful situations simulating combat. Thus, further studies are warranted prior to assessing the usefulness of this approach.

Supplementation with certain AAs, notably TYR and BCAAs, may play a useful role under stressful conditions; however, studies on the BCAAs are very preliminary in nature. Further studies on TYR are warranted, as its effectiveness has been indicated under circumstances simulating certain aspects of combat situations.

The chronic diet of an individual will influence his or her response to supplemental AAs, especially if the effect is mediated by the CNS. This impact of chronic diet is secondary to changes in plasma AA levels and competition at the blood-brain barrier for uptake into the CNS.

Finally, to maximize and maintain the effectiveness of supplemental AAs, they should not be administered with meals and should be provided on an intermittent basis. Consumption of protein-containing foods in combination with the supplemented AAs may not produce the desired change in plasma AA profiles, especially if CNS uptake of the supplemented AAs is desired. Furthermore, continued elevated plasma levels of the supplemented AAs may result in induction of its catabolic enzymes. Hence, intermittent dosing schedules should be developed to circumvent this.

REFERENCES

Anderson G.H., and E.T.S.Li 1987 Protein and amino acids in the regulation of quantitative and qualitative aspects of food intake. Int. J. Obes. 11(suppl. 3):97–108.

Barkeling, B., S.Rossner, and H.Bjorvell 1990 Effects of a high-protein meal (meat) and a high-carbohydrate meal (vegetarian) on satiety measured by automated computerized monitoring of subsequent food intake, motivation to eat and food preferences. Int. J. Obes. 14:743–751.

Blomstrand E., P.Hassmen, B.Ekblom, and E.A.Newsholme 1991 Administration of branched-chain amino acids during sustained exercise-effects on performance and on plasma concentration of some amino acids. Eur. J. Appl. Physiol. 63:83–88.

Deijen J.B., M.L.Heemstra, and J.F.Orlebeke 1989 Dietary effects on mood and performance. J. Psychiatr. Res. 23:275–283.

Diaz E., G.R.Goldberg, M.Taylor, J.M.Savage, D.Sellen, W.A.Coward, and A.M.Prentice 1991 Effects of dietary supplements on work performance in Gambian laborers. Am. J. Clin. Nutr. 53:803–811.

Federation of the American Societies for Experimental Biology, Life Sciences Research Office 1992 Safety of amino acids used as dietary supplements. Center for Food Safety and Applied Nutrition. FDA Contract No. 223–88–2124, Task No. 8.

Food and Agriculture Organization of the United Nations/World Health Organization/United Nations University 1985 Energy and Protein Requirements. Report of a Joint FAO/WHO/UNU Expert Consultation. Geneva, WHO Technical Report Series No. 724. Geneva: World Health Organization.

Glanville N.T., and G.H.Anderson 1985 The effect of insulin deficiency, dietary protein intake and plasma amino acids on brain amino acid levels in rats. Can. J. Physiol. Pharmacol. 10:603–610.

Harper A.E., N.J.Benevenga, and R.M.Wohlhueter 1970 Effects of ingestion of disproportionate amounts of amino acids. Physiol. Rev. 50:428–558.

Health and Welfare, Canada 1990a Nutrition Recommendations: The Report of the Scientific Review Committee. Ottawa, Ontario, Canada: Supply and Services Canada.

1990b Report of the Expert Advisory Committee on Amino Acids. Ottawa, Ontario, Canada: Drugs Directorate, Health Protection Branch, Department of National Health and Welfare.

Henriksson, J. 1991 Effect of exercise on amino acid concentrations in skeletal muscle and plasma. J. Exp. Biol. 160:149–165.

Li, E.T.S., and G.H.Anderson 1982 Meal composition influences subsequent food selection in the young rat. Physiol. Behav. 29:779–783.

National Research Council 1980 Recommended Dietary Allowances, 9th ed. Report of the Food and Nutrition Board, Committion on Life Sciences, Washington, D.C.: National Academy Press.

1985 Nutrient Adequacy: Assessment Using Food Consumption Surveys. Report of the Subcommittee on Criteria of Dietary Evaluation, Food and Nutrition Board, Commission on Life Sciences, National Research Council. Washington, D.C.: National Academy Press.

Peters J.C., and A.E.Harper 1985 Adaptation of rats to diets containing different levels of protein: Effects on food intake, plasma and brain amino acid concentrations and brain neurotransmitter metabolism. J. Nutr. 115:382–398.

Shwery, M.M. 1989 Effect of Chronic Dietary Protein Concentration on the Neurochemical Response to Tryptophan Administration. M.Sc. Thesis. University of Toronto, Toronto, Ontario, Canada.

Smoak B.L., A.Singh, B.A.Day, J.P.Morton, S.B.Kyle, S.J.Pepper, and P.A.Deuster 1988 Changes in nutrient intakes of conditioned men during a 5-day period of increased physical activity and other stresses. Eur. J. Appl. Physiol. 58:245–251.

Spring B., O.Maller, J.Wurtman, L.Digman, and L.Cozolino 1982-1983 Effects of protein and carbohydrate meals on mood and performance: Interactions with sex and age. J. Psychiatric Res. 17:155–167.

Spring B., J.Chiodo, M.Harden, M.J.Bourgeois, J.D.Mason, and L.Lutherer 1989 Psychobiological effects of carbohydrates. J. Clin. Psychiatry 50 (Suppl.):27–33.

Tarnopolsky M.A., J.D.MacDougall, and S.A.Atkinson 1988 Influence of protein intake and training status on nitrogen balance and lean body mass. J. Appl. Physiol. 64:187–193.

Tarnopolsky M.A., S.A.Atkinson, J.D.MacDougall, B.B.Senor, P.W.R.Lemon, and H. Schwarcz 1991 Whole body leucine metabolism during and after resistance exercise in fed humans. Med. Sci. Sports Exerc. 23:326–333.

Wagenmakers A.J., J.H.Brookes, J.H.Coakley, T.Reilly, and R.H.Edwards 1989 Exercise-induced activation of the branched-chain 2-oxo acid dehydrogenase in human muscle. Eur. J. App. Physiol. 59:159–167.

Wurtman R.J., F.Hefti, and E.Melamed 1981 Precursor control of neurotransmitter synthesis. Pharmacol. Rev. 32:315–335.

DISCUSSION

JOHN MILNER: I have a couple of comments. First, with regard to the toxicity studies that have been done, a lot of those old studies by Jessie Greenstein and others showed that for simultaneous supplementations of arginine, you might want to think in terms of that being a scavenger for the toxicity, because a lot of that relates to ammonia. You did not describe at all the effect of nitric oxide as being a regulator of growth hormone, insulin, or glucagon. Did you comment on that? I am not sure that I know that well enough either.

CAROL GREENWOOD: No, someone else is probably a bit more familiar with that.

GILBERT LEVEILLE: Carol Greenwood, on one of your slides toward the end where you were looking at tryptophan, it seemed like you reached the maximum at 75 mg/kg or whatever it was. Is that the case? There was no statistical difference between the last two treatments.

CAROL GREENWOOD: You are quite right, when you look at the data for animals fed in the low protein diet, brain TRP levels were identical when both 75 and 100 mg/kg of TRP were administered intraperitoneally. This, however was not the case for animals fed the high protein diet where changes in brain TRP were observed across all doses of TRP administered. On first observation, it may suggest that with the lower protein diet, the brain uptake carrier was saturated with 75 mg/kg TRP and hence higher TRP doses would not be effective in further increasing brain TRP levels. This could be consistent with any carrier-mediated process. Nevertheless, we have not reproduced this observation and hence it would not be appropriate to draw any firm conclusions at this time.

WILLIAM BEISEL: I know that when you use arginine and a number of other amino acids you can get hormone responses. I have seen no strong data that show when you give them orally that you get these responses. From tests we have done in our lab, we cannot show any responses with high levels of amino acids with supplements and the growth hormone process.

CAROL GREENWOOD: I know that arginine is a powerful secretagogue for a variety of hormones, including growth hormone. Indeed it can be used clinically as a test for pituitary function. Neverthless, you must remember that in these clinical tests, arginine is given on an acute basis. It would not be surprising that with chronic exposure to arginine that its catabolism would be increased so that in the long term, circulating arginine levels would be within a normal range and that chronic arginine feeding or administration would not result in chronic elevations in plasma hormone levels. Thus it may not be surprising that you do not see an effect with chronic AA treatment.

JOHN IVY: In looking at these data, I am always puzzled with high-protein diets, particularly in studies done in rats. This was done under conditions of adequate hydration.

CAROL GREENWOOD: Yes.

EDWARD HORTON: In situations like feeding military troops, you always have a relative state of dehydration. Has anyone looked at the relative impact of water availability in these kinds of studies, particularly the high-protein diets or high/amino/acid supplementation?

CAROL GREENWOOD: I do not know of any studies looking specifically at compensatory changes in water intake in association with chronic feeding of high protein diets. This is a very important point, particularly in reference to the combat situation where water availability may be severly limited. Nevertheless, there have been numerous studies examining changes in water consumption in association with AA supplementation. For example, studies in Harvey Anderson's laboratory in which they were looking at different mixtures of AA demonstrate that some, but not all, AA stimulate water intake when water availability is unlimited. These studies, however, examined the effect of acute administration of AA and the demands for additional fluid intake to allow for appropriate volumes of urine excretion when AA are administered chronically has not been examined to the best of my knowledge. This may indeed represent a contra-indication for AA supplementation especially in desert-like conditions where adequate hydration is already a problem.

WILLIAM BEISEL: During certain stresses with muscle, there is a breakdown and a release of amino acids. Does that sort of thing happen when somebody takes a large amount of tryptophan?

CAROL GREENWOOD: Yes, it does. You see tryptophan being metabolized by alternate pathways. You also see those kinds of things happening normally with hormone fluctuations in women associated with menstrual cycle activity, so we do see activation of those types of pathways, although I think the important thing that perhaps philosophically has not been addressed is that we have been talking a lot in terms of looking at carbohydrate supplementation associated with exercise. Yet, I think it is clear that, no matter what you are going to do, you are also going to get a lot of things occurring during that period and that, presumably, the amino acids are providing a skeleton in terms of that glucose.

We have not talked at all about the need for protein to replenish those amino acids that were metabolized during that exercise period, so that while the strategy may still indeed be appropriate of looking at carbohydrate loading to support the exercising time, one looks, in terms of replenishment, at the end of it not only in terms of water and electrolytes but perhaps also proteins in general or mixtures of amino acids in particular. Those would be the precursors that one would predict during that period, and that would be a time that would be more appropriate for a supplement.

JOHN IVY: I do not believe that as long as you have sufficient carbohydrates, for instance, amino acids are going to be used very much.

CAROL GREENWOOD: I agree with you in terms of providing optimal nutrients to the muscle during a bout of exercise in an adequately nourished individual. However, I think that when you look at an individual under a chronic stressful situation, that you also need to consider the impact of chronic demands. As stated before, it is highly likely that individuals in the combat situation will not be consuming adequate calories to meet their individuals in the combat situation will not be consuming adequate calories to meet their energy demands and that they will be experiencing repeated periods of prolonged exercise. Under these circumstances, AA may become important energy substrates to the muscle and it may be important to determine whether gucogenic AA have been depleted under these circumstances and whether repleting the AA pool is necessary.

JOHN IVY: I think the major glucogenic precursors during exercise is lactate coming ultimately from breakdown.

EDWARD HORTON: I think this is a very important area. Just to add to what John is saying, I did not mention it in terms of the changes that are going on during postexercise recovery. John Devlin in our group has really looked at glucose and amino acid metabolism during the first 14 hours of postexercise recovery, and John mentioned that you continue to get lactate output from nonexercising muscles if you do cycle exercise and forearm balance studies—there is continued lactate output, actually, insulin resistance, in the nonexercising muscles—so that insulin does not stimulate glucose uptake. The lactate appears to be coming from continued glycogen breakdown.

In addition to that, you also get continued alanine output, and so there is amino acid oxidation going on during the postexercise recovery period with continued alanine. So I think your point is very well taken, that we should be providing the substrates for gluconeogenesis and rebuilding glycogen stores after exercise to both carbohydrate and amino acid.

ROBERT NESHEIM: If a person is eating a regular meal following that, it seems to me you are probably taking care of that.

CAROL GREENWOOD: I would guess so. I mean, I think that under an energy replete situation, protein probably is not an issue. However, in a combative situation where the troops are not eating sufficient food, then I think the whole ballpark changes in terms of the questions that one may want to ask.

15

Tyrosine and Stress: Human and Animal Studies

Harris R.Lieberman[1]

INTRODUCTION

In a variety of combat scenarios, enhancement or prevention of stress-induced decrements in mental performance would be desirable. The use of nutrients to enhance performance may be one strategy for increasing the combat effectiveness of soldiers. Providing even a small edge in effectiveness by using a comparatively benign nutritional intervention could, in theory, significantly improve performance on the battlefield, reduce casualties, and conserve critical material resources. In the classic combat scenario, fear, loss of sleep, and exposure to harsh environmental conditions can be expected to produce substantial decrements in performance. In other situations, such as sentry duty or vehicle operation, boredom and sleepiness can reduce vigilance and cause critical errors. A nutrient that is useful in all circumstances would be of the greatest value as a performance-enhancing ration component. However, it is more likely that a substance that is beneficial in one scenario will have no effect in another scenario or will even have adverse effects if used inappropriately. Therefore, it is likely that the choice of a food constituent

[1] Harris R.Lieberman, U.S. Army Research Institute of Environmental Medicine, ATTN: SGRD-UE-OPN, Natick, MA 01760–5007

or constituents will depend on both the environment and the operational demands of the mission in which it will be used.

One nutrient that may prevent performance decrements caused by exposure to highly stressful environmental or operational conditions is the amino acid tyrosine. This substance is the precursor of several key brain neurotransmitters and may protect against the severe mental fatigue associated with exposure to life-threatening stressors that can occur in combat and certain other critical military operations. Tyrosine does not appear to have the stimulant-like activity of caffeine, so it is not likely to be useful in situations in which performance is degraded by boredom or sleepiness.

BACKGROUND

Tyrosine, a large neutral amino acid (LNAA) normally present in protein-containing foods, is the precursor of the catecholamine (CA) neurotransmitters dopamine (DA), norepinephrine (NE), and epinephrine. When it is systemically administered in pharmacologic quantities, it can, under highly stressful conditions, increase brain CA concentration and turnover (Gibson and Wurtman, 1978; Wurtman et al., 1974, 1981). There are no known adverse effects from tyrosine administration. Also, because tyrosine is normally present in substantial quantities in ordinary foods and is rapidly metabolized, its administration is unlikely to have long-term toxicity or unwanted side effects. In fact, since tyrosine exerts its effects only when a localized deficiency state exists, its effects appear to be system specific and present only when needed, such as when local CA stores are expended. Therefore, tyrosine's actions are likely to be more specific than those of most drugs, but perhaps less potent.

Precursor Coupling

The availability of tyrosine is rate-limiting for the synthesis of its neurotransmitter products only when a higher than normal level of transmitter release by catecholaminergic neurons is occurring. When CA-containing neurons are firing frequently and therefore releasing more transmitter (DA or NE), they may require more of the precursor (tyrosine) that is the substrate for transmitter synthesis. Frequent neuronal firing may enhance the kinetic properties of tyrosine hydroxylase, causing this rate-limiting, CA-synthesizing enzyme to be more susceptible to control by this amino acid or may deplete the tyrosine pools within nerve terminals (Lovenberg et al., 1975; Weiner et al., 1978).

The ability of tyrosine supplementation to enhance the synthesis of CAs in and their release from rapidly firing neurons but not from relatively quiescent cells has been demonstrated by using a variety of experimental manipulations (for a review, see Milner and Wurtman [1986]). Tyrosine administration increases brain levels of the norepinephrine metabolite methoxyhydroxyphenylethylgylcol sulfate (MHPG-SO_4) in cold-stressed rats (Gibson and Wurtman, 1978) and in the brains of spontaneously hypertensive rats (Sved et al., 1979) but not in those of control, normotensive animals. Increases in MHPG-SO_4 levels after tyrosine treatment have also been observed in rats stressed by tailshock (Lehnert et al., 1984a,b; Reinstein et al., 1984). Dopaminergic metabolism also appears to be accelerated by tyrosine administration (Brady et al., 1980).

Catecholamines and Stress

The observation that the function of catecholaminergic neurons can be precursor dependent is the basis for the hypothesis that tyrosine mitigates the adverse effects of acute stress, because such neurons regulate, in part, the behavioral, cardiovascular, and neuroendocrine consequences of stress. It is well established that the noradrenergic neurons of the locus ceruleus and hypothalamus participate in the regulation of a variety of functions that are altered during acute stress. Alertness, attention, activity, anxiety levels, blood pressure, and the secretion of certain hormones are all controlled, at least in part, by these neurons (Antelman and Caggiula, 1977; Gray, 1982; Murphy and Redmond, 1975; Stone, 1975). Certain dopaminergic neurons also appear to participate in the regulation of some of these functions.

There is a great deal of evidence demonstrating that CA-containing neurons play a key role in the regulation of arousal level and anxiety. Data from animal neurochemical and behavioral studies, from animal and human psychopharmacology, and also from clinical observations all contribute to the complex literature that exists on this topic. Because of the diversity of this literature and the extraordinary difficulties associated with any attempt to establish the neurochemical substrate of complex behavioral-cognitive states, such as anxiety, helplessness, and depression, there are many controversial issues in this area. However, in attempts to integrate the diverse data, investigators are in agreement on many key issues (Gray, 1982; Stone, 1975). For example, it is agreed that when animals are subjected to acute stress, especially when the stress cannot be avoided and is highly aversive, an array of behavioral, cardiovascular, neuroendocrine, and neurochemical changes are present (for a review, see Stone [1975]). It appears that the neurochemical substrate for this syndrome is, at least in part, the depletion of readily available central NE stores. Stressful conditions that can deplete central NE stores include cold, heat, restraint, exercise, and footshock (Stone, 1975). Acutely stressed animals become less responsive to their environment, explore less, are less aggressive and more submissive, cannot learn as readily, and generally seem debilitated (Maier and Seligman, 1976; Rapaport and Maier, 1978. The term *learned helplessness* has been applied to certain aspects of this syndrome because animals fail to respond appropriately (escape or avoid) to aversive stimuli when they are given the opportunity to do so (Maier and Seligman, 1976; Maier and Jackson, 1979; Minor et al., 1984; Weiss et al., 1976). This phenomenon has been used to model human clinical depression and posttraumatic stress disorder (Gray, 1982; van der Kolk et al., 1985).

The effects of acute stress are not limited to learning and similar behaviors, but rather, impairments in these behaviors are representative of a broad range of behavioral deficits. The underlying factor that characterizes most of the changes induced by acute stress appears to be inhibition of both spontaneous and stimulus-dependent behaviors. Acutely stressed animals, for the most part, regardless of the specific nature of the stress, generally appear to be unable to function. Not only are complex stimulus-dependent behaviors like aggression, learning, and exploration depressed, but even eating and sleep are disturbed. With the appearance of such behavioral deficits (Gray, 1982; Stone, 1975), brain NE turnover increases substantially and NE stores are depleted. (When the stress is chronic, more complex changes in NE function take place.) It is widely believed that catecholaminergic neurons participate directly in the onset of certain aspects of this acute stress-induced syndrome, which has, in fact, been termed *noradrenergic helplessness* (for a comprehensive review, see Gray [1982]).

The critical role that noradrenergic systems play in this behavioral syndrome is supported by several lines of evidence, including the effects that various pharmacologic interventions known to modify CA transmission have on behavior. Catecholaminergic agonists, for example, tricyclic antidepressants, monoamine oxidase inhibitors (MAO-I), and levodopa (a precursor of dopamine and NE and an intermediate metabolite of tyrosine), acutely reverse some of the negative consequences of stress in animals (Anisman and Sklar 1979; Glazer et al., 1975; Sherman et al., 1979). Also, CA antagonists, for example, inhibitors of tyrosine hydroxylase and dopamine-ß-hydroxylase, impair performance in avoidance or escape tasks. Drugs that primarily block the synthesis of NE, like FLA-63, also produce escape deficits, as do dopamine receptor blockers like haloperidol and pimozide. However, brain dopamine levels are more resistant to stress than brain NE levels (Gray, 1982; Stone, 1975).

Acute Behavioral Consequences of Combat

Little is known about the acute effects of combat and similar life-threatening stressors on human brain function. There is a large, mostly anecdotal literature on the effects of combat on mental processes. Many popular books and articles, as well as military histories, refer to the adverse consequences of combat stress on the performance of soldiers on the battlefield. In one of the few research studies conducted in a combat situation, the affect of Special Forces soldiers in an isolated outpost, deep in enemy territory during the earlier stages of the war in Vietnam, was assessed (Bourne et al., 1968). The primary symptom among these seasoned soldiers was hostility toward higher authorities at headquarters. Among these elite troops, anxiety and depression were not especially elevated. In one of the few laboratory studies that addressed the issue, Villoldo and Tarno (1984) modeled combat using battlefield noise (including simulated ordnance detonations), temperature extremes, chemical protective clothing, and a variety of other physical and psychological stressors. In that study, the subjects' performance on a variety of standardized tests of mental performance were significantly degraded.

Efforts have also been made to formally describe the acute behavioral syndrome that occurs among some soldiers as a consequence of exposure to combat. It has been termed combat stress reaction (CSR), and its principal symptoms are anxiety, fear of death, helplessness, crying, and tiredness. Sleep is also disturbed (Solomon et al., 1989). The behavioral manifestations of the CSR syndrome appear to resemble the helplessness syndrome described in animals. It is likely that the underlying alterations in brain CA function documented in animals subjected to acute stress are also present in humans exposed to the life-threatening stress that characterizes combat.

In many battles, casualties from the CSR syndrome have been extremely high. For example, in Okinawa during World War II, CSR casualties among U.S. soldiers made up 48 percent of all wounded-in-action U.S. battlefield casualties. For the 60 days following D-Day (June 6, 1944) in France, 40 percent of battlefield casualties were due to CSR. On some battlefields, such as the early stages of the 1973 Arab-Israeli war, casualties that resulted from CSR actually exceeded those that resulted from enemy fire (Flora, 1985). These severe losses of personnel that occur during intense combat and that are attributable to CSR indicate that an intervention that would reduce such casualties would be of great benefit. Several recent review articles have discussed the use of tyrosine as a potential countermeasure to improve performance during highly stressful military operations (Owasoyo et al, 1992; Salter, 1989).

TYROSINE AND ACUTE STRESS: STUDIES IN ANIMALS

Many drugs, like the tricyclic antidepressants or MAO-I's, that enhance central catecholaminergic transmission and that are highly effective for the treatment of human depression (after they have been administered for several weeks) have numerous acute and chronic side effects. Their acute side effects, such as drowsiness and impaired cognitive performance (Baldessarini, 1985; Curran, 1992), largely preclude their use under any circumstance in which performance enhancement is the desired outcome. Other drugs that are used to treat human anxiety disorders and acutely reduce anxiety, such as the benzodiazepines, produce acute side effects, such as drowsiness, reduced ability to maintain vigilance, and impaired memory (Koelega, 1989; McNair, 1973). Therefore, one strategy for developing performance-enhancing ration components should emphasize utilization of a nutrient that can increase catecholaminergic activity with minimal side effects.

One nutritional strategy to reduce the consequences of acute stress could be use of the dietary precursor of the CAs, tyrosine. In a number of studies, administration of tyrosine, either systemically just prior to initiation of the stress or as a dietary supplement, has been shown to partially protect animals from both the neurochemical and the behavioral consequences of the stress (Brady et al., 1980; Lehnert et al., 1984a,b; Lieberman et al., 1992; Luo et al, 1992; Rauch and Lieberman, 1990). After acute stress, animals pretreated with tyrosine more actively engage in a variety of normal behaviors in their environment compared with untreated but stressed control animals. Also, unlike stressed control animals not receiving tyrosine, the brain NE levels in treated animals were not depleted (Lehnert et al., 1984a,b).

In several of these studies (Lehnert et al., 1984a,b), tailshock was used to produce acute stress in rats. Following 60 min of such shocks, animals were permitted to recover for 15 min and were then placed in an open-field, hole poke apparatus. After observing their spontaneous behaviors for the next 10 min, the rats were euthanized and their brains were removed. Exposure to this experimental stress paradigm significantly decreased (by approximately 80 percent) open-field locomotor activity and several other spontaneous behaviors, such as rearing and hole poking, in stressed rats compared with the behaviors of unstressed control animals. However, in another group of animals that were given a diet supplemented with tyrosine and that were stressed, the frequency of these spontaneous behaviors did not differ significantly from those in the unstressed control animals. Increased dietary tyrosine apparently protected these animals from the behavioral inhibition produced by the stressor, presumably by augmenting noradrenergic, but also perhaps dopaminergic, neurotransmission (Lehnert et al., 1984a). When a similar study was conducted with rats given single intraperitoneal doses of tyrosine (200 mg/kg of body weight) or placebo immediately prior to tailshock, tyrosine also protected the animals from the acute behavioral depression induced by the stress (Lehnert et al., 1984b). In both of those studies, among the stressed but untreated animals, declines in NE levels of 30 to 40 percent were noted in specific brain regions, such as the hypothalamus, locus coeruleus, and hippocampus. Both studies of Lehnert and colleagues reported that tyrosine administration blocked this depletion. Tyrosine also increased NE turnover in specific regions of the brain of stressed animals, as measured by regional differences in brain MHPG-SO_4 levels.

Tyrosine has also been shown to facilitate several other types of animal behavior under stressful conditions. For example, it has been found to restore normal levels of aggressive behavior in animals that are subjected to cold-water stress (Brady et al., 1980). Additionally, in a stressful behavioral procedure sometimes considered to be a learned helplessness paradigm and used to screen drugs for their antidepressant activities (the Porsolt swim test [Porsolt et al., 1978]), significant dose-related potentiation of escape behavior following tyrosine administration has been observed (Gibson et al., 1982). The Porsolt test is conducted by placing the animal in a cylinder containing cold water for 3 min and assessing the duration of time that they spend actively swimming versus the amount of time that they maintain a characteristic immobile posture. Animals pretreated with tyrosine and phenylalanine (which is metabolized to tyrosine) continued to swim significantly longer than placebo-treated controls.

Studies conducted at the U.S. Army Research Institute of Environmental Medicine (USARIEM) have replicated and extended these initial studies in animals. In one series of studies (Luo et al., 1992, Rauch and Lieberman, 1990), cold-induced stress was used to produce decrements in performance. In another study, hypobaric hypoxia was the primary stressor (Lieberman et al., 1992). In the initial study of cold-induced stress (Rauch and Lieberman, 1990), rats were pretreated with 400 mg of tyrosine per kg, and their core body temperature was lowered to 30°C by immersing the animals in a cold-water bath for approximately 30 min. The Porsolt swim test was then used to assess the effects of tyrosine and cold-induced stress. As shown in Figure 15–1, the mean duration of immobility in this task increased as the core body temperature was reduced. This demonstrates that as the intensity of cold-induced stress increases, animals are less responsive to the environment. Figure 15–2 shows that when rats were pretreated with tyrosine, the duration of immobility declined significantly. In fact, tyrosine restored performance to the normal level typically observed in animals not exposed to cold-induced stress. Luo et al. (1992) replicated the findings of Rauch and Lieberman (1990) and demon

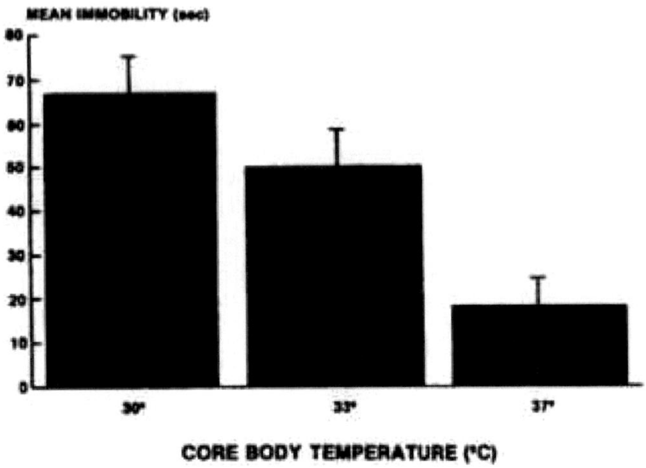

FIGURE 15–1 Changes in mean duration of immobility (in seconds) assessed in the Porsolt swim test (Porsolt et al., 1978) as a function of core body temperature. As core body temperature was reduced, the swim time decreased. Results are expressed as mean±standard error of the mean. Source: Rauch and Lieberman (1990), used with permission.

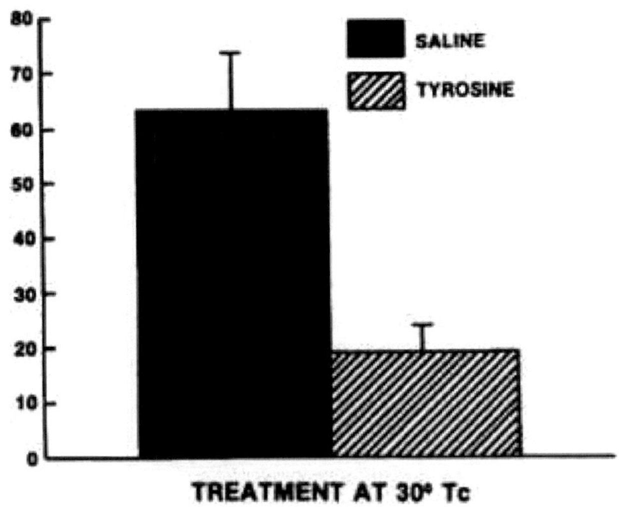

FIGURE 15–2 Effect of tyrosine (400 mg/kg given intraperitoneally) pretreatment on duration of immobility in the Porsolt swim test. Just prior to testing, the core body temperature (Tc) was lowered to 30°C. When rats were pretreated with tyrosine, the duration of immobility significantly decreased compared with that of placebo-treated rats. Results are expressed as mean ±standard error of the mean. Source: Rauch and Lieberman (1990), used with permission.

strated that the effects of tyrosine on cold-stressed animals are dose dependent (Figure 15–3).

Studies examining the effects of tyrosine on rats and humans subjected to cold-induced stress have also been conducted by the Naval Medical Research Institute (Shurtleff et al., 1992; see also Chapter 16). These studies support the hypothesis that tyrosine protects against the adverse effects of acute cold-induced stress on memory consolidation (see Chapter 16).

In another animal study conducted at USARIEM, tyrosine reversed the adverse effects of acute exposure to hypobaric hypoxia (Lieberman et al., 1992). In that study, rats were exposed to a simulated altitude of 5,950 m (19,500 ft) for 8 h. Performance was assessed by the Morris water maze, a test of spatial learning and memory (Brandeis et al., 1989) at 2 and 6 h into the exposure. A total of 400 mg of tyrosine per kg was administered intraperitoneally on two occasions: at 1.5 and 5.5 h after the start of exposure to hypoxia. This task requires animals to learn to find and remember the location of a hidden platform in a tank of water. Since the platform is not visible to the

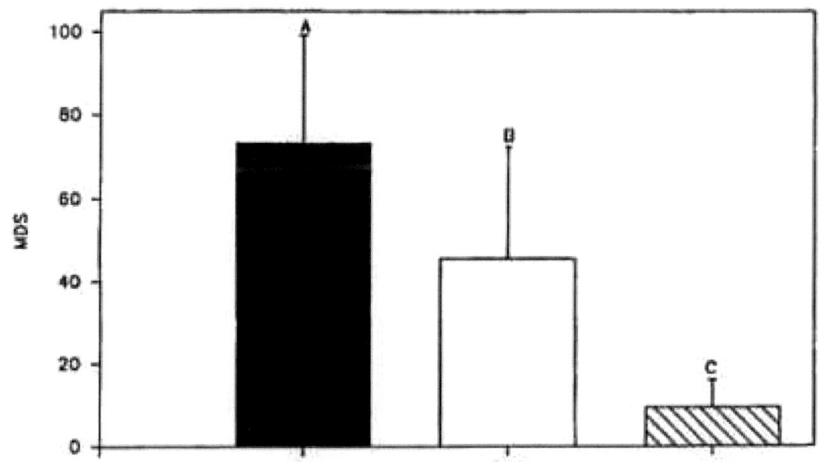

FIGURE 15–3 Effect of two doses of tyrosine (TYR; 200 and 400 mg/kg given intraperitoneally) on the duration of immobility in the Porsolt swim test (Porsolt et al., 1978). Prior to testing, the core body temperature was lowered to 30°C. The data shown here demonstrate that the effects of tyrosine on cold-stressed animals are dose dependent. Values are expressed as mean difference scores (MDS), which equals hypothermia immobility time minus normothermia immobility time. Results are expressed as mean±standard error of the mean. Letters (A-C) identify conditions that are significantly different one from another ($P \leq 0.5$).

animal, spatial cues must be employed. Although hypoxia itself clearly impairs learning and memory, the water maze task probably increases the stressfulness of the situation. When this task is used to assess performance, animals are exposed to an unusual environment in which they are required to swim to escape. In addition, the task may produce thermal stress that would contribute to the overall stressfulness of the situation. The combination of hypoxia and other stressors clearly impaired performance on this task; tyrosine reduced the decrements in performance related to working (short-term) memory (Figure 15–4).

Tyrosine has also been shown to have other potentially beneficial effects in stressful environments. For example, its acute administration can lower blood pressure in spontaneously hypertensive rats that are subjected to stressful testing conditions (Sved et al., 1979) and raise blood pressure in animals made hypotensive by blood loss, which is a model of hemorrhagic shock (Conlay et al., 1981, 1985). Tyrosine also decreases the vulnerability of the canine heart to ventricular fibrillation in a dose-dependent manner and may therefore pre

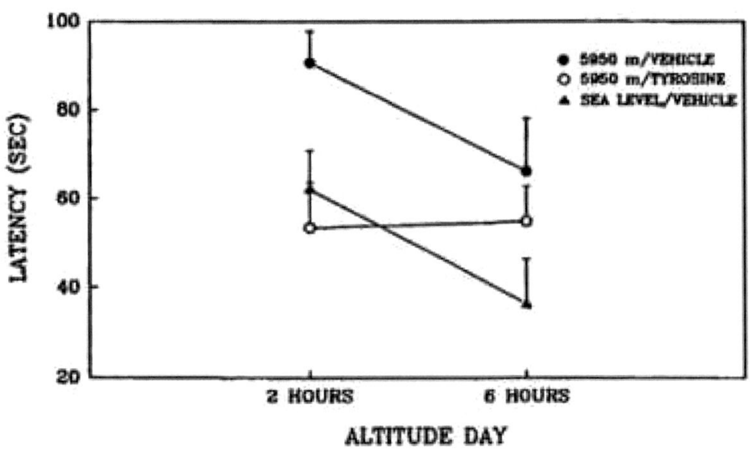

FIGURE 15–4 Effects of tyrosine and vehicle on working (short-term) memory as assessed by the Morris water maze. Rats were exposed to hypobaric hypoxia (5,950 m) or sea level conditions. A total of 400 mg of tyrosine per kg was administered intraperitoneally on two occasions: at 1.5 and 5.5 h after the start of exposure to hypoxia. Hypoxia clearly impaired performance on this task and tyrosine reduced the decrements in performance, as assessed by the latency to locate the hidden platform. Results are expressed as mean±standard error of the mean.

vent sudden, stress-induced cardiac arrest (Scott et al., 1981). It may also have beneficial effects on the neuroendocrine response to stress, since tyrosine blocks the rise in plasma corticosterone levels that occurs after unavoidable stress (Reinstein et al., 1985). It has been reported that animals who successfully cope with avoidable stress by escaping have lower levels of plasma corticosterone than animals that fail to cope (Swenson and Vogel, 1983). Some of these effects may be of particular value on the battlefield, especially tyrosine's ability to increase blood pressure in models of hemorrhagic shock.

These observations taken together suggest that tyrosine, or any treatment that potentiates CA neurotransmission without significant side effects, may be useful for treating many of the adverse consequences of severe acute stress in humans. Presumably, combat and other operations in which soldiers are exposed to life-threatening danger are situations in which tyrosine or other catecholaminergic agonists may have some beneficial effects.

TYROSINE AND ACUTE STRESS: STUDIES IN HUMANS

Tyrosine has been administered to normal human subjects in only a few studies, although it may have beneficial effects on the mood states of certain subgroups of depressed patients (Gelenberg et al., 1983). In studies with normal males, no significant behavioral effects of tyrosine administered orally at a dose of 100 mg/kg of body weight were noted (Lieberman et al., 1983). However, subjects in that study did not experience experimental stressors, and it is under stressful conditions that tyrosine would be expected to have its positive effects on behavior.

Hypobaric Hypoxia

The first study in which the behavioral effects of tyrosine were examined in humans subjected to acute stress was conducted at USARIEM (Banderet and Lieberman, 1989). The experimental stressor was acute exposure (4 h) to a combination of hypobaric hypoxia (4,200 and 4,700 m [13,800 and 15,500 ft]) and cold (15°C [60°F]). A double-blind, placebo-controlled crossover design was used, and mood, symptoms, and mental performance were assessed by using a battery of standardized behavioral tests. Exposure of humans to such simulated altitudes rapidly produces numerous adverse changes. Cognitive performance is significantly impaired on a wide variety of simple and complex aspects of behavior. Simultaneously, mood state is adversely affected, and a series of typical symptoms appear, such as headache, lightheadedness, nausea, and general malaise. There are considerable individual differences in the patterns and severities of these symptoms (for a review, see Banderet and Burse [1991]). Exposure to the secondary stressor, an ambient air temperature of 15°C, would not be expected to produce similar impairments in performance but certainly contributed to the overall stressfulness of the environment. In this study, tyrosine was administered as a total oral dose of 100 mg/kg of body weight over a 40-min period in two equal portions. There were substantial decrements in many of the parameters assessed among the volunteers in that study due to exposure to the stressors, and there were significant individual differences in the severities and patterns of the deficits. When these differences were accounted for, tyrosine appeared to have robust effects on those individuals whose performances on a given behavioral task were most severely affected. Tyrosine significantly mitigated many of the decrements in symptoms, mood, and performance induced by these stressors (Figures 15–5 to 15–7, respectively), including functions believed to be regulated by catecholaminergic neurons such as vigilance, alertness, and anxiety (Banderet and Lieberman, 1989).

To replicate and extend these findings, a second study was conducted at USARIEM (Lieberman et al., 1990). In that follow-up study, the duration of exposure to hypobaric hypoxia was extended to 7 h, a simulated altitude of 4,700 m was used, and the ambient air temperature was held at 17°C. Two oral doses of tyrosine were tested: 85 and 170 mg/kg. As in the previous study (Banderet and Lieberman, 1989), each treatment was given as a divided dose. The results of the second study were similar to those of the first study. Tyrosine significantly reduced impairments on many of the same performance-, mood-, and symptom-dependent variables among those individuals whose performances of the particular measure were most affected. However, the effects did not appear to be dose dependent.

Acute Cardiovascular Stress

The effects of tyrosine on humans exposed to acute stress have also been examined at the U.S. Air Force Armstrong Laboratory. In a double-blind, placebo-controlled crossover study, the effects of tyrosine on individuals subjected to an acute cardiovascular stressor, lower body negative pressure (LBNP), were assessed (Dollins et al., 1990; Lieberman et al., 1991). LBNP is a technique that is used to simulate gravitational stress (orthostasis) by exposing the lower body to subatmospheric pressures. This causes blood and interstitial fluids to pool in the lower extremities because of decreased venous return and increased sympathetic drive (Bonde-Petersen et al., 1984). Subjects exposed to LBNP initially respond with decreased blood pressure and increased heart rate. These changes continue until the cardiovascular system cannot maintain homeostasis, and blood pressure and heart rate fall precipitously. At this stage consciousness is lost if the LBNP exposure is not terminated. LBNP was generated in the Armstrong Laboratory study by placing subjects in a specially constructed airtight chamber from the waist down. A vacuum was then applied to the chamber and subjects were exposed to two consecutive 40-min LBNP sessions separated by a brief break. The maximum negative pressure was −50 mm Hg. When tyrosine, at a dose of 100 mg/kg, was administered orally over a 1 h period (in two 50-mg/kg oral boluses), subjects were able to maintain higher pulse pressures (Figure 15–8). In addition, changes in auditory-evoked potentials suggestive of increased central nervous system activity were also observed as a consequence of tyrosine administration (Figure 15–9).

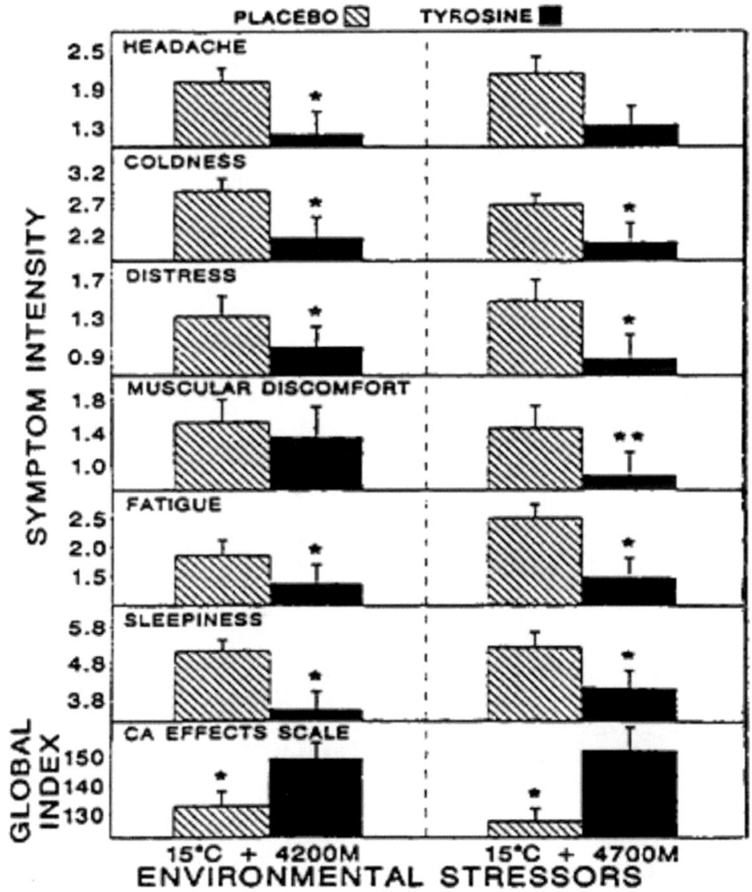

FIGURE 15–5 Effects of tyrosine treatment on a variety of parameters assessed with self-reported symptom questionnaires. The experimental stressor was a 4 h exposure to a combination of hypobaric hypoxia (4,200 m and 4,700 m) and cold (15°C). Asterisks indicate the level of statistical significance (*, $P<0.05$; **, $P<0.01$). Results are expressed as mean±standard error of the mean. CA, catecholamine. Source: Banderet and Lieberman (1989), used with permission.

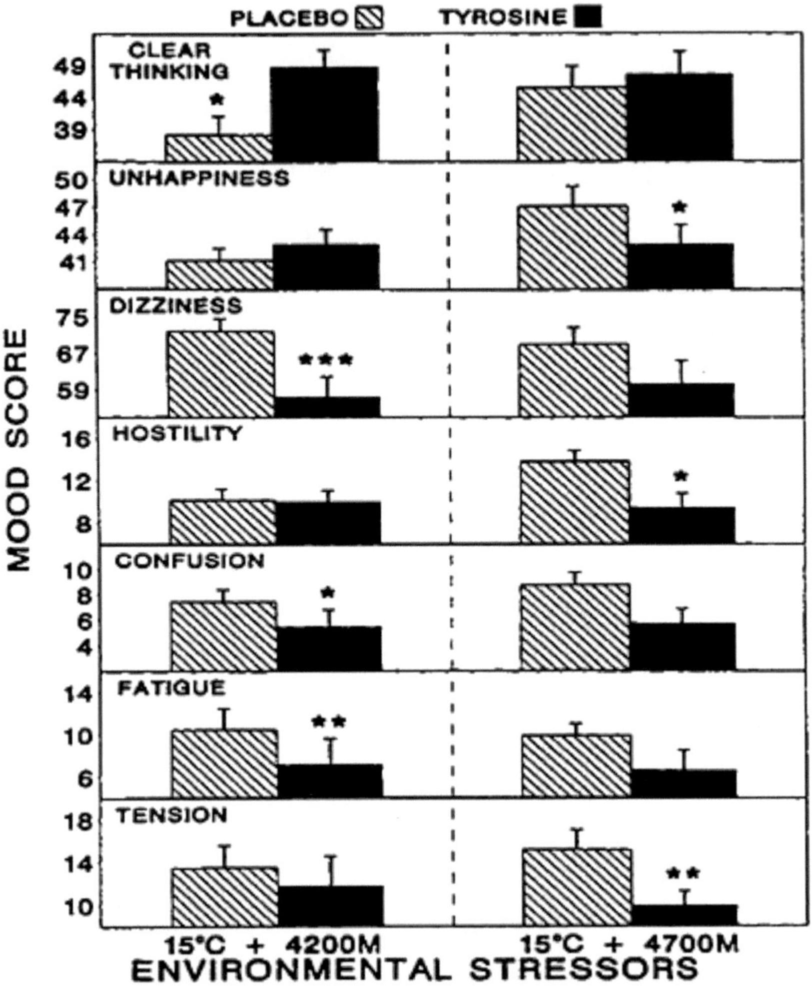

FIGURE 16–6 Effects of tyrosine treatment on mood. The experimental stressor was a 4-h exposure to a combination of hypobaric hypoxia (4,200 and 4,700 m) and cold (15°C). Asterisks indicate the level of statistical significance (*, $P<0.05$; **, $P<0.01$; ***, $P<0.001$). Results are expressed as mean±standard error of the mean. Source: Banderet and Lieberman (1989), used with permission.

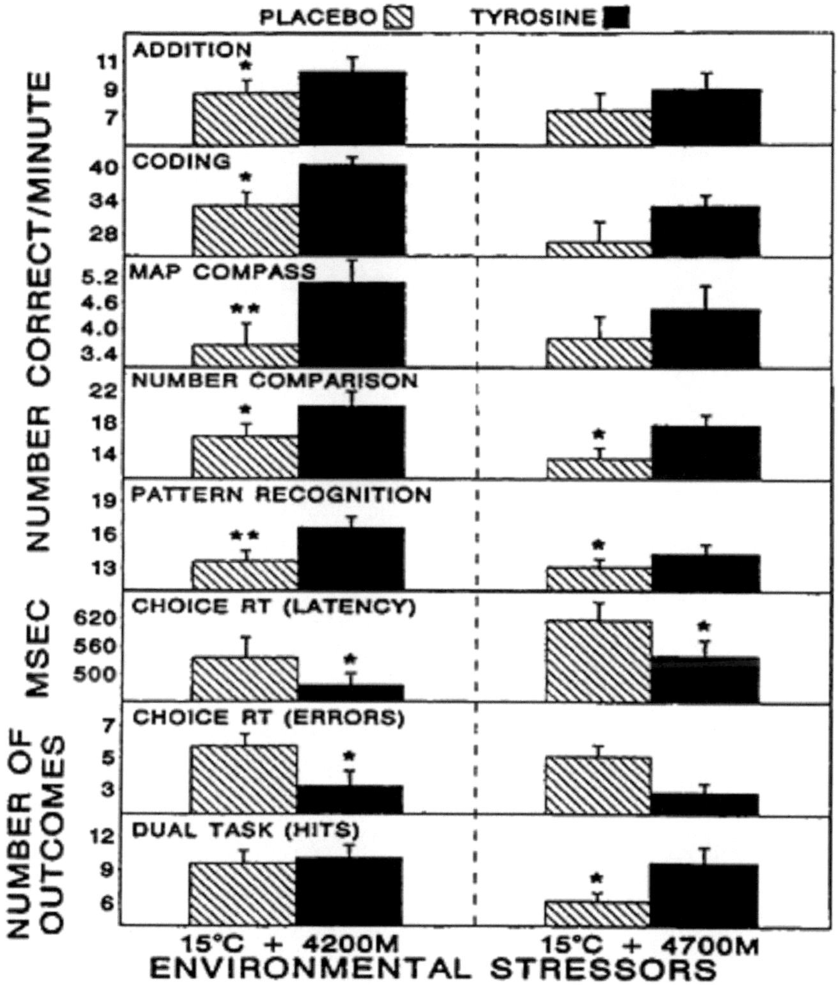

FIGURE 15–7 Effects of tyrosine treatment on cognitive, reaction time (RT), and vigilance performance. The experimental stressor was a 4-h exposure to a combination of hypobaric hypoxia (4,200 and 4,700 m) and cold (15°C). Asterisks indicate the level of statistical significance (*, P<0.05; **, P<0.01). Results are expressed as mean±standard error of the mean. Source: Banderet and Lieberman (1989), used with permission.

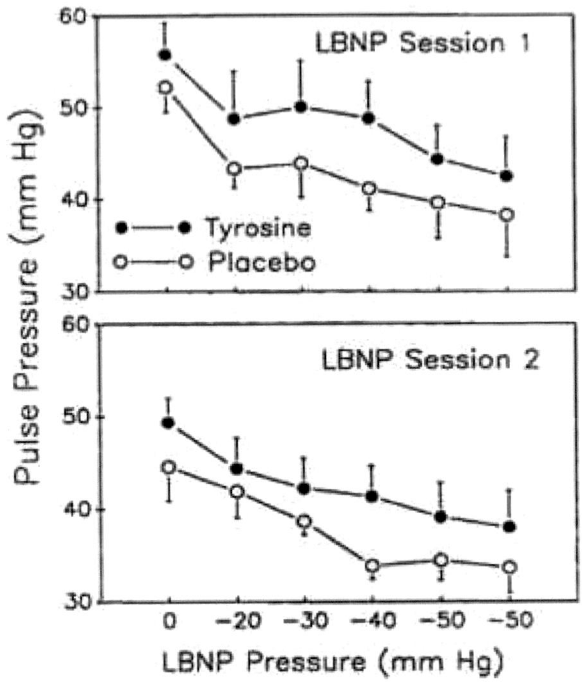

FIGURE 15–8 Change in mean±standard error of the mean, pulse pressure following treatment with 100 mg of tyrosine per kg of body weight. The experimental stressor was exposure to lower body negative pressure (LBNP).

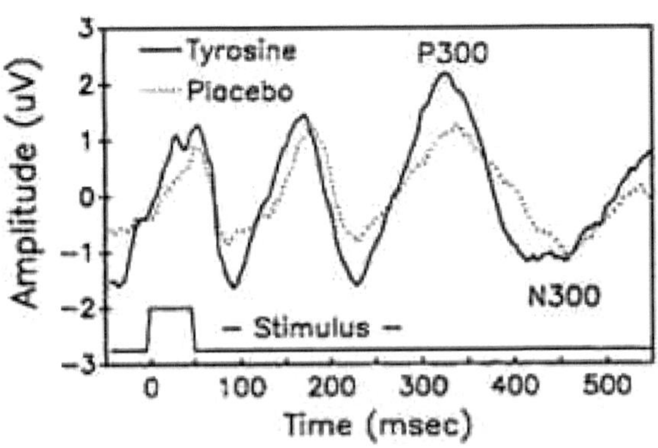

FIGURE 15–9 Change in mean amplitude of middle latency auditory evoked potential (P 300 and N 300 waves during exposure to lower body negative pressure (LBNP) stress. Subjects were treated with a total of 100 mg of tyrosine or placebo per kg of body weight.

CONCLUSIONS

Results of the studies discussed above and research presented elsewhere in this volume (see Chapter 16) suggest that the amino acid tyrosine may have beneficial effects on humans and other animals that are subjected to acute stressors. The adverse effects of hypoxia, cold, lower body negative pressure, and psychological stresses have all been reduced by treatment with tyrosine. This amino acid may have protective effects on behavioral and cardiovascular parameters because it prevents the depletion of central and peripheral catecholamines caused by acute stress. Since a variety of environmental and psychological stressors appear to deplete catecholamines, tyrosine may have wide application as a performance-enhancing ration component (PERC). However, the currently available data cannot be considered to be definitive in establishing that tyrosine should be added to a combat ration. Key issues that must be addressed by additional research include the utility of tyrosine in combat or similar situations, the generalizability of tyrosine's effects across different stressors, the appropriate dose, and in particular, whether tyrosine should be used acutely or as a routine part of the diet.

Tyrosine can be expected to be beneficial only when the stress is severe. Intense combat and similar highly stressful military operations are therefore the situations in which tyrosine could have the greatest benefit to the armed forces. A variety of considerations, however, including ethical concerns, make it difficult to test tyrosine in a realistic manner. Previous attempts to use psychological manipulations to generate stress have not shown tyrosine to be beneficial, presumably because the stress was not sufficiently intense or prolonged (H.R.Lieberman and G.Garfield, unpublished observations). It is therefore essential that studies with this nutrient continue in animals in conjunction with studies in humans. Such studies should use environmental stressors, combinations of environmental and operational stressors, or sustained exposures to stressors. Attempts to develop a suitable human model of combat stress that can be used to evaluate tyrosine and other PERCs are also necessary.

In addition to tyrosine, a variety of other nutrients have been discussed as potential PERCs. Currently, the food constituent with the most clearly demonstrated ability to enhance behavioral performance is caffeine (for recent reviews, see Lieberman [1992] and Penetar [Chapter 20, this volume]). The circumstances in which caffeine has its clearest effects on performance are, in many respects, quite different from those in which tyrosine would be expected to be useful. Caffeine appears to improve performance when individuals are engaged in long-duration, boring activities such as driving or sentry duty. Tyrosine appears to enhance performance when acute stress degrades function. If development of both compounds as PERCs continues, then different types of rations, or specially labeled supplements within rations, may be needed, depending on the operational situation. Caffeine would not be expected to have beneficial effects in high-stress scenarios, and since it can have adverse effects on sleep, it would not be advisable to add it to rations as a generic supplement. Although no adverse effects of tyrosine have been demonstrated, the apparent requirement for it to be used in high doses may preclude its use except in a specially identified form. The consumption of reduced levels of rations during combat, especially during its most stressful periods such as initial exposure to enemy action (Popper et al., 1984), also suggests that tyrosine could best be provided in a combat ration as a special stress-reduction item, perhaps in combination with an easily digested carbohydrate. Carbohydrate may facilitate tyrosine's uptake into the brain and could also provide the needed energy under such circumstances (Wurtman et al., 1981).

In summary, the critical issues that should be addressed in studies in animals and/or humans include the following:

- Demonstrate the generalizability of tyrosine's effects across a wider range of stressors.
- Establish the dose-response function for tyrosine's beneficial effects.
- Assess the risks and benefits of acute versus chronic administration of tyrosine.
- Determine whether tyrosine has efficacy in chronic stress paradigms.
- Determine the safety of tyrosine administration.
- Determine the most appropriate method for using combinations of PERC-type rations.

ACKNOWLEDGMENTS

The author thanks MAJ Mary Mays for her helpful comments on earlier versions of this chapter.

REFERENCES

Anisman, H., and L.Sklar 1979 Catecholamine depletion in mice upon reexposure to stress: Mediation of the escape deficits produced by inescapable shock. Comp. Physiol. Psychol. 93:610.

Antelman, S.M., and A.R.Caggiula 1977 Norepinephrine-dopamine interactions and behavior. A new hypothesis of stress-related interactions between brain norepinephrine and dopamine is proposed. Science 195:646.

Baldessarini, R.J. 1985 Drugs and the treatment of psychiatric disorders. Pp. 387–445 in The Pharmacological Basics of Therapeutics, 7th ed., A.G.Gilman, L.S.Goodman, T.W.Rall, and F.Murad, eds. New York: Macmillan Publishing Co.

Banderet, L.E., and R.L.Burse 1991 Effects of high terrestrial altitude on military performance. Pp. 233–254 in The Handbook of Military Psychology, R.Gal and D.Mangelsdorff, eds. New York: Wiley.

Banderet, L.E., and H.R.Lieberman 1989 Treatment with tyrosine, a neurotransmitter precursor, reduces environmental stress in humans. Brain Res. Bull. 22:759–762.

Bonde-Petersen, F., M.Suzuki, and N.J.Christensen 1984 Cardiovascular and hormonal responses to bicycle exercise during lower body negative pressure. Adv. Space Res. 4(12):31–33.

Bourne, P.G., W.M.Coli, and W.E.Datel 1968 Affect levels of ten special forces soldiers under threat of attack. Psych. Rep. 22:363–366.

Brady, K., J.W.Brown, and J.B.Thurmond 1980 Behavioral and neurochemical effects of dietary tyrosine in young and aged mice following cold-swim stress. Pharmacol. Biochem. Behav. 12:667–674.

Brandeis, R., Y.Brandys, and S.Yehuda 1989 The use of the Morris water maze in the study of memory and learning. Int. J. Neurosci. 48:29–69.

Conlay, L.A., T.J.Maher, and R.J.Wurtman 1981 Tyrosine increases blood pressure in hypotensive rats. Science 212:559–560.

Conlay, L.A., T.J.Maher, and R.J.Wurtman 1985 Tyrosine accelerates catecholamine synthesis in hemorrhaged hypotensive rats. Brain Res. 333:81–84.

Curran, H.V. 1992 Antidepressant drugs, cognitive function and human performance. Pp. 319–336 in Handbook of Human Performance, Vol. 2, Health and Performance, A.P.Smith and D.M.Jones, eds. Boston: Academic Press.

Dollins, A B., L.P.Krock, W.F.Storm, and H.R.Lieberman 1990 Tyrosine decreases physiological stress caused by lower body negative pressure (LBNP). Aviat. Space Environ. Med. 61:491.

Flora, D. 1985 Battlefield Stress: Cause, Cures and Counter Measures. Report No. ACSC-85–3232. Fort Leavenworth, Kans.: Army Command and General Staff College.

Gelenberg, A.J., J.D.Wojcik, C.J.Gibson, and R.J.Wurtman 1983 Tyrosine for depression. J. Psychiatr. Res. 17(2):175.

Gibson, C.J., and R.J.Wurtman 1978 Physiological control of brain norepinephrine synthesis by brain tyrosine concentration. Life Sci. 22:1399–1406.

Gibson, C.J., S.M.Deikel, S.N.Young, and Y.M.Binik 1982 Behavioral and biochemical effects of tryptophan, tyrosine and phenylalanine in mice. Psychopharmacology 76:118–121.

Glazer, H.I., J.M.Weiss, L.A.Pohorecky, and N.Miller 1975 Monoamines as mediators of avoidance-escape behavior. Psychosom. Med. 37:535.

Gray, J.A. 1982 The Neuropsychology of Anxiety. Oxford: Clarendon Press.

Koelega, H.S. 1989 Benzodiazepines and vigilance performance: A review. Psychopharmacology 98:145–156.

Lehnert, H., D.K.Reinstein, B.W.Strowbridge, and R.J.Wurtman 1984a Neurochemical and behavioral consequences of acute, uncontrollable stress: Effects of dietary tyrosine. Brain Res. 303:215–223.

Lehnert, H., D.K.Reinstein, and R.J.Wurtman 1984b Tyrosine reverses the depletion of brain norepinephrine and the behavioral deficits caused by tail-shock stress in rats. Pp. 81–91 in Stress: The Role of the Catecholamines and Other Neurotransmitters, E.Usdin, R.Kvetnansky, and J.Axelrod, eds. New York: Gordon and Beach.

Lieberman, H.R. 1992 Caffeine. Pp. 49–72 in Handbook of Human Performance, Vol. 2, Health and Performance, A.P.Smith and D.M.Jones, eds. Boston: Academic Press.

Lieberman, H.R., S.Corkin, B.J.Spring, J.H.Growdon, and R.J.Wurtman 1983 Mood, performance, and pain sensitivity changes induced by food constituents. J. Psychiatr. Res. 17(2):135–145.

Lieberman, H.R., L.E.Banderet, and B.Shukitt-Hale 1990 Tyrosine protects humans from the adverse effects of acute exposure to hypoxia and cold. Soc. Neurosci. Abstr. 16:272.

Lieberman, H.R., A.B.Dollins, and R.J.Wurtman 1991 Strategies to sustain and enhance performance in stressful environments: The effects of tyrosine pre-treatment on lower body negative pressure stress. Air Force Office of Scientific Research Report TR-90–0403, AD A221224 Bolling Air Force Base, Washington, D.C.: Air Force Office of Scientific Research.

Lieberman, H.R., B.Shukitt-Hale, S.Luo, J.A.Devine, and J.F.Glenn 1992 Tyrosine reduces the adverse effect of hypobaric hypoxia on spatial working memory of the rat. Soc. Neurosci. Abstr. 18:715.

Lovenberg, W., E.S.Bruck, and I.Hanbauer 1975 ATP, cyclic AMP, and magnesium increase the affinity of rat striatal tyrosine hydroxylase for its cofactor. Proc. Natl. Acad. Sci. USA 72:2955–2958.

Luo, S., L.Villamil, C.J.Watkins, and H.R.Lieberman 1992 Further evidence tyrosine reverses behavioral deficits caused by cold exposure. Soc. Neurosci. Abstr. 18:716.

Maier, S.F., and R.L.Jackson 1979 Learned helplessness: All of us were right (and wrong): Inescapable shock has multiple effects. In Psychology of Learning and Motivation 13, G.H.Bower, ed. New York: Academic Press.

Maier, S.F., and M.E.P.Seligman 1976 Learned helplessness: Theory and evidence. J. Exp. Psychol. 105:3.

McNair, D.M. 1973 Antianxiety drugs and human performance. Arch. Gen. Psychiatry 29:611.

Milner, J.P., and R.J.Wurtman 1986 Catecholamine synthesis: Physiological coupling to precursor supply. Biochem. Pharmacol. 35:875–881.

Minor, T.R., R.L.Jackson, and S.F.Maier 1984 Effects of task-irrelevant cues and reinforcement delay on choice-escape learning following inescapable shock: Evidence for a deficit in selective attention. J. Exp. Psych. 10:543.

Murphy, D.L., and D.E.Redmond 1975 The catecholamines: Possible role in affect, mood and emotional behavior in man and animals. Pp. 73–117 in Catecholamines and Behavior, A.J.Freidhoff, ed. New York: Plenum Press.

Owasoyo, J.O., D.F.Neri, and J.G.Lamberth 1992 Tyrosine and its potential use as a countermeasure to performance decrement in military sustained operations . Aviat. Space Environ. Med. 63:364–369.

Popper, R.D., G.J.Smits, H.L.Meiselman, J.Moy, and H.B.Masor 1984 Eating in combat: A survey of how much and what foods U.S. Marines eat in action. U.S. Army Natick Research, Development and Engineering Center Technical Report TR-85–010. Natick, Mass.: U.S. Army Research Institute of Environmental Medicine.

Porsolt, R.D., G.Anton, N.Blavet, and M.Jalfre 1978 Forced swimming in rats: Hypothermia, immobility and the effects of imipramine. Eur. J. Pharmacol. 47:379–391.

Rapaport, P.M., and S.F.Maier 1978 Inescapable shock and food-competition dominance in rats. Animal Learning Behav. 6:160.

Rauch, T.M., and H.R.Lieberman 1990 Tyrosine pretreatment reverses hypothermia induced behavioral depression. Brain Res. Bull. 24:147–150.

Reinstein, D.K., H.Lehnert, and R.J.Wurtman 1984 Tyrosine prevents behavioral and neurochemical correlates of an acute stress in rats. Life Sci. 34:2225–2231.

1985 Dietary tyrosine suppresses the rise in plasma corticosterone following acute stress in rats. Life Sci. 37:2157–2163.

Salter, C. 1989 Dietary tyrosine as an aid to stress resistance among troops. Milit. Med. 154:144–146.

Scott, N.A., R.A.DeSilva, B.Lown, and R.J.Wurtman 1981 Tyrosine administration decreases vulnerability to ventricular fibrillation in the normal canine heart. Science 211:727–729.

Sherman, A.D., G.L.Allers, F.Petty, and F.A.Henn 1979 A neuropharmacologically-relevant animal model of depression. Neuropharmacology 18:891.

Shurtleff, D., J.R.Thomas, J.Schrot, K.Kowalski, R.Harford, M.O.Thornton, P.A.Shea, and M.Malik 1992 Tyrosine reverses a cold-stress-induced memory deficit in humans. Soc. Neurosci. Abstr. 18:1210.

Solomon, Z., M.Mikulincer, and R.Benbenishty 1989 Combat stress reaction—clinical manifestations and correlates. Milit. Psychol. 1:35–47.

Stone, E.A. 1975 Stress and catecholamines. Pp. 31–71 in Catecholamines and Behavior, A.J.Freidhoff, ed. New York: Plenum Press.

Sved, A.F., J.D.Fernstrom, and R.J.Wurtman 1979 Tyrosine administration reduces blood pressure and enhances brain norepinephrine release in spontaneously hypertensive rats. Proc. Natl. Acad. Sci. USA 76:3511–3514.

Swenson, R., and W.Vogel 1983 Plasma catecholamine and corticosterone as well as brain catecholamine changes during coping in rats exposed to stressful footshock. Pharmacol. Biochem. Behav. 18:689–693.

Van der Kolk, B., M.Greenberg, H.Boyd, and J.Krystal 1985 Inescapable shock, neurotransmitters and addiction to trauma: Toward a psychobiology of post traumatic stress. Biol. Psychiatry 20:314–325.

Villoldo, A., and R.L.Tarno 1984 Measuring the performance of EOD equipment and operators under stress. Naval Explosive Ordnance Disposal Technology Center, NAVEODTECHCEN Technical Report T-270, AD-B083850L, San Francisco, Calif: Frederick Burk Foundation Research Center.

Weiner, N., F.L.Lee, E.Dreyer, and E.Barnes 1978 The activation of tyrosine hydroxylase in noradrenergic neurons during acute nerve stimulation. Life Sci. 22:1197–1216.

Weiss, J., H.Glazer, and L.Pohorecky 1976 Coping behavior and neurochemical changes: An alternative explanation for the original 'learned helplessness' experiments. Pp. 141–173 in Animal Models in Human Psychobiology, G.Serban and A.King, eds. New York: Plenum Press.

Wurtman, R.J., F.Larin, S.Mostafapour, and J.D.Fernstrom 1974 Brain catechol synthesis: Control by brain tyrosine concentration. Science 185:183–184.

Wurtman, R.J., F.Hefti, and E.Melamed 1981 Precursor control of neurotransmitter synthesis. Pharmacol. Rev. 32:315–335.

DISCUSSION

EDWARD HORTON: I am fascinated by the hypoxia studies, having spent a couple of summers myself up on Mount Logan studying and experiencing acute mountain sickness. I was wondering whether you have looked at the possible peripheral effects of tyrosine? For example, have you monitored arterial blood gas and looked at pCO_2 [partial carbon dioxide pressure] and pH because they have big effects on cerebral blood flow as well.

HARRIS LIEBERMAN: Our studies were designed to study the behavioral effects of tyrosine. In our first study, we did look at blood pressure and heart rate and did not see any changes associated with the administration of tyrosine, but we did not focus on those indicators in particular because they are such crude measures of the effect of hypoxia.

JOEL GRINKER: I have two questions. Have you done any other studies, and would you expect to see a threshold effect with dose-response work?

HARRIS LIEBERMAN: As the answer to the first question, have you done studies on other neurotransmitters, yes, we focused on acetylcholine initially and norepinephrine as well. The data for the other neurotransmitters are not complete at this point, and I cannot present any information on that. The other question had to do with dose-response studies. Unless I have other information, I would always assume that a dose-response function rather than a step function will be found.

JOEL GRINKER: I just wanted some clarification as to what the feeding paradigm that you referred to in the tyrosine study was, and when you said there was a significant factor, what you meant. You mentioned the feeding paradigm.

HARRIS LIEBERMAN: We always gave tyrosine by injection. Richard Wurtman and Henrik Lehnert did studies in which they fed tyrosine in the diet and found effects. I believe they gave it for a week in advance of the study, or at least several days. Dick Wurtman could probably give you more detail on that. Does this answer your question?

JOEL GRINKER: No, I think it was your dependent measures that you were talking about.

HARRIS LIEBERMAN: Oh, that was Tim Maher, and I would rather he would comment on that.

TIMOTHY MAHER: We made rats hyperphagic by removing food for 4 h and then tested the effects of a number of compounds alone or in combination with tyrosine. Although tyrosine had no effect on food intake, it significantly potentiated the effects of these factors.

16

Tyrosine and Glucose Modulation of Cognitive Deficits Resulting from Cold Stress

Stephen T.Ahlers,[1] John R.Thomas, John Schrot, and David Shurtleff

INTRODUCTION

COLD STRESS AND WORKING MEMORY

Research at the Naval Medical Research Institute on the effects of nutritional components on performance has centered primarily on alleviation of cold-induced impairment of short-term or working memory by the catecholamine precursor tyrosine and the simple sugar glucose. Efforts have focused on measures of working memory specifically, since research has shown that working memory is uniquely susceptible to disruption by cold stress. This does not imply that other cognitive abilities are not deleteriously affected by exposure to cold stress. Indeed, it is well established that impaired

[1] Stephen T.Ahlers, Thermal Stress/Adaptation Program, Naval Medical Research Institute, Bethesda, MD 20889–5607

cognitive function results from exposure to cold-induced stress that induces core hypothermia (Coleshaw et al., 1983a,b; Webb, 1984). Rather, research at the Naval Medical Research Institute has focused on the effects of exposure to cold air stress that does not result in an obvious drop in core temperature, as determined by standard thermometry methods. Under these conditions, exposure to cold ambient air (2–5°C) for periods of even as short as 1 h produces reliable and robust impairment of working memory, as determined by a delayed matching-to-sample (DMTS) test (Thomas et al., 1989, 1991a).

Figure 16–1 displays a diagram of a typical trial on the DMTS procedure used to test human subjects. At the beginning of the trial, a subject is presented with a sample stimulus matrix on a computer screen for 2 s. The screen is then blanked for a randomly determined delay of 2, 8, or 16 s. Following the delay the subject is presented with the original sample matrix and another matrix that differs slightly in that the color of one square is reversed. For a correct response, the subject must match the original sample stimulus. A typical session consists of 90 trials and takes approximately 30 min to complete. Subjects perform the DMTS task in the last 30 min of a 60-to 90-min exposure session in which the ambient temperature of the environmental chamber is either 4° or 23°C. The effect of exposure to cold stress on

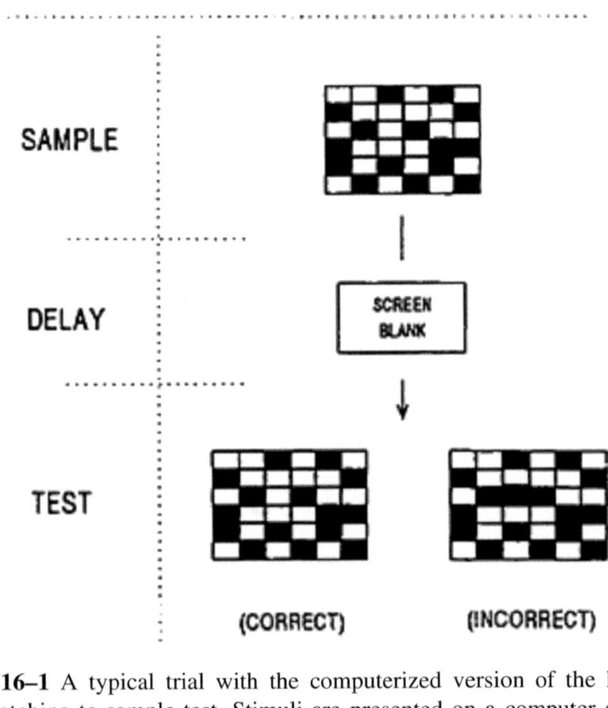

FIGURE 16–1 A typical trial with the computerized version of the human delayed matching-to-sample test. Stimuli are presented on a computer screen, and subjects respond appropriately on a keyboard.

DMTS task performance in humans is depicted in Figure 16–2. When subjects perform the task under normothermic conditions there is a gradual decrease in matching accuracy as the delay between the termination of the sample stimulus and the presentation of the comparison stimulus is increased. During exposure to cold-induced stress, this descending slope function is increased substantially, indicating that exposure to cold air causes the information in an individual's working memory to be forgotten more quickly.

It is important to note that matching accuracy at the 2-s delay was unimpaired by the cold stress. The fact that cold stress did not decrease matching accuracy at the 2-s delay might be interpreted to indicate that moderate levels of exposure to cold stress does not impair the ability of an individual to encode the stimulus into memory, but specifically affects memory retention over time. In cases in which performance at the shorter delay times is also decreased, i.e., the *y* intercept is reduced, it is generally agreed that the initial encoding of information into short-term memory is impaired (Bushnell, 1990). Ahlers et al. (1993) recently observed that a longer exposure to cold

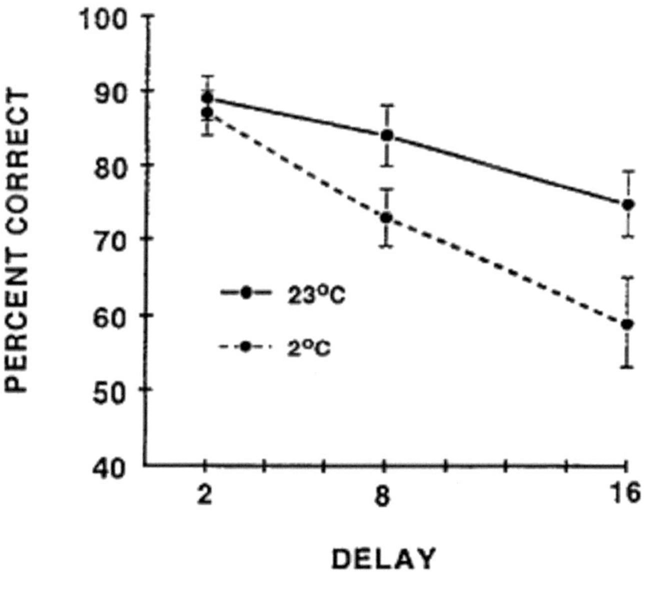

FIGURE 16–2 Matching accuracy of human subjects performing the delayed matching-to-sample task during exposure to ambient temperatures of 23° and 4°C. Delay is measured in seconds.

stress often produces impaired performance after both short and long delays. Changes in the *y* intercept (encoding) and in the slope function (retention) may reflect distinct neurobiological processes which, as described below, appear to influence the conditions in which nutritional factors ameliorate cold-induced memory decrements.

To elucidate the basic mechanisms that underlie the cold-induced memory deficit and to test prospective agents that could alleviate these effects, an animal model was developed in which rats performed a DMTS task. Although there are obvious procedural differences in the human and rat versions of the DMTS task, it is interesting to note that the decay of information over time function in short-term memory is similar in both species over a relatively brief retention interval at a normal temperature (23°C) (Figure 16–3). More striking perhaps is the similarity in the performance of humans and rats during exposure to cold-induced stress. Since rats show cold-induced impairment of working memory similar to what is observed in human subjects exposed to cold stress, initial studies of pharmacological treatments to improve performance during cold stress used this animal model.

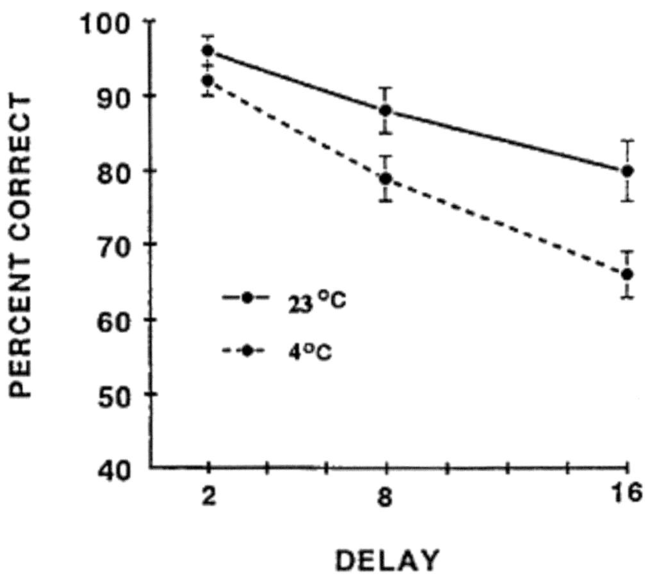

FIGURE 16–3 Matching accuracy of rats performing the delayed matching-to-sample task during exposure to ambient temperatures of 23° and 2°C. Delay is measured in seconds. Source: Thomas et al. (1991a), used with permission.

TYROSINE EFFECTS ON COLD-INDUCED MEMORY IMPAIRMENT

As shown by the extensive work by Wurtman, Lieberman, and others, administration of the catecholamine precursor tyrosine can alleviate many of the deleterious effects of acute stress by increasing the amount of catecholamine neurotransmitter depleted by a stressful event (Banderet and Lieberman, 1989; Lehnert et al., 1984; Rauch and Lieberman, 1990; Reinstein et al., 1984). Although previous studies have demonstrated that exposure to ambient cold air stress increases the turnover rate of catecholamines, which could possibly deplete neuronal stores (Gibson and Wurtman, 1978), there was still uncertainty whether the deficit in working memory that they observed was due to a stress effect that could be reversed with tyrosine or whether the deficit was derived from a direct temperature effect on neural function. The reason for this was that although the cold-induced impairment of working memory appeared to occur in the absence of core hypothermia, as determined with standard rectal thermistor probes. A study by Ahlers et al. (1991) indicated that the cold-induced memory deficit may in fact be due to a direct effect on brain temperature and, thus, may have very little to do with activation of stress pathways. They found that during exposure to cold air, the temperature in the hippocampus, a key brain structure involved in the modulation of working memory, was decreased by 1°C compared with the temperature when the DMTS task was performed during normothermic conditions. This finding added some weight to the suggestion that subtle temperature gradients in the brain may underlie many cold-induced deficits in cognition (Pozos, 1986). Because of the uncertainty regarding the nature of the cold-induced deficit in working memory, investigators examined the effects of the stress- activating hormone corticotropin-releasing factor (CRF) in the rodent model system. There were at least two compelling reasons for using CRF to examine the effects of stress on working memory. First, CRF produces the release of brain catecholamines (Dunn and Berridge, 1987; Lenz et al., 1987). Second, administration of CRF has been shown to produce behavioral deficits that are attenuated by pretreatment with tyrosine (Ahlers et al., 1992).

Cold-Induced Amnesia as a Stress Effect

Administration of CRF produced dose- and delay-dependent impairments (Figure 16–4). Low doses of CRF (0.1 and 0.3 μg) decreased DMTS task accuracy at the long delays, whereas the 1.0-μg dose of CRF decreased DMTS task accuracy across all of the delays. The pattern of impaired DMTS performance with observed increasing doses of CRF is similar to the impair ment observed with increasing exposure to cold air stress. This suggested that the impairment of working memory may in fact be due to activation of stress pathways that would produce a sustained release and an eventual depletion of endogenous brain catecholamines.

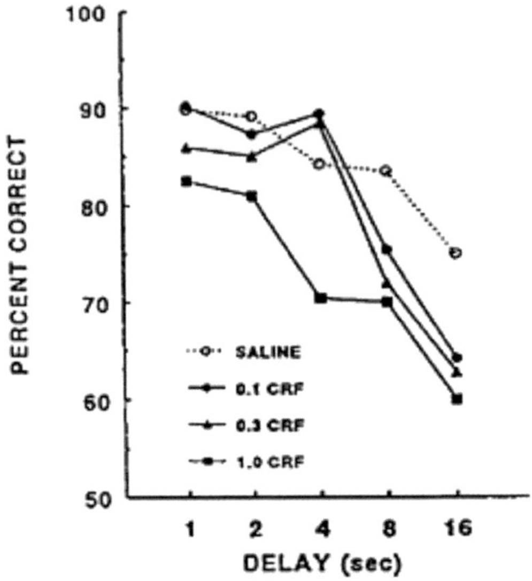

FIGURE 16–4 Effects of corticotropin-releasing factor (CRF; in micrograms) on the delayed matching-to-sample task matching accuracy in rats. Rats were administered CRF or saline intracerebroventiculary 30 min prior to the test session.

Initial Studies with Tyrosine

Because the impairment of working memory caused by cold-induced stress may in fact result from activation of the stress response system that could deplete catecholamine stores, Shurtleff et al. (1993) initially investigated whether administration of tyrosine would alleviate the cold deficit in rats exposed to cold ambient air-induced stress. The doses of tyrosine used ranged from 50 to 200 mg/kg of body weight and were administered approximately 30 min prior to the cold exposure. The results of the study with a rodent model (Shurtleff et al, 1993) indicated that tyrosine partially alleviated the deficit in matching accuracy.

Given the success in reducing the cold-induced memory impairment in rats, the emphasis was shifted to examine the effects of tyrosine in human subjects exposed to cold stress in the environmental chamber at the Naval Medical Research Institute, Bethesda, Maryland (Shurtleff, et al., 1994). In that study, administration of 150 mg/kg of tyrosine completely reversed the cold-induced memory impairment. What was particularly relevant in this finding was that tyrosine was most effective under conditions in which there was a substantial cold-induced decrement only at the longest delay time (16 s). These data clearly indicate that tyrosine effectively blocks an impairment in working memory when cold-induced stress specifically affects memory retention, i.e., in a situation in which accuracy was impaired only at the long delay.

Tyrosine Studies During Field Operations in the Cold

Once the tyrosine-induced alleviation of a cold-induced impairment of working memory in the laboratory chamber with humans was demonstrated, the next logical step was to determine whether tyrosine pretreatment would be beneficial in field situations with military personnel operating in a cold environment. Figure 16–5 shows the effects of tyrosine pretreatment on military personnel under field conditions. In this situation, military personnel were performing maneuvers in a cold weather environment in which the ambient temperature was −20°C. After spending nearly all day performing operations in the cold, half of the personnel were given 75 mg/kg of tyrosine and the other half were given a placebo. The subjects performed the DMTS task 1 h after ingestion of the placebo or tyrosine. In personnel given tyrosine

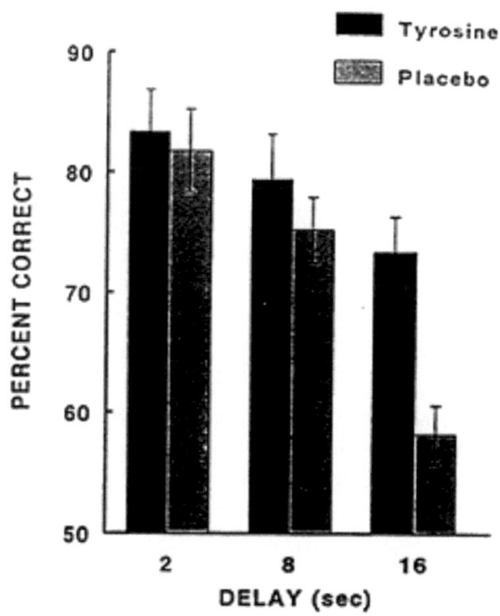

FIGURE 16–5 Effect of tyrosine pretreatment on military personnel. Tyrosine or placebo was administered to military personnel during cold weather field exercises prior to performing the delayed matching-to-sample task.

there was a substantial improvement in task accuracy at the 16-s interval compared with that in the subjects given the placebo. These results were very similar to the effects of tyrosine observed in the environmental chamber study.

The finding that tyrosine was efficacious during field studies is significant in two ways. First, it demonstrates the effectiveness of tyrosine under operational conditions most similar to conditions for which it might ultimately be recommended and used. Second, but no less significant, it validates the observation that working memory is impaired when military personnel perform duties during exposure to cold air stress. When taken together with previous research demonstrating tyrosine's beneficial effects in military personnel under a variety of stressful conditions with several different test parameters (Banderet and Lieberman, 1989), it is clear that tyrosine administration is capable of improving cognitive performance in military personnel exposed to cold stress.

The Effects of Tyrosine on Cold-Induced Impairment in Timing

In the original observation demonstrating the effects of moderate cold stress on working memory in rats, Thomas et al. (1991a) observed that in addition to a deficit in matching accuracy, rats' latencies to respond to the test stimulus decreased, whereas their latencies to respond to the sample stimulus were unchanged. In humans performing the DMTS task during cold exposure in an environment of 4°C, sample response times were slower, and test response latencies were shorter (Thomas et al., 1989). Collectively, these findings indicate that a concomitant effect of the cold-induced impairment of short-term memory may be an alteration in the speed with which cognitive operations are performed. Recent data are consistent with the notion that cold-induced stress might modulate the internal clock speed. During exposure to cold air stress, the rate of response in rats performing a differential reinforcement of low rate (DRL) procedure, which requires subjects to time their responses to a fixed time interval, increased substantially (Thomas et al., 1991b).

Although the degree to which a decrement in timing and impairment of working memory produced by exposure to cold stress may reflect some common physiological dysfunction has yet to be elucidated, investigators have examined whether tyrosine would also ameliorate the effects of cold stress exposure on timing behavior. For this experiment, rats trained on the DRL procedure were administered tyrosine during exposure to cold and normothermic environments. These data are shown in Figure 16–6. Increasing doses of the catecholamine precursor attenuated the increase in the rate of DRL responding during cold stress. The two highest doses of tyrosine essentially normalized the rats' ability to meet the requirements for the DRL procedure. These results indicate that administration of tyrosine completely blocked cold-induced changes in response timing.

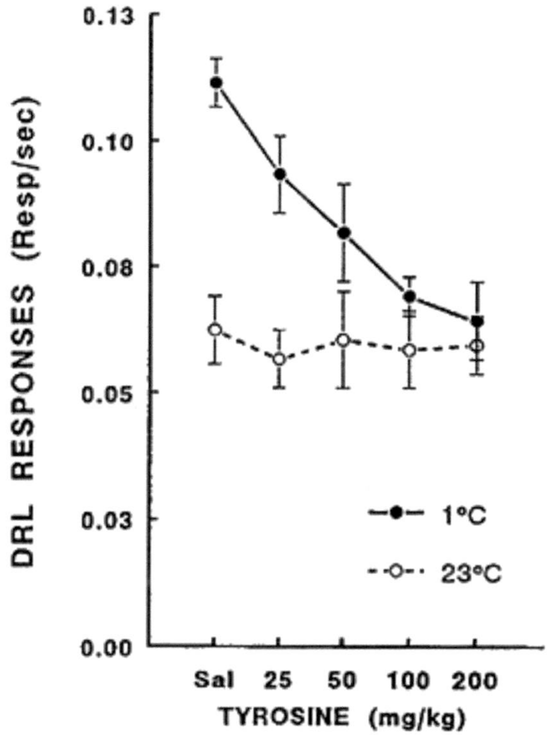

FIGURE 16–6 Effects of tyrosine administration on cold-induced increases in differential reinforcement of low rate (DRL) procedure in rats exposured to ambient temperatures of 23° and 1°C. Sal=saline.

Conclusions and Recommendations Regarding the Use of Tyrosine

The observation that tyrosine alleviates cold-induced impairment of working memory and timing behavior is consistent with the demonstrated efficacy of tyrosine in a variety of test situations with both human and animal subjects. Of particular relevance to the recommendation that tyrosine might be given to deployed military personnel are the findings of Banderet and Lieberman (1989), who have also demonstrated the efficacy of tyrosine in human subjects. Their findings demonstrate that tyrosine can reverse a number of the neuropsychological and emotional effects of the combined stresses of exposure to cold and high altitudes. Tyrosine has been found to block effectively the cold-induced deficits in working memory observed in humans both in the laboratory and in military field operations in cold weather. Taken together, these studies indicate that tyrosine certainly has potential as a nutritional component for improving the compromised performance of military personnel operating under stressful conditions (Owasoyo et al.,1992; Salter, 1989).

Situations in Which Tyrosine is Less Effective

As encouraging as these results with tyrosine may be, some caution is warranted since investigators have found that tyrosine is not universally effective in ameliorating performance decrements resulting from cold-induced stress. For example, administration of tyrosine is less effective in individuals with cold-induced learning deficits measured by a repeated acquisition (RA) task. In the RA procedure, subjects are required to learn a new sequence of appropriate responses on a daily basis. In contrast to the DMTS procedure, the RA task places a much greater demand on an individual's ability to learn new information. For this reason, it takes many trials for an individual to learn the new sequence and makes the RA task particularly sensitive in revealing learning (encoding) deficits. In laboratory and field studies, exposure to cold-induced stress consistently impairs an individual's ability to learn new information using the RA task, such that subjects make more errors over the course of a session. In studies in both humans and rats, tyrosine has not demonstrated consistent effects in modifying cold-induced decrements in the ability to learn a new response sequence as part of the RA task.

Tyrosine and Chronic Stress

The potential restrictions on circumstances in which tyrosine is effective in modifying a stress effect highlight the more general concern of defining the conditions in which tyrosine most effectively blocks stress-induced impairments. Clearly, more focused research is needed to determine these situations before it is recommended as a nutritional supplement for military personnel. Another important consideration for agents such as tyrosine is whether the efficacy may change as a function of the duration that subjects are exposed to cold temperatures. Quite apart from a concern for potential shifts in a tyrosine dose-response curve is the question of whether there might be conditions in which tyrosine administration would be less beneficial or even harmful to the health and safety of the personnel who would use it.

Several studies in individuals with chronic stress have shown that there are significant changes in the synthesis and disposition of endogenous catecholamines in the central nervous system (CNS) that could affect the pharmacodynamics of tyrosine. For example Nisenbaum et al. (1991) have shown that animals chronically exposed to the cold show a greater increase in NE release in the rodent hippocampus during acute restraint stress, as measured by in vivo microdialysis. In subsequent studies, Nisenbaum and Abercrombie (1992) demonstrated augmented release of NE in rats exposed to chronic cold-induced stress is due to a significant increase in the amount of tyrosine hydroxylase (TH), the rate-limiting enzyme for the synthesis of the catecholamines. These findings suggest that the effects of tyrosine in the brains of individuals who have been exposed to cold-induced stress for a long duration may be considerably altered.

There is still another concern about what effects tyrosine might have in chronically stressed organisms. In a recent study, Ahlers and Salander (1993) demonstrated that the acute disruptive effects of CRF are lessened considerably when CRF is administered chronically. What is particularly relevant to the use of tyrosine is the fact that a recent study by Melia and Duman (1991) demonstrated that chronic administration of CRF produces a dramatic increase in TH in the locus ceruleus. These studies indicate that chronic stress produces enduring alterations in the noradrenergic and CRF stress response systems. These changes, while adaptive, may also be the physiological antecedent conditions that lead to stress-induced pathological disease states (Chrousos and Gold, 1992; Stone, 1987). Significant alterations in the noradrenergic and CRF systems in individuals with chronic stress may not only modify the effects of tyrosine, but they may also be modified by the presence of tyrosine. These observations underscore the need for additional information on how tyrosine may modulate, or be modulated by, chronic stress.

Conditions in Which Tyrosine Would Be Contraindicated

Although tyrosine may have positive or negative effects in the CNS, depending upon situational factors, there is also the possibility that supplemental tyrosine might augment untoward peripheral actions of catecholamine release under conditions of cold stress. This has yet to be examined empirically. It is well established that peripheral NE is released in significant amounts during cold stress (Thomas et al., 1990). This drives the vasoconstriction response and helps to shunt blood to the core and maintain body temperature. There is some evidence that hypertension brought about by stress experienced in a cold environment may potentiate peripheral vasoconstrictive mechanisms and thus predispose military personnel to cold-induced vasoneuropathy such as nonfreezing cold injury or frostbite injury (Sampson, 1984). Before tyrosine is given to troops in the field, it will be important to determine whether it has any augmented effect on peripheral vasoconstriction during exposure to cold stress.

GLUCOSE EFFECTS ON COLD-INDUCED MEMORY IMPAIRMENT

The use of glucose as a nutritional factor for enhancing working memory during cold-induced stress was a result of studies demonstrating its effectiveness in improving learning and memory rather than from the development of treatments to specifically alleviate stress. Glucose has been shown to enhance memory and to alleviate memory deficits resulting from a variety of conditions (see Gold [1991] for a review). Although a majority of studies demonstrating the enhancing effects of glucose on memory have focused on the modulation of long-term memory, several reports have shown that glucose can also enhance working memory as well (Means and Fernandez, 1992; Ragozzino and Gold, 1991; Stone et al., 1991). Because of its reported effectiveness, the DMTS task (Thomas et al., 1991a) was used to examine the effects of glucose administration on the cold-induced impairment of working memory in rats. In that study, the exposure to the cold air stress produced an impairment of matching accuracy at all of the delays (Figure 16–7).

Recall from the previous discussion that when cold induces a decrease in matching accuracy at the short delays, the effect of cold on working memory is considered to be at least partially derived from an inability to initially encode information. This is of particular importance since the effects of glucose on cold-induced impairment of matching accuracy in rats are specific to only the short delays. Doses of glucose of between 10 and 100 mg/kg of body weight completely blocked the cold-induced impairment in accuracy at the 1- and 2-s delays. At the 4-s delay, all but the lowest glucose dose alleviated the decrease in matching accuracy resulting from exposure to cold stress. Although there appeared to be some improvement in performance at the 8-s delay with glucose, this did not reach statistical significance. Glucose did not alleviate the cold-induced decrement at the 16-s delay. There was no detectable improvement in performance with glucose administration in that study when rats performed in an ambient temperature of 23°C (data not shown). This was likely due to the fact that rats were at an asymptotic level of performance, especially at the short delay intervals when glucose appeared to be most effective in rats exposed to cold stress.

If the glucose preferentially modulates working memory processes by enhancing encoding, then one would expect there to be a greater effect of glu cose in a procedure that is more sensitive to encoding deficits. For this reason, the effects of glucose were examined by using the RA procedure, in which rats are required to learn a novel response sequence each day. The data showing the effects of a 50-mg/kg dose of glucose on the number of errors within a test session as a function of cold stress are depicted in Figure 16–8. In a procedure in which the acquisition of the response sequence is protracted over multiple trials, glucose not only decreased the number of errors across the session during cold stress, but it also produced fewer errors during exposure to 23°C.

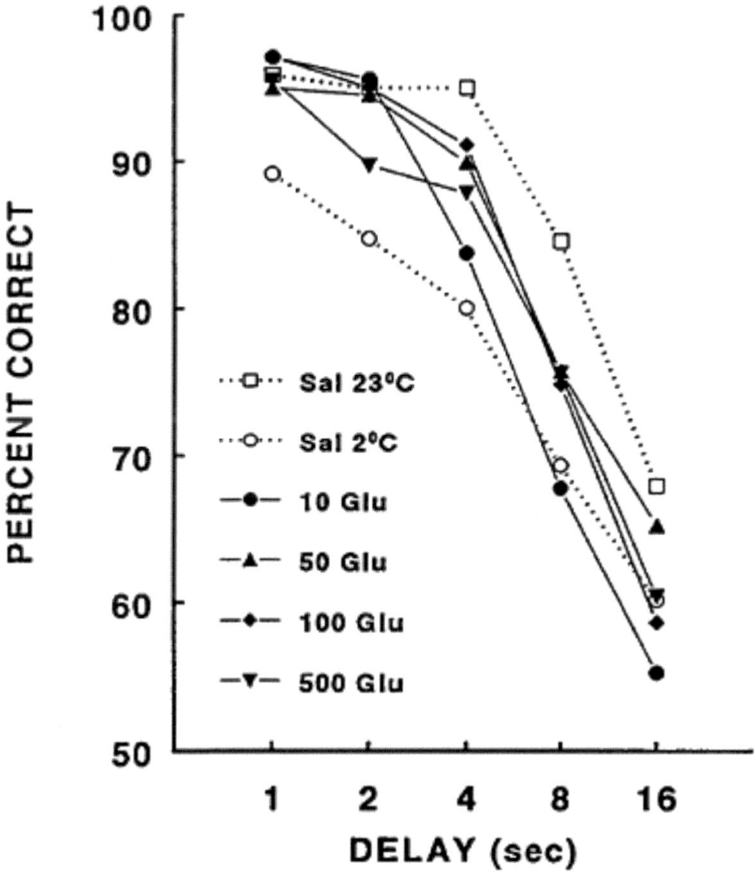

FIGURE 16–7 Glucose effects on performance impairment when rats are exposed to cold, stress (2°C). Sal=saline; Glu=glucose. Source: Ahlers et al. (1993), used with permission.

Several interesting aspects of these data are worth considering. First, when utilizing the RA procedure, glucose was effective in alleviating a cold-induced decrement in performance, whereas tyrosine had marginal efficacy, at least in rats. In the case of impairment of working memory resulting from exposure to cold stress, glucose would appear to modulate the encoding of information, whereas tyrosine would appear to affect the retention of already encoded information over time. Second, administration of glucose improved performance under nonstressed conditions. This situation is quite different from the effects of tyrosine, which is effective only during stress.

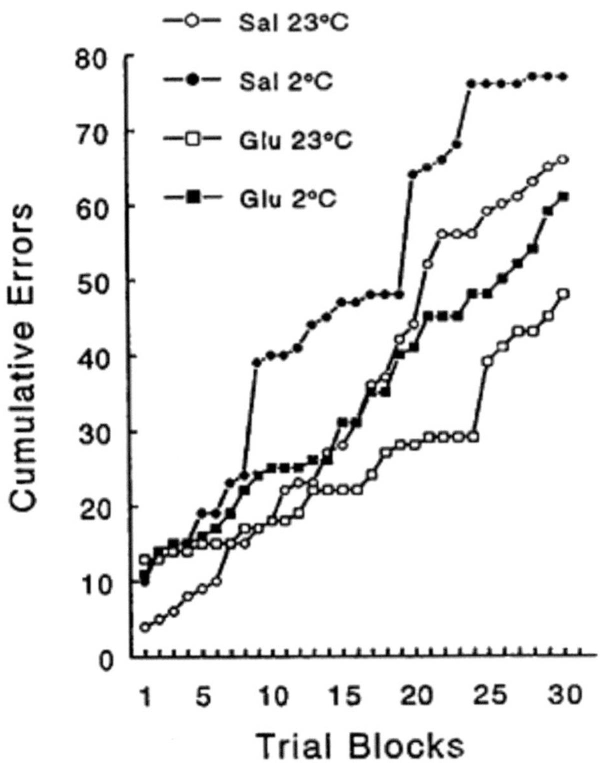

FIGURE 16–8 Effects of administration of 50 mg/kg of glucose on the number of errors committed in the repeated acquisition procedure during exposure to 23° and 2°C. Sal=saline; Glu= glucose.

Mechanisms of Action of Glucose on Working Memory

The cold-induced encoding observed when rats perform the DMTS task is similar to the effects of scopolamine, an acetylcholine (ACh) antagonist, on similar tests of working memory in rats (Bushnell, 1990). This is important since one of the proposed mechanisms for the effects that glucose has on memory is an increase in ACh levels when glucose acts as precursor to acetylcoenzyme A (Gold, 1991; Messier et al., 1991). Support for the fact that glucose modulates working memory by this type of mechanism is found in several studies demonstrating that glucose alleviates the impairment of performance produced by a cholinergic blockade (Ragozzino and Gold, 1991; Stone et al., 1991).

Another possible mechanism of action of glucose for the enhancement of performance during cold-induced stress may stem from a direct increase in glucose-mediated metabolism in specific regions of the brain. Reduced glucose utilization in those regions of the brain associated with working memory is correlated with impaired performance (Gage et al., 1984). If brain temperature were an indication of metabolic activity and glucose uptake, then the observation that the cold-induced impairment of working memory is associated with a 1°C decrease in hippocampal temperature (Ahlers et al., 1991) may have relevance to the effects of glucose on the cold-induced deficit. It is possible that administration of glucose offsets the reduction in metabolic activity and brain temperature and thus attenuates the cold-induced decrement.

Although the mechanism of action of glucose on working memory during cold stress is not known, it is fair to say that there is an abundance of data to support the notion that glucose plays an important modulatory role in cognitive processes. In addition, there has been recent speculation, supported by experimental data, that many of the putative cognition enhancers, i.e., nootropic drugs, which might be recommended for use in improving cognitive performance in military personnel, produce their beneficial effects by increasing the availability and uptake of glucose in the CNS (Wenk, 1989).

Conclusions and Recommendations Regarding Glucose as a Cognition Enhancer

The results of studies with glucose indicate that, as a nutritional component, it has the potential to enhance the performance of military personnel in operational environments. Like tyrosine, however, the circumstances in which glucose is effective in blocking a stress-induced impairment need further study.

CONCLUSIONS

- Studies have demonstrated that as nutritional supplements, tyrosine and glucose improve particular components of working memory during cold stress. A particularly important aspect of the research with tyrosine is the demonstration that it is effective in alleviating performance decrements in military personnel working under operational cold stress conditions.
- Under most circumstances, the demonstration of tyrosine efficacy in these situations would be the prelude to recommending that tyrosine be added as a staple in the diet when personnel are likely to operate under stressful conditions.

- As promising as tyrosine is, however, more research is needed to examine the effects of tyrosine in terms of how the whole organism is affected by tyrosine administration, especially under conditions of chronic stress.
- Progress with glucose as a performance enhancer during cold-induced stress is not as advanced as progress with tyrosine. The logical next step for glucose is to examine its effects in military personnel in studies in controlled environmental chambers and in field exercises and to consider its effects under acute and chronic stress conditions as well.
- In addition, given that treatments with such compounds as tyrosine and glucose may have distinct neurological effects, studies should examine the interaction of these agents when administered in combination, since, in all probability, no one treatment is likely to be universally effective in all situations.

ACKNOWLEDGMENTS

The authors gratefully acknowledge the input of Patricia M.Thornton. This research was supported by Naval Medical Research and Development Command Research and Technology Work Units 61152N.MR00001.001.1383, 62233N. MM33C30.004–1002, and 63706NM0095.004.1008.

The experiments with rats were conducted according to the principles set forth by the National Research Council (1986).

REFERENCES

Ahlers, S.T., and M.K.Salander 1993 Chronic administration of corticotropin releasing factor (CRF) results in tolerance to the suppression of performance observed with acute administration. Pharm. Biochem. Behav. 44:375–380.

Ahlers S.T., J.R.Thomas, and D.L.Berkey 1991 Hippocampal and body temperature changes in rats during delayed matching-to-sample performance in a cold environment. Physiol. Behav. 50:1013–1018.

Ahlers, S.T., M.K.Salander, D.Shurtleff, and J.R.Thomas 1992 Tyrosine pretreatment alleviates suppression of schedule-controlled responding produced by corticotropin releasing factor (CRF) in rats. Brain Res. Bull. 29:567–571.

Ahlers, S.T., D.Shurtleff, J.Schrot, J.R.Thomas, and F.Paul-Emile 1993 Glucose attenuates cold-induced impairment of delayed matching-to-sample performance in rats. Psychobiology 21:87–92.

Banderet, L.E., and H.K.Lieberman 1989 Treatment with tyrosine, a neurotransmitter precursor, reduces environmental stress in humans. Brain Res. Bull. 22:759–762.

Bushnell, P.J. 1990 Modelling working and reference memory in rats: Effects of scopolamine on delayed matching-to-position. Behav. Pharm. 1:419–427.

Chrousos, G.P., and P.W.Gold 1992 The concepts of stress and stress system disorders: Overview of physical and behavioral homeostasis. J. Am. Med. Assoc. 267:1244–1252.

Coleshaw, S.R.K., H.M.Davis, W.R.Keatinge, R.N.M.VanSomeren, and A.H.Wolff 1983a Memory registration at mildly depressed deep body temperatures. J. Physiol. 325:58.

Coleshaw, S.R.K., R.N.M.VanSomeren, A.H.Wolff, H.M.Davis, and W.R.Keatinge 1983b Impaired memory registration and speed of reasoning caused by low body temperature. J. Appl. Physiol. 55:27–31.

Dunn, A.J., and C.W.Berridge 1987 Corticotropin-releasing factor administration elicits a stress-like activation of cerebral catecholaminergic systems. Pharmacol. Biochem. Behav. 27:685–691.

Gage, F.H., P.A.T.Kelly, and A.Bjorklund 1984 Regional changes in brain glucose metabolism reflect cognitive impairments in aged rats. J. Neuroscience 4:2856–2865.

Gibson, C.J., and R.J.Wurtman 1978 Physiological control of brain norepinephrine synthesis by brain tyrosine concentration. Life Sci. 22:1399–1406.

Gold, P.E. 1991 An integrated memory system: From blood to brain. Pp. 391–418 in Peripheral Signaling of the Brain: Role in Neural-Immune Interactions and Learning and Memory, R.C.A. Frederickson, J.L.McGaugh, and D.L.Felten, eds. Lewiston, N.Y.: Hogrefe & Huber Publishers.

Lehnert, H., D.K.Reinstein, B.W.Strowbridge, and R.J.Wurtman 1984 Neurochemical and behavioral consequences of acute, uncontrollable stress: Effects of dietary tyrosine. Brain Res. 303:215–223.

Lenz, H.J., A.Raedler, H.Greten, and M.R.Brown 1987 CRF initiates biological actions within the brain that are observed in response to stress. Am. J. Physiol. 252(Reg. Integr. Comp. Physiol.):R34–R39.

Means, L.W., and T.J.Fernandez 1992 Daily glucose injections facilitate performance of a win-stay water-escape working memory task in mice. Behav. Neurosci. 106:345–350.

Melia, K.R., and R.S.Duman 1991 Involvement of corticotropin-releasing factor in chronic stress regulation of the brain noradrenergic system. Proc. Nat. Acad. Sci. USA 88:8382–8386.

Messier, C., T.Durkin, O.Mrabet, and C.Destrade 1991 Contribution of hippocampal acetylcholine synthesis to the memory-improving action of glucose. Pp. 473–477 in Peripheral Signaling of the Brain: Role in Neural-Immune Interactions and Learning and Memory, R.C.A.Frederickson, J.L.McGaugh, and D.L. Felten, eds. Lewiston, N.Y.: Hogrefe & Huber Publishers.

National Research Council 1986 Guide for the Care and Use of Laboratory Animals. Institute of Laboratory Animal Resources. Washington, D.C.: National Academy Press.

Nisenbaum, L.K., and E.D.Abercrombie 1992 Enhanced tyrosine hydroxylation in hippocampus of chronically stressed rats upon exposure to a novel stressor. J. Neurochem. 58:276–281.

Nisenbaum, L.K., M.J.Zigmond, A.F.Sved, and E.D.Abercrombie 1991 Prior exposure to chronic stress results in enhanced synthesis and release of hippocampal norepinephrine in response to a novel stressor. J. Neurosci. 11(5):1478–1484.

Owasoyo, J.O., D.F.Neri, and J.G.Lamberth 1992 Tyrosine and its potential use as a countermeasure to performance decrement in military sustained operations. Aviat. Space Environ. Med. 63:364–369.

Pozos, R.S. 1986 Cold stress and its effects on neural function. Pp. 25–35 in Human Performance in the Cold, G.A.Laursen, R.S.Pozos, and F.Hempel, eds. Bethesda, Md.: Undersea Medical Society.

Ragozzino, M.E., and P.E.Gold 1991 Glucose effects on mecamylamine-induced memory deficits and decreases in locomotor activity in mice. Behav. Neural Biol. 56:271–282.

Rauch, M.T., and H.R.Lieberman 1990 Tyrosine pretreatment reverses hypothermia-induced behavioral depression. Brain Res. Bull. 24:147–150.

Reinstein, D.K., H.Lehnert, N.A.Scott, and R.J.Wurtman 1984 Tyrosine prevents behavioral and neurochemical correlates of an acute stress in rats. Life Sci. 34:2225–2231.

Salter, C.A. 1989 Dietary tyrosine as an aid to stress resistance among troops. Milit. Med. 154:144–146.

Sampson, J.B. 1984 Anxiety as a factor in the incidence of combat cold injury: A review. Milit. Med. 149:89–91.

Shurtleff, D., J.R.Thomas, S.T.Ahlers, and J.Schrot 1993 Tyrosine ameliorates a cold-induced delayed matching-to-sample performance decrement in rats. Psychopharmacology. (Berl.) 112:228–232

Stone, E.A. 1987 Brain noradrenergic mechanisms in models of depression. Pp. 263–277 in Hormones and Depression, U.Halbreich, ed. New York: Raven Press.

Stone, W.S., B.Walser, S.D.Gold, and P.E.Gold 1991 Scopolamine- and morphine-induced impairments of spontaneous alternation performance in mice: Reversal with glucose and with cholinergic and adrenergic agonists. Behav. Neurosci. 105:264–271.

Thomas, J.R., S.T.Ahlers, J.F.House, and J.Schrot 1989 Repeated exposure to moderate cold impairs matching-to-sample performance. Aviat. Space Environ. Med. 60:1063–1067.

Thomas, J.R., S.T.Ahlers, J.Schrot, J.F.House, K.F.Van Orden, M.M.Winsborough, R.L. Hesslink, and S.B.Lewis 1990 Adrenergic response to cognitive activity in a cold environment. J. Appl. Physiol. 68:962–966.

Thomas, J.R., S.T.Ahlers, and J.Schrot 1991a Cold-induced impairment of delayed matching in rats. Behav. Neural Biol. 55:19–30.

Thomas, J.R., S.T.Ahlers, and D.Shurtleff 1991b Thermal stress modulates temporal patterns of responding on a multiple DRL-FR schedule. Physiol. Behav. 50:437–442.

Webb, P. 1984 Impaired performance from prolonged mild body cooling. Pp. 391–400 in Underwater Physiology, A.J.Bachrach and M.M.Matzen, eds. Bethesda, Md.: Undersea Medical Society.

Wenk, G.L. 1989 An hypothesis on the role of glucose in the mechanism of action of cognition enhancers. Psychopharmacology 99:431–438.

DISCUSSION

JOHN MILNER: I have a question dealing with multiple exposures to tyrosine. I am concerned that on the basis of Harris Lieberman's information about the interaction of tyrosine with some drugs, amphetamines in particular, one might, in fact, be looking at some inducible types of enzyme problems, that the response might occur once but it might not occur a second time. Do you have any information on that?

STEPHEN AHLERS: Our studies with tyrosine are replicated several times for each subject, so we do not use one dose of tyrosine; we use several doses two or three times and then use the aggregate data for analysis.

JOHN FERNSTROM: So there is no diminished response?

STEPHEN AHLERS: There is no diminishing of tyrosine's efficacy when it, in fact, works. I assume Harris Lieberman has found the same thing.

HARRIS LIEBERMAN: We have administered tyrosine repeatedly in the course of studies and have not seen any evidence that there is a diminution in effect. If you are talking about the chronic administration that Steve Ahlers was talking about at the end of his discussion [Chapter 16]—and I believe Carol Greenwood also referred to the possibility of potentiating this type of enzyme—then there may be an issue with chronic administration. Actually, your point had to do more with chronic stress than with chronic administration.

STEPHEN AHLERS: Exactly. A chronically stressed organism is probably a different organism. By the way, those changes were not transient; the tolerance to CRF persisted for 3 to 6 months.

GILBERT LEVEILLE: I have a concern that is somewhat analogous to John Fernstrom's, and it is really one of safety as we think about using materials such as tyrosine. Most of the paradigms that we have seen are the use of single bolus administrations to look for an effect. But Harris Lieberman mentioned eventually putting tyrosine in rations, and we know how these substances can be readily abused. What do we know about the toxicology of something like tyrosine administered at these dose levels?

STEPHEN AHLERS: I do not think there is much in terms of toxicology. Very rarely do you see an effect of tyrosine by itself, although we saw some effects, but I am not sure what caused those effects.

HARRIS LIEBERMAN: My response is the same as Steve Ahlers. I am not aware of anything like that with tyrosine.

STEPHEN AHLERS: Yes.

CHANDON PRASAD: And also, the cold ambient temperature is a problem. Therefore, the implication would be the release of corticotropin-releasing factor. Have you tried to give the corticotropin-releasing factor antagonist and really prove it?

STEPHEN AHLERS: That is one of our next experiments. That is actually the reason we used CRF to induce the stress response, to get around the potentially confounding differences involved with the administration of physical stressors. You are quite right, the potential of the corticotropin-releasing factor antagonist to block the effects of cold stress is very important. It is our next study.

17

Carbohydrates, Protein,, and Performance

Bonnie J.Spring,[1] *Regina Pingitore, and Jen Schoenfeld*

INTRODUCTION

Investigators have shown great interest in diets that can optimize performance in the workplace, the athletic field, and military combat situations (Kanarek and Marks-Kaufman, 1991; Lieberman, 1989; Logue, 1986; Spring, 1986). Among the candidate food constituents that might enhance performance, carbohydrates have long been accorded a special place. For example, since 1985, carbohydrates have commandeered the largest share of the U.S. Army Research Institute of Environmental Medicine's research effort on performance-enhancing food components, absorbing 60 percent of the research effort (see Chapter 3). This chapter discusses the effects of carbohydrates on mood, cognitive performance, satiety, and physical endurance. The information presented here suggests that behavioral effects are systematically influenced by the caloric and macronutrient compositions of the meal, especially by its ratio of carbohydrate to protein; by the time of day it is consumed; by individual differences, including the temperament and usual eating habits of the

[1] Bonnie J.Spring, Department of Psychology, University of Health Sciences, The Chicago Medical School, N. Chicago, IL 60064

consumer; and by the surrounding psychological context, including the influences of motivation and stress.

THE HEURISTIC IMPORTANCE OF FOLK WISDOMS

Ironically, two folk beliefs have supplied much of the impetus behind research on carbohydrates and behavior (Spring and Alexander, 1989). One folk wisdom prescribes how to acutely achieve peak performance, suggesting that ingestion of simple sugars can attain this objective. The other specifies how to attain performances that need to be elicited long after eating or sustained at a high level for a prolonged period of time. Conventional wisdom endorses the use of complex carbohydrates for that objective, suggesting that they support optimal performances that stably endure. Both folk beliefs share an assumption that fluctuations in plasma glucose levels parallel and mediate the emergence of peaks and troughs in physical and mental performance. Ordinarily, one would cursorily skim over folk wisdoms and proceed rapidly to the scientific theories that have guided research on diet and behavior. In this case, however, folk wisdoms have exerted the more powerful formative influence; therefore, this chapter describes them in some detail.

Simple Sugars

Popular wisdom holds that the energy needed to achieve a stellar performance is as accessible as the nearest candy bar (Dufty, 1975). Nearly 75 percent of Americans regard sugar as a source of quick energy, according to nationwide attitudinal surveys (Fischler, 1987). The simple carbohydrates in sweet snack foods are touted to generate a burst of stamina—the "sugar buzz"—that parallels and directly results from a steep rise in plasma glucose levels. By extrapolation from the metaphor that blood sugar energizes metabolic processes, sugar becomes the presumptive energizer of behavioral processes as well (Spring and Alexander, 1989). Empirical support for the proposition that an acute rise in plasma glucose levels translates to increased mental energy is minimal at best (Gonder-Frederick et al., 1989; Spring et al., 1987). As described later, at least within the bounds of normoglycemia, this particular proposition is probably best regarded as the reification of a metaphor.

A corollary to the folk wisdom that simple sugars offer a quick pick-me-up is the conviction that the benefits are short-lived (Dufty, 1975). Perhaps because many Americans are Puritans at heart, folk beliefs threaten that few benefits can be gleaned without a cost. In the case of simple carbohydrates and performance, that cost is "reactive hypoglycemia": an alleged sudden plummeting of plasma glucose levels that occurs because the initially steep rise in plasma glucose level triggers insulin overproduction (Harris, 1924). In folk wisdom, at least, the extreme glucose fluctuations that result from eating simple sugars propel the performer on a roller coaster ride from superproductivity to collapse. The fact that reactive hypoglycemia is far too rare a clinical condition (Permuth, 1976) to explain the modal performance characteristics of average individuals is problematic for this theory. The proposition that a less exaggerated fall in glucose within the normoglycemic range could have adverse functional consequences remains unsupported, although much research on carbohydrates and behavior has been guided by this assumption (Prinz et al., 1980; Virkkunen, 1986).

Complex Carbohydrates

Folk wisdom's dietary preventive against peaks and troughs in plasma glucose levels is ingestion of complex carbohydrates. By delaying and blunting both the rise and the fall of the plasma glucose concentration, starches are assumed to ensure a sustained source of metabolic energy, allegedly yielding stabler performance. Unlike the assumption that simple sugars commonly provoke reactive hypoglycemia, folk wisdoms about complex carbohydrates have at least some empirical support. Some starches, such as bread, do have lower glycemic indices than some simple carbohydrates, such as glucose (Jenkins et al., 1981). On the other hand, the glycemic indices for other starches, like potato, are virtually the same as that for glucose (Crapo, 1984). These findings, combined with evidence that parameters like fiber content, food form, digestibility, cooking method, and eating rate critically influence the glycemic response, have challenged the generalization that complex carbohydrates reliably engender lower glycemic indices than simple sugars do (Crapo, 1984).

It also remains unclear whether, at some interval after eating, higher glucose levels translate into better performances. Although some findings support this inference (Pollitt et al., 1981), others do not (Cromer et al., 1990). Nonetheless, a considerable research effort has aimed to promote stably high levels of performance by identifying diets that prolong the tail of the glucose curve, yielding moderate, sustained glucose elevations long after eating. Tests of large bolus doses or intermittent doses of complex carbohydrates, as well as doses that incorporate fiber and even protein (Arvedson et al., 1969), have all been justified on this basis.

DEFINING THE TARGET BEHAVIORS: MOOD, PERFORMANCE, SATIETY

What behaviors promote success in the military combat environment, and what dietary interventions will best support them? Stereotyped images of war suggest that the skills needed to succeed in military combat closely resemble the physical capabilities needed to excel in sports requiring physical endurance. Indeed, even today, military training places heavy emphasis on developing physical strength, stamina, and endurance. On the other hand, the nature of military operations has changed so greatly that, especially in combat situations, many contemporary soldiers work not from the trenches but, rather, from the seats of heavily computerized vehicles. Perhaps even more than previously, today's combat environment is as likely to tax mental and emotional wherewithal as it is to strain physical endurance. Characteristic of the combat situation are demands to generate complex cognitive or psychomotor performances under conditions of boredom, physical discomfort, prolonged sleep deprivation, or severe emotional distress. Because sensorimotor and cognitive performances are essential to all domains of military operations during war or peacetime, they are given primacy in this chapter. Because it may be necessary for long intervals to elapse between eating occasions, satiety is briefly discussed. Finally, the chapter touches peripherally upon physical endurance because that topic is addressed by other contributors to this volume.

Mood: An Underrated Outcome

Mood has been underrated and performance has been overrated as indices of dietary influences on behavior. Although it can be argued that tests of mood assess subjective, unverifiable phenomena, mood scores are highly correlated with cognitive performance, especially under extreme circumstances. Consider the findings of Bugge et al. (1979), who assessed mood and cognitive performance among Norwegian military cadets who underwent 4 days of nearly continuous sleep deprivation in addition to caloric restriction. Scores on tests of coding, logical reasoning, and letter cancellation deteriorated markedly under these conditions. Furthermore, correlation coefficients between performance and mood ranged between $r=0.85$ and 0.90 for positive mood and between $r=-0.86$ and −0.94 for negative mood. These findings suggest that under highly adverse circumstances, tests of mood and cognitive performance convey virtually the same information.

Of potentially greater importance are contexts in which mood and performance convey different information. Under ordinary circumstances, most performance tests yield only coarse indicators of organismic burden or stress.

This is because few sensorimotor or information processing tasks are so demanding of cognitive resources that they utilize full cognitive capacity (Kahneman, 1973; Wickens, 1984). Because reserve or ancillary resources are available to be allocated to whatever task is at hand, performance can remain unimpaired long after distress is evident in other functional spheres including affective state and physiological homeostasis. Indeed, the experience has been that, whereas mood reliably reflects the effects of caloric deprivation, sensorimotor and cognitive performances are insensitive to caloric restriction, except under conditions that impose an additional burden (Spring et al., 1992). Two added burdens that make caloric deprivation deficits become visible are stress or demands for continuous performance without allowing recuperative time between tasks. It is suspected that these conditions elicit deficits because they drain spare capacity and thus unmask deterioration that would otherwise not be visible.

To illustrate how insensitive performance indicators can be, consider the findings of Diaz et al. (1991), who studied the productivities of two groups of Gambian subsistence farmers during the hungry season as they worked to build a road. The farmers' work was to shovel gravel into wheelbarrows, wheel it 1.5 km to the road, unload the gravel, and repeat the cycle for 8 h. Farmers were studied under two feeding conditions: one supplying an unlimited supply of energy-dense foods; the other supplying insufficient calories to match energy expenditures. The caloric restrictions were sufficient to cause significant weight loss. Nonetheless, work productivity was unaffected: no effects could be detected on the total number of loads transported, the number of loads per working hour, or the amount of time per load. The authors attribute these results to a motivational incentive so powerful that it overrode the effects of severe energy deficit: the men were paid $0.63 per load, a generous wage by local standards.

The results of Diaz et al. (1991) can be explained by resource models, which propose that motivation, interest, and effort actually increase functional performance capacity (Kahneman, 1973). A more telling interpretation comes, perhaps, by analogy to Sholem Aleichom's story about the man who decided to save money by feeding his horse only once per day. The horse still pulled the cart just as before. Then, to save more money, the man chose to feed the horse only three times per week. Still, the horse pulled the cart. Finally, the man decided to feed the horse only once a week. The horse died. "What a shame," said the man, "just when the horse finally got used to eating three times a week!" One could infer, as the man did, that no problem existed until the horse died, but this would be the wrong conclusion. The correct conclusion is that the horse's performance was an insensitive measure of the adverse effects of caloric restriction, since the horse could still walk even when it was starving to death. To the extent that performance lags behind in reflecting adverse effects of dietary or other strictures, it is useful to have more sensitive early warning signs of impending decline. Subjective fatigue or dysphoria may offer such a potential.

Mood state can also serve as a proxy variable for *approach motivation,* an attribute that can profoundly influence combat performance. A soldier's early proactive response to potential danger can make the difference between an averted disaster and a tragic loss of life. In anecdotal accounts of friendly fire accidents presented at the conference on which this volume is based, a common denominator was that the soldier had been aware of present danger but had not acted because of fatigue, lethargy, or hesitancy. If, in that state of failure to spontaneously "go the extra mile," the recruit had been required to perform a cognitive task, he or she could probably have done so without error. The performance task would, thus, not capture highly salient information about the soldier's state: i.e., his or her lowered motivation to spontaneously initiate action of his or her own accord. Subjective fatigue can have profound motivational consequences in the combat environment.

CARBOHYDRATES AND FATIGUE

The authors' interest in dietary effects on mood stemmed from an initial study that compared the behavioral responses of 184 healthy adult men and women to a sucrose-rich, high-carbohydrate, low-protein meal versus those to a high-protein meal (Spring et al., 1983). Contrary to the popular wisdom that sugar is activating, the female subjects reported fatigue, and the male subjects reported calmness after eating carbohydrates. The gender difference was interpreted as evidence of a more intense but similar mood in women, because gender differences in average body weight render the carbohydrates in the fixed-size meal a proportionately higher dose for women.

In subsequent studies, a high-carbohydrate meal, given in sufficient quantity and eaten at lunchtime, was also found to trigger fatigue in men to a greater extent than an isocaloric protein meal did (Lieberman et al., 1986a; Spring et al., 1986). Moreover, the carbohydrate-rich meal did not need to be rich in simple carbohydrates to engender fatigue; a high-starch, protein-poor lunch also triggered greater fatigue than a protein-rich lunch.

Mechanisms: Opioids? Hypoglycemia? Serotonin?

Spring and colleagues (1989) studied three mechanisms that might explain the fatiguing effects of a high-carbohydrate meal. In a repeated-measures design, healthy adult women ate a standard breakfast in the laboratory and were assessed before and after fasting through the noon hour or eating one of three lunches that were provided in counterbalanced order. The protein lunch was 318.8 g of turkey breast plus mayonnaise, supplying 780 kcal, 105.0 g of protein, and 33.3 g of fat. The carbohydrate and balanced lunches each consisted of six sweet, cookie-type lunch bars. The carbohydrate lunch supplied 799 kcal, 105 g of carbohydrate, 0.7 g of protein, and 42.7 g of fat. The balanced lunch, offering carbohydate to protein in approximately a 3/1 ratio, supplied 774 kcal, 76.0 g of carbohydrate, 27.7 g of protein, and 40 g of fat. Self-reported fatigue and plasma glucose, serum insulin, and plasma amino acid concentrations for each condition are shown in Figures 17–1 to 17–4, respectively.

Sweet Taste

One hypothesis was that both the carbohydrate and the balanced lunches would have comparable calming effects on mood because both were sweet and would, therefore, presumably exert similar effects on endogenous opioids (Fantino et al., 1986; Getto et al., 1984; Morley et al., 1981). Inspection of Figure 17–1 shows that this hypothesis was incorrect. The carbohydrate meal

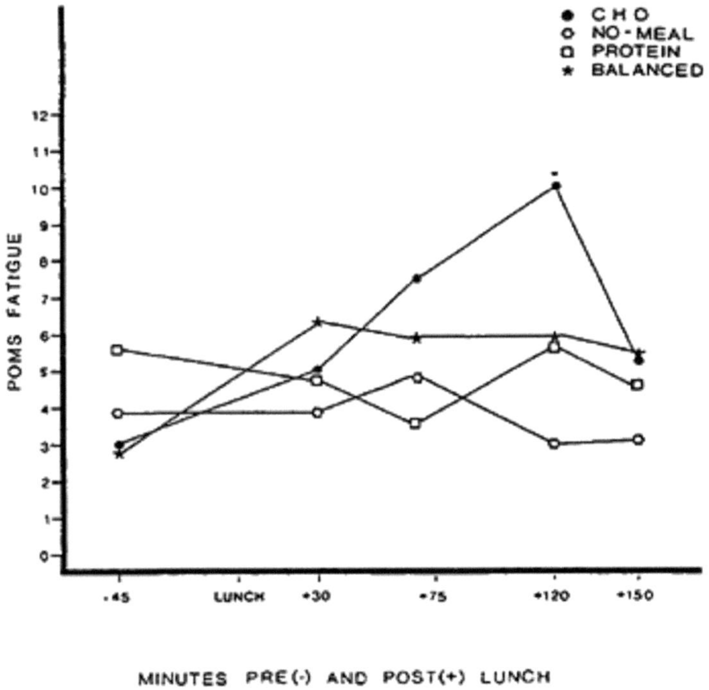

FIGURE 17–1 Fatigue reported on the Profile of Mood States (POMS) before and after eating a high-carbohydrate, low-protein lunch (CHO); a high-protein, low-carbohydrate lunch (PROTEIN); a balanced lunch containing both carbohydrate and protein (BALANCED); or fasting (NO-MEAL). SOURCE: Spring et al. (1989), used with permission.

was the only lunch that triggered a significant increase in fatigue, which occurred about 2 h after eating. In spite of their hedonic similarity to the carbohydrate cookies, the balanced cookies did not trigger fatigue.

Reactive Hypoglycemia

The next hypothesis was that if reactive hypoglycemia is responsible for carbohydrate-induced fatigue, then drowsiness should be greatest after the carbohydrate lunch and should occur in temporal proximity to an overproduction of insulin and a sharp decline in plasma glucose to hypoglycemic levels. The carbohydrate lunch did indeed trigger fatigue. As Figure 17–3 shows, however, the fatiguing effect of the carbohydrate meal could not be explained by a unique effect on insulin, because both the carbohydrate and the balanced lunches produced roughly comparable insulin responses. Furthermore, as Figure 17–2 shows, fatigue after the carbohydrate lunch could not be attributed to hypoglycemia because the plasma glucose level remained elevated at the time when fatigue occurred. The findings do not rule out the possibility that drowsiness after a carbohydrate meal could be triggered by a declining level of plasma glucose rather than by an aberrant insulin response or an absolute

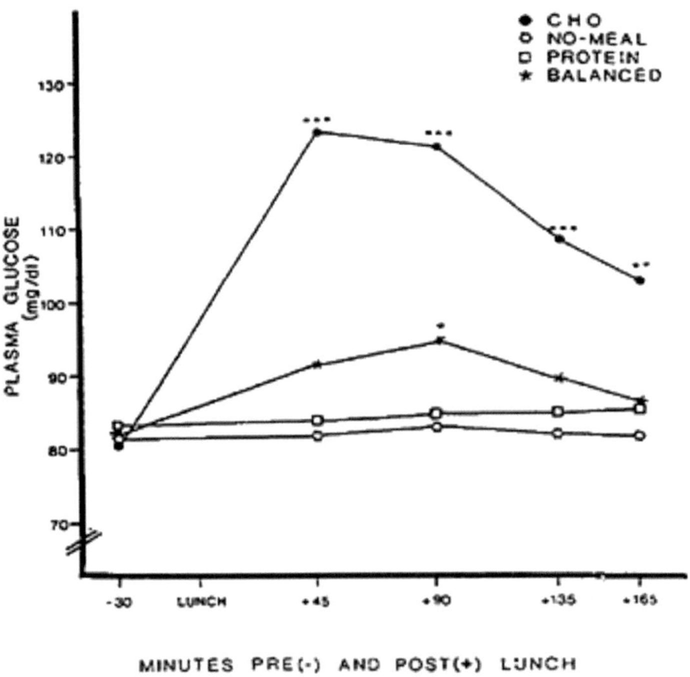

FIGURE 17–2 Plasma glucose (in milligrams per deciliter) before and after eating a high-carbohydrate, low-protein lunch (CHO); a high-protein, low-carbohydrate lunch (PROTEIN); a balanced lunch containing both carbohydrate and protein (BALANCED); or fasting (NO-MEAL).
SOURCE: Spring et al. (1989), used with permission.

hypoglycemic level of glucose. The results are, however, incompatible with a simple explanation on the basis of reactive hypoglycemia.

Plasma Amino Acids

A final hypothesis was that fatigue after eating carbohydrates results from effects on plasma amino acids, which, in turn, influence the synthesis and release of brain serotonin. Consumption of a high-carbohydrate, protein-poor meal increases the ratio of plasma tryptophan to other large neutral amino acids, which predicts increased brain tryptophan influx (Fernstrom and Wurtman, 1971). Since tryptophan is the precursor of serotonin and since the enzymes that catalyze serotonin synthesis are not fully saturated, serotonin synthesis is substrate dependent. An increase in brain tryptophan influx therefore leads to an increase in both brain serotonin synthesis and release, insofar as the latter is indexed by the cerobrospinal fluid (CSF) levels of 5-hydroxyindoleacetic acid (5-HIAA), serotonin's major metabolite (Fernstrom and Wurtman, 1972; Wurtman et al., 1980; Yokogoshi et al., 1987). Because

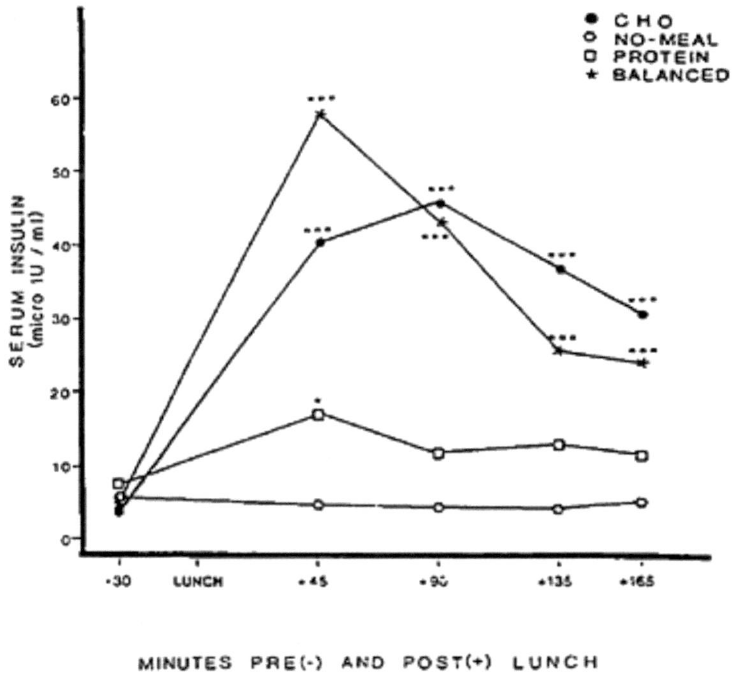

FIGURE 17–3 Serum insulin (micro-international units per milliliter) before and after eating a high-carbohydrate, low-protein lunch (CHO); a high-protein, low-carbohydrate lunch (PROTEIN); a balanced lunch containing both carbohydrate and protein (BALANCED); or fasting (NO-MEAL). SOURCE: Spring et al. (1989), used with permission.

serotonergic midbrain raphe neurons play a role in initiating the onset of sleep (Hartmann and Greenwald, 1984), drowsiness is a likely accompaniment of increased serotonin synthesis in a healthy brain. As Figure 17–4 shows, the high-carbohydrate, low-protein lunch did significantly increase the ratio of plasma tryptophan to the other large neutral amino acids that share the same transport system across the blood-brain barrier. Moreover, consistent with the hypothesis, fatigue did emerge at about the same time that the tryptophan ratio increased, although it remains unclear why fatigue dissipated even though the ratio remained elevated.

Thus far, carbohydrate-induced fatigue has emerged consistently and is most plausibly explained by the serotonin hypothesis. Neither the sweetness of lunches, nor their effects on insulin, nor their absolute effects on glucose predicted whether meals would induce fatigue. On the other hand, drowsiness occurred reliably about 2 h after a carbohydrate-rich, virtually protein-free lunch, and fatigue appeared in parallel with a rise in the tryptophan ratio.

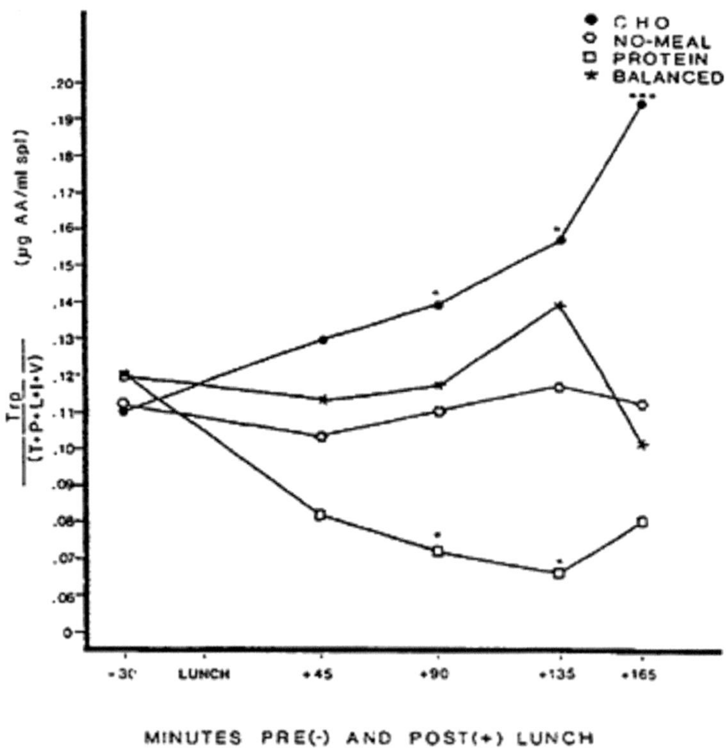

FIGURE 17–4 Ratio of plasma tryptophan (Trp) to the sum of plasma tyrosine (T), phenylalanine (P), leucine (L), isoleucine (I), and valine (V) before and after eating a high-carbohydrate, low-protein lunch (CHO); a high-protein, low-carbohydrate lunch (PROTEIN); a balanced lunch containing both carbohydrate and protein (BALANCED); or fasting (NO-MEAL). AA, amino acids. SOURCE: Spring et al. (1989), used with permission.

Breakfast Versus Lunch

Recently, the research emphasis has shifted from the midday lunch context to the study of breakfast. The results of three studies are described only briefly because they are not yet published. In a nutshell, the results suggest that there are both commonalities and differences between the manner in which carbohydrates affect mood in the morning versus the early afternoon. The core difference is that macronutrient effects are displayed across a different diurnal context. At noontime all meals exceeding about 300 cal tend to engender some fatigue. In healthy adults, both protein-rich and protein-deficient, carbohydrate-rich meals cause some drowsiness, but the latter cause greater drowsiness (cf. Rosenthal et al., 1989; Spring et al., 1983). In the morning, the diurnal pattern is reversed. Among regular breakfast eaters, a breakfast of any macronutrient composition tends to lessen fatigue in comparison with the baseline, whereas fasting leaves the person as drowsy as upon awakening. The relative activating impact of the macronutrients is, however, the same as it is at lunchtime. As breakfast, a protein-rich meal has a greater antifatiguing action than does a protein-poor, carbohydrate-rich meal.

Because of the different diurnal background, tests of carbohydrate effects on mood would be expected to produce somewhat different outcomes when the experimental meals are served as lunch rather than as breakfast. A carbohydrate test meal served as lunch should produce greater fatigue than fasting or than an isocaloric protein meal. A carbohydrate test meal served as breakfast should produce less fatigue than fasting but less activation than a protein test meal.

The Balanced Meal Threshold

To increase the plasma tryptophan ratio, a meal must be both carbohydrate-rich and protein-poor. Considerable effort has been devoted to determining just how rich in carbohydrate and how poor in protein a meal must be in order to elevate the plasma tryptophan ratio. In fasted rats, a meal containing 70–75 percent of an insulin-secreting carbohydrate increases the plasma tryptophan ratio, whereas a meal containing 25 percent carbohydrate fails to do so (Yokogoshi and Wurtman, 1986). In addition to being abundant, a carbohydrate must also be insulin-secreting (e.g., glucose, sucrose, and dextrose) if it is to elevate the tryptophan ratio. In contrast, fructose, the sugar that predominates in fruits, has a relatively weak effect on insulin. Consequently, a high-carbohydrate breakfast chiefly comprising fruit juice, even if sweetened by sucrose, fails to increase the plasma tryptophan ratio (Teff et al., 1989).

A protein-rich meal decreases the tryptophan ratio probably by contributing much larger quantities of large neutral amino acids other than tryptophan to the bloodstream. Moreover, a protein-rich meal has been found to decrease CSF tryptophan and 5-HIAA levels (Perez-Cruet et al., 1972). Proteins, however, differ in how effectively they suppress a carbohydrate-induced rise in the plasma tryptophan ratio. For example, in rats, whereas 5 percent casein or 10 percent peanut meal or gelatin fully blocks the rise triggered by a 70 percent carbohydrate meal, 10 percent lactalbumin fails to do so, and 10 percent egg white does so only partially (Yokogoshi and Wurtman, 1986).

For humans, how little protein blocks a carbohydrate-induced rise in the tryptophan ratio, creating what is, from the perspective of this ratio, a balanced meal? To answer this question, Teff and colleagues (1989) served healthy male subjects breakfast puddings containing either 0, 4, 8, or 12 percent protein. They also studied a conventional breakfast of Danish pastry and coffee, in which protein was about 10 percent the amount of carbohydrate. The ratio of plasma tryptophan to other large neutral amino acids was determined before and 2 h after each breakfast. The results are shown in Table 17–1.

Teff and colleagues (1989) found that only the pure carbohydrate breakfast elevated the plasma tryptophan ratio significantly. The 4 percent protein breakfast also elevated the ratio, although not significantly. On the other hand, breakfasts, including Danish pastry, that contained at least 8 percent protein actually lowered the tryptophan ratio slightly.

Overview of Studies on Carbohydrates and Fatigue

If increased brain tryptophan influx and serotonin synthesis is the mechanism that causes drowsiness after a high-carbohydrate meal, then carbohydrate meals that actually increase the tryptophan ratio should be the ones most likely to induce fatigue. In other words, meals that contain less than 4 percent protein should be the ones most likely to cause drowsiness. Table 17–2 presents an overview of studies that tested whether a high-carbohydrate meal induces postmeal fatigue.

Inspection of Table 17–2 indicates that carbohydrate-induced fatigue was observed most reliably in studies that used a test meal containing 0 percent protein. In contrast, fatigue was not consistently detected following carbohydrate meals that were of more balanced composition, containing more than 4 percent protein. It is also noteworthy that only one of three studies of breakfast observed carbohydrate-induced fatigue. As discussed earlier, for regular breakfast eaters, a morning meal is more likely to have activating than sedating effects.

TABLE 17–1 Effect of Dietary Treatments on Plasma Amino Acid Ratios

Breakfast Content	Treatment Time	Trp/LNAA
Protein		
0 percent	Pre	0.133±0.029
	Post	0.168±0.042*
4 percent	Pre	0.129±0.030
	Post	0.140±0.026
8 percent	Pre	0.144±0.025
	Post	0.135±0.029
12 percent	Pre	0.122±0.025
	Post	0.112±0.017
Danish pastry	Pre	0.132±0.026
	Post	0.129±0.025

NOTES: Values are given as the mean±standard deviation of 10 determinations (Tukey's test). The data revealed that only the 0 percent protein meal caused a significant change in the tryptophan ratio (q=4.73, p<0.05). Treatment time is pre-or postmeal. Trp, tryptophan; LNAA, large neutral amino acids (tyrosine, phenylalanine, leucine, isoleucine, and valine); *, P<0.05.
SOURCE: Teff et al. (1989), used with permission.

Military Applications

Carbohydrate-rich, protein-poor foods could intentionally be applied to engender fatigue in troops required to go to sleep at unusual hours. It is likely that this application would be most effective in the afternoon and possibly evening hours but would not be recommended for morning usage. Whereas most spontaneously selected meals would incorporate too much protein to be useful soporifics, macronutrient control would be possible in rations used to induce sleep in military personnel.

Individual Differences in Affective Response to Carbohydrates

Individual differences characterize the affective response to carbohydrates. In contrast to the fatiguing effects just described, individuals with certain

TABLE 17–2 Studies Testing Whether a Carbohydrate Meal Induces Greater Fatigue than a Protein Meal or Fasting Control

Study	Meal Time	Percent Protein	Result
Hartmann et al., 1977	Evening	0	Yes
Spring et al., 1983	Breakfast	0	Yes
	Lunch	0	Yes
Spring et al., 1989	Lunch	0	Yes
Lieberman et al., 1986a	Lunch	0	Yes
Lieberman et al., 1986b	Lunch	0	Yes
Rosenthal et al., 1989	Lunch	0	Yes
Thayer, 1987	Afternoon	<4	Yes
	Evening	<4	Yes
	Morning	<4	No
Wurtman et al., 1989	Evening	5.4	No
Lieberman et al., 1989	Breakfast	<13.0	No
	Evening	<13.0	Yes
Smith et al., 1988	Lunch	27.0	No

NOTE: The control condition(s) varied across studies and was either an isocaloric, higher-protein meal or fasting. Studies are arrayed according to percent protein in the carbohydrate test meal and the time of the test meal. Findings are categorized according to whether carbohydrate-induced fatigue was greater than that in the control condition (Yes) or the same or directionally less than that in the control condition (No).

conditions experience activation and reduction of depression or anxiety after eating carbohydrates. The activating and mood-enhancing effects of carbohydrates have been observed in patients with seasonal affective disorder (Rosenthal et al., 1989), obese individuals who snack preferentially on carbohydrate-rich foods (Lieberman et al., 1986b), and females with premenstrual distress syndrome (Wurtman et al, 1989). Shared features of these clinical conditions include dysphoric mood and weight management difficulties arising from overeating of high-carbohydrate snacks.

Carbohydrates and Satiety

If extended time periods must elapse between eating occasions, carbohydrate-rich, protein-poor meals have a liability in that they are not very satiating. A widely replicated finding is that, weight for weight, protein is substantially more satiating than carbohydrate (Blundell and Hill, 1988). The greater satiating power of protein is both immediate and sustained. A protein-rich meal leaves a greater sensation of fullness at the end of a meal than does an isocaloric carbohydrate-rich meal (Spring et al., 1983). Furthermore, the satiating effect carries over until the next meal. For example, Teff et al. (1989) found that a high-protein breakfast with only half the energy value of a high-carbohydrate breakfast exerted an equipotent satiating effect on lunchtime food selections.

Carbohydrates and Mood: Conclusions

Several conclusions can be made about the effects of carbohydrates on mood.

- A high-carbohydrate meal that is lacking in protein is followed by more fatigue than occurs after a meal higher in protein.
- Diurnal differences characterize the effects of carbohydrates in the morning versus those in the early afternoon. After a high-carbohydrate, low-protein lunch, fatigue increases more than after a higher-protein lunch. After a high-carbohydrate, low-protein breakfast, fatigue decreases less than after a higher-protein breakfast.
- The fatiguing effects of carbohydrate emerge most reliably when meals contain less than 4 percent protein.
- Individual differences characterize the affective response to carbohydrate. In certain clinical conditions characterized by dysphoric mood, weight management difficulties, and heightened snacking on carbohydrate-rich foods, carbohydrate has activating, antidysphoric effects.
- Weight for weight, carbohydrate is less satiating than protein.

CARBOHYDRATES AND COGNITIVE PERFORMANCE

As was the case for mood, cognitive performance is affected differently by carbohydrates taken at breakfast, at lunch, and as snacks. Therefore, these contexts are considered separately.

Breakfast

The next section on lunch discusses the postmeal dips in performance that are engendered by eating. At breakfast, however, the picture is different. The only group of subjects who have been found to show a postmeal dip in performance after eating breakfast are individuals who regularly skip breakfast (Richards, 1972). Some evidence indicates that military personnel who regularly eat breakfast exhibit greater physical fitness than those who do not (Trent and Conway, 1988). Since breakfast is one component of any appropriate meal plan that the military will implement to ensure health and fitness, the comments below pertain only to individuals who regularly eat breakfast.

A large body of research has examined whether skipping breakfast has adverse effects on the late-morning performance of cognitive tasks and whether meals of particular composition are differentially effective in preventing cognitive decline. Data are most extensive for young children, with some evidence supporting (Pollitt et al., 1981, 1983) and other evidence contradicting (Simeon and Grantham-McGregor, 1989) the hypothesis that, for healthy youngsters, skipping breakfast engenders late-morning impairment on cognitive tests. Findings for adolescents are more consistently negative, with most studies failing to find adverse effects of fasting on late-morning cognitive test scores (Arvedson et al., 1969; Cromer et al., 1990; Dickie and Bender, 1982a,b). Few studies have been carried out with adults, but in those studies that have been done in adults, decreased work output emerges reliably, and attentional or cognitive difficulties emerge intermittently (Daum et al., 1950; Tuttle et al., 1949, 1950).

Several factors influence whether late-morning performance impairments occur after skipping breakfast. First, the adverse cognitive effects of fasting are especially likely to occur in those who have a prior or current history of malnourishment (Simeon and Grantham-McGregor, 1989). Second, skipping breakfast is more likely to impair the performance of those who usually eat breakfast (Richards, 1971, 1972). Third, emotional and/or physical stress and continuous time pressure increase the likelihood that late-morning impairments will appear on tests of complex cognitive functions. Eating a breakfast of any composition works against the emergence of late-morning performance deficits, and when differences between meals are found, cognitive performance is better after the higher-protein breakfast (Spring et al., 1992).

Lunch

A large variety of cognitive performances, including vigilance, reaction time, sorting, and arithmetic, show a steady increase during the course of daylight hours (Blake, 1971). This trend is marred by a temporary decline in efficiency in the middle of the day. Some have argued that the midday decline, which has become known as the "postlunch dip," is of entirely endogenous origins (Hildebrandt et al., 1974), but there is increasing evidence that the deterioration in performance is caused at least partly by eating lunch (Smith and Miles, 1986b). The slight plateauing of the body temperature curve that is evident in early to midafternoon (Blake, 1971) may signify a vulnerable period in the diurnal rhythm, especially in contrast to the strong morning upswing. A heavy lunch is one burden that can apparently make midday performance liabilities become manifest.

Figure 17–5 shows the findings of Craig et al. (1981) for the percent drop in efficiency on a visual discrimination task after the lunch interval for students who consumed a three-course lunch versus those who fasted. Whereas a significant impairment in perceptual discrimination occurred as a function of eating lunch, the ability to discriminate was unchanged among those who skipped lunch. The magnitude of the decline was approximately a 10 percent change in performance efficiency, about comparable to the degree of impairment that would occur after missing a night of sleep (Craig, 1986). Various studies show that the postlunch dip is at a maximum 1–3 h after lunch and dissipates afterward (Craig et al., 1986; Spring et al., 1986).

Moderating Variables

Several factors moderate the magnitude and even the occurrence of the postlunch dip in performance. One of the more powerful influences is the number of calories consumed at the lunchtime meal, which, in turn, exerts its effect in interaction with usual lunchtime eating habits. Figure 17–6 shows Craig and Richardson's (1989) finding for the percent change in omission errors on a sustained-attention task as a function of the size of the subject's usual lunch and the size of the experimental meal. The results indicate that a big three-course lunch of about 1,380 cal significantly increased errors on the attentional task. Moreover, the largest drop in performance was found for subjects who were accustomed to eating a light lunch. In contrast, a light lunch of less than 300 cal did not cause a postlunch dip in performance.

The macronutrient composition of the meal also influences the likelihood that a lunch will elicit a postlunch dip and affects the magnitude of performance deterioration that will be observed. Carbohydrate-rich, protein-poor meals elicit greater performance deterioration than do isocaloric protein-rich

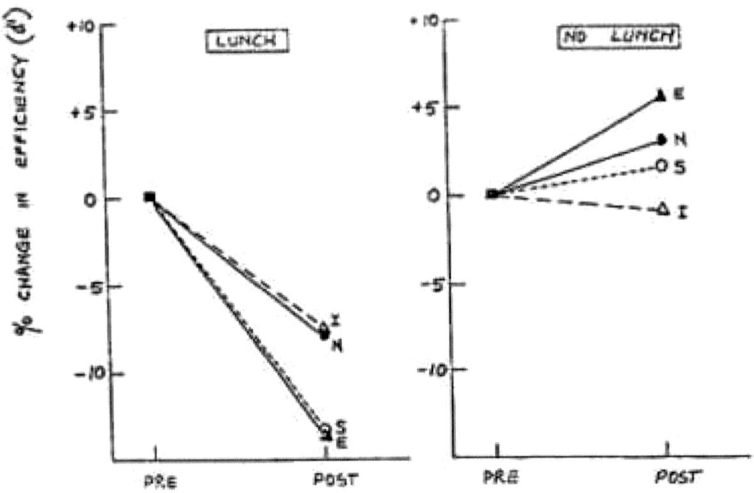

FIGURE 17–5 Afternoon drop in performance (expressed as a percentage of the morning perceptual discrimination efficiency) in lunch and no lunch groups for subjects scoring above and below the median on Eysenck Personality Inventory Introversion (I), Extraversion (E), Neuroticism (N), and Stability (S) scales. SOURCE: Craig et al. (1981), with permission.

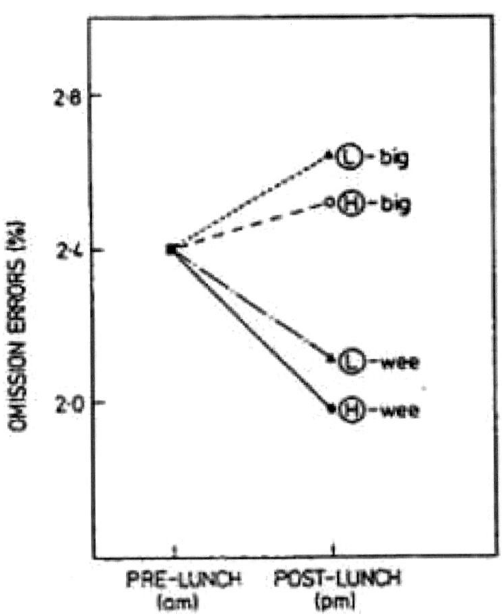

FIGURE 17–6 Postlunch percent omission errors on a sustained attention task relative to the undifferentiated prelunch covariate as a function of whether the subject usually eats a light (L) or heavy (H) lunch and whether the experimental lunch is large (big) or small (wee). SOURCE: Craig and Richardson (1989), with permission.

meals (Lieberman et al., 1986a; Simonson et al., 1948; Spring et al., 1983, 1986). A low-protein, high-carbohydrate lunch tends to induce slowing of reaction time, vigilance impairments, and decrements in sustained attention, but it does not augment susceptibility to distraction (Spring, 1984). Like their effects on mood, it is likely that the different effects of carbohydrate and protein lunches on performance will be observed for moderate-calorie meals (ranging between 300 and 1,000 kcal) and for the carbohydrate test meals that contain less than 4 percent protein. On the other hand, Smith et al. (1988) found different performance effects of larger meals that varied in their macronutrient compositions, even though all meals contained a mixture of carbohydrate and protein. Smith and colleagues reported that higher-carbohydrate meals containing either starch or sugar slowed reactions to peripheral visual stimuli, whereas higher-protein meals enhanced susceptibility to distraction.

There are also individual differences in susceptibility to the postlunch dip as a function of personality. As Figure 17–5 shows, Craig et al. (1981) found that the magnitude of the postlunch performance deterioration was greatest in stable extroverts, who can be considered to be underaroused and to have low levels of the anxiety trait. This result is consistent with findings from other studies (Smith and Miles, 1986a).

Skipping Lunch

Whether by design or happenstance, research on breakfast has focused on the relatively delayed effects of skipping the meal, whereas research on lunch has focused on the relatively acute effects of eating the meal. Given that it is sometimes necessary to skip lunch, it is worthwhile to ask whether skipping lunch results in adverse effects later in the afternoon, perhaps as a function of energy insufficiency.

Very little research has addressed skipping lunch, but two studies are available. In a laboratory setting, Kanarek and Swinney (1990) found only modest negative consquences of skipping lunch: subjects' reading times were slowed. In a field setting, Lisper and Eriksson (1980) found the more pronounced adverse effects of skipping lunch that are shown in Figure 17–7. Their subjects drove for 8 h on four occasions, taking a rest break after 4 h. The experimenters varied the rest period—short (15 min.) or long (60 min.)—and whether the subjects were permitted to eat a hot lunch. The dependent measure, speed on a subsidiary reaction time test taken while driving, is an excellent measure of the reserve capacity available to be allocated to the driving task if needed. As the data in Figure 17–7 indicate, skipping lunch had an adverse effect on performance. By the end of the drive, subjects' response times were slower if they had skipped lunch; i.e., they had less available spare capacity to dedicate to driving. Lisper and Eriksson's findings also illustrate another important phenomenon: that food does not operate in a psychological vacuum. As Figure 17–7 shows, on the day of the long pause without food, performance had deteriorated even before the lunch break. Apparently, subjects were anticipating a long, depriving wait in the middle of their 8-h drive. This finding serves as an important reminder that a meal is more than just a source of calories that reverse or prevent energy deficits. Food is also an an important psychological incentive that can enhance motivation and, hence, performance capacity.

Snacks

Carbohydrate-rich, protein-poor snacks are more likely to be eaten in the late afternoon than at any other time of day except evenings (Lieberman et al., 1989), yet no data characterize their effects on performance at that time of day. Snacks are one of the few eating vehicles likely to supply less than 5 percent protein. Carbonated beverages, graham crackers, and some cupcakes, cookies, and candies are examples of such foods. Lisper and Eriksson (1980) found late-afternoon performance deterioration that appeared to be related to energy insufficiency. To the extent that these subtle cognitive deficits are similar in

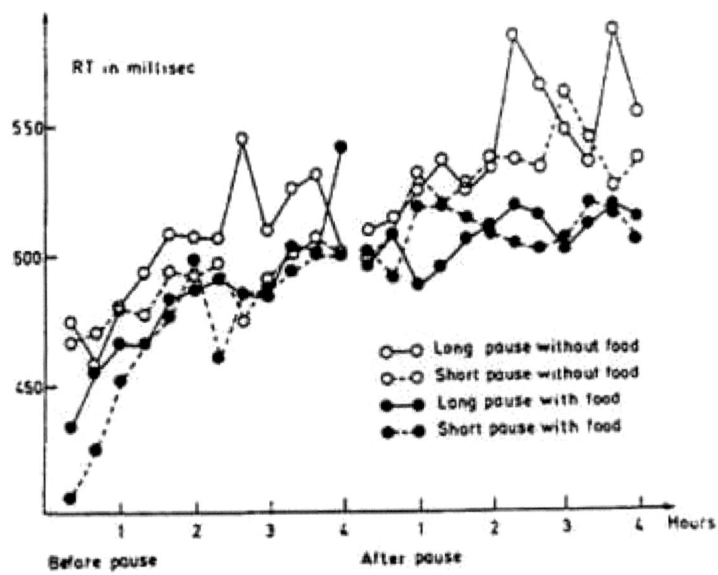

FIGURE 17–7 Changes in arithmetic means of reaction time (RT) over successive hours of driving before and after a rest break or food. SOURCE: Lisper and Eriksson (1980).

form and origin to the late-morning difficulties seen after skipping breakfast, it is plausible that late-afternoon snacking could enhance performance. Indeed, Kanarek and Swinney (1990) found support for this possibility. In their study, a calorie-rich snack improved performance on tests of sustained attention and complex cognitive functions compared with the performance after drinking a very low calorie diet soda. No differences were found between the effects of a confectionary snack versus those of a yogurt, but both snacks were balanced, containing more than 25 percent protein.

Glucose and Memory

In a series of studies of humans, Gold and colleagues report that ingesting a drink sweetened with glucose improves the memory performance of elderly subjects to a greater extent than does a saccharin-sweetened drink (Gonder-Frederick et al., 1987; Hall et al., 1989; Manning et al., 1990). They interpret their data to suggest that aging is associated with impaired brain uptake of glucose from blood, which can be attenuated by increasing circulating blood glucose levels in these subjects.

It is possible that relatively pure carbohydrate solutions have unique effects in young and elderly individuals. Nonetheless, it is striking that in the very large literature on the effects of sugars upon childrens' cognitive performance, there are a few reports of adverse effects (Goldman et al., 1986; Rosen et al., 1988), an abundance of reports of no discernible effects (cf. reviews by Spring and Alexander [1989] and Spring et al., [1987]), and no published reports of beneficial effects.

Another interpretation of the findings of Gold and colleagues is possible. In all of that group's published studies, the procedure has been to test patients after an overnight fast. In other words, the glucose load has served as a form of breakfast, and the saccharin load has served as a form of continued fasting. Additionally, because blood was drawn, the experimental paradigm includes the kind of stressors that can invoke cognitive impairments under morning fasting conditions. If this interpretation is correct, then the glucose load enhances memory in comparison with fasting only because it contains calories. If so, on the basis of the literature reviewed earlier in the section entitled "Breakfast," an isocaloric high-protein load should enhance cognitive performance to a comparable or greater extent.

Conclusions about Carbohydrates and Cognitive Performance

In summary, several generalizations can characterize the effects of carbohydrates on cognitive performance at breakfast, lunch, and snacks.

- In the morning, eating usually improves cognitive performance in comparison with fasting. The adverse effects of skipping breakfast are more likely to be observed under time pressure and stress and for regular breakfast eaters. High-protein breakfasts are more satiating than low-protein breakfasts and are somewhat more effective in sustaining late-morning performance.
- Performance on complex tasks tends to deteriorate in the early afternoon. The postlunch dip appears to be partly due to diurnal fluctuations and partly due to caloric intake. A higher than normal caloric intake exacerbates the postlunch dip, as does protein intake of less than 4 percent. Individuals differ in their susceptibilities to the postlunch dip, and psychological influences can moderate the impact of nutritional factors on performance.
- The research literature on sugar and childrens' performance provides no support for the hypothesis that a sugar-rich snack improves performance. Some literature describing studies in adults suggests that snacks can improve rich performance, but the extent to which macronutrient composition influences the degree of benefit is not well understood.

CARBOHYDRATES AND PHYSICAL ENDURANCE

Thus far, in describing cognitive performance, the argument has been advanced that any benefit of carbohydrates is limited, is largely restricted to contexts in which foods break a fast or reverse caloric insufficiencies, and is less than what would be achieved by substituting or augmenting the diet with protein. The picture changes drastically when examining physical performance, however, with a high-carbohydrate diet becoming the regimen of choice.

A diet high in carbohydrates has clear-cut benefits in the case of moderate-to high-intensity, long-endurance activities. The mechanism underlying these benefits is relatively straightforward, in that there is a direct relationship between the intensity and duration of exercise and glucose utilization by the muscles. The advantages of a high-carbohydrate diet are most evident for rigorous long-endurance activities and for individuals who are in good physical condition. The benefits include postponement of fatigue, improved performance time, and improved work output. Not only is a low-fat, high-carbohydrate diet needed to bolster glycogen supplies, but there is also a need to replenish plasma glucose levels during the activity, preferably via solutions comprising glucose polymers. Wright et al. (1991), for example, obtained the best results in terms of both power output and time to exhaustion by a combination of carbohydrate feeding before and during exercise.

CONCLUSIONS AND RECOMMENDATIONS

- The most promising indications for high-carbohydrate, low-protein foods are as soporific agents or as part of a regimen to enhance fitness for rigorous, long-endurance physical exercise.
- Findings suggest that meals that contain a mixture of protein and carbohydrate exert more beneficial effects on cognition than do meals that are virtually protein-free. Very little is known, however, of what balance between carbohydrate and protein is actually optimal for performance.
- Important differences exist between the behavioral effects of foods ingested at various times of day. Therefore, it is essential that any new ration or experimental food be tested in the diurnal contexts in which it will be used.
- There are encouraging data to suggest that snacks may offer a vehicle for enhancing cognitive performance at intervals between meals. One could even speculate that intermittent snacks might offer an alternative to meals, especially for troops that are in transit. Anecdotal accounts also suggest that soldiers in combat are more willing to eat snacks than to eat full meal rations. Both because of their appeal and because of their positive effects on performance, snacks warrant additional research. Virtually nothing is known about what macronutrient composition would make an ideal snack, and there are conflicting interpretations of the potential cognitive benefits of pure carbohydrate (glucose) snacks or meals.
- One could argue that research on diet and behavior in the military environment has overemphasized either simple cognitive or sensorimotor performances or physical performance. These domains of behavior may fail to capture other subtle and functionally very significant characteristics, such as motivation to spontaneously undertake or persist at activities, stress tolerance, or sociability. Additional work is warranted to develop sensitive measures of motivational and affective states and coping abilities to determine how these are affected by diet.
- Eating is considerably more than a process of consuming calories and macronutrients. The motivational, sociocultural, and interpersonal aspects of eating in the combat environment warrant additional attention.

REFERENCES

Arvedson, I., G.Sterky, and K.Tjernstrom 1969 Breakfast habits of Swedish schoolchildren: Effect of protein content. J. Am. Diet Assoc. 55:257–261

Blake, M.J.F. 1971 Temperament and time of day. Pp. 109–148 in Biological Rhythms and Human Performance, W P.Colquhoun, ed. London: Academic Press.

Blundell, J.E., and A.J.Hill 1988 On the mechanism of action of dexfenfluramine: Effect on alliesthesia and appetite motivation in lean and obese subjects. Clin. Neuropharmacol. 11 (Suppl. 1):S121–S134.

Bugge, J F., P.K.Opstad, and P.M.Magnus 1979 Changes in the circadian rhythm of performance and mood in healthy young men exposed to prolonged heavy physical work, sleep deprivation and caloric deficit. Aviat Space Environ. Med. 50:663–668.

Craig, A. 1986 Acute effects of meals on perceptual and cognitive functioning. Nutr. Rev. 44 (Suppl.):163–171.

Craig, A., and E.Richardson 1989 Effects of experimental and habitual lunch-size on performance, arousal, hunger and mood. Int. Arch. Occup. Environ. Health 61:313–319.

Craig, A., K.Baer, and A.Diekmann 1981 The effects of lunch on sensory-perceptual functioning in man. Int. Arch. Occup. Environ. Health 49:105–114.

Crapo, P. 1984 Theory versus fact: The glycemic response to foods. Nutr. Today March 19 (April:6–11)

Cromer, B.A., K.J.Tarnowski, A.M.Stein, P.Harton, and D.Thornton 1990 The school breakfast program and cognition in adolescents. Dev. Behav. Pediatr. 11:295–300.

Daum, K., W.W.Tuttle, C.Martin, and L.Myers 1950 Effect of various types of breakfasts on physiologic response. J. Am. Diet. Assoc. 26:503–509.

Diaz, E., G.R.Goldberg, M.Taylor, J.M.Savage, D.Sellen, W.A.Coward, and A.M.Prentice 1991 Effects of dietary supplementation on work performance in Gambian laborers. Am. J. Clin. Nutr. 53:803–811.

Dickie, N.H., and A.E.Bender 1982a Breakfast and performance. Human Nutr. Appl. Nutr. 36A:46–56.

1982b Breakfast and performance in school children. Br. J. Nutr. 48:483–496.

Dufty, W. 1975 Sugar Blues. New York: Warner Books.

Fantino, M., J.Hosotte, and M.Apfelbaum 1986 Opioid antagonist, naltrexone, reduces preference for sucrose in humans. Am. J. Physiol. 251(1,II):R91–R96.

Fernstrom, J.D., and R.J.Wurtman 1971 Brain serotonin content: Increase following ingestion of carbohydrate diet. Science 174:1023–1025.

1972 Brain serotonin content: Physiological regulation by plasma neutral amino acids. Science 178:414–416.

Fischler, C. 1987 Attitudes toward sugar and sweetness in historical and social perspective. In Sweetness, J.Dobbing, ed. New York: Springer-Verlag.

Getto, C.J., D.T.Fullerton, and I.H.Carlson 1984 Plasma immunoreactive beta-endorphin response to glucose ingestion in human obesity. Appetite 5:329–335.

Goldman, J.A., R.H.Lerman, J.H.Contois, and J.N.Udall 1986 Behavioral effects of sucrose on preschool children. J. Abnormal Child Psychol. 14:565–577.

Gonder-Frederick, L., J.L.Hall, J.Vogt, D.J.Cox, J.Green, and P.E.Gold 1987 Memory enhancement in elderly humans: Effects of glucose ingestion. Physiol. Behav. 41:503–504.

Gonder-Frederick, L.A., D.J.Cox, S.A.Bobbitt, and J.W.Pennebaker 1989 Mood changes associated with blood glucose fluctuations in insulin-dependent diabetes mellitus. Health Psychol. 8:45–59.

Hall, J.L., L.A.Gonder-Frederick, W.W.Chewning, J.Silveira, and P.E.Gold 1989 Glucose enhancement of memory in young and aged humans. Neuropsychologia 27:1129–1138.

Harris, S. 1924 Hyperinsulinism and dysinsulin. J. Am. Med. Assoc. 83:729–733.

Hartmann, E., and D.Greenwald 1984 Tryptophan and human sleep: An analysis of 43 studies. Pp. 297–304 in Progress in Tryptophan and Serotonin Research, H.G.Schlossberger, W.Kochen, B.Kinzen, and H.Steinhart, eds. New York: Walter de Gruyter.

Hartmann, E., C.L.Spinweber, and J.Fernstrom 1977 Diet, amino acids and sleep. Sleep Res. 6:61.

Hildebrandt, G., W.Rohmert, and J.Rutenfranz 1974 Twelve and 24 hr rhythms in error frequency of locomotive drivers and the influence of tiredness. Int. J. Chronobiol. 2:175–180.

Jenkins, D., T.Wolever, R.Taylor, H.Barker, H.Fielden, J.Baldwin, A.Boling, H.Newman, A.Jenkins, and D.Goff 1981 Glycemic index of foods: A physiological basis for carbohydrate exchange. Am. J. Clin. Nutr 34:362–366.

Kahneman, D. 1973 Attention and Effort. Englewood Cliffs, N.J.: Prentice-Hall.

Kanarek, R., and R.Marks-Kaufman 1991 Nutrition and Behavior. New York: Van Nostrand.

Kanarek, R.B., and D.Swinney 1990 Effects of food snacks on cognitive performance in male college students. Appetite 14:15–27.

Lieberman, H.R. 1989 Cognitive effects of various food constituents. Pp. 251–272 in Handbook of the Psychophysiology of Human Eating, R.Shepard, ed. New York: John Wiley.

Lieberman, H.R., B.Spring, and G.S.Garfield 1986a The behavioral effects of food constituents: Strategies used in studies of amino acids, protein, carbohydrate and caffeine. Nutr. Rev. 44:61–69.

Lieberman, H.R., J.Wurtman, and B.Chew 1986b Changes in mood after carbohydrate consumption among obese individuals. Am. J. Clin. Nutr. 45:772–778.

Lieberman, H.R., J.J.Wurtman, and M.H.Teicher 1989 Aging, nutrient choice, activity and behavioral responses to nutrients. Ann. N.Y. Acad. Sci. 561:196–208.

Lisper, H.O., and B.Eriksson 1980 Effects of the length of a rest break and food intake on subsidiary reaction-time performance in an 8-hour driving task. J. Appl. Psychol. 65:123–126.

Logue, A.W. 1986 The Psychology of Eating and Drinking. New York: W.H.Freeman and Company.

Manning, C.A., J.L.Hall, and P.E.Gold 1990 Glucose effects on memory and other neuropsychological tests in elderly humans. Psychol. Sci. 1:307–311.

Morley, J.E., A.S.Levine, D.M.Brown, and B.S.Handwerger 1981 Evidence for in-vivo and in-vitro modulation of the opiate receptor by glucose. Soc. Neurosci. Abstr. 7:854.

Perez-Cruet, J., A.Tagliamonte, P.Tagliamonte, and G.L.Gessa 1972 Changes in brain serotonin metabolism associated with fasting and satiation in rats. Life Sci. 11:31–39.

Permuth, M.A. 1976 Postprandial hypoglycemia. Diabetic Care 25:719–733.

Pollitt, E., K.L.Leibel, and D.Greenfield 1981 Brief fasting, stress and cognition in children. Am. J. Clin. Nutr. 34:1526–1533.

Pollitt, E., N.L.Lewis, C.Garza, and R.J.Shulman 1983 Fasting and cognitive function. J. Psychiatric Res. 17:169–174.

Prinz, R.J., W.A.Roberts, and E.Hantman 1980 Dietary correlates of hyperactive behavior in children. J. Consult. Clin. Psychol. 48:760–769.

Richards, M.M.C. 1971 The effect of nutrition state on performance. Dissertation for Diploma in Nutrition, Dunn Nutritional Laboratory, University of Cambridge.

Richards, M.M.C. 1972 Studies on breakfast and mental performance. Nutrition 26:219–223.

Rosen, L.A., S.R.Booth, M.E.Bender, M.L.McGrath, S.Sorrell, and R.S.Drabman 1988 Effects of sugar (sucrose) on children's behavior. J. Consult. Clin. Psychol. 56:583–589.

Rosenthal, N.E., M.J.Genhart, B.Cabellero, F.M.Jacobsen, R.G.Skwerer, R.D.Coursey, S. Rogers, and B.Spring 1989 Psychobiological effects of carbohydrate- and protein-rich meals in patients with seasonal affective disorder and normal controls. Biol. Psychiatry 25:1029–1040.

Simeon, D.T., and S.Grantham-McGregor 1989 Effects of missing breakfast on the cognitive functions of school children of differing nutritional status. Am. J. Clin. Nutr. 49:646–653.

Simonson, E., J.Brozek, and A.Keys 1948 Effects of meals on visual performance and fatigue. J. Appl. Psychol. 1:270–278.

Smith, A., and C.Miles 1986a Acute effects of meals, noise and nightwork. Br. J. Psychol. 77:337–387.

Smith, A.P., and C.Miles 1986b The effects of lunch on cognitive vigilance tasks. Ergonomics 29:1251–1261.

Smith, A., S.Leekam, A.Ralph, and G.McNeill 1988 The influence of meal composition on post-lunch changes in performance efficiency and mood. Appetite 10:195–203.

Spring, B. 1984 Recent research on the behavioral effects of tryptophan and carbohydrate. Nutr. Health 3:55–67.

1986 Effects of foods and nutrients on the behavior of normal individuals. Pp. 1–47 in Nutrition and the Brain, Vol. 7, R.J.Wurtman and J.Wurtman, eds. New York: Raven Press.

Spring, B., and B.L.Alexander 1989 Sugar and hyperactivity: Another look. Pp. 231–249 in Handbook of the Psychophysiology of Human Eating, R.Shepard, ed. New York: John Wiley.

Spring, B., O.Maller, J.Wurtman, L.Digman, and L.Cozolino 1983 Effects of protein and carbohydrate meals on mood and performance: Interactions with sex and age. J. Psychiatric Res. 17:155–167.

Spring, B., H.Lieberman, G.Swope, and G.S.Garfield 1986 Effects of carbohydrates on mood and behavior. Nutri. Rev. 44:51–60.

Spring, B., J.Chiodo, and D.Bowen 1987 Carbohydrates, tryptophan and behavior: A methodological review. Psychol. Bull. 102:234–256.

Spring, B., J.Chiodo, M.Harden, M.Bourgeois, J.Mason, and L.Lutherer 1989 Psychobiological effects of carbohydrates. J. Clin. Psychiatry 50 (Suppl. 5):274–333.

Spring, B., R.Pingitore, M.Bourgeois, K.Kessler, and E.Bruckner 1992 The effects and non-effects of skipping breakfast: The results of three studies. Report presented at the Annual Meeting of the American Psychological Association, Washington, D.C.

Teff, K.L., S.N.Young, L.Marchand, and M.I.Botez 1989 Acute effect of protein or carbohydrate breakfasts on human cerebrospinal fluid monoamine precursor and metabolite levels. J. Neurochem. 52:235–241.

Thayer, R.E. 1987 Energy, tiredness, and tension effects of a sugar snack versus moderate exercise. J. Personality Social Psychol. 52:119–125.

Trent, L.K., and T.L.Conway 1988 Dietary factors related to physical fitness among navy shipboard men. Am. J. Health Promotion 3:12–25.

Tuttle, W.W., M.Wilson, and K.Daum 1949 Effect of altered breakfast habits on physiologic response. J. Appl. Physiol. 1:545–559.

Tuttle, W.W., K.Daum, L.Myers, and C.Martin 1950 Effect of omitting breakfast on the physiologic response of men. J. Am. Diet. Assoc. 26:332–335.

Virkkunen, M. 1986 Reactive hypoglycemic tendency among habitually violent offenders. Nutr. Rev. 44(Suppl):94–103.

Wickens, C.D. 1984 Processing resources in attention. Pp. 63–102 in Varieties of Attention, R. Parasuraman and D.R.Davies, eds. Orlando: Academic Press.

Wright, D.A., W.M.Sherman, and A.R.Dernbach 1991 Carbohydrate feedings before, during, or in combination improve cycling endurance performance. J. Appl. Physiol. 71 1082–1088.

Wurtman, J.J., A.Brzezinski, R.J.Wurtman, and B.Laferrere 1989 Effect of nutrient intake on premenstrual depression. Am. J. Obstet. Gynecol. 161:1228–1234.

Wurtman, R.J., F.Hefti, and E.Melamed 1980 Precursor control of neurotransmitter synthesis. Pharmacol. Rev. 32:315–335.

Yokogoshi, H., and R.J.Wurtman 1986 Meal composition of plasma amino acid ratios: Effect of various proteins or carbohydrates, and of various protein concentrations. Metabolism 35:837–842.

Yokogoshi, H., T.Iwata, K.Ishida, and A.Yoshida 1987 Effect of amino acid supplementation to low protein diet on brain and plasma levels of tryptophan and brain 5-hydroxyindoles in rats. J. Nutr. 117:42–47.

DISCUSSION

RICHARD JANSEN: That was certainly an excellent review. It makes some order out of chaos. Putting this research together with your previous research, you have high carbohydrates producing a subjective feeling of fatigue. But in the context of exercise, high carbohydrate levels lengthen how long the athlete can perform.

BONNIE SPRING: To some extent, I think you are noting it is the difference between subjective and objective findings. I also think we need to acknowledge some very different uses of the term *performance.* I think we have created a lot of confusion for ourselves by using the generic term *performance* as if the same thing is being captured by the task of doing mental work at a desk and the task of running a marathon. I think that these two kinds of work are so totally different that it is hard to generalize from one to the other.

RICHARD JANSEN: Even physical performances that require prolonged endurance demands tremendous mental effort to create the motivation to keep on going and to monitor internal and external cues.

BONNIE SPRING: You raise another interesting empirical question. I have never seen a study that looked at complex decision making while somebody was running a marathon. I'll bet it would not be too hard to conduct such a study, but I do not know anybody who has done that. I wonder if there might actually be an incompatibility between carbohydrate loading and complex cognitive functioning contrary to what you suggest. I am not sure that we can assume that athletes are really at their mentally most agile while they are running. They may feel great, but I do not know what their mental performance is. There may also be independent reasons why carbohydrate loading benefits endurance performance. For example, carbohydrates may exert pain-suppressing effects, by enhancing brain tryptophan influx.

JOHN IVY: We did a study 5 years ago and I never published the mental aspects of the study, but we had individuals go through an exhaustive workout—about 50 percent maximum oxygen consumption—which took about 4 or 4.5 h. We gave them a mental test prior to the start of the workout again at the point of exhaustion. They actually did better after they were exhausted than they did prior to the exercise.

RICHARD WURTMAN: What was the test?

JOHN IVY: It was a mathematical test. They had to do so many calculations in a set period of time. We had two groups: one in which pre-loaded with carbohydrates and one which did not, and no difference in results between the two groups was found.

EDWARD HORTON: I think what Bonnie Spring has brought up here is that you use the definition of fatigue very differently when you are talking about muscular fatigue versus mental fatigue, but I think that the issues of what happens when you are exercising and how well your brain works are very important questions to investigators.

A number of studies have looked at the effect of physical conditioning programs on mood and self-image and things like that, which brings up yet another question, which is how do carbohydrates affect one's performance differently if one is physically conditioned than when one is not conditioned. So there are many interactions that would be very interesting to investigate.

BONNIE SPRING: There is also interesting literature on the carbohydrate loading protocols that, in the old days, involved a period of carbohydrate deprivation prior to carbohydrate loading. People following those protocols tended to get very irritable and cranky during the phase of carbohydrate deprivation.

ELDON ASKEW: How important do you think the type of snack would be in the military context of meals, skipped meals, or missed meals during the day? It might be possible to find a snack but not find a meal. Do you think we might find a performance enhancement?

BONNIE SPRING: I think you might find that a snack enhances performance if it reverses a performance impairment that was caused by caloric deprivation. When performance deficits appear as a result of caloric deprivation, for example, after skipping breakfast, those effects show up most clearly when an individual is under stress. The point has been made repeatedly that in the laboratory you do not come near the level of stress you are going to find in the field. So if performance in the field is undermined by *both* caloric depreivation and profound levels of stress, performance decrements should be observable and at least partially reversible by provision of calories. Snacks might also be the solution to the fact that you cannot get people in the field to eat a whole meal. Maybe you could get them to consume adequate caloric intake via a snack at every 4-h intervals.

DAVID SCHNAKENBERG: We have many fixed training scenarios, maybe operational scenarios, that will try to go to a point where you are going to go to battle. You may have forced marches but the commanders, if they know what they are doing, will indulge a break at a certain time for personal leave or a water break because you want everyone to drink, to remain hydrated. We have not yet given doctrine to say that while you are drinking also break out and eat a small, 200-to-300 calorie food bar. We could obviously compose it to be high in carbohydrates, high fat, or mixed, but if we had some good thoughts in terms of how to design a realistic experimental situation and look at some important endpoints, we could come up with some answers as to whether it really makes a difference. We know it makes a difference if they drink and maybe change their socks, but we have not yet really convinced people to eat because it will deliver a benefit.

PATRICK DUNNE: I am a former athlete and I would suggest looking at a different athletic context. Most of your exercise physiology studies are done on single, individual athletes, so the whole issue of coupling performance to group decision making does not happen. But how about studies on team sports where you have 70 percent $\dot{V}_{O_2\ max}$ [maximal oxygen uptake] while playing basketball, and there is a lot of group decision making involved? Maybe individuals playing team sports are better models for military performance than the maxed-out marathoner. We must also look at the impact of the exercise on the person who has fatigue but whose catecholamine system is also turned on, which is a more complex interaction. I know it is easier to study one system at a time, but you are going to get your answers in the interactions.

RICHARD WURTMAN: A test is now underway by the Boston Celtics. They are going to test what I guess Steve Ahlers was talking about. The evidence that when you run a marathon, the plasma choline level before the marathon and of course the original concern that it might impair neuromuscular transmission might diminish acetylcholine production in muscles, but if you are creating plasma choline, you are also affecting brain acetylcholine levels. The Boston Celtics have bezen testing it, and they allege that in the fourth quarter they do better.

18

Structured Lipids: An Overview and Comments on Performance Enhancement Potential

Ronald J.Jandacek[1]

INTRODUCTION

This examination of the role of structured lipids in performance enhancement defines structured lipids and compares their properties and metabolism with those of typical long-chain dietary fats. The potential use of structured lipids in diets intended to enhance performance is examined in this chapter in light of the current understanding of fat metabolism and the relatively small amount of information now available on the specific use of structured lipids in performance enhancement.

The primary focus of research with structured lipids has been in the areas of parenteral and enteral nutritional regimens for the stresses caused by surgery, burns, and trauma. A review of results of these uses of structured lipids is included in this chapter to give a complete picture of the metabolism of structured lipids.

[1] Ronald J.Jandacek, Research Chemist, Procter & Gamble Co., Miami Valley Laboratories, P.O. Box 398707, Cincinnati, OH 45239–8707

Investigations into the use of structured lipids to enhance physical performance in normal subjects have been limited to the replacement of typical fats or carbohydrates by the significant fatty acid component of structured lipids: medium-chain fatty acids. These few studies are summarized, and their results are discussed.

This chapter first discusses the metabolism of typical long-chain triacylglycerol (LCT) fats. It then compares the metabolism and properties of medium-chain fatty acids and medium-chain triacylglycerols (MCTs) with those of LCTs. Structured lipids are then defined, and their uses in enteral and parenteral nutrition are reviewed. Finally, the data from the use of MCTs in exercise trials are reviewed and discussed.

THE METABOLISM OF TYPICAL LCT FATS

Most of the fats in the human diet are triacylglycerol compounds, which are glycerol esters of fatty acids with 12 to 18 carbon atoms. A class of triacylglycerols that occurs occasionally in natural fats and oils has been made synthetically by esterification of glycerol with a mixture of long-chain fatty acids (12–18 carbon atoms) and of medium-chain fatty acids (6–10 carbon atoms). The metabolism of these mixed fatty acid triacylglycerols, known as *structured lipids,* has been compared with that of typical LCTs (Figure 18–1).

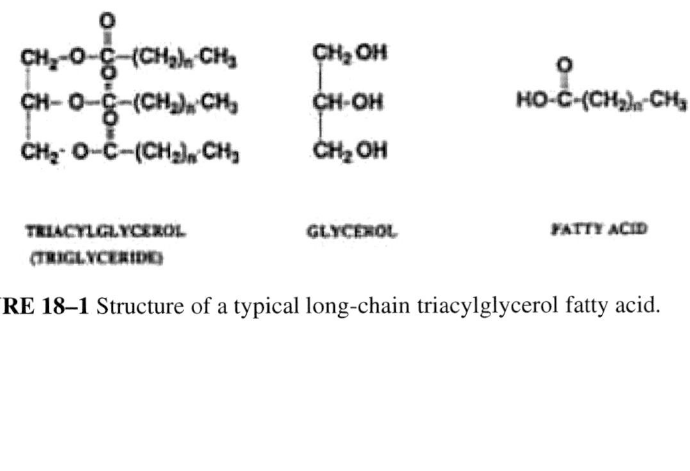

FIGURE 18–1 Structure of a typical long-chain triacylglycerol fatty acid.

To assess the metabolism of structured lipids, it is useful to review the areas of fat metabolism in which structured lipids may differ significantly from normal fats.

The utilization of typical LCT fats begins with ingestion and transit to the stomach where a gastric or lingual lipase begins to catalyze the hydrolysis of a small fraction of the fat to diacylglycerol and free fatty acid (Hamosh et al., 1975). This hydrolysis may be more important in the infant than in the adult.

Fat is released into the small intestine more slowly than water-miscible substances, and here most of the fat is digested and absorbed. The coarse emulsion of fat is converted into a much finer dispersion of oil droplets through mechanical mixing and the reduction of interfacial tension as bile salts, and phospholipids are introduced through gallbladder contraction.

This dispersion of fat greatly increases the interfacial area where pancreatic lipase can act to catalyze the hydrolysis of the triacylglycerol into the 2-monoacylglycerol and fatty acids from the 1 and 3 positions of the glycerol. These digestion products become part of mixed micelles of bile salts and phospholipid—molecular aggregates that are compatible with theaqueous milieu of the intestine but that contain lipophilic components. These mixed micelles are responsible for the transport of fatty acids and 2-monoacylglycerol through the aqueous medium to the intestinal mucosal cell. Micellar transport also facilitates the transport of the fat digestion products through an unstirred water layer that hinders the absorption of hydrophobic compounds (Figure 18–2).

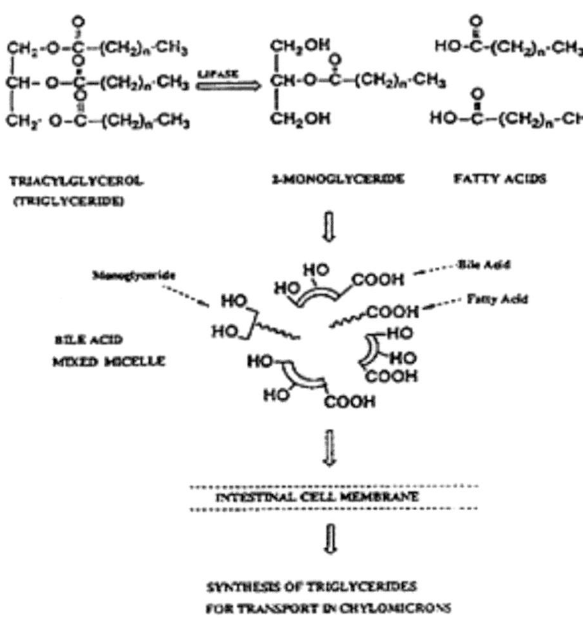

FIGURE 18–2 Lipase-catalyzed hydrolysis of triacylglycerol and the micellar dissolution and transport of the resulting fatty acids and 2-monoacylglycerol products.

It is important to note that the fat must be hydrolyzed before it can be absorbed. There is no absorption through the assimilation of intact oil droplets by pinocytosis (Cardell et al., 1967).

Although pancreatic lipase hydrolyzes fat only in the 1 and 3 positions of the molecule, it is nevertheless possible for fatty acids in the 2 position of the triacylglycerol to be hydrolyzed. This apparent violation of the specificity of pancreatic lipase occurs because of the relative instability of both the 2-monoacylglycerol and the 1,2-diacylglycerol (Crossley et al., 1959). These molecules rearrange by migration of the fatty acid in the 2 position to the 1 or 3 position, which is readily hydrolyzed by lipase (Figure 18–3). This rearrange

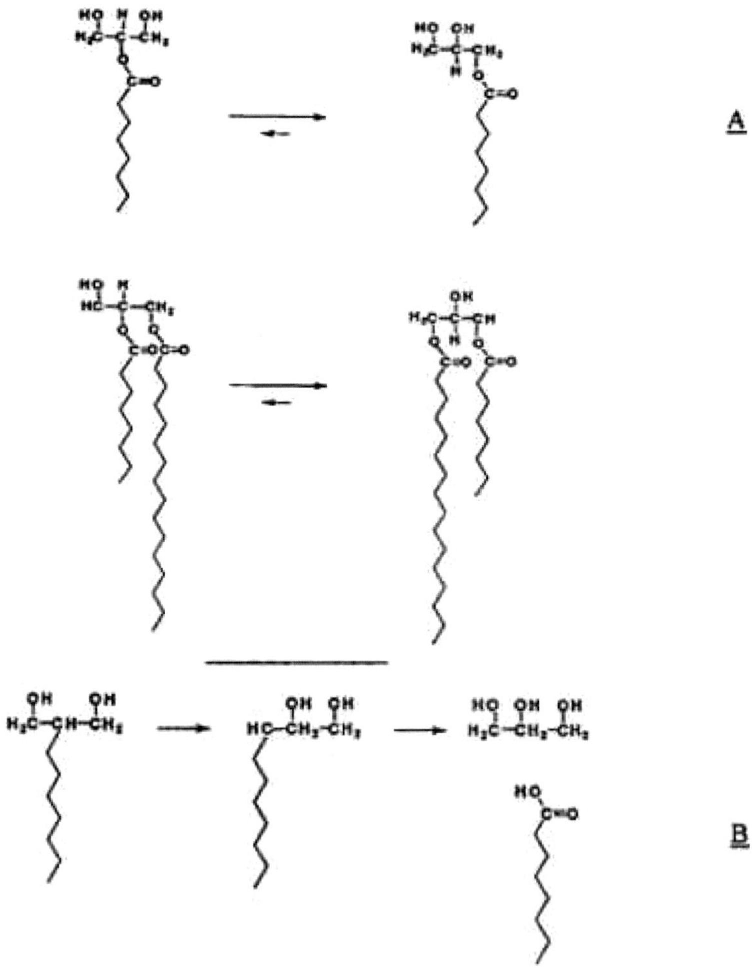

FIGURE 18–3 **(A)** Rearrangement of 2-monoacylglycerol and 1,2-diacylglycerol. **(B)** Effect of acyl migration on the hydrolysis of acylglycerols.

rangement is more rapid when the fatty acid is either a short-chain one or an unsaturated one, and a portion of the 2-position fatty acids may be absorbed as fatty acids rather than as monoacylglycerols (Benzonana et al., 1964).

In the enterocyte of the intestinal wall, high concentrations of fatty acids and monoacylglycerols are undesirable, and these compounds are rapidly converted into less toxic species, a triacylglycerol similar to that which was ingested. The 2 position of the ingested LCT is essentially maintained in the newly synthesized triacylglycerol. The fat is combined with a small amount of protein and phospholipid and is packaged in a chylomicron particle that is transported via the lymph into the blood circulation. These chylomicrons encounter lipoprotein lipase during the initial circulation, and their triacylglycerol compounds are hydrolyzed to form fatty acids that are available for utilization by the peripheral tissue. The chylomicron remnants and remaining fat are removed from the circulation by the liver for conversion into very-low-density lipoprotein.

A COMPARISON OF MEDIUM- AND LONG-CHAIN FATTY ACIDS

Medium-Chain Fatty Acids

Fat digestion and absorption change markedly with fatty acids that contain fewer than 12 carbon atoms. There is evidence that lauric acid, with 12 carbon atoms, partly follows the absorption pattern for long-chain fatty acids and partly follows that for the 6–8- and 10-carbon fatty acids, generally classified as medium-chain fatty acids (Bragdon and Karmen, 1960) (Figure 18–4). The atypical (compared with long-chain fatty acids) digestion, absorption, and metabolism of caproic (hexanoic), caprylic (octanoic), and capric (decanoic) acids are the source of the unique properties of structured lipids. A summary of these properties lays the foundation for a review of structured lipids.

Medium-chain triacylglycerols (MCTs) were first introduced to human nutrition more than three decades ago by V.K.Babayen, who was exploring ways to utilize the medium-chain fatty acids that were a by-product of the production of lauric acid from coconut oil (Senior, 1968). MCTs were prepared with these fatty acids by esterification with glycerol. Caprylic and capric acids together make up 13 percent of the fatty acids in coconut oil, and triacylglycerols made only of caprylic and capric acids account for somewhat less than 1 percent of the total oil. Thus, small amounts of MCTs have been consumed by humans for many centuries, and MCTs prepared by esterification of medium-chain fatty acids and glycerol were assumed to be generally recognized as safe. Studies of MCTs have included the early investigations of digestion and absorption and more recent experiments on parenteral nutrition (Bach and Babayen, 1982).

It was found that MCTs are well utilized in cases of pancreatic insufficiency that hinder the digestion and absorption of typical long-chain triacylglycerols (LCTs). Although there is some evidence that MCTs could be absorbed as intact molecules in the absence of pancreatic lipase (Clark, 1968), hydrolysis possibly takes place during the absorption of most MCTs. MCTs differ markedly from LCTs in intestinal hydrolysis in that they are hydrolyzed at a much higher rate than the LCTs (Jandacek, 1987). This rapid hydrolysis is the key event that provides the unique behavior both of MCTs and of structured lipids. MCTs are readily hydrolyzed, and their digestion products are caprylic acid, capric acid, and the 2-monoacylglycerols of these acids. One can postulate that a rapid rearrangement of the 2-monoacylglycerol to the 1-monoacylglycerol (Figure 18–3B) takes place in the small intestine so that lipase catalyzes the nearly complete hydrolysis of the MCTs. It is also possible that the 1,2-diacylglycerol produced in the stomach by gastric lipase is rearranged to the 1,3-diacylglycerol in the small intestine and is then completely hydrolyzed.

The rapid hydrolysis of MCTs may in part result from the ease of removal of reaction products from the oil-water interface where the lipase is active. This prevention of rate-slowing product buildup depends on the solubilization and transport of fatty acids and monoacylglycerols by bile salt micelles in the hydrolysis of LCTs in the intestine. Although micelles may be somewhat involved in the removal of MCT digestion products, many of these products

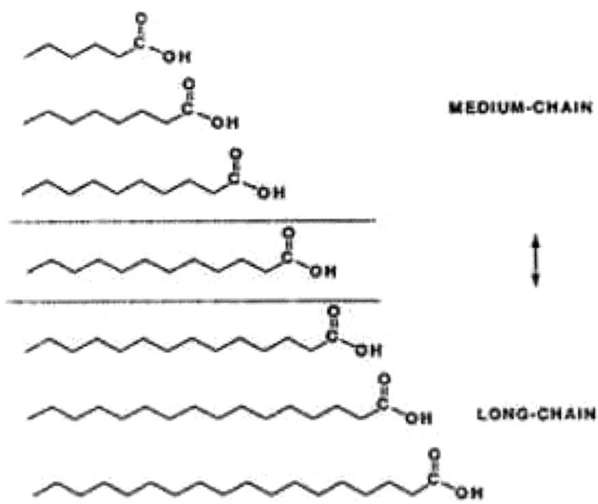

FIGURE 18–4 Description of fatty acids of various lengths. Medium-chain generally refers to fatty acids of 6, 8, or 10 carbon atoms. Long-chain fatty acids have 14 or more carbon atoms. Lauric acid (12 carbon atoms) can behave like both classes of fatty acids.

products are removed by a fast, nonmicellar dissolution in the aqueous medium of the small intestine (Figure 18–5). The products are transported to and through the unstirred water layer coating the intestinal cell membrane without dependence on micellar dissolution.

The ingestion of MCTs as a bolus does not stimulate contraction of the gallbladder, and it does not raise the plasma cholecystokinin level in the manner in which it occurs following LCT ingestion (Hopman et al., 1984; Isaacs et al., 1987). Intestinal cramping and diarrhea were observed after the MCT bolus (Hopman et al., 1984); however, the general acceptance of MCTs in mixed meals suggests amelioration by other nutrients or a development of tolerance.

MCTs are also quite distinct from LCTs in the next step in the metabolic pathway. After absorption into the intestinal mucosal cell, LCT digestion products are reassembled into newly synthesized LCTs, packaged into chylomicrons, and transported via the lymph into the blood. MCT fatty acids are only sparingly found in the lymph, and there they are found only as a trace component of a mixed triacylglycerol with two long-chain fatty acids and one medium-chain fatty acid. The aqueous solubility of the MCT fatty acids causes them to enter the portal circulation bound to albumin for direct transport to the liver (Hashim, 1968) (Figure 18–6). This first encounter of MCT fatty acids

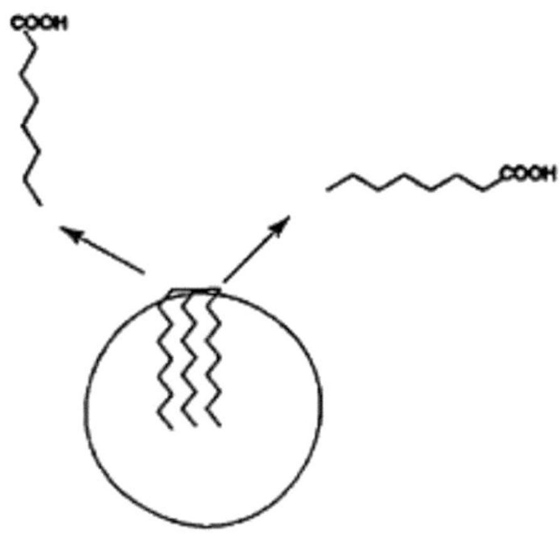

NON-MICELLAR TRANSPORT OF MCT HYDROLYSIS PRODUCTS

FIGURE 18–5 Nonmicellar (monomeric) dissolution and transport of medium-chain fatty acids contribute to the rapid digestion and absorption of fats containing medium-chain fatty acids.

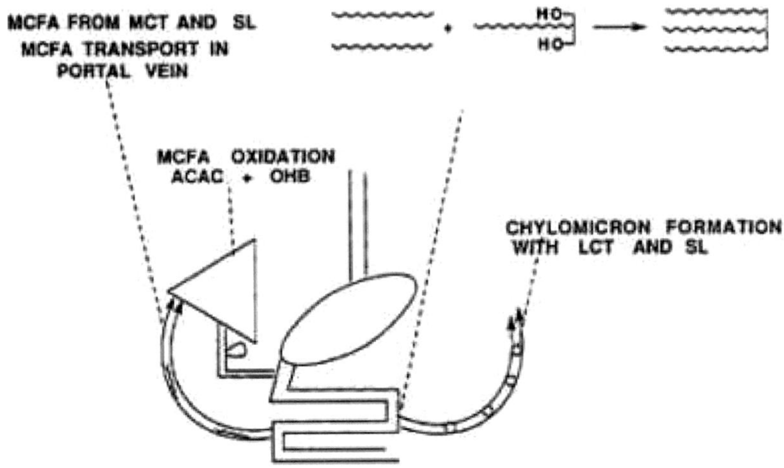

FIGURE 18–6 Medium-chain fatty acids (MCFA) are transported in the portal vein and oxidized to form acetoacetate (ACAC) and ß-hydroxybutyrate (OHB). Long-chain fatty acids and 2-monoacylglycerol form triacylglycerols in the enterocyte and are transported as chylomicrons in the lymph. (LCT, long-chain triacylglycerol; MCT, medium-chain triacylglycerol; SL, structured lipid; OH, hydroxyl).

with the liver is an important deviation from LCT metabolism, where the LCTs in chylomicrons reach the liver only after a significant portion has been hydrolyzed by lipoprotein lipase for delivery of fatty acids to peripheral tissues.

It is generally accepted that the oxidation of fatty acids is facilitated by carnitine, which transports the fatty acid as an acylcarnitine into mitochondria. It has also been widely accepted that carnitine does not play a significant role in the transport of medium-chain fatty acids; however, there is now some evidence for carnitine's involvement in the metabolism of MCTs (Rossle et al., 1990). Measurements of the levels of short-chain and long-chain acylcarnitine in the blood after infusion of a mixed MCT-LCT emulsion showed an increase in short-chain carnitine. This increase is consistent with the fact that oxidation of medium-chain fatty acids depends in part on carnitine but does not imply carnitine's role in their transport.

The difference between long-chain and medium-chain fatty acid metabolism continues in the mitochondria. There is a large body of evidence that shows medium-chain fatty acids to be preferentially oxidized in comparison with long-chain fatty acids. Scheig compared the oxidation of [1-^{14}C] palmitic acid and [1-^{14}C]octanoic acid in rat tissues (Scheig, 1968). In the liver, kidney, diaphragm, heart, brain, and perirenal fat-pad, the extent of oxidation of octanoic acid to $^{14}CO_2$ was higher than that of palmitic acid. The difference in the liver was approximately sevenfold. The epididymal fat-pad showed the same trend, but the difference was not significant. Complementary to this observation was the extent of lipid synthesis in each of these tissues. In all examined tissues except the perirenal fat-pad, more lipid was synthesized from palmitic acid than from octanoic acid, with more than a 10-fold difference seen in the liver.

The oxidation of MCTs results in the production of ketones (Yeh and Zee, 1976) when fat is the principal fuel for the body, as in those receiving very-low-carbohydrate diets. The level of ketone production seen after MCT ingestion is generally far less than the high levels that are cause for concern in patients with diabetic ketosis. It has been suggested that the production of ketone bodies from MCTs is of benefit in stress situations, since they can provide ketones as an energy source for extrahepatic tissue (Birkhahn, 1988; Maiz et al., 1984).

Comparison of the dietary thermogenesis resulting from meals containing LCTs and MCTs yielded results that further distinguished the metabolism of the fats on the basis of chain length. Hill and coworkers fed subjects liquid formula diets containing 150 percent of estimated energy requirements with 40 percent of calories as fat for 1 week in a double-blind crossover regimen (Hill et al., 1989). The thermal response to the MCTs was nearly twice that to the LCTs after 5 days of feeding (12 ± 1.3 percent versus 6.6 ± 1.0 percent) of ingested energy. The authors concluded that a principal component of this thermal effect of MCT-containing food was the energy expended in lipogenesis from the caloric excess of the MCTs. The lipogenesis from MCTs is an inefficient process with little elongation of the octanoate and, principally, the production of the acetate that is used in the de novo synthesis of fatty acids.

The feeding of MCTs to animals results in virtually no deposition of octanoic and decanoic acids in the carcass or adipose tissue (Jandacek et al., 1991). Rather, palmitic acid is the dominant species.

In addition to the metabolic differences between MCTs and LCTs, there are some noteworthy physical differences. The energy content (bomb calorimetry) of MCTs is approximately 8 kcal/g, in comparison with 9 kcal/g for LCTs because a higher fraction of the carbon atoms in MCTs is already bonded to oxygen and cannot be further oxidized. In the physical properties that are of importance in food preparation and consumption, MCTs are quite similar to unsaturated vegetable oils. They are, however, measurably less stable at frying temperatures and have a flash point that is markedly lower than those of typical vegetable oils (Yang, 1989). This difference results from the higher volatility of the oil and the traces of lower-molecular-weight products produced during frying.

Given their palatability and their relatively high caloric content when compared with those of carbohydrate and protein, MCTs have been utilized as substitutes for LCTs in the diets of patients with metabolic disorders that limit the consumption of traditional LCT fats. MCTs can be used to provide the hedonic benefit and the caloric density of fat in a meal and have been successfully used in the nutritional management of pancreatic insufficiency (Holt, 1968; Huang, 1968). However, MCTs do not provide essential fatty acids, which are particularly crucial in children. MCTs are valuable in the nutritional treatment of alcoholic pancreatitis and cholestatic liver disease; both of which decrease the concentration of bile acids below their critical micellar concentration.

MCTs have also been used in patients with elevated blood triglycerides resulting from an inability to clear chylomicrons from their plasma. The MCTs can again provide the calories and palatability of fat, but they do not contribute to the formation of chylomicrons and therefore reduce the postprandial lipid levels in the blood (Furman, 1968).

MCTs are currently commercially available as an over-the-counter drug in neat form. MCTs are also included in infant formula that is formulated to provide well-absorbed energy to premature infants who have poorly developed systems of fat digestive enzymes. In Europe, MCTs are sold commercially as the fat component of a diet margarine and in neat form as a salad oil for special dietary purposes.

Other Dietary Fatty Acids

Some recent studies with structured lipids in the diets of patients experiencing trauma-induced stress have centered not only on the mediumchain fatty acid component of the structured lipid but also on the long-chain fatty acid moiety. In particular, structured lipids with omega-3 fatty acids have been synthesized and investigated, so a review of the properties of this class of fatty acids is relevant to an understanding of structured lipids.

The omega terminology for fatty acids is based on the number of carbon atoms from the terminal methyl carbon to the first double bond of the hydrocarbon chain. Omega-3 fatty acids, also called N-3 fatty acids, have a double bond three carbons from the terminal methyl group. The omega-3 fatty acids that have been the focus of hundreds of metabolic studies in the last decade are those found in marine oils, eicosapentaenoic and docosahexaenoic acids (EPA and DHA, respectively). The convenience of the omega terminology is seen in the elongation and desaturation pathways for the synthesis of fatty acids in animals. The omega-3 fatty acids are precursors for other omega-3 fatty acids, and similarly, omega-6 fatty acids are precursors for elongated and desaturated omega-6 fatty acids. α-Linolenic acid is a precursor for DHA and EPA (Figure 18–7).

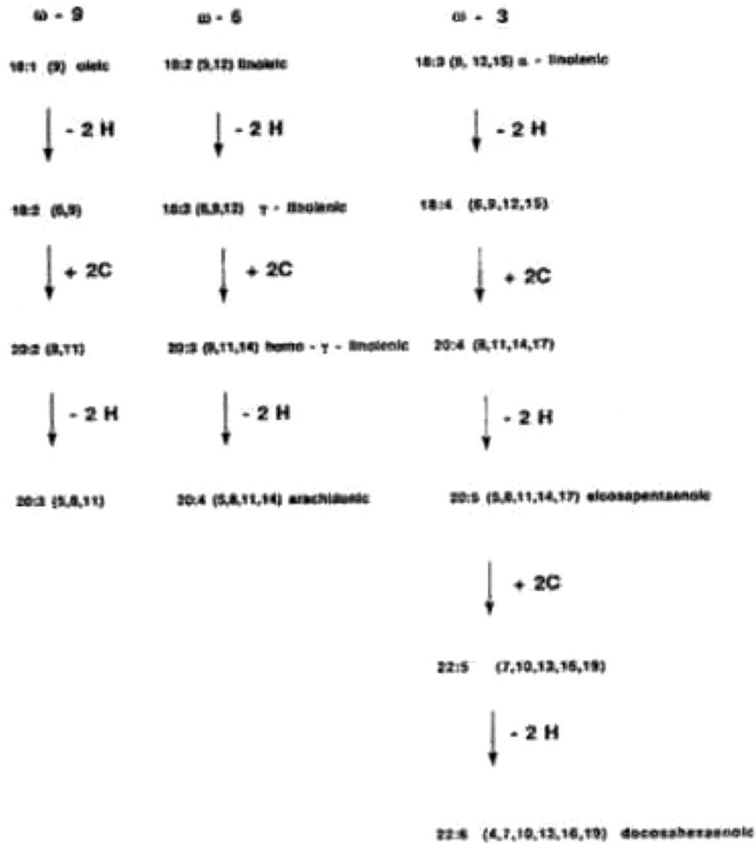

FIGURE 18–7 The metabolism of omega-9, omega-6, and omega-3 fatty acids.

The well-established effects of the addition of significant quantities of EPA and DHA to the diet are a reduction in plasma triglyceride levels and a decreased tendency for platelet aggregation. The latter effect has been shown to be a result of changing the eicosanoid levels that influence aggregation, in particular the levels of thromboxane and prostacyclin. This effect on eicosanoids presumably reflects the displacement of arachidonic acid by DHA in cell membrane phospholipids. Since arachidonic acid is the precursor for proaggregatory eicosanoids, a reduction in arachidonic acid levels and competition for enzymes by DHA alter prostaglandin and leukotriene levels. The inflammatory responses mediated by eicosanoids are also presumably altered by dietary DHA and EPA.

Since arachidonic acid is the precursor for most prostaglandins and leukotrienes, their production might also be altered by manipulation of the dietary level of the precursor to arachidonic acid, linoleic acid (both of these are omega-6 fatty acids). Linoleic acid is clearly established as an essential fatty acid that is a dietary requirement for good health (Holman, 1971; Innis, 1991). A level of linoleic acid that provides approximately 1 percent of energy is probably sufficient for normal growth and health. Relatively high levels of linoleic acid have generally been considered beneficial for health because of an association with reduced levels of total and low-density lipoprotein cholesterol. There is, however, a relatively recent concern that an excess of dietary linoleic acid may be detrimental because it raises the levels of arachidonic acid and its eicosanoid products. The essential fatty acid requirement has therefore been reexamined, with general acceptance of a requirement for omega-3 fatty acids as well as linoleic acid. There is also the possibility that under certain stress situations, minimization of linoleic acid's activity through an appropriate dietary omega-3/omega-6 fatty acid ratio may be beneficial. Some studies with structured lipids have followed this general hypothesis (Teo et al., 1991).

DEFINITION OF STRUCTURED LIPIDS

The preceding review of the properties of medium-chain triacylglycerols (MCTs) is important to an understanding of the materials that have become known as structured lipids. Structured lipids are fats that are synthesized from mixtures of long-chain and medium-chain fatty acids (Figure 18–8), and indeed, it is the presence of the medium-chain fatty acids that differentiates structured lipids from typical long-chain triacylglycerols (LCTs). As discussed below, the features that differentiate MCTs from LCTs are included in part in the properties of the structured lipids. These differences include the rates of lipase-catalyzed hydrolysis, oxidation, and lipogenesis. They have resulted in interesting therapeutic potentials for the structured lipids.

As mentioned earlier, structured lipids are not new to the human gastrointestinal system, since a calculation based on the approximation of a random distribution of medium- and long-chain fatty acids would indicate that approximately 16 percent of triacylglycerols in butterfat and 38 percent of triacylglycerols in coconut oil have the compositions of MML and MLL, where M and L signify medium- and long-chain fatty acids, respectively.

Among the first examinations of fat that was enriched with structured lipids was work reported in the mid-1950s and early 1960s. Mattson and coworkers showed that fats made from acetic acid and long-chain fatty acids (acetin fats) sustained growth in rats (Mattson et al., 1956). Fernandes and colleagues transesterified octanoic acid with olive oil to make a "capryl olive oil" in which octanoic acid was 46 percent of the fatty acids (Fernandes et al., 1962). Clement and coworkers showed that mixed butyrate and LCTs were hydrolyzed by human pancreatic lipase (Clement et al., 1962), and Jensen and colleagues studied the hydrolysis of triacylglycerols made with long-chain fatty acids and either butyrate or caproate (Jensen et al., 1962). In general, those studies showed that the hydrolysis of triacylglycerols comprising mixed short-or medium-chain fatty acids with long-chain fatty acids was similar to that of all LCTs. The absorption of the medium-chain fatty acids was found to be by a route other than the lymphatic system in those studies. No utility or benefit of dietary structured lipids was apparent from those early reports.

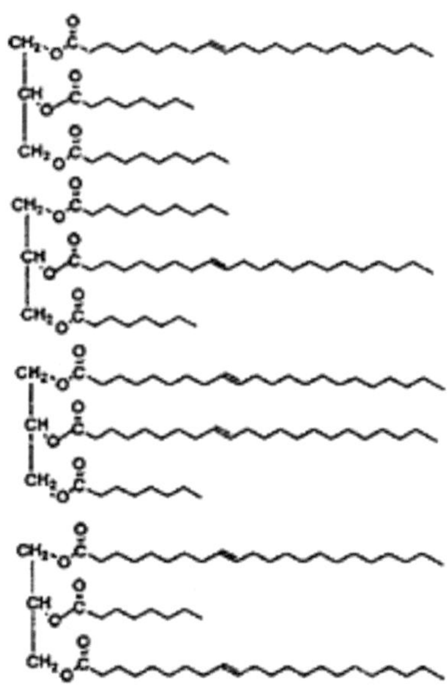

FIGURE 18–8 Triacylglycerols of structured lipids include randomly arranged medium- and long-chain structures. Examples of the principal components are shown.

STRUCTURED LIPIDS IN ENTERAL AND PARENTERAL NUTRITION

A second look at the mixed long- and medium-chain triacylglycerols that were to become known as structured lipids took place in the early 1980s. The potential application of these fats resulted from the experience with fat in total parenteral nutrition (TPN) formulations. Two decades of the use of fat in TPN formulations had demonstrated its advantages, including the provision of essential fatty acids and a high caloric density with a small osmotic load. Although the development of the process and the emulsifiers used for emulsification of soybean oil in these formulations allowed the use of a fat in TPN formulations, the metabolism of fat infused intravenously differs from that of orally ingested fat in some important ways. These differences are determined by the relationship of the physical chemistry of a fat dispersion to its metabolism.

An orally ingested LCT is hydrolyzed in the lumen of the small intestine and is reassembled in the enterocyte into a triacylglycerol that has approximately the same composition as and a structure similar to that of the ingested fat. This absorbed fat is made compatible with the aqueous phases of the lymphatic and blood systems by packaging the triacylglycerol into a chylomicron—a particle that is 75.0–1,000.0 nm in diameter with a hydrophilic shell of protein and phospholipid and a core of triacylglycerol and cholesterol ester. The chylomicron comprises 80–95 percent triacylglycerol by weight.

There is evidence that the emulsified fat in TPN formulations does not follow the same rates of hydrolysis and uptake by peripheral tissue as does the orally ingested fat in chylomicrons. The difference in the rates of uptake of infused chylomicrons and infused artificial emulsions by liver and adipose tissue has been shown in rats (Mattson and Jandacek, 1991; Waddell et al., 1954; Johnson et al., 1990). The reticuloendothelial system of the liver is affected by infused emulsions, as evidenced by the decreased clearance of injected particles in humans (Jensen et al., 1990).

Fats that are rapidly hydrolyzed by lipase, and in particular by lipoprotein lipase, might be expected to be advantageous for use in parenteral fat emulsions. Two approaches have been taken to provide a more nearly physiological rate of hydrolysis: formulations that blend MCTs with LCTs in a mixture of the two fats and formulations based on structured lipids. These formulations were originally intended to deliver essential fatty acids and provide well-utilized energy.

The most extensive exploration of the effects of structured lipids has been in TPN and enteral feeding formulations in trauma, burn, and infection stress models. Although such studies are not directly related to the potential use of structured lipids in the enhancement of performance, they are the principal source of data related to the nutrition biochemistry of structured lipids. Since the end product of structured lipids in TPN or enteral feeding formulations or in a potentially performance-enhancing diet is the fatty acid, studies of medium chain fatty acids in enteral and TPN formulations are also of relevance.

A summary of studies that are representative of the application of structured lipids and MCTs in TPN and enteral feeding stress models is presented in Table 18–1. Investigations of the enteral and oral use of structured lipids have sought to utilize two potential benefits. The first is the end result of nitrogen sparing in stressed organisms. The nitrogen sparing presumably would result from the facile absorption of the fatty acids of the structured lipid, the relatively high caloric density (and low osmolality) of the nutrient formulation, and the utilization of the medium-chain fatty acids as energy sources. The production of ketones (acetoacetate and ß-hydroxybutyrate) from the medium-chain fatty acids could presumably directly deliver energy sources for utilization by muscle tissue. Three of these studies (DiMichele et al., 1988, 1989; Teo et al., 1989) support this possibility, although the advantage of a structured lipid over a physical mixture of MCTs and LCTs is not always evident, as shown in the nitrogen balance equivalence of the structured lipid and the MCT-LCT mix in the study of DiMichele and colleagues (1989).

The study by Teo and colleagues (1991) suggests that a structured lipid synthesized to include the omega-3 fatty acids, eicosapentaenoic acid (EPA) and docosahexaenoic acid (DHA), can be beneficial by reducing lactic acidosis. The authors suggest that the eicosanoid-mediated vasoactive effects of the omega-6 fatty acids were diminished by the omega-3 fatty acids in the structured lipid. In that study the omega-3 structured lipid was not compared with a structured lipid that was low in omega-6 fatty acids, such as one formulated from a vegetable oil with a high level of oleic acid.

The second potential benefit would apply in patients with insufficient lipase, as in the case of pancreatic obstruction in patients with cystic fibrosis. Structured lipids could hydrolyze as readily as MCTs and could reduce the level of pancreatic lipase required for hydrolysis and absorption of the fatty acids. The advantage of structured lipids over MCTs in this application would be the absorption of essential fatty acids as well as medium-chain fatty acids. Hubbard, McKenna, and colleagues compared the absorption of linoleic acid from structured lipids with that from safflower oil (Hubbard and McKenna, 1987; McKenna et al., 1985). The advantage of structured lipids was not clear in their study subjects, although there was a time lag in the appearance of linoleic acid in the subjects' blood after ingestion of a safflower oil-containing meal but not after ingestion of a structured lipid with linoleic acid. Since lipase-catalyzed hydrolysis of triacylglycerol splits the 1- and 3-position fatty acids, a structured lipid with medium-chain fatty acids in these positions would seem appropriate for use in patients with pancreatic insufficiency. The hydrol

TABLE 18-1 Summary of Studies Investigating the Potential of Structured lipids as a Source of Calories and Essential Fatty Acids in Enteral and Parenteral Nutrition

Route of Delivery and Study	Species	Method	Type of Fat	Results
Enteral and oral delivery				
McKenna et al. (1985)	Cystic fibrosis patients	Normal diet	SL (25 percent 18:2), SL (40 percent 18:2), safflower oil, safflower oil emulsion	Absorption of linoleate delayed after safflower oil compared with that after SL
Hubbard and McKenna (1987)	Cystic Fibrosis Patients	Normal Diet	SL (sunflower), safflower oil	Absorption of linoleate delayed after safflower compared with that after SL
Jandacek et al. (1987)	Rat intestinal pancreatic insufficiency model	Intestinal infusion	Specific SL and LCT analog	SL absorption higher than that of long-chain analog
DiMichele et al. (1986)	Rat, 30 percent burn	Enteral (gastrostomy)	MCT, LCT, SL (from dairy fat), SL (from safflower oil)	Nitrogen balance positive and highest in both SL groups; protein synthesis highest in dairy SL; serum albumin lowest in LCT
DiMichele et al. (1989)	Rat, 30 percent burn	Enteral (gastrostomy)	MCT, LCT, SL, MCT-LCT mix	Serum albumin higher in SL, MCT; Nitrogen balance higher in SL, mix
Teo et al. (1989)	Rat, 30 percent burn	Enteral (gastrostomy)	SL (fish oil), safflower oil	SL increased nitrogen balance, liver protein synthesis
Teo et al. (1991)	Guinea pig, endotoxin infusion	Oral feeding 6 weeks prior to infusion	SL (MCT-fish oil), safflower oil	Hyperlactatemia less with SL

Parenteral delivery				
Hamaway et al. (1985)	Rat femoral fracture and *Escherichia coli* implant	TPN, 4 days	MCT-LCT mix, fat-free LCT	Bacteria in blood highest with fat-free and LCT
	Rat injected with radio-labeled *Escherichia coli*	TPN, 4 days	MCT-LCT mix, fat-free LCT	Liver uptake of label highest with MCT-LCT mix
Sobrado et al. (1985)	Guinea pig, burn, radio-labeled bacteria injected	TPN	LCT, MCT, SL	At 75 percent of nonprotein energy, lung uptake of bacteria highest with LCT; at 50 percent, no difference
Jensen et al. (1990)	Human ^{99}TC-sulfur colloid injection	TPN	Continuous LCT, intermittent LCT, intermittent MCT-LCT mix	RES cleared colloid decreased by intermittent LCT
Nakagawa et al. (1991)	Rat	TPN, fat as 10 and 20 percent of nonprotein energy	Fat-free, MCT, LCT, SL (specific structure) MCT-LCT mix	Hepatic lipid higher with fat-free and MCT; lowest was LCT and SL; nitrogen balance lowest in MCT
Mitsuyoshi et al. (1992)	Rat injected with streptozocin and given ^{14}C-glucose	TPN	Fat-free, LCT, MCT, LCT-MCT mix, SL	Highest $^{14}CO2$ and ketones in SL group

NOTE: SL, structured lipids; LCT, long-chain triacylglycerols; MCT, medium-chain triacylglycerols; TPN, total parenteral nutrition; ^{99}Tc, technetium-99; RES, reticuloendothelial system.

lysis rate and absorption of such a compound (2-linoleoyl-1,3-dioctanoyl glycerol) was found to be markedly higher than those of a typical LCT (Jandacek et al., 1987).

Whether or not this specific structure is advantageous will require further comparisons with randomly arranged structured lipids. The rapid migration of fatty acids in the 2 position of monoacylglycerols and diacylglycerols to the equilibrium 1, and 3 positions may result in a rapid hydrolysis rate for randomly arranged structured lipids as well as for those with the medium-chain fatty acids in the 1 and 3 positions. For example, the hydrolysis of a triacylglycerol molecule from a randomly arranged structured lipid such as 1-linoleoyl-2,3-dioctanoyl glycerol would first form the 1-linoleoyl-2-octanoyl glycerol (diacylglycerol). Diacylglycerols with short or unsaturated fatty acids in the 2 position rapidly rearrange to the 1,3-diacylglycerol. This rearrangement would create a molecule with the medium-chain fatty acid in the lipase-accessible 3 position. After hydrolysis of this molecule, the octanoic acid and the 1-monoacylglycerol would be available for absorption. The importance of this process occurring in the intestine (or in blood, with lipoprotein lipase) would depend on the relative rates of hydrolysis, absorption, and rearrangement.

In light of the topic of this chapter, it should be noted that the investigations of the enteral feeding of structured lipids have used stressed animals. No advantages have been demonstrated in healthy animals. The comparisons of the absorption of fats from the intestine have been made with animal models or patients with insufficient pancreatic lipase. There has not been an investigation or hypothesis that supports an advantage for structured lipids in the nutrition of normal subjects with a normal concentration of lipase, which is far in excess of that required for normal fat consumption (Kasper, 1970).

The studies of the use of structured lipids in parenteral nutrition have generally demonstrated that structured lipids do not overload the reticuloendothelial system when compared with LCTs (Jensen et al., 1990; Sobrado et al., 1985). It is not clear, however, that there is an advantage when structured lipids are compared with a physical mixture of LCT and MCT (Hamawy et al., 1985; Nakagawa et al., 1991). The MCT-LCT mix has been included in a total parenteral nutrition (TPN) formulation that is marketed in Europe.

MEDIUM-CHAIN FATTY ACIDS IN EXERCISE STUDIES

The studies that are of most relevance to the topic of performance enhancement have not utilized structured lipids but have utilized MCTs. A review of those studies is of value, however, since normal, healthy subjects readily change a structured lipid into its fatty components. The lumen of the intestine experiences the intact structured lipid triacylglycerol, but the metabolic fate of the structured lipid will be the same as that of a mixture of MCTs with LCTs since lipase-catalyzed hydrolysis presents the enterocyte with the same products (Figure 18–9). Essential fatty acid absorption would be expected to be the same regardless of whether the dietary fat comprised a physical mixture of MCTs and safflower oil or a structured lipid made from MCTs and safflower oil.

The general hypothesis for the benefit of MCTs in performance enhancement is that of the possibility of sparing glycogen from utilization during exercise through rapid oxidation of the medium-chain fatty acids for fuel. After digestion and absorption, the medium-chain fatty acids become a fuel that quickly reaches the liver and provides energy through mitochondrial oxidation. The production of acetoacetate and ß-hydroxybutyrate from fatty acid oxidation would be delivered as an energy source for muscle and would potentially diminish glycogen utilization. An extrapolation of this hypothesis would be to predict increased endurance since the utilization of glycogen would be delayed during a continuous period of work.

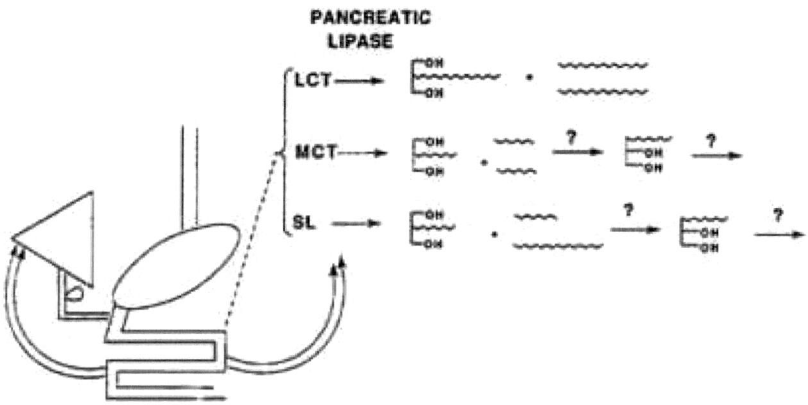

FIGURE 18–9 In the lumen of the small intestine, long-chain fatty acids and 2-monoacylglycerol are produced and absorbed. Medium-chain triacylglycerols (MCTs) and structured lipids (SLs) are hydrolyzed and probably rearranged to allow further hydrolysis. Structured lipids hydrolyze to give the same products that would be formed from mixtures of long-chain triacylglycerols (LCTs) and medium-chain triacylglycerols. OH, hydroxyl groups.

Another potential benefit of the use of MCTs in place of carbohydrate would be the avoidance of the insulin elevation and possible hypoglycemia during exercise that follows a high-carbohydrate meal. Again, the use of medium-chain fatty acids instead of glucose for fuel could result in this effect.

Although these hypotheses seem to be a reasonable mechanism for a metabolic benefit for medium-chain fatty acids resulting from MCTs or structured lipids, there has been no consistent experimental support for their validity. Table 18–2 summarizes the studies that have compared MCTs with other fuels during exercise.

These studies have consistently shown a modest increase in circulating ketone bodies after ingestion of MCT-containing meals. MCT was shown in one study to blunt the increased insulin levels that occurred after ingestion of an isocaloric amount of carbohydrate, but during exercise the carbohydrate was preferentially oxidized compared with the MCTs (Howald and Decombaz, 1983). Another study did not show a reduction of insulin levels when MCTs replaced carbohydrate (Ivy et al., 1980). There was no evidence that MCTs would spare glycogen, and as a result, there was also no evidence that MCTs would extend the time to exhaustion.

These studies therefore do not provide support for the use of MCTs in the enhancement of work and exercise performance. The direct extrapolation of this conclusion to structured lipids is appropriate since the only unique fuel provided by structured lipids is the medium-chain fatty acid component. Medium-chain fatty acids from structured lipids follow the same digestion and absorption process as medium-chain fatty acids from MCTs (Webb and Sanders, 1991).

A clue to the inability of MCTs to spare glycogen is seen in a study in which dietary MCTs significantly enhanced dietary thermogenesis when MCTs were in excess of energy needs and compared with LCTs (Hill et al., 1989). That study raised the possibility that this thermogenesis represents energy that is uncoupled from phosphorylation so as to generate heat without work. The conversion of medium-chain fatty acids to long-chain fatty acids involves the energy-consuming process of the synthesis of fatty acids from acetate groups.

OTHER CONSIDERATIONS OF MCTS AND STRUCTURED LIPIDS

MCT, MCT-LCT mixes, and structured lipids may provide benefits in a nutritional regimen as part of the treatment for the stresses caused by burn injury, surgery, and infection, but there is currently little support for their use in performance enhancement. There are some other applications of the unique metabolic behaviors of precursors of medium-chain fatty acids.

With regard to the development of chronic illness, there is evidence that MCTs do not contribute to the promotion of tumors that is seen with long-chain fatty acid triacylglycerols in experimental animals that have been challenged with a carcinogen (Cohen and Thompson, 1987). This putative benefit may result from the lower caloric density of MCT or from the minimal deposition of fatty acids in the adipose tissues of MCT-fed animals.

The use of MCTs in the nutritional treatment of lipase insufficiency continues to be a viable regimen. In addition, the use of structured lipids with appropriate levels of essential fatty acids may ensure the maintenance or development of a healthful essential fatty acid status.

Another interesting property of structured lipids is the ability to combine desirable physical and metabolic properties in a triacylglycerol. The formulation of a structured lipid with medium-chain fatty acids and behenic acid (22 carbons, saturated), a high-melting-point fatty acid, yields a material (caprenin) that is similar in texture and melting behavior to cocoa butter (Webb and Sanders, 1991). This hedonic benefit is coupled with hydrolysis in the intestine to produce medium-chain fatty acids and a high-melting-point species of behenic acid—the fatty acid, its soap, or the monoglyceride. The behenic compounds, because of their insolubilities and high melting points, are poorly absorbed from the intestine and are excreted. Behenate absorption from caprenin has been shown to be about 30 percent of that ingested, so the caloric density of this structured lipid is approximately 5 kcal/g, or 55 percent of the 9 kcal of typical LCTs per g. The material is therefore a unique, low-calorie substitute for cocoa butter.

A technological development may produce another generation of structured lipids that have so far received little attention. Immobilized lipases have been successfully used in the synthesis of triacylglycerols with fatty acids in specific positions of the triacylglycerol structures. This process is presumably able to provide commercial quantities of specific structured triacylglycerols, and it is now possible to synthesize structured lipids with positional specificity (Jensen et al., 1987). Compounds such as the 1,3-dioctanoyl or 1,2-didecanoyl structured lipids should be available in quantity if research discloses some unique benefits attributable to these structures.

CONCLUSIONS AND RECOMMENDATIONS

Structured lipids are triacylglycerols synthesized from mixtures of long-chain fatty acids and medium-chain fatty acids. Structured lipids and medium-chain triacylglycerols (MCTs) have been shown to provide benefits in their applications in parenteral and enteral nutrition in the sparing of nitrogen and maintenance of reticuloendothelial system function in patients

TABLE 18-2 Summary of Studies of MCT Metabolism During Exercise

Study	Method	Diet	Results
Decombaz and Roux (1980)	Rats on treadmill	Corn oil, MCT, glucose, water	MCT increased ketone levels; glycogen utilization was the same in all groups; time to exhaustion was the same in all groups
Ivy et al. (1980)	Humans at 70 percent of maximum oxygen consumption	Fasting, MCT, LCT, carbohydrate	Percentage of energy from lipid was the same with MCT, LCT, and carbohydrate; MCTs did not alter the pattern of preferential oxidation of carbohydrate during exercise; serum glucose and insulin levels were similar for all groups during exercise
Decombaz et al. (1983)	Humans at 60 percent of maximum oxygen consumption	MCT, maltodextrins (carbohydrate)	Glycogen decrease was the same for MCT and carbohydrate
Howald and Decombaz (1983)	Humans at 60 percent of maximum oxygen consumption	MCT, maltodextrins	Carbohydrate was oxidized more than MCT during exercise; MCT oxidized during rest period; MCTs reduced insulin peak
Sabatin et al. (1987)	Humans at 60 percent of maximum oxygen consumption	MCT, LCT, glucose, fasting	No change in time to exhaustion; glucose was 80 percent oxidized; MCT was 45 percent oxidized, and LCT was 9 percent oxidized

Auclair et al. (1988)	Rats on treadmill	MCTs, LCTs, glucose, water	MCT reduced insulin levels; ketone levels were lowest with glucose; muscle and liver glycogen levels were highest with glucose
Sabatin et al. (1989)	Rats on treadmill	Carbohydrate, LCTs, MCTs, high protein	MCT was equivalent to LCT for blood glucose, free fatty acids, and glycerol; MCT was greater than LCT for ketone body levels; MCT, LCT ketone bodies were greater than others; muscle glycogen levels were similar in all groups; liver glycogen of the MCT group was lowest
Sabatin et al. (1991)	Rats on treadmill	Glucose, MCTs, LCTs	Exercise decreased food intake in rats; food intake was decreased by LCT and MCT at 3–6 h and 0–3h, respectively

NOTE: MCT, medium-chain triacylglycerols; LCT, long-chain triacylglycerols.

stressed by burns, surgery, and trauma. These fats can also provide energy and essential fatty acids in an absorbable form to patients with lipase insufficiency. However, there is inadequate evidence to support the use of structured lipids or MCTs to enhance exercise performance.

Specific Recommendations

- Examinations of MCTs in exercise studies have attempted to show a reduction in glycogen depletion by prefeeding of MCTs. There have apparently not been studies of the use of MCTs or structured lipids in glycogen repletion. Although there would not seem to be an advantage over dietary carbohydrate in this regard, there are no data to confirm or refute this possibility.
- The studies with MCTs in exercise have generally utilized a high-exertion model. The possible sparing of glycogen by MCTs or structured lipids has not been addressed at moderate levels of work output.
- It is possible that the thermogenesis provided by MCTs in overfeeding could have some utility in a low-temperature environment. If this application of MCTs is beneficial, then structured lipids may provide advantages over MCTs by lessening the gastrointestinal distress resulting from the MCT bolus.
- Any benefits that may be discovered for MCTs in normal, healthy individuals may be better provided by structured lipids. The reduced gastrointestinal distress and the production of medium-chain fatty acids by the digestion of structured lipids suggest that structured lipids would provide the same nutrients in a more acceptable form.
- The chronic ingestion of structured lipids with appropriate levels of omega-3 and omega-6 essential fatty acids may provide optimum health in terms of platelet aggregation, inflammatory reactions, and the promotion of cancer. Any studies of structured lipids in this context should include comparisons with other optimum fats such as those containing high levels of oleic acid or with low-fat diets.
- If high-fat diets are desirable, as in the case of minimizing ration volume, then structured lipids might be advantageous compared with normal long-chain triacylglycerols (LCTs). The stomach emptying of structured lipids would be expected to be faster than that of LCTs and slower than that of MCTs. An optimum balance of caloric density and postprandial digestion might be provided.

REFERENCES

Auclair, E., P.Satabin, E.Servan, and C.Y.Guezennac 1988 Metabolic effects of glucose, medium-chain triglyceride and long-chain triglyceride feeding before prolonged exercise in rats. Eur. J. Appl. Physiol. 57:126–131.

Bach, A.C., and V.K.Babayen 1982 Medium-chain Triglycerides; an update. Am. J. Clin. Nutr. 36:950–952.

Benzonana, G.B., B.Entressangles, G.Marchis-Mouren, L.Pasero, L.Sarda, and P.Desnuelle 1964 Further studies on pig pancreatic lipase. Pp. 141–154 in Metabolism and Physiological Significance of Lipids, R.M.C.Dawson and D.N.Rhodes, eds. New York: Wiley.

Birkhahn, R.H. 1988 Invited comment: The role of synthetic compounds in clinical nutrition. J. Parenter. Enteral Nutr. 9:559–565.

Bragdon, J.H., and A.Karmen 1960 The fatty acid composition of chylomicrons of chyle and serum following the ingestion of different oils. J. Lipid Res. 1:167–170.

Cardell, R.R., S.Badenhausen, and K.R.Porter 1967 Intestinal triglyceride absorption in the rat. J. Cell Biol 34:123–155.

Clark, S.B. 1968 Limiting factors in maximal steady state absorption of medium chain triglycerides. Pp. 69–95 in Medium Chain Triglycerides, J.R.Senior, ed. Philadelphia: University of Pennsylvania.

Clement, G., J.Clement, and J.Bezard 1962 Action of human pancreatic lipase on synthetic mixed symmetrical triglycerides of long-chain acids and butyric acid. Biochem. Biophys. Res. Commun. 8:238–242.

Cohen, L.A., and D.O.Thompson 1987 The influence of dietary medium chain triglycerides on rat mammary tumor development. Lipids 22:455–461.

Crossley, A., I.P.Freeman, B.J.F.Hudson, and J.H.Pierce 1959 Acyl migration in diglycerides. J. Chem. Soc. No volume:760–764.

Decombaz, J., and L.Roux 1980 Glycogen utilization in exercise after increased plasma fatty acids or ketone bodies. Int. J. Vitam. Nutr. Res. 50:210–211.

Decombaz, J., M.J.Arnaud, H.Milon, H.Moesch, G.Philippossian, A.L.Thelin, and H.Howard 1983 Energy metabolism of medium-chain triglycerides versus carbohydrate during exercise. Eur. J. Appl. Physiol. 52:9–14.

DiMichele, S.J., M.D.Karlstad, V.K.Babayan, N.Istfan, G.L.Blackburn, and B.R.Bistrian 1988 Enhanced skeletal muscle and liver protein synthesis with structured lipid in enterally fed burned rats. Metabolism 37:787–795.

DiMichele, S.J., M.D.Karlstad, B.R.Bistrian, N.Istfan, V.K.Babayan, G.L.Blackburn 1989 Enteral nutrition with structured lipid: Effect on protein metabolism in thermal injury. Am. J. Clin. Nutr. 50:1295–1302.

Fernandes, J., J.H.Van de Kamer, and H.A.Weijers 1962 The absorption of fats studied in a child with chylothorax. J. Clin. Invest. 34:1026–1036.

Furman, R.H. 1968 Effects of medium-chain length triglycerides on serum lipids. Pp. 51–61 in Medium Chain Triglycerides, J.R.Senior, ed. Philadelphia: University of Pennsylvania.

Hamawy, K.J., L.L.Moldawer, M.Georgieff, and A.J.Valicente 1985 The effect of lipid emulsions on reticuloendothelial system function in the injured animal. J. Parenter. Enteral Nutr. 9:559–565.

Hamosh, M., H.L.Klaeveman, R.O.Wolf, and R.O.Scow 1975 Pharyngeal lipase and digestion of dietary triglyceride in man. J. Clin. Invest. 55:908–913.

Hashim, S.A. 1968 Studies of medium chain fatty acid transport in portal blood. Pp. 81–90 in Medium Chain Triglycerides, J.R.Senior, ed. Philadelphia: University of Pennsylvania.

Hill, J.O., J.C.Peters, D.Yang, T.Sharp, M.Kaler, N.Abumrad, and H.L.Greene 1989 Thermogenesis in humans during overfeeding with medium-chain triglycerides. Metabolism 38:641–648.

Holman, R.T. 1971 Essential fatty acid deficiency. Prog. Chem. Fats Other Lipids 9:279–348.

Holt, P.R. 1968 Studies of medium chain triglycerides in patients with differing mechanisms for fat malabsorption. Pp. 97–107 in Medium Chain Triglycerides, J.R.Senior, ed. Philadelphia: University of Pennsylvania.

Hopman, W.P.M., J.B.M.J.Janasen, G.Rosenbusch, and C.Lamers 1984 Effect of equimolar amounts of long-chain triglycerides and medium-chain triglycerides on plasma cholecystokinin and gallbladder contraction. Am. J. Clin. Nutr. 39:356–359.

Howald, H., and J.Decombaz 1983 Nutrient intake and energy regulation in physical exercise. Experientia 44:77–88.

Huang, N.N. 1968 Medium chain triglycerides in cystic fibrosis. Pp. 207–217 in Medium Chain Triglycerides, J.R.Senior, ed. Philadelphia: University of Pennsylvania.

Hubbard, V.S., and M.C.McKenna 1987 Absorption of safflower oil and structured lipid preparations in patients with cystic fibrosis. Lipids 22:424–441.

Innis, S.M. 1991 Essential fatty acids in growth and developmnent. Prog. Lipid Res. 30:39–103.

Isaacs, P.E.T., S.Ladas, I.C.Forgacs, R.H.Dowling, S.V.Ellam, T.E.Adrian, and S.R.Bloom 1987 Comparison of effects of ingested medium- and long-chain triglycerides on gallbladder volume and release of cholecystokinin and other gut peptides. Dig. Dis. Sci. 32:481–486.

Ivy, J.L., D.L.Costill, W.J.Fink, and E.Maglischo 1980 Contribution of medium and long chain triglyceride intake to energy metabolism during prolonged exercise. Int. J. Sports Med. 1:15–20.

Jandacek, R.J., J.A.Whiteshide, B.N.Holcombe, R.A.Volpenhein, and J.D.Taulbee 1987 The rapid hydrolysis and efficient absorption of triglyceride with octanoic acid in the 1 and 3 position and long-chain fatty fatty acid in the 2 position. Am. J. Clin. Nutr. 45:940–945.

Jandacek, R.J., J.A.Whiteside, B.N.Holcombe, C.M.Kuehlthau, J.C.Peters, and J.D. 1991 Taulbee Reduced storage of eicosapentaenoic and docosahexaenoic acids in the weanling rat. J. Nutr. Biochem. 2:142–149.

Jensen, G.L., E.A.Mascioli, D.L.Seidner, N.W.Istfan, A.M.Domnitch, K.Selleck, V.K.Babayen, G.L.Blackburn, and B.R.Bistrian 1990 Parenteral infusion of long- and medium-chain triglycerides and reticuloendothelial function in man. J. Parenter. Enteral Nutr. 14:467–471.

Jensen, R.G., J.Sampugna, R.M.Parry, and T.L.Forster 1962 Absence of fatty acid specificity during lipolysis of some synthetic triglycerides by ß-esterase preparations from milk. J. Dairy Sci. 45:842–847.

Jensen, R.G., D.R.Galluzo, and B.Huge-Jensen 1987 Specificity of free and immobilized lipases from *Mucor miehi.* J. Am. Oil Chem. Soc. 64:644.

Johnson, R.C., S.K.Young, R.Cotter, L.Lin, and W.B.Rowe 1990 Medium-chain-triglyceride lipid emulsion: Metabolism and tissue distribution. Am. J. Clin. Nutr. 52:502–508.

Kasper, H. 1970 Faecal fat excretion, diarrhea, and subjective complaints with highly dosed oral fat intake. Digestion 3:321–320.

Maiz, A., K.Yamazaki, J.Sobrado, V.K.Babayen, L.L.Moldawer, B.R.Bistrian, and G.L. Blackburn 1984 Protein metabolism during total parenteral nutrition (TPN) in injured rats using medium-chain triglycerides. Metabolism 33:901–915.

Mattson, F.H., and R.J.Jandacek 1991 Distribution among tissues of intravenously administered sucrose octaoleate. Lipids 26:750–753.

Mattson, F.H., J.C.Alexander, F.J.Baur, and H.H.Reller 1956 Short-term feeding studies on acetin fats. J. Nutr. 59:277–285.

McKenna, M.C., V.S.Hubbard, and J.G.Bieri 1985 Linoleic acid absorption from lipid supplements in patients with cystic fibrosis with pancreatic insufficiency and in control subjects. J. Pediatr. Gastroenterol. Nutr. 4:45–51.

Mitsuyoshi, K., Y.Hiramatsu, M.Nakagawa, M.Yamamura, K.Hioki, and M.Yamamota 1992 Effect of structured lipids as energy substrate after hepatectomy in rats with streptozocin-induced diabetes. Nutrition 8:41–46.

Nakagawa, M., Y.Hiramatsu, K.Mitsuyoshi, M.Yamamura, K.Hioki, and M.Yamamato 1991 Effect of various lipid emulsions on total parenteral nutrition-induced hepatosteatosis in rats. J. Parenter. Enteral Nutr. 15:137–143.

Rossle, C., Y.A.Caroentier, M.Richelle, W.Dahlan, N.P.D'attelis, P.Furst, and D.H.Elwyn 1990 Medium-chain triglycerides induce alterations in carnitine metabolism. Am. J. Physiol. 258:E944–E947.

Satabin, P., P.Portero, G.Defer, J.Brecout, and C.Guezennec 1987 Metabolic and hormonal responses to lipid and carbohydrate diets during exercise in man. Med. Sci. Sports Exerc. 19:218–223.

Satabin, P., B.Bois-Joyeux, M.Chanez, C.Y.Guezennec, and J.Peret 1989 Effects of long-term feeding of high-protein or high-fat diets on the response to exercise in the rat. Eur. J. Appl. Physiol. 58:583–590.

Sabatin, P., E.Auclair, E.Servan, C.L.Achagiotis and C.Y.Guezennec 1991 Influence of glucose, medium- and long-chain triglyceride gastric loads and forced exercise on food intake and body weight in rats. Physiol. Behav. 50:147–150.

Scheig, R. 1968 Hepatic metabolism of medium chain fatty acids. Pp. 39–49 in Medium Chain Triglycerides, J.R.Senior, ed. Philadelphia: University of Pennsylvania.

Senior, J.R. 1968 Introductory remarks by the chairman. Pp. 3–7 in Medium Chain Triglycerides, J.R. Senior, ed. Philadelphia: University of Pennsylvania.

Sobrado, J., M.L.Moldawer, J.J.Pomposelli, E.A.Mascioli, V.K.Babayen, B.R.Bistrian, and G.L. 1985 Blackburn Lipid emulsions and reticulo-endothelial function in healthy and burned guinea pigs. Am. J. Clin. Nutr. 42:855–863.

Teo, T.C., S.J.DeMichele, K.M.Selleck, V.K.Babayan, G.L.Blackburn, and B.R.Bristrian 1989 Administration of structured lipid composed of MCT and fish oil reduces net protein catabolism in enterally fed burned rats. Ann. Surg. 210:100–107.

Teo, T.C., K.M.Selleck, J.M.F.Wan, J.J.Pomposelli, V.K.Babayen, G.L.Blackburn, and B.R. Bristrian 1991 Long-term feeding with structured lipid composed of medium-chain and N-3 fatty acids ameliorates endotoxic shock in guinea pigs. Metabolism 40:1152–1159.

Waddell, W.R., R.P.Geyer, E.Clarke, and F.J.Stare 1954 Function of the reticuloendothelial system in removal of emulsified fat from the blood. J. Physiol. 177:747–750.

Webb, D.R., and R.A.Sanders 1991 Caprenin 1. Digestion, absorption, and rearrangement in thoracic duct-cannulated rats. J. Am. Coll. Toxicol. 10:325–340.

Yang, D.K. 1989 Tailored triglycerides having improved autoignition characteristics. U.S. Patent 4,832,975.

Yeh, Y.Y., and P.Zee 1976 Relationship of ketosis to metabolic changes induced by acute medium-chain triglyceride feeding in rats. J. Nutr. 106:58–67.

DISCUSSION

GILBERT LEVEILLE: The exercise phenomenon has not been greatly studied but I would think that during aerobic exercise, when tissues would be in a relatively anaerobic state, one would predict that medium-chain triglycerides (MCTs) would be no better and, possibly, could be worse than long-chain fatty acids. And this would not prevent the depletion of glycogen. That is what people found, but apparently, no one looked at the effect of medium-chain triglycerides or structured lipids in a situation with a more moderate exercise level.

RONALD JANDACEK: I have not seen that.

GILBERT LEVEILLE: That would be the situation in which it should have a beneficial effect.

ELDON ASKEW: On the effect of medium-chain triglycerides on thermogenesis, is this simply that the MCTs have a higher specific dynamic action? Is that what you are referring to there?

ELDON ASKEW: Nothing, though, on a substituted normal-calorie diet?

RONALD JANDACEK: No.

STEVEN ZEISEL: You touched in it during your talk, but could you go over the evidence that omega-3 fatty acid pretreatment seems to moderate the response to endotoxin? We know that if you are using MCT, it would be the same.

RONALD JANDACEK: Not MCT. There were two studies by Teo and the Harvard group. Again, I do not think that the mechanism is very clear, other than the mechanism for those with a vasoactive effect, these omega-3 fatty acids and also an effect on the eicosanoids, that the omega-3 fatty acids do reduce the eicosanoid production that is normally seen from omega-6 fatty acids or arachidonic acid.

CAROLE GREENWOOD: Question about cholesterol metabolism and structured lipids.

RONALD JANDACEK: I do no think that it is. There are a couple of studies with octanoic acid. G.L.Crozier showed that octanic acid is a substrate for cholesterol synthesis. But I do not know where the break in chain length is.

WILLIAM BEISEL: On the basis of what we predict from just Clyde Beany's studies with acid, do you predict that the structured lipids will be able to deliver the omega-3 or omega-6 fatty acids to generate predictable changes in the cell wall, phagocytic cells, or lymphocytes. Has any of that been done?

RONALD JANDACEK: Not with structured lipids. I think the advantage is that if you make a specific structured lipid, you can define exactly what your omega-3 fatty acid level is. There is one patent by F.Mendy in France showing some oxidative stabilization of these long-chain, highly unsaturated fatty acids by putting the medium-chain in the 1 and 3 positions. I do not know whether he proved that or not, but if that is the case, that may be an advantage because certainly the lack of hedonic benefits of fish oil fatty acids is clear.

19

Choline: Human Requirements and Effects on Human Performance

Steven H.Zeisel[1]

INTRODUCTION

Choline is an essential component of the human diet and is important for the normal functioning of all cells (Zeisel and Blusztajn 1994). As such, it has great potential for use as a dietary modulator of human performance. Several mechanisms can explain how these effects are mediated. Acetylcholine synthesis can be influenced by the availability of choline; it is an important neurotransmitter controlling such diverse neural functions as memory and control of muscle function. Choline-phospholipids are extremely important structural elements of cells and are essential for the normal processing of dietary fat. Recently, researchers have begun to understand that choline-phospholipids also are transducers of signals from the exterior of cells to the nucleus. This signaling mechanism is so important and is so widely

[1] Steven H.Zeisel, Department of Nutrition, School of Public Health and School of Medicine, University of North Carolina, Chapel Hill, NC 27599–7400

distributed that its manipulation by changing the diet is likely to be a powerful tool for improving human performance.

Choline is present in some form in all cells, predominantly as one of the choline-phospholipids phosphatidylcholine, lysophosphatidylcholine, choline plasmalogen, platelet-activating factor, or sphingomyelin. All of these are essential components of all membranes (Zeisel, 1990). The importance of choline as a nutrient was first appreciated during the pioneering work on insulin when the association between a low-choline diet and fatty infiltration of the liver was recognized (Best and Huntsman, 1935). The term *lipotropic* was coined to describe choline and the other substances that prevent the deposition of fat in the liver.

Until recently, choline was considered a dispensable nutrient for humans because there is an endogenous pathway for the de novo biosynthesis of the choline moiety (Bremer and Greenberg, 1961). In addition, the demand for choline is modified by the rate of growth of an individual and by complex interrelationships between choline and the nutrients methionine, folic acid, and vitamin B12 (lipotropes) (Zeisel, 1988). However, it is known that human cells grown in culture have an absolute requirement for choline (Eagle, 1955), and recent studies have established that choline is indeed an essential nutrient for normal humans when methionine is not available in excess of requirements (Zeisel et al., 1991) (see discussion below).

DIETARY SOURCES OF CHOLINE

Calculations of dietary choline intake are based on estimates of the free choline and phosphatidylcholine contents of foods (Engel, 1943; Food and Nutrition Board, 1973; McIntire et al., 1944; Weihrauch and Son, 1983; Zeisel et al., 1986). Measurements of the lysophosphatidylcholine, glycerophosphocholine, and phosphocholine contents of rat tissues (Pomfret et al., 1989) show that these choline-containing compounds are also present in high concentrations in many tissues (e.g., the concentrations of each of these three esters in rat muscle were approximately 100 nmol/g.) Thus, the foods eaten by humans probably also contain significant amounts of these esters of choline. In addition, the choline concentrations in tissues rise postmortem. For these reasons, choline intake (especially unesterified choline intake) is probably greatly underestimated.

In addition to the naturally occurring choline in foods, significant amounts are added as dietary supplements. Choline chloride and choline bitartrate are listed in the *Code of Federal Regulations* as nutrients and/or dietary supplements that are generally recognized as safe (Federation of American Societies for Experimental Biology, 1975). More than 5,000 kg of choline chloride and more than 12,000 kg of choline bitartrate were used in the manufacture of foods in 1970 (Federation of American Societies for Experimental Biology, 1975). Most of the choline added to foods was found in infant formulas (Federation of American Societies for Experimental Biology, 1975).

On the basis of these data and reasonable estimates of food intake, total choline intake in the adult human (as free choline and the choline in phosphatidylcholine and other choline esters) is greater than 700–1,000 mg/day (Federation of American Societies for Experimental Biology, 1981; Zeisel, 1981). When humans were switched from a diet of normal foods to a defined diet containing 500 mg of choline (750 mg of choline chloride), Zeisel and colleagues (1991) observed that plasma choline and phosphatidylcholine concentrations decreased in most subjects. This suggests that normal dietary intake of choline exceeds 500 mg. Consumption of choline is higher in humans who ingest phosphatidylcholine (also called *lecithin*) as a dietary supplement (the capsules or granules sold over the counter are usually only 35 percent phosphatidylcholine).

Plasma choline concentrations in fasting subjects vary from 7 to 20 μM, with the plasma of most adult human subjects having concentrations of 10 μM, whereas plasma phosphatidylcholine concentrations are approximately 1–1.5 mM (Aquilonius et al., 1975; Sheard et al., 1986; Zeisel et al., 1980, 1991). Liver phosphocholine is the most labile pool of choline and seems to be the most sensitive indicator of choline nutriture (Pomfret et al., 1990). In the adult human, serum choline concentrations fluctuate modestly (increase 1.5-fold) when common choline-containing foods are ingested (Zeisel et al., 1980). Total body stores of choline in humans can be estimated on the basis of measurements of choline pool concentrations in animal tissues; it is estimated that a 70-kg human contains more than 5 mmol of free choline (500 mg) and more than 300 mmol of choline (30 g) in esterified form (Zeisel et al., 1991).

The only source of choline other than from the diet is from the de novo biosynthesis of phosphatidylcholine catalyzed by phosphatidylethanolamine-*N*-methyltransferase (PeMT). This enzyme synthesizes phosphatidylcholine via sequential methylation of phosphatidylethanolamine by using *S*-adenosylmethionine as a methyl donor (Blusztajn et al., 1979; Ridgway and Vance, 1987; Zeisel, 1981). Most PeMT activity is found in the liver (Bjornstad and Bremer, 1966).

CHOLINE AND METHYL GROUP METABOLISM

The demand for choline as a methyl donor is probably the major factor that determines how rapidly a diet deficient in choline induces pathology. The pathways of choline and 1-carbon metabolism intersect at the formation of methionine from homocysteine (Figure 19–1) (Finkelstein et al., 1982; Mudd and Poole, 1975; Wong and Thompson, 1972). Methionine is regenerated from homocysteine in a reaction catalyzed by betaine: homocysteine methyltransferase, in which betaine, a metabolite of choline, serves as the methyl donor (Finkelstein et al., 1982). The only alternative mechanism for regeneration of methionine is via a reaction catalyzed by 5-methyltetra-hydrofolate:-homocysteine methyltransferase, which uses a methyl group generated de novo from the 1-carbon pool (Finkelstein et al., 1982, 1988). Methionine is converted to *S*-adenosylmethionine in a reaction catalyzed by methionine adenosyl transferase. *S*-Adenosylmethionine is the active methylating agent for many enzymatic methylations.

A disturbance in folate or methionine metabolism results in changes in choline metabolism and vice versa. During choline deficiency, the hepatic choline concentration decreases rapidly (Zeisel et al., 1989). At the same time, hepatic *S*-adenosylmethionine concentrations are decreased (Barak et al., 1982; Poirier et al., 1977; Shivapurkar and Poirier, 1983; Zeisel et al., 1989). It has been suggested that the availability of methionine limits *S*-adenosylmethionine synthesis during choline deficiency because the 5-methyltetrahydrofolate:-homocysteine methyltransferase reaction alone cannot fulfill the total requirement for methionine, and the betaine-dependent remethylation of homo

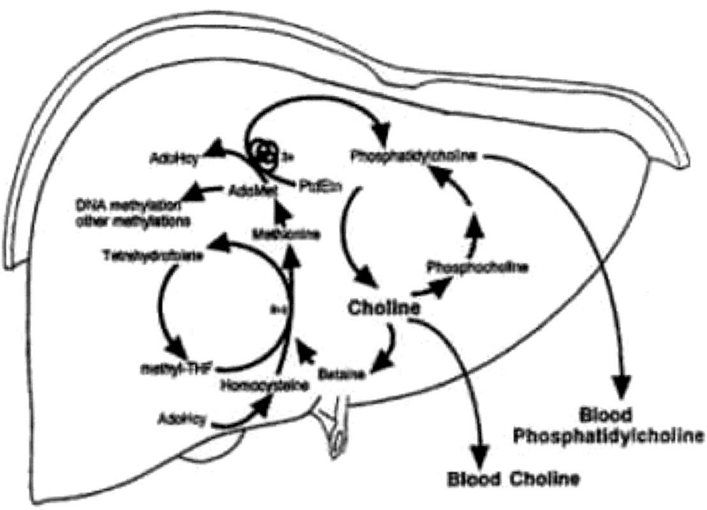

FIGURE 19–1 Choline, folate, and methionine metabolism are closely interrelated. AdoHcy, *S*-adenosylhomocysteine; AdoMet, *S*-adenosylmethionine; PtdEtn, phosphatidylethanolamine; THF,

cysteine is limited by the availability of betaine (Finkelstein et al., 1982). Choline deficiency is also associated with inhibition of hepatic glycine-*N*-methyltransferase activity, which is believed to be important for the removal of excess *S*-adenosylmethionine from the liver (Cook et al., 1989). Betaine concentrations in the livers of choline-deficient rats are markedly diminished (Barak and Tuma, 1983; Finkelstein et al., 1982; Wong and Thompson, 1972), as are total folate concentrations (Horne et al., 1989).

Methotrexate, which is widely used in the treatment of cancer, psoriasis, and rheumatoid arthritis, limits the availability of methyl groups by competitively inhibiting dihydrofolate reductase, a key enzyme in intracellular folate metabolism. When 1-carbon metabolism is poisoned, the only alternative to choline as a source of methyl groups for regeneration of methionine is lost. Hepatic choline, phosphocholine, *S*-adenosylmethionine, and betaine concentrations are diminished after treatment with methotrexate (Barak and Kemmy, 1982; Barak et al., 1984; Freeman-Narrod et al., 1977; Pomfret et al., 1990; Svardal et al., 1988). Folate metabolism is also altered in choline-deficient rats (Horne et al., 1989; Selhub et al., 1991), which is reflected by the greater residence time of folate molecules within liver.

REQUIREMENT FOR CHOLINE IN HUMANS

In the rat (Lombardi, 1971), hamster (Handler and Bernheim, 1949), guinea pig (Tani et al., 1967), pig (Blair and Newsome, 1985; Fairbanks and Krider, 1945), dog (Best and Huntsman, 1932; Hershey and Soskin, 1931), monkey (Hoffbauer and Zaki, 1965), trout (Ketola, 1976), quail (Ketola and Young, 1973), and chicken (Ketola and Nesheim, 1974), choline deficiency results in liver dysfunction. Extremely large amounts of lipid (mainly triglycerides) accumulate in the liver during choline deficiency (Blusztajn and Zeisel, 1989; Lombardi, 1971; Lombardi et al., 1968; Yao and Vance, 1988, 1989), beginning within hours to days after rats are started on a choline-deficient diet (daCosta et al., 1993). Triacylglycerol accumulation occurs because it is secreted from liver as very-low density lipoprotein (VLDL), and phosphatidylcholine is a required component of VLDL (Yao and Vance, 1988, 1989).

Healthy humans fed a choline-deficient diet for 3 weeks developed biochemical changes consistent with choline deficiency (Zeisel et al., 1991). Subjects were admitted to the Clinical Research Center at Boston University School of Medicine and were constantly observed for 5 weeks. During the first week all subjects consumed the same choline-containing diet. During the middle 3 weeks of the study the control group continued on the choline-containing diet while the choline-deficient group consumed the same diet without choline. During the fifth week all subjects consumed the choline-containing diet. Humans ingesting a choline-deficient diet for 3 weeks had diminished plasma choline and phosphatidylcholine concentrations, as well as diminished erythrocyte membrane phosphatidylcholine concentrations. Serum alanine transaminase activity, a measure of hepatocyte damage, increased significantly when a choline-deficient diet was ingested. This experiment establishes a requirement for choline in the diets of normal humans.

Humans with Special Needs for Choline

Choline deficiency may be of clinical importance in several groups of individuals. Humans running a marathon have lower blood choline concentrations after the run than before the run (Conlay et al., 1986). Supplementation with choline before and during a 32-km (20-mile) run prevented this drop in plasma choline and improved the subjects' run times by 5 min (Sandage et al., 1992). The reasons for this drop in choline are undefined and might not reflect the utilization of choline but the redistribution of choline as fluid pools shift during exertion.

The demand for choline in normal adults is likely to be smaller than the demand for choline in infants, because large amounts of choline must be used to make phospholipids in growing organs (Zeisel, 1990). The observed changes that occurred in choline-deficient adult humans might have been greater if growing children were studied. Malnourished humans, in whom stores of choline, methionine, and folate have been depleted (Chawla et al., 1989; Sheard et al., 1986), are also more likely than healthy adult subjects to need dietary choline. Fatty liver develops in obese rats in which 90 percent of their small intestine was bypassed. Choline supplementation prevented this, and choline-deficient diets in such animals exacerbated the accumulation of fat in the liver (Kaminski et al., 1980). Amino acid-glucose solutions used in the total parenteral nutrition of humans contain no choline (Chawla et al., 1985; Sheard et al., 1986). The lipid emulsions used to deliver extra calories and essential fatty acids during parenteral nutrition contain choline in the form of phosphatidylcholine (a 20 percent emulsion contains 13.2 μmol/ml), and humans treated with parenteral nutrition required 1,000–1,700 μmol (approximately 800–1,360 mg) of choline-containing phospholipid per day during the first week of parenteral nutrition therapy to maintain plasma choline levels (Sheard et al., 1986). Burt et al. (1980) reported that plasma choline concentrations were decreased in patients receiving parenteral nutrition at the same time that liver dysfunction was present. Conditions that enhance hepatic triglyceride synthesis (such as carbohydrate loading) increase the requirement for choline for the export of triglyceride from liver (Carroll and Williams, 1982). Thus, treatment of malnourished patients with high-calorie parenteral nutrition solutions at a time when choline stores are depleted might enhance the likelihood of hepatic dysfunction. When supplemental choline (in the form of lecithin) was administered during parenteral nutrition in humans, plasma choline levels returned to normal, and the incidence of hepatic dysfunction and steatosis diminished (Buchman et al., 1992). Subjects treated with placebo did not get better. These observations, that humans fed very-high-calorie diets develop fatty liver that can be alleviated by choline treatment, may be of relevance to designers of very-high-calorie rations for soldiers.

OTHER MECHANISMS WHEREBY CHOLINE INFLUENCES CELLULAR FUNCTION

As discussed earlier, choline is required for two types of signaling mechanisms that are fundamental modulators of the functions of many cells. It is a precursor for the widely distributed neurotransmitter acetylcholine, and it is a precursor for choline-phospholipids, which play a vital role in the regulation of transmembrane signaling.

Cholinergic Neurotransmission in the Brain

Only a small fraction of dietary choline is acetylated, catalyzed by the activity of choline acetyltransferase (Haubrich et al., 1975b; White and Cavallito, 1970). Choline acetyltransferase is highly concentrated in the terminals of cholinergic neurons (Malthe and Fonnum, 1972), but it is also present in such non-nervous system tissues as the placenta (Rama Sastry and Henderson, 1972). The availability of choline and acetyl-coenzyme A (acetyl-CoA) influence choline acetyltransferase activity (Cohen and Wurtman, 1975, 1976; Haubrich et al., 1974, 1975a). In the brain it is unlikely that choline acetyltransferase is saturated with either of its substrates, so that choline (and possibly acetyl-CoA) availability determines the rate of acetylcholine synthesis (White and Wu, 1973). Some investigators report that administration of choline or phosphatidylcholine results in the accumulation of acetylcholine within brain neurons (Haubrich et al., 1974, 1975a; Cohen and Wurtman, 1975, 1976), whereas others observe that such acceleration of acetylcholine synthesis by choline administration can be detected only after pretreatments with agents that cause cholinergic neurons to fire rapidly (Miller et al., 1989; Trommer et al., 1982; Wecker, 1986, 1988; Wecker and Dettbarn, 1979; Wecker et al., 1989). Increased brain acetylcholine synthesis is associated with an augmented release into the synapse of this neurotransmitter. A temporal dissociation between choline administration and effects on brain acetylcholine synthesis and release has been observed (Trommer et al., 1982). The choline taken up by the brain may first enter a storage pool (perhaps the phosphatidylcholine in membranes) before being converted to acetylcholine.

Pharmacological amounts (5–20 g) of supplemental choline characteristically have been administered to alter cholinergic neurotransmission. Choline chloride supplementation (500 mg/kg of body weight in drinking water) increased the number of dendritic spines in the cerebral cortexes of old mice (Bertoni-Freddari et al., 1985; Mervis et al., 1985). In these same animals, memory, as assessed by learning performance, was improved by choline supplementation (Bartus et al., 1980). Choline supplementation during both pre- and postnatal development had long-term enhancing effects on spatial memory in rats, and this improvement was still detected in adults who were treated as infants (Meck et al., 1989). In those studies, effects were detected as late as 8 months after treatment; these changes have now been shown to persist beyond 26 months of age (W.H.Meck, Columbia University, personal communication, 1993). Choline supplementation during the perinatal period led to a significant reduction in both the number of working memory errors and the number of reference memory errors made both during acquisition and at steady-state performance.

The mechanism for this effect of choline on brain function has not been elucidated. Adult rats treated perinatally with choline had increased muscarinic receptor densities as measured by [^{3}H]quinuclidinyl benzilate binding in both the hippocampus and the frontal cortex when compared with those of untreated littermates (Meck et al., 1989). Levels of choline acetyltransferase in the hippocampus were significantly lower in choline-treated rats, although there was no significant change in their levels in the frontal cortex (Meck et al., 1989). Acetylcholine neurotransmission is important for memory in normal humans and rodents (Bartus et al., 1982), and acetylcholine synthesis can be driven by the increased availability of choline (Blusztajn and Wurtman, 1983). Increased choline can enhance activity in the basal forebrain cholinergic system, thereby leading to improved memory function in a variety of species, including rats, mice, mollusks, and humans (Barry and Gelperin, 1982; Bartus et al., 1980; Sahley et al., 1986; Sitaram et al., 1978a,b). Choline may influence brain function via its effects on phospholipid biosynthesis (Schmidt and Wecker, 1981; Wecker, 1986, 1990). These observations suggest that the effects of choline on brain function, mediated by increased cholinergic neurotransmission or by changes in brain membrane and structures, may be a performance-enhancing effect of choline that can be exploited when designing rations for soldiers.

Neuromuscular Junction

Administration of choline increases acetylcholine (ACh) synthesis and release in peripheral neurons (muscle, adrenal, and heart cholinergic neurons) (Wurtman et al., 1980). Choline availability directly influences ACh synthesis and release at the neuromuscular junction. Definitive demonstration of this has been obtained by using the isolated phrenic nerve-diaphragm preparation (Bierkamper and Goldberg, 1980). The phrenic nerve was stimulated at 7 Hz (0.2 ms, 0.6 V), and release of ACh was measured and compared with spontaneous release (no stimulation). Physiological variations in choline in the perfusing medium (0–60 μM) resulted in marked changes in ACh release. In the absence of choline, electrical stimulation of the nerve for 1 h evoked a mean release of 5.13 ±0.62 pmol/min. In the presence of 30 or 60 μM choline, choline-stimulated release increased to 6.75±0.07 and 9.78±1.67 pmol/min, respectively. These changes were highly significant ($P<0.01$).

Humans fed a choline-deficient diet for 3 weeks (see earlier discussion) (Zeisel et al., 1991) were tested electromyographically for muscle conduction velocity while exerting a constant force with their anterior tibialis muscle. As fatigue began, conduction velocity diminished. The slope of decay of conduction velocity was more than two times faster in those given a choline-deficient diet than in controls (S.Zeisel, unpublished data, 1993).

The effects of choline on peripheral cholinergic parasympathetic neurotransmission are also significant. Intravenous choline administration (8–32 mg/kg) produces a sharp fall in blood pressure in rats (Singh, 1973) but not in cats (40 mg/kg of body weight intravenously [Kapp et al., 1970]). Oral administration of choline (10 g/day) had a slight hypotensive effect in humans (Boyd et al., 1977). Choline could be acting by increasing vagal tone to the heart or by dilating arterioles. Although added choline increases acetylcholine release in in vitro preparations of heart (Loffelholz, 1981), changes in the cardiac rate have not been observed in healthy humans treated with choline.

The urinary bladder muscle is also controlled by parasympathetic cholinergic neurotransmission. Bladders isolated from choline-deficient animals showed a 46 percent increase in the maximum response to acetylcholine compared with those from animals with normal levels of choline, whereas bladders from animals on choline-enriched diets showed a 15 percent decrease in maximum contractile response. The results are consistent with the hypothesis that muscarinic receptors are down-regulated to compensate for the increased parasympathetic activity associated with choline-enriched diets and up-regulated to compensate for the decreased parasympathetic activity associated with choline-deficient diets (Wallace et al., 1985)

Choline and Signal Transduction

Current Concepts of Signal Transduction

Signals are transmitted across membranes via a highly interactive cascade of molecular events (Figure 19–2). In the simplest form, an extracellular sensor detects a signal and transmits this message into the interior of the cell via a protein phosphorylation cascade to a final component that acts as a transcriptional regulator. Phospholipids act as vital elements in transmembrane signaling. Agonist-induced hydrolysis of phosphatidyl-inositol bisphosphate linositides (PtdIns) has been established as a major mechanism for transmitting messages into the interior of cells via protein phosphorylation cascades, which ultimately regulate gene transcription. There is a growing body of evidence that choline phospholipids (phosphatidylcholine, sphingomyelin, and their metabolites) are also important mediators and modulators of transmembrane signaling. These functions may explain how choline phospholipids influence normal physiological processes as well as a diverse group of pathological processes.

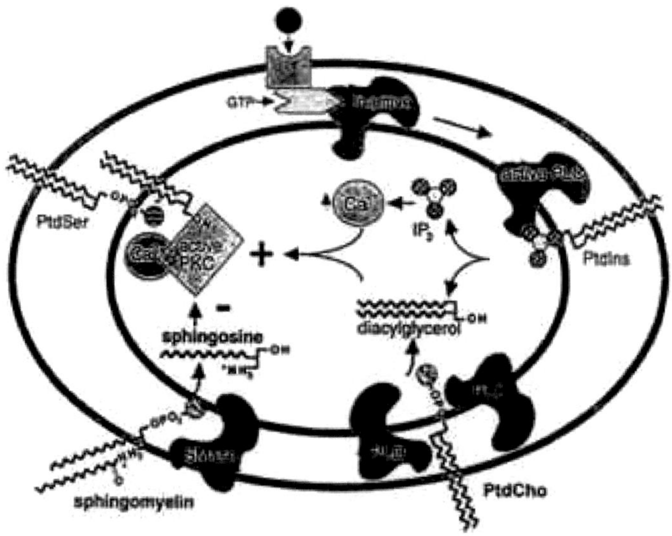

FIGURE 19–2 Choline-phospholipids and signaling. Activation of receptor results in the subsequent activation of phospholipases (PLC, phospholipase C; PLD, phospholipase D), which hydrolyze phosphatidylinositol bisphosphate (PtdIns) and phosphatidylcholine (PtdCho). Diacylglycerol and inositol-1,4,5-trisphosphate (IP_3) are generated. These second messengers activate protein kinase C (PKC). Subsequent hydrolysis of sphingomyelin generates sphingosine and ceramide, which are inhibitors of PKC and act to terminate signaling. SMase, sphingomyelinase; PtdSer, phosphatidylserine; OH, hydroxyl group; NH_3^+, ammonium ion Ca^{2+}, calcium ion; GTP, guanoisne triphosphate; OPO_2, phosphate.

Hundreds of messengers whose effects are mediated by hydrolysis of phospholipids have been identified. An incomplete list includes acetylcholine (M_1 receptor), norepinephrine (α_1), epinephrine (α_1), dopamine, histamine (H_1 receptor), serotonin, vasopressin, angiotensin II, cholecystokinin, gastrin, pancreozymin, substance P, bradykinin, thromboxane, thrombin, collagen, platelet-activating factor, secretagogues, growth factors, and most mitogens. For many of these messengers, the receptor-ligand interaction leads to altered conformation of the receptor so that it can activate a GTP (guanosine diphosphate)- binding protein (G protein). In the inactive state, GDP (guanosine triphosphate) is bound to the complex. Activation triggers replacement of GDP with GTP. The activated G protein stimulates the next effector protein in the signal cascade. The GTPase activity intrinsic to the α subunit eventually hydrolyzes GTP, ending the signal (Meldrum et al., 1991).

The activation of the G protein results in the subsequent activation of phospholipase C (PLC) activity within the plasma membrane. The PLCs are a family of phosphodiesterases that hydrolyze the glycerophosphate bond of intact phospholipids to generate 1,2-*sn*-diacylglycerol (DAG) and an aqueous soluble head group. It is believed that specific receptors couple to specific PtdIns-PLC isotypes (Meldrum et al., 1991). In a similar manner, specific receptors appear to be linked to activation of specific phosphatidlycholine-PLCs (Exton, 1990) (see discussion below).

The action of PLC triggers the next event in the signal cascade, which is the activation of protein kinase C (PKC; serine-threonine kinases). The first step in PKC activation is the formation of a enzyme-calcium ion (Ca^{2+})-phospholipid complex. The products generated by PtdIns-PLC include inositol-1,4,5-trisphosphate (IP_3) and DAG. IP_3 is a water soluble product that acts to release calcium from stores in the endoplasmic reticulum. This increase in cytosolic calcium makes more calcium available for binding to PKC isotypes that are Ca^{2+} dependent (PKCsα, ß1/2, and γ; PKCs δ, ε, ζ, θ and η lack the calcium-binding C2- domain of PKC and therefore are not calcium dependent; Stabel and Parker, 1991). Calcium increases the tightness of association of these PKCs with the membrane, thereby increasing membrane occupancy. This facilitates binding of DAG, which, as described earlier, is the other product of PLC activity. The DAG-PKC complex approaches the membrane more closely, placing the kinase in a pocket of negatively charged phosphatidylserine head groups, into which Ca^{2+} is attracted. Thus, DAG increases the affinity of PKC for calcium. Normally, PKC is folded so that an endogenous pseudosubstrate region on the protein is bound to the catalytic site, thereby inhibiting activity. The combination of DAG and Ca^{2+} causes a conformational change in PKC, causing flexing at a hinge region so as to withdraw the pseudosubstrate and unblock the PKC catalytic site. The appearance of diacylglycerol in membranes is usually transient, and therefore, PKC is activated only for a short time after a receptor has been stimulated.

The events that occur downstream from PKC are just beginning to be characterized. Serine-threonine kinases and tyrosine kinases catalyze phosphorylation events distal to PKC. These phosphorylation cascades serve to enhance amplification of the original signal. Clearly, PKC signals impinge on several known intracellular control circuits (Stabel and Parker, 1991). The targets for phosphorylation by PKC include receptors for insulin, epidermal growth factor, and many of the proteins involved in the control of gene expression, cell division, and cell differentiation (Nishizuka, 1986; Weinstein, 1990). It is likely that a plethora of PKC targets will be studied in the next few years.

Choline Phospholipids and Signal Transduction

The hydrolysis of phosphatidylcholine (PtdCho) occurs in response to a range of agonists, some of which activate PtdCho-specific PLCs and phospholipase D (PLD; PLD generates phosphatidic acid and choline) (Exton, 1990). PtdCho hydrolysis can act to sustain a message that was initially transmitted via inositide breakdown. Sustained activation of PKC is essential for triggering cell differentiation and proliferation (Nishizuka, 1992). PtdCho breakdown can generate second messengers independent of PtdIns breakdown. This is important, because several isotypes of PKC are activated by DAG in the absence of an increase in intracellular calcium (see earlier discussion) (Stabel and Parker, 1991). The fatty acid species in PtdCho are different from those in PtdIns; therefore, the diradylglycerols generated from each will differ. PtdCho is made up of different molecular species, including ester-, ether- and vinyl-linked species. Further diversity exists, because the acyl chain structure can vary greatly. Therefore, hydrolysis of PtdCho can generate multiple species of diradylglycerols. The predominant components of diradylglycerol in tissues are the ester-linked 1,2-diacyl species and the 1-alkyl-2-acyl glycerols (ether-linked 1-*O*-alkyl-2-acyl and vinyl-linked 1-*O*-alk-1'-enyl-2-acyl species). These subclasses of DRGs may differ in their ability to activate PKC (Bass et al., 1989; Cabot and Jaken, 1984; Daniel et al., 1988; Dawson and Cook, 1987; Ford et al., 1989; Heymans et al., 1987). It is possible that the DRGs generated from PtdCho are recognized by special isotypes of PKC, which act in a different domain than does inositide-stimulated PKC, and this may provide a mechanism to maintain signal specificity.

Other products of PtdCho hydrolysis, such as phosphatidic acid, lysophosphatidylcholine (lysoPtdCho), and free fatty acids also are second messengers (Besterman et al., 1986; Exton, 1990). Phosphatidic acid can act as a mitogen (Wakelam et al., 1991). LysoPtdCho stimulates PKC activity (Nishizuka, 1992), but it is a membrane-lytic detergent with potential toxic effects. LysoPtdCho generation is important in chemotaxis, relaxation of smooth muscle, and activation of T lymphocytes (Nishizuka, 1992). Phospholipase A_2 (PLA_2) generates free fatty acids from PtdCho. It is activated by many agonists including tyrosine kinase activators (epidermal growth factor and platelet-derived growth factor) and PKC activators (Nishizuka, 1992). Arachidonic acid, which is generated by PLA_2, can be a precursor for lipoxygenase- or cyclo-oxygenase generated products (Stabel and Parker, 1991). Oleic and arachidonic acids are able to activate soluble PKC but not membrane-bound PKC (Khan et al., 1992). This may be important for differential activation of the separate isotypes of PKC.

Although PtdCho hydrolysis generates a series of messengers that sustains the PKC phosphorylation cascade, the choline-phospholipid sphingomyelin (SM) is hydrolyzed to generate messengers that terminate the cascade. The hydrolysis of SM by sphingomyelinase (which produces ceramide and phosphocholine from SM) is activated by multiple agonists, including 1α,25-dihydroxyvitamin D_3, tumor necrosis factor, and γ interferon (Merrill, 1992). Ceramide is a potent inhibitor of cell growth as well as a promoter of cell differentiation. Its metabolite, sphingosine, is a potent inhibitor of PKC and acts by blocking DAG activation (Merrill and Stevens, 1989). Lysosphingomyelin is also formed during the hydrolysis of SM (see Figure 19– 2) and inhibits PKC (Hannun and Bell, 1989). The synthesis of SM from ceramide and PtdCho generates DAG (Figure 19–2), but it is not known whether this DAG is delivered to a subcellular location where it is available for PKC activation. At present it is suspected that a major function for receptor-mediated activation of sphingomyelinase is the generation of products that stop the signaling cascade.

Choline and Carcinogenesis

Choline deficiency is an excellent example of how choline can influence PKC signal transduction. Choline is the major dietary source for labile methyl groups, and its metabolism is interrelated with methionine and folate metabolism; choline deficiency depletes all of these methyl donors (Zeisel, 1990). Choline is the only single nutrient for which dietary deficiency is associated with the development of cancer (Newberne and Rogers, 1986).

As discussed before, during choline deficiency, secretion of triglyceride (TG) is inhibited. This causes TG and DRG to accumulate (daCosta et al., 1993), and this accumulation is associated with significant increases in PKC activity in hepatic plasma membranes. There is a stable activation of PKC, an increase in the total PKC pool in the cell, or both (daCosta et al., 1993), with changes in several PKC isotypes (at 6 weeks of choline deficiency, the amounts of PKCs α and δ are increased 2-fold and 10-fold, respectively). The accumulation of DAG and the subsequent activation of PKC within the liver during choline deficiency may be the critical abnormality that eventually contributes to the development of hepatic cancer in these animals. Several lines of evidence indicate that cancers might develop secondary to abnormalities in PKC-mediated signal transduction (Weinstein, 1990). It is interesting that choline deficient rats not only have a higher incidence of spontaneous hepatocarcinoma but that they are also markedly sensitized to the effects of administered carcinogens (Newberne and Rogers, 1986). Perturbed PKC signal transduction may lower the threshold dose of carcinogen needed to initiate the development of cancers.

CONCLUSIONS AND RECOMMENDATIONS

- Choline is an essential nutrient for humans and can affect human performance via multiple mechanisms. Of immediate practical application in the design of rations is choline's use for the handling and packaging of lipid within the liver. Rations must be formulated to be calorically dense (high fat), and the calories administered to troops are much higher than those ingested by the normal population. This high-calorie diet should increase demands for choline to package lipid within liver.
- In the near term, it appears reasonable to explore choline's ability to enhance muscle function in individuals performing strenuous exercise. The data indicating efficacy are preliminary and need to be carefully replicated before changes in ration compositions are implemented.
- Finally, the ubiquitous role that phosphatidylcholine plays in transmembrane signaling suggests that significant enhancement of human performance might be obtained through dietary manipulation of such signaling. Several drug companies are actively pursing the identification of pharmacologic agents that can be used to manipulate transmembrane signaling. A significant investment in basic research on dietary interactions with cell signaling needs to be made before practical applications to human rations can be recommended. The very potent effects already demonstrated for dietary modulation of cell signaling (carcinogenesis) suggest that any investment made on such basic research would be worthwhile.

ACKNOWLEDGMENTS

Some of the work described here was supported by grants from the National Institutes of Health (AG-09525 and RR-00046) and the American Institute for Cancer Research.

REFERENCES

Aquilonius, S.M., G.Ceder, T.U.Lying, H.O.Malmlund, and J.Schuberth 1975 The arteriovenous difference of choline across the brain of man. Brain Res. 99:430–433.

Barak, A.J., and R.J.Kemmy 1982 Methotrexate effects on hepatic betaine levels in choline-supplemented and choline-deficient rats. Drug Nutr. Interact. 1:275–278.

Barak, A.J., and D.J.Tuma 1983 Betaine, metabolic by-product or vital methylating agent? Life Sci. 32:771–744.

Barak, A.J., H.C.Beckenhauer, and D.J.Tuma 1982 Use of *S*-adenosylmethionine as an index of methionine recycling in rat liver slices. Anal. Biochem. 127:372–375.

Barak, A.J., D.J.Tuma, and H.C.Beckenhauer 1984 Methotrexate hepatotoxicity. J. Am. Coll. Nutr. 3:93–96.

Barry, S.R. and A.Gelperin. 1982 Exogenous choline augments transmission at an identified cholinergic synapse in terrestrial mollusk *Limax maximus*. J. Neurophysiol. 48:439–450.

Bartus, R.T., R.L.Dean, J.A.Goas, and A.S.Lippa 1980 Age-related changes in passive avoidance retention: Modulation with dietary choline. Science 209:301–303.

Bartus, R.T., R.Dean, B.Beer, and A.S.Lippa. 1982 The cholinergic hypothesis of geriatric memory dysfunction. Science 217:408–414.

Bass, D.A., L.C.McPhail, J.D.Schmitt, S.Morris-Natschke, C.E.McCall and R.L.Wykle 1989 Selective priming of rate and duration of the respiratory burst of neutrophils by 1,2-diacyl and 1-*O*-alkyl-2-acyl diglycerides. Possible relation to effects on protein kinase C. J. Biol. Chem. 263:19610–19617.

Bertoni-Freddari, C., R.F.Mervis, C.Giuli, and C.Pieri 1985 Chronic dietary choline modulates synaptic plasticity in the cerebellar glomeruli of aging mice. Mech. Aging Dev. 30:1–9.

Best, C.H., and M.E.Huntsman 1932 The effects of the components of lecithin upon the deposition of fat in the liver. J. Physiol. 75:405–412.

1935 Effect of choline on liver fat of rats in various states of nutrition. J. Physiol. 83:255–274.

Besterman, J.M., V.Duronio, and P.Cuatrecasas. 1986 Rapid formation of diacylglycerol from phosphatidylcholine: A pathway for generation of a second messenger. Proc. Natl. Acad. Sci. 83:6785–6789.

Bierkamper, G.G., and A.M.Goldberg 1980 Release of acetylcholine from the vascular perfused rat phrenic nerve hemidiaphragm. Brain Res. 202:234–237.

Bjornstad, P., and J.Bremer 1966 In vivo studies on pathways for the biosynthesis of lecithin in the rat J. Lipid Res. 7:38–45.

Blair, R., and F.Newsome 1985 Involvement of water-soluble vitamins in diseases of swine. J. Animal Sci. 60:1508–1517.

Blusztajn, J.K., and R.J.Wurtman 1983 Choline and cholinergic neurons. Science 221:614–620.

Blusztajn, J.K., and S.H.Zeisel 1989 1,2-*sn*-Diacylglycerol accumulates in choline-deficient liver. A possible mechanism of hepatic carcinogenesis via alteration in protein kinase C activity? FEBS Lett. 243:267–270.

1979 Synthesis of lecithin (phosphatidylcholine) from phosphatidylethanolamine in bovine brain. Brain Res. 179:319–327.

Blusztajn, J.K., S.H.Zeisel, and R.J.Wurtman 1985 Developmental changes in the activity of phosphatidylethanolamine *N*-methyltransferases in rat brain. Biochem. J. 232:505–511.

Boyd, W.D., W.J.Graham, G.Blackwood, I.Glen, and J.McQueen 1977 Clinical effects of choline in Alzheimer senile dementia. Letter. Lancet 2:711.

Bremer, J., and D.Greenberg 1961 Methyl transfering enzyme system of microsomes in the biosynthesis of lecithin (phosphatidylcholine) . Biochim. Biophys. Acta 46:205–216.

Buchman, A.L., M.Dubin, D.Jenden, A.Moukarzel, M.H.Roch, K.Rice, J.Gornbein, M.E. Ament, and C.D.Eckhert 1992 Lecithin increases plasma free choline and decreases hepatic steatosis in long-term total parenteral nutrition patients. Gastroenterology 102:1363–1370.

Burt, M.E., I.Hanin, and M.F.Brennan 1980 Choline deficiency associated with total parenteral nutrition. Lancet 2:638–639.

Cabot, M.C., and S.Jaken 1984 Structural and chemical specificity of diradylglycerols for protein kinase C activation. Biochem. Biophys. Res. Commun. 125:163–169.

Carroll, C., and L.Williams 1982 Choline deficiency in rats as influenced by dietary energy somics. Nutr. Rep. Inter. 25:773.

Chawla, R.K., C.J.Berry, M.H.Kutner, and D.Rudman 1985 Plasma concentrations of transsulfuration pathway products during nasoenteral and intravenous hyperalimentation of malnourished patients. Am. J. Clin. Nutr. 42:577–584.

Chawla, R.K., D.C.Wolf, M.H.Kutner, and H.L.Bonkovsky 1989 Choline may be an essential nutrient in malnourished patients with cirrhosis. Gastroenterology 97:1514–1520.

Cohen, E.L., and R.J.Wurtman 1975 Brain acetylcholine: Increase after systemic choline administration. Life Sci. 16:1095–1102.

1976 Brain acetylcholine: Control by dietary choline. Science 191:561–562.

Conlay, L.A., R.J.Wurtman, K.Blusztajn, I.L.Coviella, T.J.Maher and G.E.Evoniuk 1986 Decreased plasma choline concentrations in marathon runners. Letter. N Engl. J. Med. 315:892.

Cook, R.J., D.W.Horne, and C.Wagner 1989 Effect of methyl group deficiency on one-carbon metabolism in rats. J. Nutr. 119:612–617.

daCosta, K.A., E.F.Cochary, J.K.Blusztajn, S.F.Garner, and S.H.Zeisel. 1993 Accumulation of 1,2-*sn*-diradylglycerol with increased membrane-associated protein kinase C may be the mechanism for spontaneous hepatocarcinogenesis in choline deficient rats. J. Biol. Chem. 268:2100–2105.

Daniel, L.W., G.W.Small, J.D.Schmitt, C.J.Marasco, K.Ishaq, and C.Piantadosi 1988 Alkyl-linked diglycerides inhibit protein kinase C activation by diacylglycerols. Biochem. Biophys. Res. Commun. 151:291–297.

Dawson, W.D. and J.S.Cook 1987 Parallel changes in amino acid transport and protein kinase C localization in LLL-PK1 cells treated with TPA or diradylglycerols. J. Cell. Physiol. 132:104–110.

Eagle, H. 1955 The minimum vitamin requirements of the L and Hela cells in tissue culture, the production of specific vitamin deficiencies, and their cure. J. Exp. Med. 102:595–600.

Engel, R.W. 1943 The choline content of animal and plant products. J. Nutr. 25:441–446.

Exton, J.H. 1990 Signaling through phosphatidylcholine breakdown. J. Biol. Chem. 265:1–4.

Fairbanks, B.W. and J.L.Krider 1945 Significance of B vitamins in swine nutrition. N. Am. Vet. 26:18–23.

Federation of American Societies for Experimental Biology 1975 Evaluation of the Health Aspects of Choline Chloride and Choline Bitartrate as Food Ingredients. PB262–654. Springfield, Va.: National Technical Information Service.

1981 Effects of Consumption of Choline and Lecithin on neurological and Cardiovascular Systems. PB82–133257. Springfield VA, National Technical Information Service.

Finkelstein, J.D., J.J.Martin, B.J.Harris, and W.E.Kyle 1982 Regulation of the betaine content of rat liver. Arch. Biochem. Biophys. 218:169–173.

Finkelstein, J.D., J.J.Martin, and B.J.Harris 1988 Methionine metabolism in mammals. The methionine-sparing effect of cystine. J. Biol. Chem. 263:11750–11754.

Food and Nutrition Board 1973 Comprehensive GRAS Survey, Usage Levels Reported for NAS Appendix A Substances (Group 1) Used in Regular Foods. Washington, D.C.: National Academy of Sciences.

Ford, D.A., R.Miyake, P.E.Glaser, and R.W.Gross 1989 Activation of protein kinase C by naturally occurring ether-linked diglycerides. J. Biol. Chem. 264:13818–13824.

Freeman-Narrod, M., S.A.Narrod, and R.P.Custer 1977 Chronic toxicity of methotrexate in rats: Partial to complete projection of the liver by choline: Brief communication. J. Natl. Cancer Inst. 59:1013–1017.

Handler, P. and F.Bernheim 1949 Choline deficiency in the hamster. Proc. Soc. Exp. Med. 72:569.

Hannun, Y.A. and R.M.Bell 1989 Regulation of protein kinase C by sphingosine and lysosphingolipids. Clin. Chim. Acta 185:333–345.

Haubrich, D.R., P.W.Wedeking, and P.F.Wang 1974 Increase in tissue concentration of acetylcholine in guinea pigs in vivo induced by administration of choline. Life Sci. 14:921–927.

Haubrich, D.R., P.F.Wang, D.E.Clody, and P.W.Wedeking 1975a Increase in rat brain acetylcholine induced by choline or deanol. Life Sci. 17:975–980.

Haubrich, D.R., P.F.Wang, and P.W.Wedeking. 1975b Distribution and metabolism of intravenously administered choline[methyl-3-H] and synthesis in vivo of acetylcholine in various tissues of guinea pigs. J. Pharmacol. Exp. Ther. 193:246–255.

Hershey, J.M. and S.Soskin. 1931 Substitution of "lecithin" for raw pancreas in a diet of depancreatized dog. Am. J. Physiol. 93:657–658.

Heymans, F., S.C.Da, N.Marrec, J.J.Godfroid, and M.Castagna 1987 Alkyl analogs of diacylglycerol as activators of protein kinase C. FEBS Lett. 218:35–40.

Hoffbauer, F.W., and F.G.Zaki 1965 Choline deficiency in the baboon and rat compared. Arch. Pathol. 79:364–369.

Horne, D.W., R.J.Cook, and C.Wagner. 1989 Effect of dietary methyl group deficiency on folate metabolism in rats. J. Nutr. 119:618–621.

Kaminski, D.L., E.J.Mueller, and M.Jellinek 1980 Effect of small intestinal bypass on hepatic lipid accumulation in rats. Am. J. Physiol. 239:G358–G362.

Kapp, J., M.J.Mahaley, and G.L.Odom 1970 Experimental evaluation of potential spasmolytic drugs. J. Neurosurg. 32:468–472.

Ketola, H.G. 1976 Choline metabolism and nutritional requirement of lake trout *(Salvelinus namaycush)*. J. Anim. Sci. 43:474–477.

Ketola, H.G., and M.C.Nesheim 1974 The influence of dietary protein and methionine levels on the requirement for choline by chickens. J. Nutr. 104:1484–1486.

Ketola, H.G., and R.J.Young 1973 The need for dietary choline by young Japanese quail. Poult. Sci. 52:2362–2363.

Khan, W.A., G.C.Blobe, and Y.A.Hannun. 1992 Activation of protein kinase C by oleic acid. J. Biol. Chem. 267:3605–3612.

Loffelholz, K. 1981 Release of acetylcholine in the isolated heart. A Review. Am. J. Physiol. 240:H431–H440.

Lombardi, B. 1971 Effects of choline deficiency on rat hepatocytes. Fed. Proc. 30:139–142.

Lombardi, B., P.Pani, and F.F.Schlunk 1968 Choline-deficiency fatty liver: Impaired release of hepatic triglycerides. J. Lipid Res. 9:437–46.

Malthe, S.D., and F.Fonnum 1972 Multiple forms of choline acetyltransferase in several species demonstrated by isoelectric focusing. Biochem. J. 127:229–236.

McIntire, J.M., B.S.Schweigert, and C.A.Elvehjem 1944 The choline and pyridoxine content of meats. J. Nutr. 28:219–223.

Meck, W.H., R.A.Smith, and C.L.Williams 1988 Pre- and postnatal choline supplementation produces long-term facilitation of spatial memory. Dev. Psychobiol. 21:339–353.

Meck, W.H., R.A.Smith, and C.L.Williams 1989 Organizational changes in cholinergic activity and enhanced visuospatial memory as a function of choline administered prenatally or postnatally or both. Behav. Neurosci. 103:1234–1241.

Meldrum, E., P.J.Parker, and A.Carozzi 1991 The Ptd-Ins-PLC superfamily and signal transduction. Biochim. Biophys. Acta 1092:49–71.

Merrill, A.H. 1992 Ceramide: A new lipid "second messenger"? Nutr. Rev. 50:78–80.

Merrill, A.H. and V.L.Stevens 1989 Modulation of protein kinase C and diverse cell functions by sphingosine- a pharmacologically interesting compound linking sphingolipids and signal transduction. Biochim. Biophys. Acta 1010:131–139.

Mervis, R., L.Horrocks, P.Demediuk, L.Wallace, D.R.Meyer, S.Beall, K.Caris, and E.Naber 1985 Neurobehavioral effects of chronic choline-containing diets on the adult and aging C57BL/6NNIA mouse brain. Ann. N.Y. Acad. Sci. 444:469–70.

Miller, L.G., D.J.Greenblatt, R.B.Roy, F.Lopez, and L.Wecker 1989 Dietary choline intake modulates benzodiazepine receptor binding and gamma-aminobutyric acid A receptor function in mouse brain. J. Pharmacol. Exp. Ther. 248:1–6.

Mudd, S.H. and J.R.Poole 1975 Labile methyl balances for normal humans on various dietary regimens. Metab. Clin. Exp. 24:721–735.

Newberne, P.M. and A.E.Rogers 1986 Labile methyl groups and the promotion of cancer. Annu. Rev. Nutr. 6:407–432. Nishizuka, Y.

1986 Studies and perspectives of protein kinase C. Science 233:305–312.

Nishizuka, Y. 1992 Intracellular signaling by hydrolysis of phospholipids and activation of protein kinase C. Science 258:607–614.

Poirier, L.A., P.H.Grantham, and A.E.Rogers 1977 The effects of a marginally lipotrope-deficient diet on the hepatic levels of *S*-adnosylmethionine and on the urinary metabolites of 2-acetylaminofluorene in rats. Can. Res. 37:744–748.

Pomfret, E.A., K.A.daCosta, L.L.Schurman, and S.H.Zeisel 1989 Measurement of choline and choline metabolite concentrations using high-pressure liquid chromatography and gas chromatography-mass spectrometry. Anal. Biochem. 180:85–90.

Pomfret, E.A., K.A.daCosta, and S.H.Zeisel. 1990 Effects of choline deficiency and methotrexate treatment upon rat liver. J. Nutr. Biochem. 1:533–541.

Rama Sastry, B.V., and G.I.Henderson 1972 Kinetic mechanisms of human placental choline acetyltransferase. Biochem. Pharmacol. 21:787–802.

Ridgway, N.D., and D.E.Vance 1987 Purification of phosphatidylethanolamine *N*-methyltransferase from rat liver. J. Biol. Chem. 262:17231–17239.

Sahley, C.L., S.R.Barry, and A.Gelperin 1986 Dietary choline augments associative memory function in Limax maximus. Neurobiol. 17:113–120.

Sandage, B.W., R.N.Sabounjian, R.White, and R.J.Wurtman 1992 Choline citrate may enhance athletic performance. Physiologist 35:236a.

Schmidt, D.E., and L.Wecker 1981 CNS effects of choline administration: Evidence for temporal dependence. Neuropharmacology 20:535–539.

Selhub, J., E.Seyoum, E.A.Pomfret, and S.H.Zeisel 1991 Effects of choline deficiency and methotrexate treatment upon liver folate content and distribution. Cancer Res. 51:16–21.

Sheard, N.F., J.A.Tayek, B.R.Bistrian, G.L.Blackburn, and S.H.Zeisel 1986 Plasma choline concentration in humans fed parenterally. Am. J. Clin. Nutr. 43:219–2–24.

Shivapurkar, N., and L.A.Poirier 1983 Tissue levels of *S*-adenosylmethionine and *S*-adenosylhomocysteine in rats fed methyl-deficient, amino acid-defined diets for one to five weeks. Carcinogenesis 4:1051–1057.

Singh, G.S. 1973 Letter: Action of choline on the rat blood pressure. Indian J. Physiol. Pharmacol. 17:125.

Sitaram, N., H.Weingartner, E.D.Caine, and J.C.Gillin 1978a Choline: Selective enhancement of serial learning and encoding of low imagery words in man. Life Sci. 22:1555–1560.

Sitaram, N., H.Weingartner, and J.C.Gillin 1978b Human serial learning: Enhancement with arecholine and choline impairment with scopolamine. Science 201:274–276.

Stabel, S., and P.J.Parker 1991 Protein kinase C. Pharmac. Ther. 51:71–95.

Svardal, A.M., P.M.Ueland, R.K.Berge, A.Aarsland, N.Aarsaether, E.P.Lonning, and H.Refsum 1988 Effect of methotrexate on homocysteine and other compounds in tissues of rats fed a normal or a defined, choline-deficient diet. Cancer Chemother. Pharmacol. 21:313–318.

Tani, H., S.Suzuki, M.Kobayashi, and Y.Kotake 1967 The physiological role of choline in guinea pigs. J. Nutr. 92:317–324.

Trommer, B.A., D.E.Schmidt, and L.Wecker 1982 Exogenous choline enhances the synthesis of acetylcholine only under conditions of increased cholinergic neuronal activity. J. Neurochem. 39:1704–1709.

Wakelam, M.J.O., S.J.Cook, S.Currie, S.Plamer, and R.Plevin 1991 Regulation of the hydrolysis of phosphatidylcholine in Swiss 3T3 cells. Biochem. Soc. Trans. 19:321–324.

Wallace, L.J., M.G.Kolta, M.C.Gerald, and R.F.Mervis 1985 Dietary choline affects response to acetylcholine by isolated urinary bladder. Life Sci. 36:1377–1380.

Wecker, L. 1986 Neurochemical effects of choline supplementation. Can. J. Physiol. Pharmacol. 64:329–333.

Wecker, L. 1988 Influence of dietary choline availability and neuronal demand on acetylcholine synthesis by rat brain. J. Neurochem. 51:497–504.

Wecker, L. 1990 Dietary choline: A limiting factor for the synthesis of acetylcholine by the brain. Adv. Neurol. 51:139–145.

Wecker, L., and W.D.Dettbarn 1979 Relationship between choline availability and acetylcholine synthesis in discrete regions of rat brain. J. Neurochem. 32:961–967.

Wecker, L., G.Cawley, and S.Rothermel 1989 Acute choline supplementation in vivo enhances acetylcholine synthesis in vitro when neurotransmitter release is increased by potassium. J. Neurochem. 52:568–575.

Weihrauch, J.L. and Y.S.Son 1983 The phospholipid content of foods. J. Amer. Oil Chem. Soc. 60:1971–1978.

Weinstein, I.B. 1990 The role of protein kinase C in growth control and the concept of carcinogenesis as a progressive disorder in signal transduction. Adv. Second Messenger Phosphoprotein Res. 24:307–316.

White, H.L. and C.J.Cavallito 1970 Choline acetyltransferase. Enzyme mechanism and mode of inhibition by a styrylpyridine analogue. Biochim. Biophys. Acta 206:343–358.

White, H.L. and J.C.Wu 1973 Kinetics of choline acetyltransferases (EC 2.3.1.6) from human and other mammalian central and peripheral nervous tissues. J. Neurochem. 20:297–307.

Wong, E.R., and W.Thompson 1972 Choline oxidation and labile methyl groups in normal and choline-deficient rat liver. Biochim. Biophys. Acta 260:259–271.

Wurtman, R.J., F.Hefti, and E.Melamed 1980 Precursor control of neurotransmitter synthesis. Pharmacol. Rev. 32:315–335.

Yao, Z.M., and D.E.Vance 1988 The active synthesis of phosphatidylcholine is required for very low density lipoprotein secretion from rat hepatocytes. J. Biol. Chem. 263:2998–3004.

1989 Head group specificity in the requirement of phosphatidylcholine biosynthesis for very low density lipoprotein secretion from cultured hepatocytes. J. Biol. Chem. 264:11373–11380.

Zeisel, S.H. 1981 Dietary choline: Biochemistry, physiology, and pharmacology. Ann. Rev. Nutr. 1:95–121.

1988 "Vitamin-like" molecules: Choline. Pp. 440–452 in Modern Nutrition in Health and Disease, 7th ed. Philadelphia: Lea & Febiger.

1990 Choline deficiency. J. Nutr. Biochem. 1:332–349.

Zeisel, S.H. and J.K.Blusztajn 1994 Choline and human nutrition Ann. Rev. Nutr. 14:269–296.

Zeisel, S.H., J.H.Growdon, R.J.Wurtman, S.G.Magil, and M.Logue 1980 Normal plasma choline responses to ingestion of lecithin. Neurology 30:1226–1229.

Zeisel, S.H., D.Char, and N.F.Sheard 1986 Choline, phosphatidylcholine and sphingomyelin in human and bovine milk and infant formulas. J. Nutr. 116:50–58.

Zeisel, S.H., T.Zola, K.A.daCosta, and E.A.Pomfret 1989 Effect of choline deficiency on *S*-adenosylmethionine and methionine concentrations in rat liver. Biochem. J. 259:725–729.

Zeisel, S.H., K.A.daCosta, P.D.Franklin, E.A.Alexander, J.T.Lament, N.F.Sheard, and A.Beiser 1991 Choline, an essential nutrient for humans. FASEB J. 5:2093–2098.

DISCUSSION

RICHARD WURTMAN: I want to congratulate you on a fine review. In the athlete study, I think that the actual choline base is only 1 gram. If it was 3 grams, I think I would know. But my question is this. If we all need 6 to 12 grams of phosphatidylcholine—and that is made up of one-eighth choline—that means we are taking in about three-quarters of a gram to a gram and a half of choline per day; suppose we decided to raise choline intake to 3 grams a day, which would not be crazy if you considered my grandfathers, both of whom, I am told, ate two eggs for breakfast each day. I think the consequence of reducing dietary cholesterol is concurrently to reduce dietary choline. My question is, what is the down side of giving people 3 grams of choline per day as opposed to the gram or gram and a half that they are getting now?

STEVEN ZEISEL: I think that our exposure to choline is greater than the amount that we eat. I agree that human deficiency studies suggest that about 500 milligrams to a gram of choline must be what normal humans eat, but we are exposed to more because reabsorbed bile phosphatidylcholine is about equal to dietary phosphatidylcholine on any single day. It is just recirculated over and over again, so that an individual is exposed to twice as much. Ingesting 3 g choline (3 times normal dietary intake) should not be harmful if you do not give this as free choline. The problem with free choline is that the absorption system from the gut is saturated at about 4 mm of choline in humans. Above that concentration, gut bacteria convert it to trimethylamine which makes you smell like a rotten fish. Choline and glycerophosphorcholine should not cause these problems because they are not broken down to free choline within the gut, and bacteria cannot utilize them to make trimethylamine.

I do not know of any studies that suggest any significant toxicity from taking 3 g of choline for a long period of time. There were a number of studies done in patients with Alzheimer's disease and controls in which they gave phosphatidylcholine at does delivering about 3 g choline per day for years and the investigators did not report low blood pressure, tachycardia, or slowed heart rate. They did not report any other major problems except for occasional depression, which is probably normal in the population being studied.

EDWARD HORTON: Steve, thank you for a very stimulating, provocative lecture. I am fascinated by the data that choline deficiency or low choline levels may be associated with easy fatigability of muscle. There is preliminary evidence, and not very strong evidence, that activation of protein kinase C may be involved in the translocation and activation of the glucose transport system of the skeletal muscle, and so it would be very interesting to look to see whether there is a defect in the glucose transport system in choline-deficient animals.

STEVEN ZEISEL: I would be glad to study this.

ALLISON YATES: Health food stores have been selling lecithin over the years, and there has not been any definitive analyses of its effects. I am not aware of any studies showing changes in people who are dosing themselves with lecithin.

STEVEN ZEISEL: Lecithin is not phosphatidylcholine. What is sold in health food stores is only about 35 percent phosphotidylcholine, and people are not taking in very significant doses when they ingest a gram of that; they are taking in 200 milligrams of phosphatidylcholine, which is probably not changing their dietary intake a whole lot. A lot of lecithin is added to manufactured foods; chocolate bars have it. That lecithin is not pure phosphatidylcholine, but rather it too is approximately 35 percent phosphatyidyl choline.

RONALD JANDACEK: The studies in prenatal rats fascinated me. The closest analogy that I can think of in human studies is a study in which the investigators studied extensively the children of mothers who were well nourished except for brief periods of time during pregnancy. Those studies probably covered all the areas you are talking about. Although it has been a long time since I read that book, I remember that the investigators saw very few behavioral effects.

STEVEN ZEISEL: Again, when you starve, you break down cells and you release phosphatidylcholine choline, so it is not the same thing as being choline deficient. I think a better model is the following: human milk contains a huge amount of choline, especially during the first few days of life. There has been a recent study of premature infants in England in which they were bottle fed human milk, which has a high choline content, or infant formula, which has about a fourfold lower choline content. They reported that IQ was significantly worse in the premature infants fed the infant formula than in those fed breast milk. I think the defferntial was 8 I.Q. points.

ROBERT NESHEIM: Does choline taste terrible? What is the problem of adding it to a food product?

STEVEN ZEISEL: Choline is added to infant formula. Most people would add it as phosphatidylcholine which does not have the bitter taste of choline.

RICHARD WURTMAN: A firm in Massachusetts sells citrus drinks, and it is now making a choline supplement in a citrus drink for use in this type of testing. I have tasted it and I cannot taste the choline. I think a good food chemist can disguise anything.

JOHN VANDERVEEN: Steve Zeisel, maybe you can help us out on a regulatory problem that has been a thorn in the side of the compliance people for years. That is, they have been insisting that the source of choline be labeled on boxes or whatever as soy lecithin. Then the industry argues that all the lecithin that is available really comes from soy and not from any other source and therefore it should only be lecithin. Is there any reason to debate the distinction?

STEVEN ZEISEL: The reason is that phosphatidylcholine does not only contain choline, it contains two fatty acids. In soy lecithin they are unsaturated fatty acids. If part of efficacy has to do with the fatty acid constituents, you would want to know the difference. One thing I did mention, right from the story of total parenteral nutrition, is that there is a study from Emory University that came out a couple of months ago in which they showed that patients treated with normal intravenous solutions with lipid emulsions developed fatty liver and liver dysfunction. The investigators found that giving phosphatidylcholine as an oral supplement completely reversed the fatty liver, and in the people given placebo, there was no reversion of fatty livers. I would suggest that total parenteral nutrition is not delivering enough choline and that these people are deficient.

DAVID SCHNAKENBERG: What mechanism are you proposing for the effect of 3 hours of exercise on plasma choline levels?

STEVEN ZEISEL: I think either muscle, being 45 percent of lean body weight, is using a great deal as a methyl donor or to make acetylcholine. It could be as simple an explanation as a shift in location of the choline pool because of water shifts.

RICHARD WURTMAN: I think you are right. It is a very good research question with several possibilities. I think some experimentation could come up with an answer just in terms of what we are doing. There has been no formal approach to this. I would like to establish if we could go to that.

DAVID SCHNAKENBERG: How big a drop is this?

RICHARD WURTMAN: We did this in a total of 45 runners in the Boston Marathon in 2 successive years. The average decrease in plasma choline level was about 45 percent, but for some of them, the level was down by about 60 percent. Everybody showed a drop. I think only 1 person out of the 45 did not show a drop, but in some the drop was small, 20 percent.

The other thing we did was to run people 5, 10, 15, and 20 miles. There was not a linear drop in plasma choline levels with distance. You do not really see much decrease at all until about 15 miles, and then between 15 and 20 miles there was a decrease. Again, I think it would be useful to determine the mechanism, because that may tell a lot about muscle physiology and body chemistry in terms of exercise. It would not be difficult, I think, to set up studies to find out.

JOHN VANDERVEEN: I am just curious. Has anyone made any estimates about the total amount of choline in the body?

STEVEN ZEISEL: Yes I have. I do not remember the exact number but as I said, I think it is about 4 percent of dry body weight.

20

Effects of Caffeine on Cognitive Performance, Mood, and Alertness in Sleep-Deprived Humans

David M.Penetar,[1] Una McCann, David Thorne, Aline Schelling, Cynthia Galinski, Helen Sing, Maria Thomas, and Gregory Belenky

INTRODUCTION

The demands and pace of continuous military operations produce sleep fragmentation and varying degrees of sleep deprivation in soldiers. The observable effects of this sleep disruption include decreased alertness, slowed thinking, lapses in attention, decreased motivation, and a performance phenomenon called the *speed-accuracy-tradeoff.* Several studies have documented performance and mood changes during periods of sleep deprivation (Babkoff et al., 1989a,b; Mikulincer et al., 1989; Thorne et al., 1983).

[1] David M.Penetar, Walter Reed Army Institute of Research, Washington, D.C. 20307–5100

There is a decline in the performance of accuracy tasks involving attention, reasoning abilities, and reaction time. Alertness decreases, and there are changes in self-reported fatigue (increases) and vigor (decreases). Sustaining optimum soldier performance relates to the prevention or amelioration of these changes. Three categories of solutions include the following: (1) *Doctrinal solutions* involve the overtraining of soldiers to perform their tasks with a minimum of cognitive effort; ensuring that soldiers are cross-trained so that crew members can substitute for each other when necessary; developing and adhering to appropriate work-rest cycles, including rotating crews as the mission permits; developing efficient leadership tactics so that unnecessary demands are not placed on subordinates; and modifying equipment and systems so that the likelihood of making errors is as small as possible. (2) *Behavioral solutions* make sure that soldiers sleep as much as they can, whenever they can (sleep discipline), while paying attention to where and how they sleep (sleep hygiene), that is, in as comfortable a position as possible, away from the noise and bustle of other soldiers and equipment. (3) *Pharmacological solutions* may be warranted in special circumstances, when adherence to doctrinal and behavioral solutions is not possible or breaks down. This last category of solutions for preventing or ameliorating sleep deprivation effects is the topic of the research reported in this chapter.

The characteristics of stimulant drugs useful in specific military situations are not only effectiveness but low therapeutic toxicity and low abuse potential, *d*-Amphetamine was tested for its ability to reverse changes in mood, alertness, and cognitive performance after an extended period of sleep deprivation (Newhouse et al., 1989). Although effective, its restricted legal status and the psychological side effects associated with long-term use, coupled with its abuse potential, almost certainly prohibit large-scale use. Caffeine is a universally available, legal, and socially accepted and used stimulant with low toxicity and low abuse potential. It is believed to reverse the performance and mood effects seen during sleep deprivation, although it has not been tested systematically.

Caffeine has a long history of use and can be found in many common foods, drinks, and medications. Although caffeine has been the subject of pharmacological studies for several decades, the mechanism of action of its effects on the central nervous system have only recently been defined as a blockade of adenosine receptors (Choi et al., 1988; Fredholm, 1985; Snyder, 1984). Extensive reviews of caffeine (Dews, 1984; Weiss and Laties, 1962) conclude that its stimulant properties are weak in comparison with those of other drugs (e.g., amphetamine) and that its effects are modest, making detection of these effects difficult and generalizations cumbersome. Dews (1984), however, states that the following three effects are clear: (1) it has the tendency to postpone sleep; (2) it reduces the degradation of performance because of fatigue and boredom; and (3) it decreases hand steadiness. The interpretation distilled from these and other reviews is that caffeine's effects are significant primarily when performance of repetitive, nonintellectual tasks is partially degraded. What is lacking in the literature and of importance to military operations is a systematic study of caffeine's effects on sleep-deprived individuals and the assessment of caffeine's effectiveness in reversing the changes caused by sleep deprivation.

EFFECTS OF CAFFEINE ON PERFORMANCE

A common method of assessing the effects of stimulant drugs is to measure individuals' reaction times on laboratory tasks. Older reviews and several recent articles failed to find that caffeine has significant effects on the reaction times of various tasks (Bruce et al., 1986; Kuznicki and Turner, 1986; Rapoport et al., 1981; Swift and Tiplady, 1988). Recently, however, caffeine has been found to significantly decrease reaction times in auditory and visual choice tasks when it was used at doses of as little as 32 mg and as great as 600 mg (Jacobson and Edgley, 1987; Lieberman et al., 1987a,b; Roache and Griffiths, 1987). Other cognitive and psychomotor skills measured by the digit-symbol substitution task, serial subtraction of numbers, addition, symbol cancellation, card sorting, signal detection, symbol copying, and number cancellation have not been found to be affected by caffeine (Bruce et al., 1986; Childs, 1978; Ghoneim et al., 1986; Lieberman et al., 1987b; Loke et al., 1985; Roache and Griffiths, 1987; Swift and Tiplady, 1988), although Battig et al. (1984) report that 300 mg of caffeine had a positive effect on a letter cancellation test.

EFFECTS OF CAFFEINE ON MOOD AND ALERTNESS

Several questionnaires and methods have been used to assess caffeine's effects on mood. Studies have shown that doses of 200 to 250 mg of caffeine elevate mood (Lieberman et al., 1987b; Swift and Tiplady, 1988) and that these effects can last for up to 3 h. Higher doses (600 mg) can produce increases in subjects self-ratings of tension or anxiety and increases in caffeine-related physical symptoms (Roache and Griffiths, 1987). Caffeine significantly affects measures of alertness and sleepiness. Doses of 100 mg and more postpone the onset of sleep (Dews, 1982; Goldstein et al., 1965), and a dose of approximately 300 mg significantly improves daytime alertness in both partially sleep-deprived and fully rested individuals, as measured by the multiple sleep latency test (Lumley et al., 1987). Walsh et al. (1990) report that 4 mg of caffeine per kg of body weight (approximately 300 mg) significantly increases latency to sleep onset at test periods throughout the night (0100 to 0500 h). This effect was seen in light and moderate caffeine users. Multiple sleep latency test results by Rosenthal et al., (1991) showed that caffeine at doses of 75 and 150 mg increases alertness whether an individual is fully rested or partially sleep deprived. Zwyghuizen-Doorenbos et al. (1990) showed that 250 mg of caffeine improved daytime alertness for at least 3 h in moderately sleepy subjects.

PHYSIOLOGICAL EFFECTS OF CAFFEINE

The literature supports the fact that caffeine has low toxicity and produces no serious physiological side effects in adults (Rall, 1985; Stavric, 1988). Caffeine's physiological effects are dependent on whether the subject is caffeine-naive or a regular user. In caffeine-naive subjects, a 250-mg oral dose increased the systolic blood pressure by 11 mm Hg (Robertson and Curatolo, 1984). The heart rate declined during the first hour after drug administration and then increased above the baseline during the second hour. Regular users who were deprived of caffeine showed a significant increase in their systolic blood pressure (4 mm Hg), whereas regular users who were not deprived of caffeine showed no significant increases. Other researchers have found no significant changes in blood pressure or heart rate even after a 500-mg oral dose (Bruce et al., 1986; Myers 1988). Newcombe et al. (1988) showed that doses of 300 to 350 mg do not affect the prevailing cardiac rhythm or rate and do not cause clinically significant ventricular or supraventricular dysrhythmias. Specific studies concerning the cardiovascular effects of caffeine at doses above 500 mg are lacking. In several studies, however, higher doses (up to 800 mg) were administered in other contexts (Chait and Griffiths, 1983; Griffiths and Woodson, 1988). Chait and Griffiths (1983) reported that one subject experienced shakiness and an upset stomach after receiving 200 mg of caffeine, and higher doses were not tested in that subject. All other subjects tolerated doses up to 800 mg well. Other clinically relevant physiological effects include the relaxation of smooth muscles (especially the bronchii) and diuresis. Respiration rate is increased by 250-mg doses in caffeine-naive users (Curatolo and Robertson, 1983). Caffeine has the ability to increase metabolic rate, but its effect on body temperature in humans has not been reported in the literature.

In summary, studies indicate that caffeine can have significant effects on mood and performance, even at relatively low doses, in non-sleep-deprived individuals and has effects on alertness in moderately sleep-deprived individuals. The following section reports the effectiveness of caffeine in reversing the alterations seen in performance, mood, and alertness following a prolonged period of sleep deprivation.

MATERIALS AND METHODS

Subjects

Fifty normal, healthy, nonsmoking, drug-free males between the ages of 18 and 32 (mean age, 23.6 years) were recruited through advertisements in college newspapers. Subjects were within normal weight limits for their height and were moderate users of caffeine (no more than 300 mg on a daily basis). After giving free and informed written consent, subjects underwent a thorough physical and laboratory examination and completed a self-assessment questionnaire for anxiety and depression (Snaith et al., 1976). Exclusion criteria included past or present major medical or psychiatric illness, positive urine drug screen, regular tobacco use, excessive caffeine use (more than 300 mg on a daily basis), questionnaire scores above 6 (out of a possible 12) for either anxiety or depression, or atypical sleeping patterns (e.g., self-reports of difficulty in falling asleep or regular involuntary early morning awakenings). Following completion of the screening procedures, the subjects were randomly assigned to one of four drug conditions: placebo (n=12), 150 mg/70 kg (n= 13), 300 mg/70 kg (n=12), or 600 mg/70 kg (n=13).[1]

Procedure

Subjects arrived in the laboratory in groups of three to four each on the evening before the sleep deprivation period began. All subjects were required to refrain from caffeine and alcohol ingestion for 72 h prior to the beginning of the study. Blood and urine samples were taken to ensure that the subjects were free of caffeine and other drugs of abuse. They were trained on a computerized performance assessment battery (Thorne et al., 1985) designed to assess several cognitive functions periodically at approximately 2-h intervals throughout the sleep deprivation period (see full description below). Eleven electrodes were attached to the scalp and face by using the international 10–20 system of electrode placement. Electroencephalograms (EEGs), electrooculograms (EOGs), and submental electromyograms (EMGs) were recorded

[1] Subjects were paid for their participation. The investigators adhered to AR 70–25 (U.S. Department of the Army, 1989) and U.S. Army Medical Research and Development Command Reg 70–25 (1989), on the use of volunteers in research.

continuously by using an 8-channel Oxford Medilog ambulatory cassette recorder. Dinner was provided between training sessions. Subjects retired at 2300 h. The sleep deprivation period began upon awakening the next morning at 0700 h (day 1). They remained awake for the next 64.5 h over a 3-day period (e.g., 0700 h Tuesday morning to 2230 h Thursday night), except for brief periods during administration of the modified Multiple Sleep Latency Tests (MSLTs). Subjects were monitored continuously by the staff to prevent unintentional sleep and were provided with books, games, movies, music tapes, conversation, and occasional brief walks to occupy them between tests.

On the morning of day 3 (at 0700 h after 48 h of sleep deprivation), a Teflon catheter was inserted into a forearm vein of each subject and was maintained with a heparin lock (heparin sodium, 20 Units/ml) to facilitate repeated drawing of blood samples before and after drug administration. At 0800 h (following 49 h of sleep deprivation), subjects were administered placebo or one of three doses of caffeine, USP anhydrous (City Chemical Corporation, New York, N.Y.). Doses were either 150, 300, or 600 mg/70 kg of body weight. Caffeine was administered orally by having the subjects drink 250 ml of an artificially sweetened lemon juice drink in which the caffeine powder was dissolved. Placebo consisted solely of the sweetened lemon juice drink. All doses were given in a double-blind manner.

Performance Measures

The computerized performance assessment battery included tests of code substitution and recall, logical reasoning, sustained attention with a mental arithmetic task (referred to as the *serial addition/subtraction task*), match-to-sample, and choice reaction time. These tasks were administered every 2 h through the sleep deprivation period and at 1, 2, 3, 4, 6, 8, 10, and 12 h after caffeine administration.

Code Substitution and Recall. A code key that paired the digits 1 through 9 in a one-to-one correspondence with letters was presented to the subjects. Below the key, a letter appeared and subjects had to press the key of the correct number. The code key disappeared after 27 pair presentations; if needed, they could see it again by pressing 0. Fifty-four pairs were presented. Recall was assessed after the subject completed the rest of the battery tasks (about 15 min later). Subjects had to press a number in response to each of nine letter presentations; no code key was available during the recall testing.

Logical Reasoning. A task of logical reasoning ability was adapted from Baddeley (1968). The letter pair AB or BA was presented along with a statement that correctly or incorrectly described the order of the letters within the pair (e.g., "B follows A" or "A is not preceded by B"). The subject decided whether the statement was true (same) or false (different) and pressed the "S" or "D" key accordingly. The 32 possible permutations were presented once each in random order.

Sustained Attention. Sustained attention ability was assessed by the serial addition/subtraction task adapted from Pauli as used by Wever (1979, 1981). The task was a machine-paced mental arithmetic task requiring sustained attention and concentration. Two randomly selected digits and either a plus or a minus sign were displayed sequentially in the same center screen location followed by a prompt symbol: (?). The subject performed the indicated addition or subtraction and entered the least significant digit of the result. If the result was negative, the subject first added 10 to it and entered the single positive digit that was the remainder. The digits and signs were each presented for 250 ms and were separated by 200 ms, with the next trial beginning 500 ms after the response. The task ended after 50 responses and typically took 3 to 4 min.

Match-to-Sample. Subjects viewed a 6-by-6 block of squares with 36 red and green squares arranged in random order (each block contained an equal number of red and green squares). This task of immediate recall allowed subjects to view the arrangements for as long as they liked and then press a key to present two choices, one of which matched the original set of squares. They were required to pick the correct matching square. Twenty trials were presented.

Reaction Time. A choice reaction time task was used to measure reaction time. The visual-motor task required subjects to press the numbered keyboard keys corresponding to numbers presented on the screen. The digits 0 through 9 appeared one at a time in the center of the screen. The stimulus remained on until a response was made. Fifty numbers were presented. This task was designed to fulfill the requirements of a standard reaction time task while closely resembling the physical requirements of the serial addition/subtraction task.

Mood Measures

Profile of Mood States. The Profile of Mood States (POMS) (McNair et al., 1981) is a 65-item adjective checklist that measures current mood states along six subscales: tension-anxiety, anger-hostility, depression-dejection, vigor-activity, fatigue-inertia, and confusion-bewilderment. Subjects rated themselves on each adjective from 1 (not at all) to 5 (extremely).

Visual Analog Scales (VAS). Subjects rated themselves with a mark along a line 100-mm in length. The lines were labeled "alert/able to concentrate," "anxious," "energetic," "feel confident," "irritable," "jittery/nervous," "sleepy," and "talkative." Additional ratings were obtained on four possible effects of sleep deprivation and caffeine administration. They were heart pounding, headache, sweaty, and upset stomach. The lines were labeled "not at all" on the left end and "extremely" on the right end.

The POMS and VAS were completed five times during the sleep deprivation period prior to drug administration at 0900 and 2000 h on days 1 and 2 and at 0600 h on the morning of day 3 (2 h before caffeine administration). POMS and VAS ratings were taken at 1, 2, 4, 8, and 12 h after drug administration.

Alertness Measures

Multiple Sleep Latency Tests. Each modified multiple sleep latency test (MSLT) was conducted by having the subjects lie in bed in a darkened, sound-attenuated room with their eyes closed. They were instructed to relax and allow themselves to fall asleep. EEGs, EOGs, and EMGs were displayed on a Grass Electroencephalograph (model 8–10D) for on-line scoring of awake versus sleep during the MSLT. An experimenter awakened a subject after 30 s of stage 2 sleep or the onset of rapid eye movement (REM). The test was terminated at 20 min if sleep had not occurred. MSLTs were conducted at 0930, 1130, 1430, 1630, 1830, and 2030 h on days 1 and 2 of the sleep deprivation period. MSLTs were conducted eight times on day 3 (at 1.5, 2.5, 3.5, 4.5, 6.5, 8.5, 10.5, and 12.5 h after drug administration).

Stanford Sleepiness Scale. For the Stanford Sleepiness Scale (SSS) (Hoddes et al., 1973), subjects selected one of seven statements that best described their current state of alertness, ranging from 1 (feeling active and vital; alert; wide awake) to 7 (almost in reverie; sleep onset soon; losing struggle to remain awake). The SSS was completed approximately every 2 h throughout the sleep deprivation period (at 0900, 1100, 1400, 1600, 1800,

2000, 2200, 2400, 0200, 0400, and 0600 h on days 1 and 2). The SSS was completed eight times on day 3 (at 1, 2, 3, 4, 6, 8, 10, and 12 h after drug administration).

Vital Signs

Measurements of blood pressure, heart rate, and oral temperature were taken at least every 2 h throughout the sleep deprivation period. After caffeine administration, measurements were taken at 15, 30, 60, 90, 120, 150, 180, and 210 min and then hourly until 13 h after drug administration.

Catecholamine and Caffeine Assays

Blood samples were collected prior to and at 15, 30, 60, and 90 min, and 2, 2.5, 3, 4, 6, 8, 10, and 12 h following drug administration. Results are reported elsewhere (Eddington et al., 1993; and Penetar et al., 1993).

Statistical Analysis

Separate two-factor repeated measures analysis of variance by using the General Linear Model (SAS Institute, Cary, N.C.) were performed for each dependent variable and POMS subscale. The two factors were group or dose and time. First, each dependent variable was analyzed for group differences and effects of the sleep deprivation period prior to the drug administration by using all measurements made prior to drug administration. Second, each dependent variable was analyzed for the effects of drug and time after drug administration by using the last value obtained prior to drug administration and all values obtained after drug administration. Statistical results thus reported for the main effects of drug dose, the main effects of time, and an interaction between these main effects. A level of $P<0.05$ was accepted as significant, with the Greenhouse-Geisser adjustment criterion used in evaluating the main effects of time and the interaction between the main effects. Significant main effects were further evaluated by the Newman-Keuls Multiple Range Test.

RESULTS

Performance Tests

For each of the tasks, three measures of performance were analyzed: accuracy (percent correct), speed (responses per unit of time), and throughput (number of correct responses per unit of time). The throughput measure takes both accuracy and speed of performance into account and was subjected to statistical testing. Significant effects of caffeine were observed on the throughput measure for the choice reaction time, serial addition/subtraction, and logical reasoning tasks (Figure 20–1 and Table 20–1).

Performance on the choice reaction time task for 8 h after drug administration in subjects who received the 600-mg dose was significantly different from that in subjects who received the placebo. The 150-mg dose improved performance for 4 h. For subjects receiving the 300-mg dose,

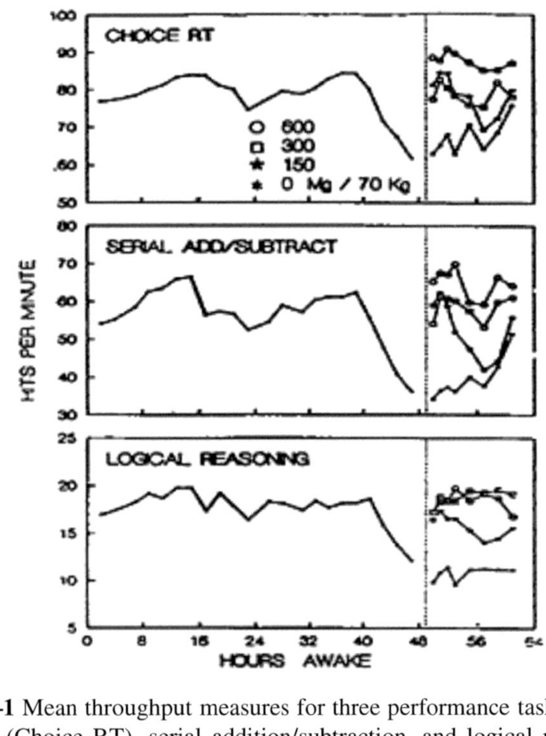

FIGURE 20–1 Mean throughput measures for three performance tasks: choice reaction time (Choice RT), serial addition/subtraction, and logical reasoning. Predrug means include data for all subjects; there were no differences between the groups prior to drug administration. Caffeine was administered after 49 h of sleep deprivation (0800 h on day 3), and testing continued for 12 h after drug administration. Note the different ordinate scales for the three tasks. Results for the 600-mg dose group were significantly different from those for the placebo group for 8 h on the choice reaction time task, for 10 h on the serial addition/subtraction task, and for the full 12 h on the logical reasoning task. See text for more details on dose and duration effects.

performance was not significantly different from that for subjects receiving the placebo at any point following administration. For the serial addition/subtraction task, all doses of caffeine significantly improved performance for 3 h. For subjects receiving the 600-mg dose, performance remained significantly better than that for subjects receiving placebo for 10 h after drug administration, with no significant differences observed among the dose groups at the final 12-h testing period. Performance on the logical reasoning task by subjects receiving the two highest doses of caffeine was significantly better than by subjects receiving placebo for the entire 12-h period. In addition, caffeine restored performance to the levels obtained after rest during this interval. Performance after administration of the 150-mg dose was significantly different from that after administration of placebo for 6 h after drug administration.

Mood Measures

The effects of sleep deprivation on mood, as measured by the POMS and VAS, are reported in more detail elsewhere (Penetar et al., 1993). Briefly, the scores of all six subscales of the POMS changed significantly as a result of the sleep deprivation. Tension [$F(5,230)=12.3$, $P<0.001$], anger [$F(5,230)= 7.42$, $P<0.001$], depression [$F(5,230)=16.4$, $P<0.001$], fatigue [$F(5,230) =97.9$, $P<0.001$], and confusion [$F(5,230)=57.4$, $P<0.001$] increased, whereas vigor decreased [$F(5,230)=87.3$, $P<0.001$]. Similarly, ratings on the VAS showed the effects of sleep deprivation. The main effects for the time before drug administration showed that alertness [$F(4,184)=103.39$, $P< 0.001$], energy levels [$F(4,184)=109.2$, $P<0.001$], confidence [$F(4,184)= 48.96$, $P<0.001$], and talkativeness [$F(4,184)=23.46$, $P<0.001$] declined, whereas irritability [$F(4,184) =20.29$, $P<0.001$] and sleepiness [$F(4,184)= 138.11$, $P<0.001$] increased.

Following caffeine administration, significant increases in the POMS vigor subscale and significant decreases in the POMS subscales of fatigue and confusion were observed (Table 20–1). Vigor ratings for all three dose groups were significantly different from those for the placebo group for 2 h after caffeine adminstration. Vigor ratings for the 600-mg dose group were 97 percent of those for subjects in the rested condition 1 h after caffeine administration and remained at 84 percent of those for subjects in the rested condition at the 2-h measurement. Conversely, fatigue ratings for all three caffeine dose groups decreased significantly for 2 h following caffeine administration. Confusion ratings in the 150-mg dose group were significantly

TABLE 20-1 Performance, Mood, and Physiology Analysis of Variance[*] Summary

	Dose	Time	Interaction
Performance Battery (throughput measure)			
Code substitution	$F(3,46) = 1.22$, $P = 0.3127$	$F(8,368) = 9.72$, $P < 0.0001$[§]	$F(24,368) = 1.47$, $P = 0.0996$
Code recall	$F(3,46) = 0.29$, $P = 0.8344$	$F(8,368) = 3.73$, $P = 0.0008$[§]	$F(24,368) = 1.40$, $P = 0.1174$
Logical reasoning	$F(3,46) = 10.07$, $P < 0.0001$[§]	$F(8,368) = 9.98$, $P < 0.0001$[§]	$F(24,368) = 1.58$, $P = 0.0748$
Serial addition/ subtraction	$F(3,46) = 16.57$, $P < 0.0001$[§]	$F(8,368) = 21.43$, $P < 0.0001$[§]	$F(24,368) = 3.35$, $P < 0.0001$[§]
Match-to-sample	$F(3,46) = 2.01$, $P = 0.125$	$F(8,368) = 4.78$, $P < 0.0002$[§]	$F(24,368) = 1.05$, $P = 0.4071$
Choice reaction time	$F(3,46) = 0.76$, $P = 0.5218$	$F(8,368) = 0.36$, $P = 0.8993$	$F(24,368) = 12.3$, $P < 0.0001$[§]
Profile of Mood States questionnaire			
Tension	$F(3,46) = 0.5$, $P = 0.6817$	$F(6,276) = 13.34$, $P < 0.0001$[§]	$F(18,276) = 1.43$, $P = 0.155$
Anger	$F(3,46) = 0.1$, $P = 0.9614$	$F(6,276) = 13.5$, $P < 0.0001$[§]	$F(18,276) = 1.8$, $P = 0.366$
Depression	$F(3,46) = 0.65$, $P = 0.5856$	$F(6,276) = 5.4$, $P < 0.001$[§]	$F(18,276) = 1.1$, $P = 0.065$
Vigor	$F(3,46) = 2.86$, $P = 0.0471$[§]	$F(6,276) = 28.18$, $P < 0.0001$[§]	$F(18,276) = 4.0$, $P < 0.0001$[§]
Fatigue	$F(3,46) = 2.03$, $P = 0.1235$	$F(6,276) = 25.74$, $P < 0.0001$[§]	$F(18,276) = 3.05$, $P < 0.001$[§]
Confusion	$F(3,46) = 1.18$, $P = 0.3284$	$F(6,276) = 22.19$, $P < 0.0001$[§]	$F(18,276) = 2.87$, $P < 0.001$[§]
Stanford Sleepiness Scale	$F(3,45) = 0.93$, $P = 0.4335$	$F(8,360) = 35.16$, $P < 0.0001$[§]	$F(24,360) = 2.91$, $P = 0.0005$[§]
Visual Analog Scales			
Alert/able to concentrate	$F(3,46) = 3.27$, $P = 0.0295$[§]	$F(6,276) = 39.34$, $P < 0.0001$[§]	$F(18,276) = 3.51$, $P < 0.0001$[§]
Anxious	$F(3,46) = 3.3$, $P = 0.0283$[§]	$F(6,276) = 2.18$, $P = 0.0632$	$F(18,276) = 0.87$, $P = 0.5914$
Energetic	$F(3,46) = 4.44$, $P = 0.0081$[§]	$F(6,276) = 23.74$, $P < 0.0001$[§]	$F(18,276) = 4.12$, $P < .0001$[§]

Feel confident	$F(3,46) = 1.44$, $P = 0.0283$§	$F(6,276) = 30.95$, $P < 0.0001$§	$F(18,276) = 3.05$, $P < 0.0001$§
Irritable	$F(3,46) = 0.98$, $P = 0.4093$	$F(6,276) = 10.88$, $P < 0.0001$§	$F(18,276) = 1.72$, $P = 0.0669$
Jittery/nervous	$F(3,46) = 3.99$, $P = 0.0132$§	$F(6,276) = 8.56$, $P < 0.0001$§	$F(18,276) = 1.74$, $P = 0.0468$§
Sleepy	$F(3,46) = 8.7$, $P < 0.0001$§	$F(6,276) = 35.97$, $P < 0.0001$§	$F(18,276) = 3.0$, $P < 0.0002$§
Talkative	$F(3,46) = 1.46$, $P = 0.2378$	$F(6,276) = 12.97$, $P < 0.0001$§	$F(18,276) = 3.18$, $P < 0.0001$§
Heart pounding	$F(3,46) = 3.26$, $P = 0.0298$§	$F(6,276) = 4.6$, $P = 0.0019$§	$F(18,276) = 0.96$, $P = 0.4842$
Headache	$F(3,46) = 0.77$, $P = 0.5146$	$F(6,276) = 1.71$, $P = 0.1501$	$F(18,276) = 0.89$, $P = 0.5523$
Sweaty	$F(3,46) = 1.72$, $P = 0.1759$	$F(6,276) = 2.69$, $P = 0.0599$	$F(18,276) = 0.67$, $P = 0.7069$
Upset stomach	$F(3,46) = 0.33$, $P = 0.8065$	$F(6,276) = 4.2$, $P = 0.0017$§	$F(18,276) = 0.76$, $P = 0.7053$
Vital Signs			
Systolic blood pressure	$F(3,46) = 1.14$, $P = 0.3442$	$F(18,828) = 4.83$, $P < 0.0001$§	$F(54,828) = 1.0$, $P = 0.4794$
Diastolic blood pressure	$F(3,46) = 0.56$, $P = 0.6465$	$F(18,828) = 7.76$, $P < 0.0001$§	$F(54,828) = 1.88$, $P = 0.0021$§
Pulse	$F(3,46) = 0.74$, $P = 0.5309$	$F(18,828) = 24.03$, $P < 0.0001$§	$F(54,828) = 0.89$, $P = 0.6295$
Oral temperature	$F(3,46) = 3.19$, $P = 0.0321$§	$F(18,828) = 20.46$, $P < 0.0001$§	$F(54,828) = 1.15$, $P = 0.2699$

†F values presented are the variance ratios generated by separate two-factor repeated measures analysis of varience (General Linear Model, SAS Institute, Gary, N.C.) where (x,y) equals the degrees of freedom for each ratio.

§Statistically significant effects.

decreased in comparison with those in the placebo group 2 h after caffeine administration.

Caffeine reversed the sleep deprivation effects reported in subjective ratings of alertness for 2 h, energy levels for 12 h, confidence for 2 h, sleepiness for 12 h, and talkativeness for 2 h following drug administration. Caffeine significantly increased self-rated anxiety for 2 h, and jitteriness or nervousness for 12 h following drug administration. Ratings of heart pounding, headache, sweatiness, and upset stomach were unaffected by caffeine.

Alertness Measures

Multiple Sleep Latency Tests

For the rested condition (day 1), mean sleep latency periods were between 16.3 and 19.9 min. Sleep deprivation significantly [$F(11,506)=202.39$, $P<0.001$] decreased latency periods to a range of 5.6 to 7 min on day 2. Significant dose [$F(3,46)=5.18$, $P<0.005$], time [$F(7,322)=5.61$, $P<0.001$] and time×dose interactions [$F(21,322)=1.99$, $P<0.05$] were observed following caffeine administration. Latency periods for the highest dose (600 mg/70 kg) group increased significantly above placebo latency periods for the placebo group (10.2 min versus 5.0 min) (Figure 20–2) and

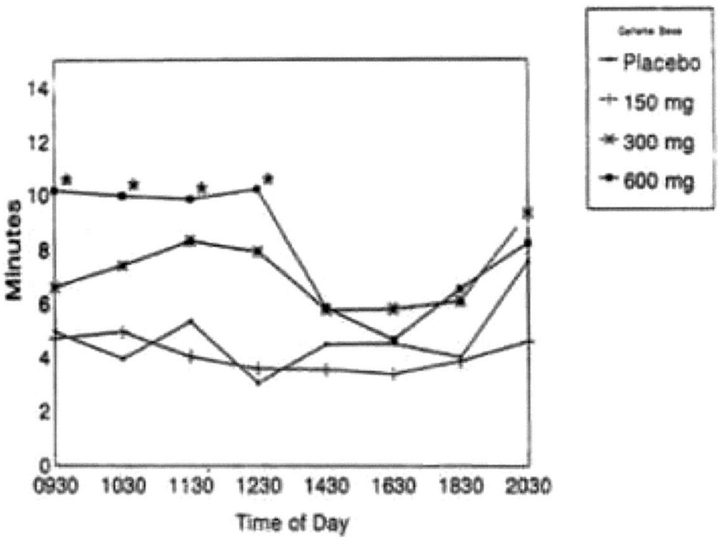

FIGURE 20–2 Latency to stage 2 sleep following caffeine administration. *, results for the 600-mg dose group were significantly different from those for the placebo group ($P<0.05$).

remained at this level for 4.5 h after drug administration. The dose of 300 mg/70 kg appeared to have effects intermediate between those of the highest dose tested and the placebo; however, these effects were not significantly different from those for the other dose groups.

Stanford Sleepiness Scale

Average values of the Stanford Sleepiness Scale increased gradually from 1.6 at 0900 h on day 1 (subjects rested) to a maximum average of 4.8 at 0600 h on the morning of day 3, indicating a significant effect of sleep deprivation (Table 20–2). Caffeine's effects were significant for 2 h after drug administration and were not dose-related (i.e., all doses were equally effective).

Vital Signs

Diastolic blood pressure and oral temperature were significantly affected by caffeine administration (Table 20–1 and Figure 20–3). At 1 h after admini

TABLE 20–2 Stanford Sleepiness Scale Scores

Time	Mean for All Subjects	Placebo	150 mg	300 mg	600 mg
Day 1 (0900 h)	1.6				
Day 2 (0900 h)	3.5				
Day 3					
0600	4.6				
0800 (drug administration)					
0900 (+1 h)		3.5	2.2*	2.4*	1.9*
1000 (+2 h)		3.8	2.2*	2.7*	2.8*
1100 (+3 h)		3.7	2.5	2.4	2.7
1200 (+4 h)		3.2	2.8	3.2	2.5
1400 (+6 h)		2.9	3.0	3.3	2.6
1600 (+8 h)		2.8	3.3	3.1	2.9
1800 (+10 h)		2.9	3.5	3.0	2.7
2000 (+12 h)		2.8	3.1	3.3	2.3

NOTE: Subjects selected one of seven statements that best described their current state of alertness, ranging from 1 (feeling active and vital; alert; wide awake) to 7 (almost in reverie; sleep onset soon; losing struggle to remain awake). There were no significant differences in scores among the groups prior to drug administration; therefore, a single mean score is reported.

*Significantly different from placebo ($P<0.05$).

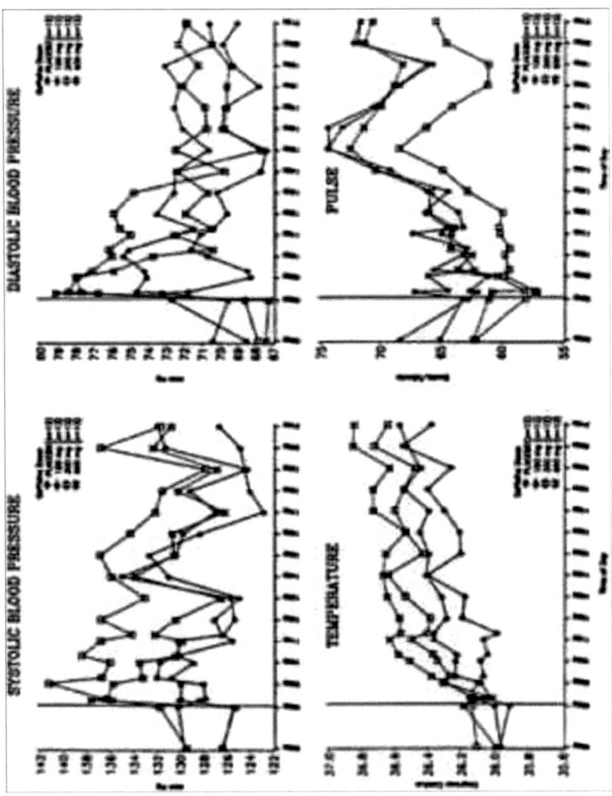

FIGURE 20–3 Time course of caffeine effects on four vital signs. Caffeine was observed to have significant effects on diastolic blood pressure (at 1 h) and oral temperature from 2 to 12 h after drug administration. See text for details.

stration, both the 300- and the 600-mg doses significantly increased diastolic blood pressure in comparison with the placebo; there were no significant differences at other time points. The 600-mg dose of caffeine significantly increased oral temperature in comparison with placebo at several measurement times after administration: 2, 2.5, 3, 4, 6, 8, and 12 h. Neither systolic blood pressure nor pulse was significantly affected.

DISCUSSION

The study described here indicates that caffeine is effective in reversing the performance degradations and the alterations in mood and alertness produced by periods of prolonged sleep deprivation. The results indicate that these beneficial effects can be long-lasting and not at the expense of serious mood or physiological side effects.

Sleep deprivation degrades cognitive performance. The effects of caffeine on performance in non-sleep-deprived volunteers have been well documented, even at the low dose levels commonly found in food and drink products (see Lieberman [1992] for a review). The study described here extends the usefulness of caffeine, showing that large doses (up to 600 mg) are effective in improving a variety of cognitive performances in sleep-deprived individuals, and outlines the time course of its effects in these individuals. The tasks used in the present study were chosen to sample a variety of cognitive abilities with varying mental demands. Choice reaction time requires little thinking but does require great accuracy and speed. The serial addition/subtraction task is a machine-paced task but has a greater mental component, whereas the logical reasoning task is self-paced and requires the greatest amount of thought for accurate responses. Caffeine produced improved performances of all three tasks, with performance returning to those of rested subjects for up to 12 h after caffeine administration. Caffeine was not observed to affect recall or code substitution tasks. In toto, these results are in concert with those presented previously (Lieberman, 1992; Roache and Griffiths, 1987) and document for the first time the relatively long-lasting effects of this drug on cognitive performance. The study described here shows that caffeine compares favorably with amphetamine in reversing the effects of sleep deprivation on cognitive performance. Using an identical sleep deprivation paradigm, Newhouse et al. (1989) showed that 20 mg of amphetamine is required to produce sustained performance improvements.

Sleep deprivation also alters mood and degrades alertness. The present study documents the fact that caffeine can have significant beneficial effects in reversing these mood changes; sleepiness and confusion declined, whereas increases in energy and confidence levels were reported. Although there were increased ratings of anxiety and jitteriness or nervousness, these effects were not severe and did not elicit complaints from the subjects. Depending on the measure, alertness, which was severely degraded by 49 h of sleep deprivation, was improved for 2 to 4.5 h, whereas self-ratings of sleepiness in groups treated with caffeine remained significantly lower than those in the placebo group for 12 h. In this regard, caffeine was not as effective as amphetamine. The alertness of amphetamine treated subjects (20 mg), as measured by sleep latency tests, was nearly restored to the levels of rested subjects for 7 h (Newhouse et al., 1989). Caffeine's effects on alertness are therefore less potent and shorter acting than amphetamine's.

Caffeine's effects on physiological measures are important for assessing its usefulness as a stimulant. The study described here shows that relatively high doses of caffeine are well tolerated by sleep-deprived individuals and that its effects are similar to those found in other studies in non-sleep-deprived subjects given lower doses than those used in the present study (Myers, 1988; Newcombe et al., 1988). Additionally, there were no changes in self-reports of other side-effects (heart pounding, headache, sweatiness, upset stomach). Of note was caffeine's observed effect on oral temperature. Oral temperature normally rises during the day, from a low in the early morning hours to a peak in the early evening hours. The subjects in the present study showed this typical response. Caffeine increased temperatures above the normal rise throughout the observation period, again revealing an important aspect of its effects and duration of action. The significance of this effect awaits further experimentation, although this type of effect has been observed previously with another stimulant, *d*-amphetamine (Newhouse et al., 1989).

RECOMMENDATIONS

- The results of the present study would seem to indicate that caffeine can be an ideal stimulant for use during military operations when performance declines secondary to sleep disruption and sleep fragmentation. Doses of 600 mg are needed to reverse severely degraded performance as a result of long periods of sleep deprivation. Presumably, lower doses (200–400 mg) would be effective in ameliorating the changes caused by shorter periods of deprivation.
- Given the legal and social acceptance of caffeine, and its low abuse potential, caffeine tablets (200 mg/tablet) should be included in food rations.
- Use of caffeine should be restricted to special situations when sleep has been unusually disrupted and for the benefit of temporarily (10–12 h) restoring alertness and sustaining performance during critical periods of military operations.

- Finally, although caffeine can temporarily sustain performance during continuous operations, it should be emphasized that no drug can substitute for adequate sleep.

ACKNOWLEDGMENTS

The authors thank the staff of the Behavioral Biology, in particular Sharon Balwinski and Kevin Peyton, for assistance in the conduct of the experiment described here. Investigators adhered to AR 70–25 and USAMRDC Reg 70–25 on the use of volunteers in research. Use of trade names does not constitute endorsement of product. The views of the authors do not purport to reflect the position of the Department of the Army or the Department of Defense.

REFERENCES

AR 70–25 1989 See U.S. Department of the Army. 1989.

Babkoff, H., M.Mikulincer, T.Caspy, R.L.Carasso, and H.C.Sing 1989a The implications of sleep loss for circadian performance accuracy. Work Stress 3:3–14.

Babkoff, H., H.C.Sing, D.R.Thorne, S.G.Genser, and F.W.Hegge 1989b Perceptual distortions and hallucinations reported during the course of sleep deprivation. Perceptual Motor Skills 68:787–798.

Baddeley, A.D. 1968 A 3-minute test based on grammatical transformations. Psychonomic Sci. 10:341–342.

Battig, K., R.Buzzi, J.R.Martin, and J.M.Feierabend 1984 The effects of caffeine on physiological functions and mental performance. Experentia 40:1218–1223.

Bruce, M., N.Scott, M.Lader, and V.Marks 1986 The psychopharmacological and electrophysiological effects of single doses of caffeine in healthy human subjects. Br. J. Clin. Pharmacol. 22:81–87.

Chait, L.D., and R.R.Griffiths 1983 Effects of caffeine on cigarette smoking and subjective response. Clin. Pharmacol. Ther. 34:612–622.

Childs, J.M. 1978 Caffeine consumption and target scanning performance. Hum. Factors 20:91–96.

Choi, O.H., M.T.Shamin, W.L.Padgett, and J.W.Daly 1988 Caffeine and theophylline analogues: Correlation of behavioral effects with activity as adenosine receptor antagonists and as phosphodiesterase inhibitors. Life Sci. 43:387–398.

Curatolo, P.W., and D.Robertson 1983 The health consequences of caffeine. Ann. Intern. Med. 98:641–653.

Dews, P.B. 1982 Caffeine. Ann. Rev. Nutr. 2:323–341.

1984 Behavioral effects of caffeine. Pp. 86–103 in Caffeine, P.B Dews, ed. New York: Springer-Verlag.

Eddington, N.D., S.I.Lugo, G.Kamimori, E.Fadiran, D.Penetar 1993 The influence of caffeine administration on *in-vivo* catecholamine pharmacodynamics in sleep deprived volunteers. Pharmacol. Res., 10:S-360

Fredholm, B.B. 1985 On the mechanism of action of theophylline and caffeine. Acta Med. Scand. 217:149–153.

Ghoneim, M.M., J.V.Hinrichs, C.K.Chiang, and W.H.Loke 1986 Pharmacokinetic and pharmacodynamic interactions between caffeine and diazepam. J. Clin. Psychopharmacol. 6:75–80.

Goldstein, A., R.Warren, and S.Kaizer 1965 Psychotropic effects of caffeine in man. I. Individual differences in sensitivity to caffeine-induced wakefulness. J. Clin. Pharmacol. Exp. Therapeutics 149:156–169.

Griffiths, R.R., and P.P.Woodson 1988 Reinforcing effects of caffeine in humans. J. Pharmacol. Exp. Ther. 246:21–29.

Hoddes, E., V.Zarcone, H.Smythe, R.Phillips, and W.Dement 1973 Quantification of sleepiness: A new approach. Psychophysiology 10:431–436.

Jacobson, B.H., and B.M.Edgley 1987 Effects of caffeine on simple reaction time and movement time. Aviat. Space Environ. Med. 58:1153–1156.

Kuznicki, J.T., and L.S.Turner 1986 The effects of caffeine on caffeine users and non-users. Physiol. Behav. 37:397–408.

Lieberman, H.R. 1992 Caffeine. Pp. 49–72 in Factors Affecting Human Performance, Vol. 2: The Physical Environment, D.Jones and A.Smith, eds. London: Academic Press.

Lieberman, H.R., R.J.Wurtman, G.G.Emde, and I.L.G.Coviella 1987a The effects of caffeine and aspirin on mood and performance. J. Clin. Pharmacol. 7:315–320.

1987b The effects of low doses of caffeine on human performance and mood. Psychopharmacology 92:308–312.

Loke, W.H., J.V.Hinrichs, and M.M.Ghonheim 1985 Caffeine and diazepam: Separate and combined effects on mood, memory, psychomotor performance. Psychopharmacology 87:344–350.

Lumley, M., T.Roehrs, D.Asker, F.Zorick, and T.Roth 1987 Ethanol and caffeine effects on daytime sleepiness/alertness. Sleep 10:306–312.

McNair, D.M., M.Lorr, and L.F.Droppleman 1981 Profile of Mood States. San Diego, Calif: Educational and Industrial Testing Service.

Mikulincer, M., H.Babkoff, T.Caspy, and H.Sing 1989 The effects of 72 hours of sleep loss on psychological variables. Br. J. Psychol. 80:145–162.

Myers, M.G. 1988 Effects of caffeine on blood pressure. Arch. Inter. Med. 148:1189–1193.

Newcombe, P.F., K.W.Renton, P.M.Rautaharju, C.A.Spencer, and T.J.Montague 1988 High-dose caffeine and cardiac rate and rhythm in normal subjects. Chest 94:90–94.

Newhouse, P.A., G.Belenky, M.Thomas, D.Thorne, H.C.Sing, and J.Fertig 1989 The effects of *d*-amphetamine on arousal, cognition, and mood after prolonged total sleep deprivation. Neuropsychopharmacology 2:153–164.

Penetar D., U.McCann, D.Thorne, G.Kaminori, G.Galinski, H.Sing, M.Thomas, G.Belenky 1993 Caffeine reversal of sleep deprivation effects on alertness and mood. Psychpharmacology, 112:359–365.

Rall, T.W. 1985 Central nervous system stimulants: The methylxanthines. Pp. 589–603 in The Pharmacological Basis of Therapeutics, A.G.Gilman, L.S.Goodman, T.W.Rall, and F.Murad, eds. New York: Macmillan Publishing Company.

Rapoport, J.L., M.Jensvold, R.Elkins, M.S.Buchsbaum, H.Weingartner, C.Ludlow, T.P. Zahn, C.J.Berg, and A.H.Neims 1981 Behavioral and cognitive effects of caffeine in boys and adult males. J. Nervous Mental Dis. 169:726–732.

Roache, J.D., and R.R.Griffiths 1987 Interactions of diazepam and caffeine: Behavioral and subjective dose in humans. Pharmacol. Biochem. Behav. 26:801–812.

Robertson, D., and P.W.Curatolo 1984 The cardiovascular effects of caffeine. Pp. 77–85 in Caffeine, P.B.Dews, ed. New York: Springer-Verlag.

Rosenthal, L., T.Roehrs, A.E.Zwyghuizen-Doorenbos, D.Plath, and T.Roth 1991 Alerting effects of caffeine after normal and restricted sleep. Neuropsychopharmacology, 4:103–108.

Snaith, R.P., G.W.K. Bridge, and M.Hamilton 1976 The Leeds scales for the self-assessment of anxiety and depression. Br. J. Psychiatry 128:156–165.

Snyder, S.H. 1984 Adenosine as a mediator of the behavioral effects of xanthines. Pp. 129–141 in Caffeine, P.B.Dews, ed. New York: Springer-Verlag.

Stavric, B. 1988 Methylxanthines: Toxicity to humans. 2. Caffeine. Fed. Chem. Toxicol. 26:645–662.

Swift, C.G., and B.Tiplady 1988 The effects of age on the response to caffeine. Psychopharmacology 94:29–31.

Thorne, D.R., S.G.Genser, H.C.Sing, and F.W.Hegge 1983 Plumbing human performance limits during 72 hours of high task load. Pp. 17–40 in Proceedings of the 24th DRG Seminar on The Human as a Limiting Element in Military Systems. Toronto: Defence and Civil Institute of Environmental Medicine.

1985 The Walter Reed performance assessment battery. Neurobehav. Toxicol. Teratol. 7:415–18.

U.S. Department of the Army. 1989 Army Regulation 70–25. "Use of Volunters As Subjects of Research". 25 October. Washington, D.C..

Walsh, J.K., M.J.Muehlbach, T.Humm, Q.S.Dickens, J.L.Sugerman, and P.K.Schweitzer 1990 Effect of caffeine on physiological sleep tendency and ability to sustain wakefulness at night. Psychopharmacology 101:271–273.

Weiss, B., and V.G.Laties 1962 Enhancement of human performance by caffeine and the amphetamines. Pharmacol. Rev. 14:1–36.

Wever, R. 1979 The Circadian System of Man. Berlin: Springer-Verlag.
1981 On varying work-sleep schedules: The biological perspective. Pp. 51–86 in The Twenty-four Hour Workday: Proceedings of a Symposium on Variations in Work-Sleep Schedules, L.C.Johnson, D.I.Tepas, W.P.Colquhoun, and M.J.Cilligan, eds. DHHS (NIOSH) Publication #81–127. Cincinnati: Department of Health and Human Services.
Zwyghuizen-Doorenbos A, T.A.Roehrs, L.Lipschutz, V.Timms, and T.Roth 1990 Effects of caffeine on alertness. Psychopharmacology 100:36–39.

DISCUSSION

HARRIS LIEBERMAN: We have some unpublished data from a couple of studies in which we did find significant effects of caffeine on mood swing. We did not use doses as low as 32 milligrams but used doses of 64 and 128 milligrams of caffeine. Effects on performance by doses lower than those are hard to detect, but over the long run, over a series of studies, my feeling is that there really are effects with low dosages, and those are the doses that we typically take in our background.

JOEL GRINKER: I was just curious whether in any of the caffeine studies or in any of the other supplement studies age has been looked at systematically as a factor. I have two thoughts, one, that in fact it might potentiate the ability of older individuals or that in fact it has less effectiveness, and I wonder if you have any comments.

DAVID PENETAR: I have here one study that related to age. Typically, these studies were done, with young, healthy males.

HARRIS LIEBERMAN: We did look at the age parameter in one of our caffeine studies, but we did not see any significant differences as a function of age or gender.

JOHN VANDERVEEN: I was curious as to the uniformity of the synthesis associated with sleep. Do you find much variation that would indicate that shortness of sleep time versus onset of sleep, etc. Are they uniform in your subjects or are they highly individualistic?

DAVID PENETAR: In terms of a rested individual?

JOHN VANDERVEEN: Yes.

DAVID PENETAR: What we do is we bring them into the study the night before and give them 9 hours of time in bed before we start the study, so at that time they are all pretty consistent in the amount of sleep that they have had.

JOHN VANDERVEEN: No, I meant the effects of caffeine on their subsequent sleep. Do you find a uniform effect in terms of delay of sleep or shortness of length of sleep, etc?

DAVID PENETAR: We did not specifically look at that because by the time they went to bed it was over 12 hours after they had received caffeine.

WILLIAM WATERS: A couple of questions. One pertaining to the onset of parameters. Did you have a look at whether or not you have any data or whether or not sleep can be induced prior to that?

DAVID PENETAR: No, I do not have any data on that. I am not sure that is reported.

WILLIAM WATERS: It could be that what you had was a referral of something that might allow it to occur. The other thing was, under the influence of caffeine, did you notice any change in the number, the length, stage one, and arousals?

DAVID PENETAR: Again, by the time our subjects went to bed, it was over 12 hours after they had received the caffeine, and we did not see any changes; there were no differences between the groups. We did monitor them. We recorded them through their sleep, and we saw no differences in sleep architecture, time of sleep, time to bed, or sleep efficiency; we saw no differences for 12 hours.

JOHANNA DWYER: I worked with a neurologist who was interested by some observations years ago, when they did a lot more electroconvulsive shock than they do now. Apparently, they used to prime the patients with caffeine, and by doing this, they could use a lower level of shock and still get the same effect. The reason I bring it up here is not because I hope anyone here is heavily into this, but rather, are there other changes in the electroencephalograms in terms of caffeine's effects that may be in addition to what we have been talking about?

DAVID PENETAR: No, I do not know.

ALLISON YATES: Just one thing. I noticed in some of the graphs that it almost looked as if at 600 milligrams the subjects might have had even a little bit better performance than they had initially in their first 24 hours. This result is important in considering enhancement of performance with normal subjects.

DAVID PENETAR: Harris, your subjects could not sleep at night.

HARRIS LIEBERMAN: Yes, two slides that you showed with my studies, the vigilance and reaction times, were for subjects who had stayed up all night the night before and who were back in the morning after the administration. Their performances were similar to those with placebos under the same conditions. I consider that to be above normal, although since caffeine is such a common component of the diet, it is hard to untangle it all.

ALLISON YATES: That is why I was wondering yesterday what the baseline levels were.

HARRIS LIEBERMAN: We typically include that as a parameter in our studies and look to see whether there are differences between moderate, low, and heavy caffeine users in their responsiveness, and in the low and moderate range there is not much difference. When you get to the real high users, you see big differences in responsiveness. That depends on the timing of administration, whether they are in a deprivation stage, or whether they are already on a lot caffeine.

ROBERT NESHEIM: Were you defining it high?

HARRIS LIEBERMAN: Average caffeine consumption is about 200 milligrams per day, which is maybe three cups of not very strong coffee. I define high for the purpose of categorizing subjects as above 400 or 500 milligrams per day.

DAVID SCHNAKENBERG: Just a couple of observations. We used to always think that members of the Army must be heavy coffee drinkers because you get that perception, but looking out in field studies where soldiers are eating rations, we found out that even though you gave a meal ready-to-eat, 90 percent of the coffee packets were returned unused. The rest of the 10 percent probably went mostly to the senior sergeants, who had a chance to stay by the talking place and make some coffee for themselves. So young soldiers in the field today are not heavy coffee drinkers. I am sure they drink plenty of caffeine if they have carbonated beverages. But most of the time carbonated beverages are not available to them in the field, although maybe in Desert Storm cans of Coke manged to get inside of the tanks anyway.

My question is, has anybody done sleep studies on evaluating caffeine using the vehicle of delivering the caffeine in the form of a cola or in the form of a coffee beverage itself?

DAVID PENETAR: A number of studies look at coffee drinking when they give caffeine. In fact, in some of the studies reported here, they took decaffeinated coffee and added caffeine to it, and the subjects drank it that way. In other studies it was either caffeine pills or caffeine powder dissolved in some drink.

DAVID SCHNAKENBERG: Can subjects get a comparable effect with the caffeinated coffee versus decaffeinated coffee? For instance, I am sure your subjects knew when they were receiving a placebo.

DAVID PENETAR: Ours was powdered caffeine dissolved in a lemon juice drink, and the lemon juice drink was very bitter. As you know, caffeine powders are very bitter, so they could not tell what they were drinking other than lemon juice drink. If they talked among themselves, they just said "oh, it is not very good, it was bitter."

WILLIAM BEISEL: So many of the emergency rations and so on seem to be candy bars with chocolate flavoring. How much of that is caffeine?

DAVID PENETAR: Milk chocolate has about 7 milligrams per ounce, whereas bakery chocolate or unsweetened chocolate has about 35 milligrams per ounce. They figure that, for example, a Hershey's candy bar has 25 to 35 milligrams per ounce, so it is not a lot, and it is less than most sodas.

21

The Role of Carnitine in Enhancing Physical Performance

Peggy R.Borum[1]

INTRODUCTION

Human muscle contains a high concentration of carnitine. The first well-documented function of carnitine was found to be facilitation of the transport of long-chain fatty acids into the matrix of the mitochondrion, which is the site for beta-oxidation. Fatty acids are an important fuel for muscle metabolism. During endurance exercise, the oxidation of fatty acids spares the use of muscle glycogen and delays the onset of fatigue. Muscle tissue cannot synthesize carnitine and thus is dependent on the transport of carnitine from the bloodstream. Blood carnitine is derived from endogenous biosynthesis in the liver and kidney and from exogenous sources in the diet.

[1] Peggy R.Borum, 409 FHSN, P.O. Box 110370, The University of Florida, Gainsville, FL 32611

There is controversy as to whether or not administration of carnitine improves exercise performance. The difference in the intensity of exercise, the training or conditioning of the subjects, the quantity of carnitine administered, the route of administration, and the timing of administration relative to the exercise have led to different experimental results (Vecchiet et al., 1990).

FUNCTIONS OF CARNITINE

Carnitine Stimulates Fatty Acid Oxidation

The impermeability of all membranes to carbon chains activated to the coenzyme A (CoA) level, as diagramed in Figure 21–1 is well recognized. The carnitine transport system consists of carnitine and three proteins that result in the transport of the carbon chain moiety of acyl-CoA across a membrane and reesterified to another CoA molecule residing on the opposite side of the membrane (Borum, 1983). As diagramed in Figure 21–2, at the completion of the action of the carnitine transport system, the carbon chain is located on the opposite side of the membrane and is esterified to a different CoA molecule.

Long-chain fatty acids activated to the CoA level were the first acylcarnitines to be documented as being transported across a membrane, as diagramed in Figure 21–3. However, the acyl-CoA may be of any chain length and may be the metabolite derived from fatty acids, carbohydrates, or amino acids. The importance of carnitine in the oxidation of medium-chain fatty acids has been discussed recently (Borum, 1992).

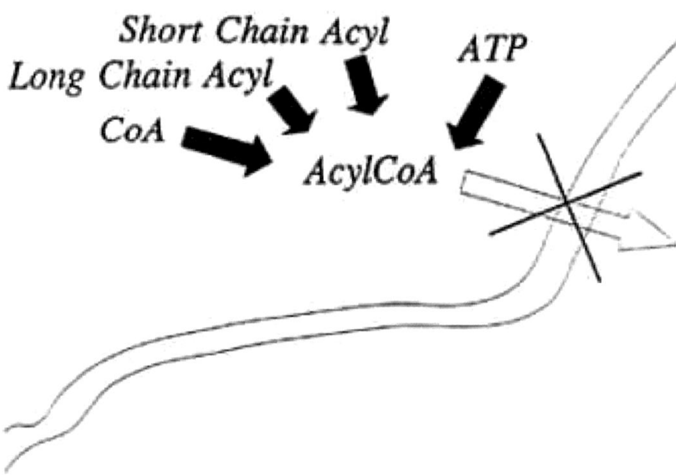

FIGURE 21–1 Acyl-coenzyme A (AcylCoA) moieties cannot penetrate membranes.

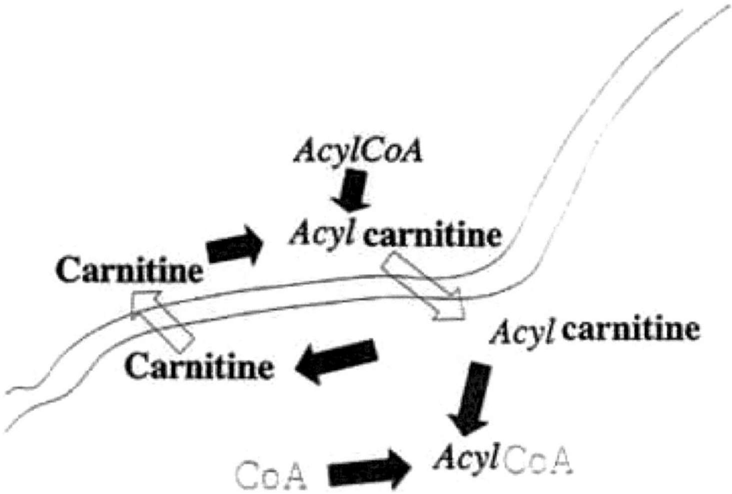

FIGURE 21–2 The carnitine transport system results in the acyl moiety of the acyl-coenzyme A (acylCoA) being transported to the opposite side of the membrane and esterified to a CoA moiety on the opposite side of the membrane.

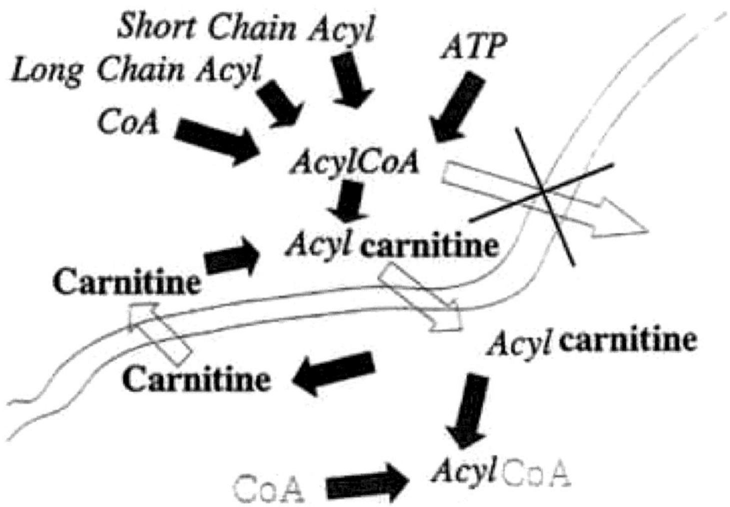

FIGURE 21–3 The carnitine transport systems function in the transport of both short-chain and long-chain acyl-coenzyme A (acylCoA) across membranes.

Carnitine Transports Acyl-CoA Across Membranes

It is clear that in beta-oxidation of long-chain fatty acids, carnitine is essential for the transport of long-chain acyl-CoA as long-chain acylcarnitine across the inner membrane of the mitochondrion. Carnitine is also essential in the transport of short-chain acyl-CoA as short-chain acylcarnitine across several membranes. During some physiological conditions, the goal of the transport process is to provide a needed substrate to the subcellular organelle where it is required. During other physiological conditions, the goal of the transport is to remove from a subcellular organelle a metabolite that is accumulating to toxic levels. In the latter condition, carnitine is functioning in a detoxification process. During exercise, carnitine is critical in providing needed substrates and in removing potentially toxic compounds.

Carnitine Prevents Accumulation of Lactate

During intense exercise, acetyl-CoA is produced at a faster rate than it can be used in the Krebs cycle. The rate-limiting factor in the Krebs cycle is frequently the availability of oxygen. During intense exercise, oxygen is limiting and the muscle produces lactate. The advantages of lactate production are that it permits the continuation of glycolysis with production of nicotinamide adenine dinucleotide, does not deplete limiting concentrations of CoA, and can be removed from the cell. The disadvantages of lactate production are that it can cause acidosis and it is a low-energy compound. An alternative pathway is for pyruvate to form acetyl-CoA, which in turn forms acetylcarnitine, which does not deplete limiting concentrations of CoA and which can be removed from the cell.

Carnitine Stimulates Utilization of Carbohydrate and Amino Acids

Since a common metabolite in the oxidation of fatty acids, amino acids, and glucose is acetyl-CoA, the role of carnitine in the transport of acetyl-CoA as acetylcarnitine across membranes places carnitine in the role of facilitating the oxidation of all three fuels used by the body.

Acylcarnitine Is a Storehouse of High Energy That Is Transportable

An important characteristic of acylcarnitine is that it is a high-energy compound, and thus, the acyl-CoA can be reformed without the use of an ATP molecule (Borum, 1986). Figure 21–4 illustrates the fact that the transport of acylcarnitine across a membrane delivers both the carbon chain and high energy (equivalent to an ATP molecule) to the new site. Thus, another advantage of the formation of acetylcarnitine rather than lactate by muscle is that high metabolic energy is preserved.

Acylcarnitine Permits Administration of High Energy

In addition to the supplementation of free carnitine, it is also possible to use acetylcarnitine and propionylcarnitine as supplements. Supplementation with the latter two compounds provides the carnitine moiety, the carbon chain moiety, and high metabolic energy. Additional research is needed to evaluate the potential benefit of supplementing individuals with a compound that potentially provides high metabolic energy.

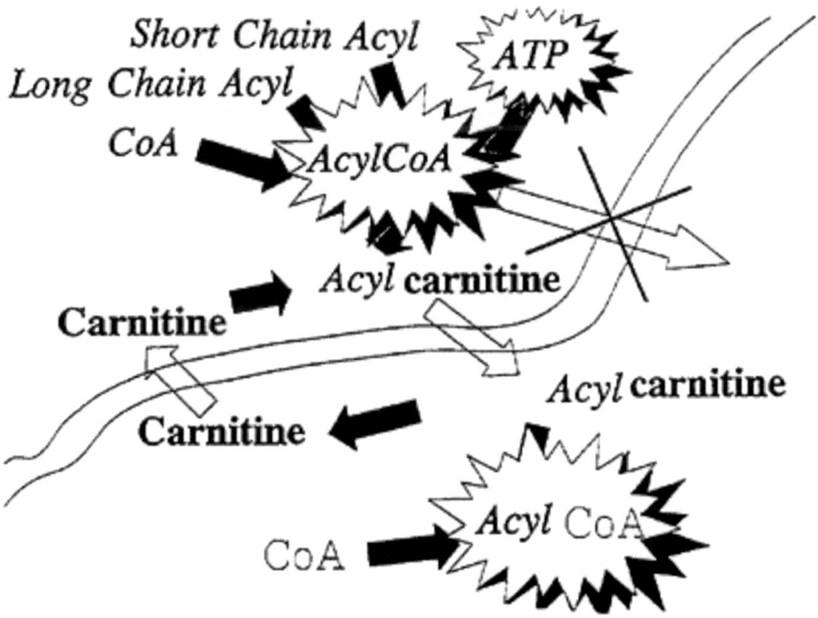

FIGURE 21–4 The carnitine transport system maintains the high energy level of the acylcoenzyme A (acylCoA), allowing the acyl-CoA to be esterified on the opposite side of the membrane without the use of an additional ATP molecule. The overall effect of the action of the carnitine transport system is the delivery of both the acyl group and high energy to the new site on the opposite side of the membrane.

ASSAY METHODS FOR CARNITINE AND ACYLCARNITINE

The most widely used assay for carnitine and acylcarnitine is the radioenzymatic assay (Borum, 1990). The assay uses radiolabeled acetyl-coenzyme A (acetyl-CoA) and an unknown amount of carnitine as substrates for the enzyme carnitine acetyltransferase and separates the radiolabeled acetylcarnitine product from the unreacted radiolabeled substrate. When alkaline hydrolysis is used to remove all acyl groups, the assay provides an excellent means of measuring total carnitine. The assay cannot be used to identify specific acylcarnitines. Although it is frequently used in combination with acid precipitation techniques to estimate long-chain acylcarnitines and short-chain acylcarnitines, investigators have found that caution must be used unless the measurement of the different fractions of acylcarnitine and free carnitine are documented to equal the total amount of carnitine measured. Specific acylcarnitines can be identified by gas chromatography-mass spectrometry techniques. The published methods require research-grade instruments and procedures that are not practical for measuring acylcarnitine levels in a large number of samples. However, ongoing work in several laboratories should permit measurement of specific acylcarnitines with bench-top instruments. These analytical techniques should greatly enhance investigators' ability to address many of the issues discussed below.

POTENTIAL USE OF CARNITINE TO ENHANCE PHYSICAL PERFORMANCE

Intensity of Exercise Affects Carnitine Metabolism

High- and low-intensity types of exercise require two qualitatively distinct states of skeletal muscle metabolism. The transition between these two metabolic states for different exercise intensities occurs at a work load approximated by the lactate threshold, which is defined as the exercise intensity at which elevated plasma lactate concentrations are first observed (Hiatt et al., 1989).

Muscle acetyl-CoA and acetylcarnitine contents increase dramatically at the onset of intense exercise. When the duration of exercise is prolonged, acetyl-CoA and acetylcarnitine contents decrease in different proportions but are maintained above resting levels at exhaustion when muscle glycogen levels are depleted. As fatigue approaches, the carbohydrate-derived acetyl-CoA content decreases at a rate more rapid than the decrease in acetylcarnitine (Spriet et al., 1992b).

Muscle carnitine metabolism does not change in a graded fashion with exercise, but only when exercise is of sufficient intensity to qualitatively alter muscle substrate metabolism. Six normal male subjects exercised on a bicycle ergometer on two separate occasions with a constant work load. Low-intensity exercise was performed for 60 min at a work load equal to 50 percent of the lactate threshold, and high-intensity exercise was performed for 30 min at a work load between the lactate threshold and the maximal work capacity for the individual (Hiatt et al, 1989).

The data in Table 21–1 show that low-intensity exercise for 60 min has no detectable effect on muscle carnitine composition, but high-intensity exercise for 10 min decreases the free carnitine concentration and dramatically increases the short-chain acylcarnitine concentration of muscle. There were only minor changes in these muscle parameters between 10 and 30 min of intense exercise. After 60 min of recovery from high-intensity exercise, the total muscle carnitine content returned to baseline values. The short-chain acylcarnitine content remained elevated and the free carnitine content was only 46 percent of the content in the resting state, reflecting a continued redistribution of the carnitine pool. The finding of a persistent change in muscle carnitine metabolism into recovery is consistent with the observation that in humans, metabolic rate and substrate utilization remain altered for several hours after exercise and may have implications for the performance of repetitive bouts of high-intensity exercise (Hiatt et al., 1989).

TABLE 21–1 Changes in Muscle Acylcarnitine Levels During Exercise (percentage of value at rest)

Carnitine Fraction	60 min of Low-Intensity Exercise	10 min of High-Intensity Exercise
Free	100	34
Short chain	100	550
Long chain	100	100
Total	100	81

SOURCE: Adapted from Hiatt et al. (1989).

The effect of exercise on plasma carnitine metabolism differed from that observed in muscle. With low-intensity exercise there were no changes in the profile of plasma carnitine with the exception of a small increase in plasma long-chain acylcarnitine. The plasma free carnitine level was increased at 15 min of high-intensity exercise but was unchanged from the values at rest during the remainder of the exercise and the recovery period. The plasma short-chain acylcarnitine concentration increased from that at rest during exercise and remained elevated 10 min into recovery before returning to baseline levels at 30 min of recovery. Compared with the large changes in muscle after 10 min of exercise, the ratio of short-chain acylcarnitine to total acid-soluble carnitine in plasma increased modestly and only after 30 min of exercise. In contrast to muscle, the ratio of short-chain acylcarnitine to total acid-soluble carnitine in plasma had normalized by 30 min of recovery (Hiatt et al., 1989).

Muscle Training Affects Nutrient Utilization During Exercise

Training of muscle may result in muscle adaptations for the metabolism of fatty acids during prolonged exercise. Six trained and six untrained human males exercised for 3 h at 60 percent of their maximal dynamic knee extension capacity. Arterial plasma free fatty acid concentrations increased over time in both groups. Fractional uptake of free fatty acids across the thigh remained unchanged over time in the trained group (15 percent) but decreased in the untrained group. Thus, the total free fatty acid oxidation was higher in the muscles of the trained group. Glucose uptake increased in both groups over time and was significantly higher in the untrained group during the last hour of exercise. Although the contribution of extracellular substrates to thigh oxidative metabolism increased during the third hour of exercise in both groups of subjects, only in the thighs of the trained group was there an increased utilization of the plasma free fatty acids (Turcotte et al., 1992).

Carnitine Affects Pyruvate Metabolism

Pyruvate oxidation was measured in intact mitochondria isolated from fresh human skeletal muscle obtained from the excision of pectoralis minor in the course of a mastectomy for breast cancer; the muscle was free of macroscopic neoplastic infiltration, however. The data listed in Table 21–2 show that pyruvate oxidation increased significantly in the presence of L-carnitine and that inhibitors of the transport of either pyruvate or carnitine across the intact membrane greatly decreased the oxidation of pyruvate (Uziel et al., 1988).

Pyruvate dehydrogenase complex activity (PDHC) was measured in mitochondria made permeable to cofactors by exposure to hypotonic medium. PDHC activity increased in the presence of L-carnitine as shown in Table 21–2. As expected, because of the use of leaky mitochondria, the addition of an inhibitor of either pyruvate transport or carnitine transport across membranes had no effect on activity. D-Carnitine, deoxycarnitine, and choline, which are structural analogs of L-carnitine, had no effect on activity. When L-carnitine was omitted, only 0.2 percent of the pyruvate oxidized was transformed to acetylcarnitine. When 1 mM carnitine was added, PDHC activity nearly doubled and 82 percent of the pyruvate oxidized was transformed to acetylcarnitine. PDHC stimulation occurred only at pyruvate concentrations greater than 0.25 mM, suggesting that carnitine and carnitine acetyltransferase can buffer the acetyl-CoA excess in human mitochondria when pyruvate is oxidized at high rates (Uziel et al., 1988).

TABLE 21–2 Pyruvate Metabolism (Percentage of Control Value)

Addition	Pyruvate Oxidation in Intact Mitochondria	Pyruvate Dehydrogenase Complex Activity
1 mM L-Carnitine	176	182
Inhibitor of pyruvate transport	6	109
Inhibitor of pyruvate transport +1 mM L-carnitine	5	ND
Inhibitor of carnitine transport	88	100
Inhibitor of carnitine transport	95	164
1mM D-Carnitine	ND	100
1 mM Deoxycarnitine	ND	103
1 mM Choline	ND	100

NOTE: ND, not determined.
SOURCE: Adapted from Uziel et al. (1988).

Ten moderately trained male subjects aged 20–30 years performed a maximal exercise test on a bicycle ergometer, beginning with a light warm-up load followed by progressive incremental increases of 50 W every 3 min. The tests were stopped when one of the following was reached: (1) achievement of theoretical maximal heart rate, (2) muscular exhaustion, or (3) onset of severe dyspnea. Three days later the test was repeated after a randomized loading of either placebo or L-carnitine (2 g) (Siliprandi et al., 1990). Ninety minutes after carnitine administration and with the subjects at rest, plasma free carnitine levels increased, and short-chain carnitine levels did not change. In both the placebo and carnitine trials, exercise decreased plasma free carnitine levels and increased plasma short-chain carnitine levels. Plasma long-chain carnitine levels did not change in any instance (Siliprandi et al., 1990).

Maximal exercise increased plasma lactate levels 15-fold and pyruvate levels 3.5-fold in the placebo trial. In each subject the increases in both lactate and pyruvate levels with maximal exercise were significantly lower after carnitine administration, in spite of the significantly greater amount of work carried out by 7 of the 10 subjects. In the carnitine trial the increase in lactate levels was lower throughout the trial, and the return to baseline levels during the 12-min recovery period was the same in both the placebo and carnitine trials. There was an inverse correlation of lactate and acetylcarnitine in plasma (Siliprandi et al., 1990).

Both free carnitine levels and short-chain carnitine levels increased in urine after carnitine administration (especially free carnitine). Exercise did not induce appreciable changes. When individual acylcarnitine levels were estimated by isotope-exchange high-pressure liquid chromatography in the placebo trial, exercise induced a significant decrease in acetylcarnitine levels and a concomitant increase in the amount of a four-carbon (C_4) compound (the authors suggested that it was isobutyrylcarnitine). After carnitine administration but with no exercise, there was a decrease in the amount of the C_4 compound. Exercise after carnitine loading showed an increase in acetylcarnitine levels and an almost disappearance of the C_4 compound. It is important to note that all these data are percentages of the total short-chain acylcarnitine and that the absolute amount of the short-chain acylcarnitine was much greater in the carnitine trial than in the placebo trial (Siliprandi et al., 1990).

The authors interpreted the increase in plasma and urinary short-chain acylcarnitine levels with carnitine administration as reflecting a washout of short-chain acyls that accumulate in tissues as the CoA ester during exercise. They suggested that in the placebo trial, pyruvate dehydrogenase was inhibited, which caused an energy crisis, and that branched-chain amino acids were used for energy, which gave rise to the C_4 compound. They suggest that, with carnitine supplementation, the branched-chain amino acids were not needed because pyruvate dehydrogenase was not so inhibited (Siliprandi et al., 1990). The authors did not address the issue of why there is a greater need for oxidation of branched-chain amino acids at rest with no carnitine supplementation than at maximal exercise with carnitine supplementation. The identification of the C_4 compound as isobutyrylcarnitine should only be considered tentative and should be further investigated.

The possible effect of supplying free fatty acids during intense exercise on carnitine metabolism and the use of carbohydrate versus fat have been investigated. Rats were randomly assigned to a no-fat or a high-fat treatment and were perfused (single pass) by using one of three conditions: (1) 10 min at rest, (2) 10 min at rest and 1 min of stimulation, and (3) 10 min at rest and

5 min of stimulation. The right hind limb was used to obtain control samples of the soleus (89 percent slow oxidative fibers and 11 percent fast oxidative-glycolytic fibers) and red gastrocnemius from the deep portion of the gastrocnemius medial head (59 percent fast oxidative-glycolytic fibers, 35 percent slow oxidative fibers; and 9 percent fast glycolytic fibers). The perfusion media contained no fat in the fat-free group and approximately 1 mM oleate in the high-fat group (Spriet et al., 1992a). It should be noted that the fatty acid profile of the perfusion medium was nonphysiological.

Oxygen uptake was similar in the fat-free and high-fat treatments at rest and during stimulation. Muscle acetylcarnitine plotted versus acetyl-CoA levels for both treatments and all conditions gave a positive linear relationship ($r = 0.82$ for red gastrocnemius and ($r = 0.70$ for soleus) (Spriet et al., 1992a).

Provision of high levels of free fatty acids while at rest increased acetyl-CoA and acetylcarnitine contents, despite an unchanged oxygen uptake, suggesting that little regulation of free fatty acid metabolism exists in skeletal muscle while at rest. Altered free fatty acid provision did not affect the increases in acetyl-CoA and acetylcarnitine during intense stimulation, suggesting that carbohydrate-derived acetyl-CoA dominates during exercise of this intensity (Spriet et al., 1992a).

Carnitine Supplementation May Increase Use of Fatty Acids During Exercise

Ten highly conditioned subjects performed a control test of 45 min of cycling at 66 percent of maximal oxygen uptake $\dot{V}_{O_2\ max}$; this was followed by 60 min of recovery in a sitting position. Each subject repeated this trial after 28 days of placebo and L-Carnitine treatment of 2 g/day (double blinded crossover design). There were no differences between the control test and the placebo test throughout the exercise and recovery periods (Gorostiaga et al., 1989).

The respiratory quotient was lower ($P > 0.05$) in carnitine-treated subjects than in placebo or control subjects during exercise. The oxygen uptake, heart rate, blood glycerol concentrations, and resting plasma fatty acid concentrations listed in Table 21–3 showed a trend toward higher values in the carnitine-treated period but was not significant at the 0.05 level (Gorostiaga et al., 1989). These observations suggest increased lipid utilization by muscle during exercise with carnitine treatment, but the data are far from dramatic.

TABLE 21–3 Exercise After Placebo or Carnitine Supplementation in the Same Subjects

Parameter	Carnitine	Placebo
RQ at last minute of exercise	0.95±0.01	0.98±0.02
Heart rate at last minute of exercise (beats/min)	178.8±2.8	176.3±3.2
$\dot{V}_{O_2\ max}$ at last minute of exercise (liters/min)	2.82±0.11	2.80±0.13
Blood glucose at 40th min of exercise (mM)	4.63±0.3	4.35±0.3
Blood glycerol at 40th min of exercise (mM)	0.238±0.03	0.198±0.03
Free fatty acid levels at rest (mM)	0.284±0.05	0.143±0.03

NOTE: Values are means±standard errors of the means. RQ, respiratory quotient; $\dot{V}_{O_2\ max}$, maximal oxygen uptake.

SOURCE: Adapted from Gorostiaga et al. (1989).

Carnitine Supplementation May Preserve Available Coenzyme A Pool

It can be calculated that during perfusion of the rat hind limb at rest, 97.7 percent (soleus) to 99.1 percent (red gastrocnemius) of the extra acetyl-CoA produced by adding free fatty acid to the perfusion medium was buffered by the formation of acetylcarnitine. Total acetylcarnitine accumulations during perfusion at rest were 5- to 2.5-fold greater than the resting CoA contents of red gastrocnemius and soleus, respectively. If there was no buffering of acetylcarnitine, the entire mitochondrial CoA store would be acetylated in 9 s in the red gastrocnemius and in 20 s in the soleus. After peak accumulation of acetylcarnitine during muscle stimulation, approximately 20 and 41 percent of the total carnitine pool would be acetylated in the soleus and red gastrocnemius, respectively (Spriet et al., 1992a).

In an experiment involving skiing uphill and downhill in difficult terrain at race pace for more than 13 h, the authors (Decombaz et al., 1992) calculated the estimated fuel cost of the exercise to be 38 MJ or 9,100 kcal. The authors assumed the following: 353 g of carbohydrate intake, 850 g of glycogen from muscles (25 kg, 3 percent glycogen), 100 g of liver glycogen, and 10 percent of energy from protein. Therefore 350 g of fat must have been oxidized. If 90 percent of the fat (1,100 nmol of free fatty acid) was oxidized in the muscle, the pool of muscle carnitine must have been acylated 13-fold during the race (1,100 mmol of free fatty acid×25 kg of muscle×3.33 mmol of total carnitine/kg of muscle) with no net loss of carnitine (Decombaz et al., 1992).

Eight subjects exercised for 3–4 min on a bicycle ergometer at work loads corresponding to 30, 60, and 90 percent of their $\dot{V}_{O_2\ max}$, The graded exercise in that investigation was very important, and investigations that use different percent $\dot{V}_{O_2\ max}$ may not be comparable. Muscle biopsy specimens were taken at rest, at the end of the work period, and after 10 min of recovery. During the incremental exercise test, there was an increase in muscle lactate levels, an increase in the levels of the active form of the pyruvate dehydrogenase complex, and an increase in both acetyl-CoA and acetylcarnitine levels, with a corresponding decrease in CoA and free carnitine levels. At work loads of 60 and 90 percent of $\dot{V}_{O_2\ max}$, the accumulation of lactate showed that the rate of pyruvate formation from glucose was higher than the catalytic rate of the pyruvate dehydrogenase complex. The accumulation of acetyl-CoA and acetylcarnitine showed that the rate of condensation of acetyl groups with oxaloacetate was less than their rate of formation (Constantin-Teodosiu et al., 1991).

The authors calculated that if the pyruvate dehydrogenase complex is fully active during exercise, the following calculations would apply to muscle (Constantin-Teodosiu et al., 1991):

- Maximum rate of pyruvate degradation during exercise=20–25 µmol/s/kg of muscle,
- CoA concentration at rest=9 µmol/kg of muscle,
- L-carnitine concentration at rest=3,600 µmol/kg of muscle, and
- the entire store of CoA in muscle could theoretically be acetylated within less than 1 s.

The high concentration of carnitine and the high levels of activity of carnitine acetyltransferase and carnitine acetylcarnitine translocase in muscle tissues enable carnitine to act as a buffer for excess acetyl-CoA production opposing the depletion of CoA. Depletion of CoA would result in the inhibition of the pyruvate dehydrogenase complex and the inhibition of oxoglutarate dehydrogenase in the citric acid cycle. It should be remembered that since acetylcarnitine is a high-energy compound, the acetyl units stored as acetylcarnitine during heavy exercise would be available if the exercise intensity decreased. Also, the acetyl unit would not require metabolic energy to re-form acetyl-CoA.

Carnitine Supplementation May Increase Work Output

Ten healthy males (moderately trained, but the authors [Vecchiet et al., 1990] did not give) $\dot{V}_{O_2\ max}$) performed three tests to maximal exercise intensity separated by 72 h. The intensity of the exercise was increased by 50 W every 3 min. The first test was performed without any treatment. The other two tests began 90 min after administration of a single oral dose of carnitine (2 g) or placebo in random order. Tests were terminated after muscular exhaustion or upon reaching the theoretical maximal heart rate (Vecchiet et al., 1990).

As exercise intensity increased, both $\dot{V}_{O_2\ max}$ and the blood lactate level increased. After carnitine treatment, all subjects tolerated similar exercise intensities but with a significant reduction of $\dot{V}_{O_2\ max}$ and the blood lactate level. When the subjects were required to exercise to their maximal capacity, 9 of the 10 subjects were able to do substantially more work in the session in which they received carnitine. Both the work output and the $\dot{V}_{O_2\ max}$ were significantly increased by carnitine pretreatment (Vecchiet et al., 1990). Other investigators have not found L-carnitine supplementation to modify either the physiological parameters or the circulating metabolites (Oyono-Enguelle et al., 1988).

Mixed-type latissimus dorsi of the dog was used to show the effect of carnitine on an in situ fatigue test. L-Carnitine appeared to improve the force of this muscle by 34 percent while the muscle was stimulated in situ. Ten mongrel dogs were used on different days with at least a 1-week interval. The musculus latissimus dorsi was trained by continuous stimulation with a frequency that was increased every 2 weeks until a frequency of 60 contractions per min was reached. An 8-min test was performed by using a pacemaker as the control test. The test was repeated after a rest period of 30 min, during which time the drug to be investigated was infused. The authors (Dubelaar et al., 1991) did not address the issue of whether the experimental design would distinguish between an effect of carnitine on exercise and an effect on the recovery period between the two exercise sessions. Drugs (saline; 0.15 mmol of L-carnitine, D-carnitine, or choline per kg of body weight) were infused at a rate of 0.15 mmol/min, and only one drug was tested in each experiment (Dubelaar et al., 1991).

When two control tests were repeated at a 30-min interval during which saline was infused, no significant change in force occurred. A third test after another 30-min rest period showed the same pattern. Administration of L-carnitine resulted in a significant increase in force throughout the second test, resulting in a significantly higher amount of work carried out by the muscle. The effect of L-carnitine on the contractile force was less pronounced in animals in which the latissimus dorsi was conditioned for 12 weeks. During this training period, the percentage of type I muscle fibers increased from 23 ±3 to 69±16 percent (Dubelaar et al., 1991).

After intravenous administration of carnitine, total plasma carnitine levels rose from 23±0.6 to 322±61 nmol/ml, but the concentration in the muscle remained the same. The structural analog choline did not improve the contraction force of the muscle. D-Carnitine decreased the contraction force significantly during the last minutes of the exercise. In the presence of high insulin levels, which is known to inhibit fatty acid oxidation, the insulin itself had no effect on contraction force, but the stimulation of the force by carnitine was no longer seen in the presence of insulin and glucose (Dubelaar et al., 1991).

Exercise May Alter Metabolic Compartmentation of Carnitine and Acylcarnitine

Eighteen cross-country skiers took part in a race in the Alps that lasted an average of 13 h and 26 min. The skiers' heart rates indicated performance at 72 percent of $\dot{V}_{O_2\ max}$. The reduced oxygen pressure at the high altitude added a hypoxic stress. Carnitine intake 2 weeks before the race was 50±4 mg/kg. The total carnitine concentration of resting muscle (vastus lateralis) was measured twice, with a 2-year interval for eight of the subjects. Muscle carnitine concentrations did not change with time and did not correlate with carnitine intake, but they showed consistent interindividual differences (Decombaz et al., 1992).

After exercise, the total muscle carnitine concentration was unaltered, but the free carnitine concentration decreased 20 percent and the short-chain carnitine concentration increased 108 percent. The correlation between the drop of one and the rise of the other was weak (r=0.23). This suggests that, in addition to acylation in situ, there may be significant interorgan exchange in the form of an efflux of free carnitine from the muscle and an influx of acetylcarnitine from the liver (where it may be raised after exercise) to the muscle. A significant finding is the stability of total carnitine levels in muscle after long and demanding periods of exercise. Therefore, the persistently elevated urinary carnitine excretion with exercise would not be at the expense of muscle carnitine. The ratio of short-chain acylcarnitine to total soluble carnitine rose from 19 to 37 percent. There was no correlation between the total carnitine concentration in muscle at rest and finishing time. There was a lack of correlation between muscle carnitine and maximal aerobic power or duration of training. This lack of correlation indicates that endurance conditioning has little effect on skeletal muscle carnitine concentrations in humans (Decombaz et al., 1992).

Seven moderately trained male subjects ages, 19–31 years; $\dot{V}_{O_2\,max}$, 3.3 to 4.3 liters/min participated in a study of prolonged (120 min) moderate-intensity exercise. The first submaximal bicycle ergometer exercise session lasted 120 min at approximately 50 percent of the individual $\dot{V}_{O_2\,max}$. After 1–2 months, a second exercise session immediately preceded by 5 days of oral L-carnitine (inner salt, 1 g 5 times per day) and 1 g of L-carnitine on the morning of the test was conducted. It should be noted that the dose was much higher than the amount of carnitine that would be expected to be obtained in the diet (Soop et al., 1988).

Blood samples were collected from the femoral arterial catheter and one of the femoral venous catheters at rest, after 40 and 120 min of exercise, and at 40 min postexercise. A continuous intravenous infusion of [^{14}C]oleic acids bound to human albumin (1.6 μCi/min) was given during the 30 min preexercise and during the last 20 min of exercise (Soop et al., 1988). The experimental design appeared to assume that the metabolism of oleic acid is indicative of the metabolism of all fatty acids. The experiment should be repeated with a labeled physiological mixture of fatty acids.

Carnitine supplementation did not influence the relation between arterial oleic acid concentration and leg uptake. During exercise there was a progressive increase in total and acylated plasma carnitine concentrations and a decrease in the concentrations of plasma free carnitine. At 40 min postexercise, there was a decline in total and acylated carnitine levels in comparison with those at 120 min, but the levels at both times were still higher than those preexercise. The ratio of acylated carnitine to free carnitine increased from preexercise values during the exercise and remained elevated at 40 min postexercise (Soop et al., 1988).

The following data concerning the release and uptake of carnitine by muscle was collected during the exercise session with no carnitine supplementation:

Free carnitine:

- Rest—no evidence of net uptake or release;
- 40 min of exercise—release almost significant;
- 120 min of exercise—significant release;
- 40 min postexercise—no net exchange.

Acylated carnitine

- Rest—no net exchange;
- 40 min of exercise—no net exchange;
- 120 min of exercise—tendency toward uptake; and
- 40 min postexercise—significant release.

The exercise-induced changes in plasma carnitine concentrations after carnitine supplementation followed the same pattern that was observed before carnitine supplementation, except that the free carnitine concentration rose in response to exercise (Soop et al., 1988).

Urinary carnitine excretion did not differ before or during exercise with no carnitine supplementation. More than 10 times as much carnitine was excreted during exercise with carnitine supplementation, and a larger percentage was found to be free carnitine (Soop et al., 1988).

As a result of the exercise-induced release of free carnitine and a simultaneous tendency toward uptake of acylated carnitine, no net exchange of total carnitine was observed during exercise. The release of free carnitine from the muscle occurred concomitantly with a decrease in the plasma free carnitine level. The level of plasma acylated carnitine rose, in spite of no evidence of a release by the leg muscle. Thus, the observed fall in plasma free carnitine levels and the rise in acylated carnitine levels in response to exercise is difficult to explain solely in terms of alterations in muscle carnitine exchange. Results suggest that during exercise, free carnitine is released from muscle and acylated at a site other than contracting muscle. The most likely site for carnitine acylation is the liver. The carnitine released from muscle during exercise is either redistributed to tissues other than muscle or accumulated in plasma, since urinary carnitine excretion was not affected by exercise (Soop et al., 1988).

Since several studies have shown no effect of carnitine supplementation on the total muscle carnitine concentration during exercise but have shown a beneficial effect of the carnitine supplementation on exercise performance, some authors speculate that there is an "extramyocytal" effect of carnitine. "The question arises whether there is a compartment in muscle other than the striated muscle cells, from which carnitine can be lost during muscle performance. The question could be rephrased, Do endothelial and/or vascular smooth muscle cells lose carnitine during muscle stimulation?" (Dubelaar et al., 1991:E192). These authors have previously shown that in cultured endothelial cells, the bulk of ATP may come from carnitine-dependent fatty acid oxidation. It is possible that the cells of the vascular wall lose carnitine because of the relative ischemia during muscle stimulation. The lesser effect of carnitine in the trained muscle is in line with this hypothesis, since the number of capillaries is known to increase by training, leading to better oxygenation and possibly preventing functional decompensation of the relatively vulnerable vascular cells (Dubelaar et al., 1991).

DIETARY INTAKE VERSUS PHARMACOLOGICAL ADMINISTRATION

Unpublished data show that most Americans consume between 50 and 100 mg of carnitine per day in their diets. Some individuals consume up to 300 mg of dietary carnitine per day. Most of the studies evaluating the effect of carnitine supplementation on exercise performance have used quantities that are severalfold higher than the typical dietary carnitine intakes. It is important to remember that the data available on the intestinal absorption and metabolic compartmentation of 100 mg of dietary carnitine may not be applicable to supplementation with pharmacological doses of carnitine. Carnitine supplementation in investigations concerning exercise have used free carnitine. Acetylcarnitine and propionylcarnitine have been used in Europe in clinical trials involving a variety of patients. The uptake of these acylcarnitine supplements by some organs may be greater than the uptake of free carnitine. Future studies should consider their use as supplements.

CONCLUSIONS AND RECOMMENDATIONS

It is clear that carnitine has an important metabolic role in the exercising muscle. However, the specific functions of carnitine and acylcarnitine and the effect of supplementation remain to be elucidated. The design of future investigations should carefully address the following issues:

- *Assay methodology*—The radioenzymatic assay is appropriate for total carnitine measurements, but it should be used with caution to measure fractions of acylcarnitines. Bench-top gas chromatography-mass spectrometry methodologies should be further developed to measure specific acylcarnitines in a large number of samples. Caution should be used in the use of a carnitine concentration value as an indicator of the carnitine status in another cell type. Plasma, red blood cells, white blood cells, urine, and muscle should all be evaluated in each investigation.
- *Chemical form of supplementation*—Published investigations concerning exercise have all used free carnitine as the chemical form that is used in supplementation. Acetylcarnitine and propionylcarnitine should be evaluated for their use in supplementation.
- *Timing of supplementation*—The time relationship of the dose of carnitine supplementation to the time of exercise has varied from investigation to investigation and may be the cause of some of the variability of the results. The time relationship of dose and exercise needs to be carefully evaluated.

- *Dose of supplementation*—In studies with carnitine supplementation, higher doses than are found in most diets have been used. The optimal dose has not be defined.
- *Physical training of subjects*—Physical training alters muscle metabolism, including the metabolism of carnitine. All investigations should use subjects who have the same level of training as the individuals for whom the data will be utilized.
- *Intensity of exercise*—The intensity of exercise alters muscle metabolism, including the metabolism of carnitine. All investigations should use the intensity of exercise for which the data will be utilized.
- *Animal studies*—Some experimental questions require techniques that are too invasive to be performed in humans and thus require animals. Although rodents have been used for most experiments in the past, they are not the best animal model because their muscle metabolism is significantly different from that of humans. Swine would be a better choice.
- *Practical requirements*—Carnitine is sufficiently stable to withstand long-term storage. It does have a bitter aftertaste, but it can be masked with citrus flavor. Carnitine has been found to be safe under most circumstances. However, more is not necessarily better, and investigations of patients with different pathophysiologies have indicated that better results can sometimes be obtained with lower doses.

REFERENCES

Borum, P.R. 1983 Carnitine. Ann. Rev. Nutr. 3:233–259.

1986 Carnitine function. Pp. 16–27 in Clinical Aspects of Human Carnitine Deficiency, P.R. Borum, ed. New York: Pergamon Press.

1990 Carnitine: Determination of total carnitine using a radioenzymatic assay. J. Nutr. Biochem. 1:111–114.

1992 Medium chain triglycerides in formula for preterm neonates: Implications for hepatic and extrahepatic metabolism. J. Pediatr. 120:S139–S145.

Constantin-Teodosiu, D., J.I.Carlin, G.Cederblad, R.C.Harris, and E.Hultman 1991 Acetyl group accumulation and pyruvate dehydrogenase activity in human muscle during incremental exercise. Acta Physiol. Scand. 143:367–372.

Decombaz, J., B.Gmuender, G.Sierro, and P.Cerretelli 1992 Muscle carnitine after strenuous endurance exercise. J. Appl. Physiol. 72:423–427.

Dubelaar, M.L., C.M.H.B.Lucas, and W.C.Hülsmann 1991 Acute effect of L-carnitine on skeletal muscle force tests in dogs. Am. J. Physiol. Endocrinol. Metab. 260:E189–E193.

Gorostiaga, E.M., C.A.Maurer, and J.P.Eclache 1989 Decrease in respiratory quotient during exercise following L-carnitine supplementation. Int. J. Sports Med. 10:169–174.

Hiatt, W.R., J.G.Regensteiner, E.E.Wolfel, L.Ruff, and E.P.Brass 1989 Carnitine and acylcarnitine metabolism during exercise in humans. Dependence on skeletal muscle metabolic state. J. Clin. Invest. 84:1167–1173.

Oyono-Enguelle, S., H.Freund, C.Ott, M.Gartner, A.Heitz, J.Marbach, F.Maccari, A.Frey, H.Bigot, and A.C.Bach 1988 Prolonged submaximal exercise and L-carnitine in humans. Eur. J. Appl. Physiol. 58:53–61.

Siliprandi, N., F.Di Lisa, G.Pieralisi, P.Ripari, F.Maccari, R.Menabo, M.A.Giamberardino, and L.Vecchiet 1990 Metabolic changes induced by maximal exercise in human subjects following L-carnitine administration. Biochim. Biophys. Acta 1034:17–21.

Soop, M., O.Bjorkman, G.Cederblad, L.Hagenfeldt, and J.Wahren 1988 Influence of carnitine supplementation on muscle substrate and carnitine metabolism during exercise. J. Appl. Physiol. 64:2394–2399.

Spriet, L.L., D.J.Dyck, G.Cederblad, and E.Hultman 1992a Effects of fat availability on acetyl-CoA and acetylcarnitine metabolism in rat skeletal muscle. Am. J. Physiol. Cell Physiol. 263:C653–C659.

Spriet, L.L., D.A.MacLean, D.J.Dyck, E.Hultman, G.Cederblad, and T.E.Graham 1992b Caffeine ingestion and muscle metabolism during prolonged exercise in humans. Am. J. Physiol. Endocrinol. Metab. 262:E891–E898.

Turcotte, L.P., E.A.Richter, and B.Kiens 1992 Increased plasma FFA uptake and oxidation during prolonged exercise in trained vs. untrained humans. Am. J. Physiol. Endocrinol. Metab. 262:E791–E799.

Uziel, G., B.Garavaglia, and S.Di Donato 1988 Carnitine stimulation of pyruvate dehydrogenase complex (PDHC) in isolated human skeletal muscle mitochondria. Muscle Nerve 11:720–724.

Vecchiet, L., F.Di Lisa, G.Pieralisi, P.Ripari, R.Menabò, M.A.Giamberardino, and N.Siliprandi 1990 Influence of L-carnitine administration on maximal physical exercise. Eur. J. Appl. Physiol. 61:486–490.

DISCUSSION

GILERT LEVEILLE: Two questions. One, when we use acetyl or propionyl carnitine as an oral supplement, do we know if it is absorbed in that form?

PEGGY BORUM: That is being looked at. There are actually clinical trials that are ongoing with acetyl and propionyl, but I do not think that the data are in yet. There is some indication that what is happening is that the acetylcarnitine that is in the gastrointestinal tract is not the same molecule that gets into the bloodstream. Acetate may be removed from acetylcarnitine in one location of the cell and acetylcarnitine resynthesized in another location using a different acetate molecule.

PART VI

Safety and Regulatory Aspects of Potential Ration Enhancement

In PART VI THE FINAL TWO CHAPTERS address the safety and regulatory aspects of potential performance-enhancing food components. The first chapter is an overview of a recent report that reviewed amino acids. The final chapter addresses the regulation of food components by the U.S. Food and Drug Administration.

22

Safety Concerns Regarding Supplemental Amino Acids: Results of a Study

Timothy J.Maher[1]

INTRODUCTION

In the late summer and fall of 1989 there suddenly appeared a number of individuals who developed eosinophilia-myalgia syndrome (EMS) associated with the use of supplemental L-tryptophan (Hertzman et al., 1990; Kamb et al., 1992). This amino acid, which has been used for many years for its pharmacological properties (e.g., as a sedative-hypnotic, analgesic, and anorexiant), was available to consumers under the guise of a "dietary supplement" in health food stores, pharmacies and grocery or department stores (Young, 1986). More than 30 individuals died and many thousands were severely injured in the United States alone as a result of exposure to what is now believed to have been a contaminant in one manufacturer's L-tryptophan. This contaminant, 1,1'-ethylene-bis (tryptophan), commonly referred to as "Peak 97" or "Peak E," was produced during the manufacture of this amino acid (Mayeno et al., 1990). A number of other impurities have since been detected in implicated

[1] Timothy J.Maher, Professor and Chairman, Department of Pharmacology, Massachusetts College of Pharmacology, 179 Longwood Avenue, Boston, MA 02115

lots of L-tryptophan, the concentrations of which varied significantly over time as the manufacturer presumably modified synthesis and/or purification conditions during its quest to produce this amino acid more efficiently.

THE FASEB/LSRO STUDY

Largely as a result of the tragic EMS epidemic that resulted from the use of L-tryptophan, the U.S. Food and Drug Administration (FDA) contracted with the Life Sciences Research Office (LSRO) of the Federation of the American Societies for Experimental Biology (FASEB) to perform an extensive review of the scientific literature to determine the safety of amino acids used as dietary supplements (Federation of the American Societies for Experimental Biology, Life Sciences Research Office, 1992). Not only was L-tryptophan use to be assessed for safety, but in addition, all the available amino acids were to be evaluated, since prolonged daily ingestion of large quantities of these compounds as dietary supplements is known to occur.

In the fall of 1990, LSRO initiated the study by first searching the extant scientific literature for reports that related to the safety of amino acids. During February 1991, LSRO sponsored an open meeting where interested parties could present information and views related to this issue (U.S. Food and Drug Administration, 1990). Eight individuals made oral presentations, and 30 individuals or organizations later submitted written materials for consideration by LSRO. Following these activities, an ad hoc expert panel consisting of nine scientists was assembled. The panel met on four occasions during the subsequent year to advise LSRO on the adequacy of the available materials and to prepare a final report. In addition to assessing safety on the basis of information in the present literature, the report also contained suggested guidelines for future safety evaluations. This report was made available in the summer of 1992 (Anderson and Raiten, 1992).

RESULTS OF THE STUDY

The use of amino acids as dietary supplements created a serious dilemma in the evaluation of safety, since these substances are used primarily by consumers for presumed pharmacological purposes or for the enhancement of physiological function rather than for any nutritional purposes. There was no evidence available in the literature indicating that a normal, healthy individual would benefit nutritionally in any way from supplementation of the diet with a single amino acid. Even in those individuals with a less than ideal diet, the practice of supplementing the diet with single amino acids was considered potentially dangerous. Additionally, the literature was replete with studies demonstrating "antinutritional" effects (i.e., depressed growth and other adverse effects) associated with the intake of imbalanced amino acid diets (Benevenga and Steele, 1984).

Products in the marketplace that were surveyed were characterized by a wide diversity of label information and generally failed to provide the required information regarding chemical composition, isomeric identification, purity, shelf-life and contraindications to use. For instance, although some labels of products containing L-phenylalanine warned patients with phenylketonuria, others failed to do so. The potential for adverse effects associated with the ingestion of this amino acid in patients with this inherited metabolic abnormality are well documented (Lenke and Levy, 1980; Matalon et al., 1991).

Although manufacturers carefully avoid legal drug claim language on labels and advertising, many product labels and advertisments clearly suggested that such products provided pharmacological rather than nutritional benefit. No reliable information was available to accurately assess the patterns of consumption of these supplements in the U.S. population. The expert panel was aware of the use of D-amino acids as dietary supplements and concluded that such a practice was clearly inappropriate because these enantiomerically related amino acids have generally been shown to provide no nutritional support for humans and, in many cases, are potent toxicants (Friedman, 1991). Concern was also expressed regarding the interaction between amino acids used as dietary supplements and over-the-counter and prescription drugs, as this constitutes an area not adequately investigated to date. There are numerous examples in the literature detailing observed or potential interactions between these amino acids and monoamine oxidase inhibitors, many antidepressants, sympathomimetic amines, and opioids (Glassman and Platman, 1969; Hull and Maher, 1990).

As part of the scope of work associated with the FASEB/LSRO investigation, some estimate of the safe upper level of intake for each individual amino acid was requested. The expert panel was unable to identify a safe upper level for any of the amino acids considered, beyond that normally found in typical proteins. Additionally, the only safe form of amino acid ingestion was considered to be via protein in the diet.

Proposed Guidelines for Safety Evaluation

As a result of the paucity of available information bearing upon the safety of amino acids used as dietary supplements, the ad hoc expert panel concluded that a systematic approach to safety testing was needed. The proposed testing should involve studies in both animals and humans and should employ a two-tiered approach. In the first tier, studies with animals should investigate the effects of acute and chronic ingestion of amino acids. Such studies would include the determination of weight changes, food intake, neurological and behavioral changes, liver function, routine blood chemistry and hematological parameters, hormonal changes, and pharmacokinetic profiles following oral administration of the amino acid with and without food in both sexes. Multiple observation points would be used throughout the studies, and various doses would be employed. The expert panel suggested doses of 3, 10, 30, and 100 times the nutritional requirements for indispensable amino acids and 3, 10, 30 and 100 times the levels permitted for protein fortification for the dispensible amino acids (21 CFR 172.320). Teratologic and developmental effects would also be ascertained simultaneously during this preliminary testing phase. On the basis of the findings of those studies and the existing literature, specialized studies would then be performed during the second tier. The second-tier studies would include functional assessment and gross pathological examinations.

Following studies in animals, acute and chronic testing in humans would be required to satisfy additional safety concerns. Growth, neurological and behavioral function, hematological parameters, pharmacokinetic profiles, and hormonal changes would be monitored following exposure to various doses of the selected amino acids. Although initial studies should be carried out in normal healthy adult volunteers, additional studies should use selected groups of individuals who might be expected to use the particular amino acid, e.g., athletes and bodybuilders. Since certain subsets of the population, e.g., infants, children, adolescents, pregnant and lactating women, and elderly individuals, might be expected to be at greater risk of adverse effects from ingestion of particular amino acids, they should be excluded from such studies. Additionally, persons with specific diseases or conditions, e.g., diabetes mellitus, endocrine disorders, hepatic disease, or other conditions, should similarly be excluded from this phase of investigation. Special precautions would be required to address safety concerns in these subgroups, and studies in these subgroups should be performed only after a reasonable degree of safety has been established.

SUMMARY AND RECOMMENDATIONS

The FASEB/LSRO report on the safety of amino acids as dietary supplements concluded the following:

- There is no nutritional rationale to the use of amino acids as dietary supplements, and such a practice can be dangerous.
- Supplemental amino acids are used for pharmacological rather than nutritional purposes.

- Currently available labeling fails to supply the required information on a routine basis.
- The extant scientific literature fails to support a safe upper limit for supplementation with any amino acid beyond that found in protein.
- There are several subsets of the population that are likely to be more sensitive to the adverse effects of amino acid supplementation.
- Systematic testing in animals and humans is required before the safety of supplemental amino acids can be adequately assessed.

It is therefore recommended by this author that any approach to the fortification of military rations with supplemental amino acids beyond those levels found in protein should be considered a pharmacological intervention and not merely a nutritional manipulation, and thus should be initiated with appropriate caution to safeguard the welfare of those who consume military rations.

REFERENCES

Anderson, S.A., and O.J.Raiten (eds.) 1992 Safety of amino acids used as dietary supplements. Bethesda, MD: FASEB.

Benevenga, N.J., and R.D.Steele 1984 Adverse effects of excessive consumption of amino acids. Annu. Rev. Nutr. 4:157–181.

Federation of the American Societies for Experimental Biology, Life Sciences Research Office 1992 Safety of amino acids used as dietary supplements. Center for Food Safety and Applied Nutrition. FDA Contract No. 223–88–2124, Task No. 8.

Food and Drug Administration 1990 Evaluation of the safety of amino acids and related products; announcement of study; request for scientific data and information; announcement of open meeting. Fed. Regist. 55:49141–49142.

Friedman, M. 1991 Formation, nutritional value, and safety of D-amino acids. Pp. 447–481 in Nutritional and Toxicological Consequences of Food Processing. New York: Plenum Press.

Glassman, A.H., and S.R.Platman 1969 Potentiation of a monoamine oxidase inhibitor by tryptophan. J. Psychiatric Res. 7:83–88.

Hertzman, P.A., W.L.Blevins, J.Mayer, B.Greenfield, M.Ting, and G.J.Gleich 1990 Association of the eosinophilia-myalgia syndrome with the ingestion of tryptophan. N. Engl. J. Med. 322:869–873.

Hull, K.M., and T.J.Maher 1990 L-Tyrosine potentiates the anorexia induced by mixed-acting sympathomimetic drugs in hyperphagic rats. J. Pharmacol. Exp. Ther. 255:403–409.

Kamb, M.L., J.J.Murphy, J.L.Jones, J.C.Caston, K.Nederlof, L.F.Horney, L.A.Swygert, H.Falk, and E.M.Kilbourne 1992 Eosinophilia-myalgia syndrome in L-tryptophan-exposed patients. J. Am. Med. Assoc. 267:77–82.

Lenke, R.R., and H.L.Levy 1980 Maternal phenylketonuria and hyperphenylalaninemia: An international survey of the outcome of untreated and treated pregnancies. N. Engl. J. Med. 303:1202–1208.

Matalon, R., K.Michals, C.Azen, E.G.Friedman, R.Koch, E.Wenz, H.Levy, F.Rohr, B. Rouse, L.Castiglioni, W.Hanley, V.Austin, and F.de la Cruz 1991 Maternal PKU collaborative study: The effect of nutrient intake on pregnancy outcome. J. Inherit. Metab. Dis. 14:371–374.

Mayeno, A.N., F.Lin, C.S.Foote, D.A.Loegering, M.M.Ames, C.W.Hedberg, and G.J.Gleich 1990 Characterization of “Peak E,” a novel amino acid associated with eosinophilia-myalgia syndrome. Science 250:1707–1708.

Young, S.N. 1986 The clinical psychopharmacology of tryptophan. Pp. 49–88 In Nutrition and the Brain, R.J.Wurtmen and J.J.Wurtman, eds. Vol. 7. New York: Raven Press.

23

Regulation of Amino Acids and Other Dietary Components Associated with Enhanced Physical Performance1

John E.Vanderveen[2]

INTRODUCTION

In the discussions in this volume of research on the use of amino acids and other dietary components to affect physical and mental performance, one question was asked repeatedly: "Is this substance a food or a drug?" Researchers and potential suppliers of these substances are motivated to ask that question because different regulations apply to drugs and foods. These differences include the labeling of the product, requirements for premarketing approval, practices required during manufacturing, the records that must be maintained during production and manufacturing, and the way in which the substance is dispensed. The question also has a profound impact on how the safety of the substance is addressed and what claim can be made for the substance in relation to disease.

The answer to the question depends on answers to a number of other questions, including what the substance is and what it contains, how it is used,

[1] The views expressed in this chapter reflect the policy of the Food and Drug Administration at the time of the CMNR Workshop in November, 1992. In the future the policy may be revised to meet legislative mandates or public health needs.

[2] John E.Vanderveen, Director, Office of Plant and Dairy Foods and Beverages, Food and Drug Administration, 200 C Street, S.W., Washington, DC 20204

what claims are being made for it, its history of use, its safety under the conditions of use, and how it is administered. The answers to these questions help to classify the substance in accordance with statutory and case law and in implementing regulations.

The Federal Food, Drug, and Cosmetic Act (FD&C Act) defines the term *food* as articles used for food or drink for humans or animals, chewing gum, and articles used as components of any other such article (United States Code §321 [f]). In case law the term *food* in the first part of this definition has been further defined as articles consumed primarily for their taste, aroma, or nutritive value (Nutrilab, Inc. vs. Schweiker, 1993). The FD&C Act defines the term *drug* as articles recognized in the official *United States Pharmacopeia,* the official *Homeopathic Pharmacopeia of the United States,* the official *National Formulary,* or supplements to any of them; (United States Code §321[a]), articles intended for use in the diagnosis, cure, mitigation, treatment, or prevention of disease in humans or animals; articles (other than food) intended to affect the structure or any function of the bodies of humans or animals; and articles intended for use as components of any articles specified above.

There is some overlap in the definitions of foods and drugs. Therefore, it is not always possible to categorize a substance as either a food or a drug without knowing how it is being used or the claims being made for it. Occasionally, a substance is both a food and a drug. For example, prescribing niacin for an individual to meet his or her nutritional needs is a nutritional function; however, if large amounts are given to lower high blood cholesterol levels, it can be argued that it is not serving as a nutrient but has an effect on a function of the body and therefore is a drug. As Timothy Maher indicated in Chapter 22, an amino acid is generally considered to be a food, but if that amino acid is marketed as a remedy for sleep disorders, depression, premenstrual syndrome, and other medical conditions, then it would be classified as a drug.

Several times during the November 1992 workshop it was suggested that a therapeutic amount of a nutrient was used, therefore, it was a drug and not a food. On one occasion it was stated another way: "The amount needed to show an effect was many times higher than human nutritional requirements and therefore was clearly a drug amount." In the early 1960s, the U.S. Food and Drug Administration (FDA) decided that the use of vitamins A and D above 150 percent of the U.S. Recommended Dietary Allowance (U.S. RDA) was a drug use. The agency argued that use of amounts of these vitamins above 150 percent of the U.S. RDA clearly had no nutritional value and the vitamins were therefore taken for their pharmacological effects. The FDA was challenged for this regulatory position, and the court ruled that just because a supplement exceeded a nutritional requirement level, there was no legal basis to declare the product a drug (The National Nutritional Foods Association and Solgar Co., Inc. vs. Food and Drug Administration, 1974).

A long-standing policy of FDA is that the route of administration may determine whether the substance is a drug or a food. According to thispolicy, foods are only consumed enterally (through the digestive tract), whereas drugs are consumed both enterally and parenterally (outside the digestive tract). In a case currently pending, a court is deciding whether the absorption of vitamin B_{12} through the nasal membranes makes the vitamin a drug. At this time, the FDA considers any substance that is injected or otherwise administered through the skin and that has a metabolic effect to be a drug.

For years, FDA's policy was to treat any label claim that purported benefits relative to a disease or condition as grounds for automatically subjecting the food to drug regulations. This position was based on the definition of a drug in the FD&C Act. It was also part of the original nutrition labeling regulations published in 1973 (Code of Federal Register, 1973). The Nutrition Labeling and Education Act of 1990 (NLEA) provided the FDA with the authority to publish regulations that would allow manufactures to provide specific health claims on food labels to describe a nutrient-disease relationship but they would not be required to call the product a drug (United States Congress, 1990). However, the provisions of the NLEA establish specific criteria as to when such claims are permitted. In brief, such claims must be based on all publicly available scientific literature, and experts knowledgeable about the relationship must substantially agree that the claim may be permitted.

In considering the issue of safety, the FD&C Act requires that a food be safe, as judged by the standard that there is reasonable certainty that no harm will be done when the food is consumed as intended. Unlike a drug, no risk-benefit standard is applied for a food. Consequently, a substance that presents some risk of harm and that is used to maintain or improve performance would likely be considered a drug and would be subject to drug regulations. Finally, use of a product that contains measurable amounts of one or more essential nutrients usually implies food status, but other factors such as safety are important overriding considerations.

Under the FD&C Act, several categories of food ingredients have a long history of safe use. In 1958, an amendment to the FD&C Act created two new categories for these food ingredients. One category was based largely on history of use and was referred to in the Act as generally recognized as safe (GRAS) (United States Code, §321[s]). Those substances in use before the passage of the 1958 amendment were automatically given GRAS status. Many, but not all, of these substances have been subjected to an affirmation process to ensure their safety at levels traditionally used in foods. The agency mounted a major effort to affirm the safety of these GRAS substances. Data on use levels were gathered by the Committee on GRAS Substances of the Food and

Nutrition Board, National Academy of Sciences; safety data were assembled by the Special Committee on GRAS Substances, which was established by the Life Sciences Research Office of the Federation of the American Societies for Experimental Biology (FASEB).

Foods not in use before 1958 can gain official GRAS status through a petition process. The petition must demonstrate that the substance is safe at the levels of intended use. For example, rapeseed oil (canola oil) with low erucic acid content was affirmed as GRAS as a result of a petition by the Canadian government (Federal Register, 1984). Regardless of how GRAS status is obtained for a substance, the determination is usually based on specific levels of use. If new uses developed for the substance require higher levels of that substance, then additional assessments must be made to gain official GRAS status for the new levels of use.

Still other substances are claimed to have GRAS status as a result of the manufacturer's self-determination. Such determinations have been made for substances with no history of use, such as some protein isolates, and new higher levels of use have been made for GRAS substances that were not part of the affirmation process. Examples of the latter are some plant gums and pectin, which are used to increase the fiber content of foods. These products are likely to remain in the marketplace as long as the agency is not confronted with a scientific basis to challenge the safety of the substance. However, any data that raise safety concerns must be addressed by sound scientific arguments; otherwise, there will be a legal basis for removing the substance from the food supply. In addition to a potentially costly recall, a manufacturer would likely be fully responsible for any harm to consumers caused by the use of the substance. A review of the safety data by an independent authoritative scientific body may lower this risk.

New food ingredients that do not fit in any of the GRAS categories are food additives (United States Code §321[s]). Approval to market a food additive is gained by submitting a petition to the FDA with sufficient data to demonstrate reasonable certainty of no harm at the intended levels of use. Regulations for food additives often differ from those for GRAS substances; greater specificity is associated with both levels and conditions of use, and new additional uses for an approved food additive automatically require a separate petition. Procedures for filing a food additive petition are included in FDA regulations. The compositions of both food additive and GRAS substances must be known, and methods must exist for analyzing the substances in foods. Food additives that have harmful contaminants such as natural toxins, heavy metals, and microorganisms will not be approved. Evidence that a food additive is free of such harmful substances must be provided as part of the petition.

Among food products, dietary supplements are subject to certain provisions of the FD&C (United States Code §350). Dietary supplements include vitamins and essential mineral supplements, other essential nutrients such as amino acids, and nonessential substances such as herbal products. In 1978, an amendment to the FD&C Act placed limitations on how the potencies of vitamins and essential mineral supplements can be regulated. This so-called Proxmire Amendment prohibits the agency from using any regulatory authorities in the FD&C except those for food additives for regulating the potencies of vitamins and mineral supplements. Essentially, the only limitations that can be imposed on these products are those associated with safety. Other types of dietary supplements are not covered by the Proxmire Amendment and therefore are subject to other food provisions of the FD&C Act relative to potency. It is important, however, that this category of food has been afforded special status relative to claims for one year under the Dietary Supplement Act of 1992 (United States Congress, 1992), and the agency is required to propose new rules for regulating these substances.

Regardless of the category to which a new substance belongs, safety data are necessary before the substance can be legally marketed. Research conducted on animals usually provides much of the data on which safety assessments are based; however, clinical data are increasingly important in situations in which a substance is intended to have an effect on body structure or function. Clinical studies conducted on an unapproved substance that will be marketed as a drug require an Investigational New Drug application (IND). An IND provides a useful mechanism for obtaining the authority to conduct tests on substances that affect body structure or function but that will eventually be marketed as a food. Obtaining an IND for such testing provides some measure of protection if problems are incurred during the research. Clearly, the sponsor will still be responsible for any harm caused by the use of the product, but acquisition of an approved IND will demonstrate an effort to comply with the law and perform such tests in a safe manner. The requirements for obtaining an IND are not complicated, especially for small clinical studies involving 50 or fewer subjects. The following must be provided: (1) data on the toxicology of the product (usually obtained from animal studies), (2) chemical data indicating the purity of the test substance, (3) procedures for obtaining informed consent for the study, (4) evidence of approval of an institutional review board, and (5) the study protocol. The FD&C Act gives FDA the authority to grant permission for clinical testing of unapproved food additives; however, no regulations have been created to implement this provision of the act.

With regard to the regulatory status of amino acids and other dietary components associated with enhanced physical performance, the agency first addressed the addition of amino acids to foods in 1945 (Food and Drug

Administration, 1945). In a Trade Correspondence, the agency indicated that such a food was considered to be a food for special dietary use and would have to be labeled to conform to applicable regulations. The agency also indicated that amino acid preparations for oral use may in some cases also be subject to the drug provisions of the act. Amino acids were listed on the original GRAS list under "nutrients and/or dietary supplements" in 1961 (Federal Register, 1961). In 1972, the agency proposed that the GRAS status of all amino acids for nutritive purposes be revoked (Federal Register, 1972). A food additive regulation was proposed, setting out the conditions under which amino acids used as food additives may be safely added to intact, protein-containing foods that were considered significant sources of dietary protein. The proposal stated that this action did not include amino acids in foods that did not contain intact protein in their original form. The FDA finalized the regulations in 1973 (Federal Register, 1973). In so doing, the agency stated that it wanted to prevent the random addition of amino acids to foods and limited the approved use of amino acids as additives to foods in which intact protein primarily occurred naturally. From 1973 to 1977, all amino acids were listed as "not GRAS" as a nutrient and/or dietary supplement and were subject to the food additive regulation. However, in 1977 the Code of Federal Regulations involving foods was recodified, and by error, L-tryptophan was listed as GRAS. At the same time, the agency seized two quantities of L-tryptophan being sold as dietary supplements on the grounds that the L-tryptophan in these supplements was an unapproved food additive. The court ruled that the claimant was entitled to rely on the GRAS list as published (Federal Register, 1993). The agency corrected the error but took no action because of other priorities. The industry maintains that those amino acids that were in the marketplace are safe and are GRAS on the basis of self-determination. The FDA's position is that amino acids cannot be GRAS because there was a determination through public rule making that supported the agency's assessment that free amino acids are not GRAS.

In 1991, the agency removed L-tryptophan supplements from the market after it was discovered that they were associated with the eosinophilia myalgia syndrome (EMS), which reportedly caused the deaths of at least 38 individuals and serious illness in more than 1,500 others (Varga, et al., 1992). Following this serious incident, the agency contracted with the Life Sciences Research Office (LSRO) of FASEB to review the existing data on the safety of all amino acids. The FASEB report that was discussed by Timothy Maher in Chapter 22 the result of that effort (LSRD, 1992) (FASEB, 1992). The FDA is reviewing the report and is considering appropriate action. Clearly, many individuals consumed L-tryptophan supplements without apparent harm. There is significant evidence that EMS may have been caused, or at least made worse, by a contaminant in the L-tryptophan supplements. Until there is clear evidence that such a contaminant was the cause of EMS, however, it would be unlawful to market L-tryptophan as a food except in accordance with the food additive regulation (Code of Federal Regulations, 1993). In light of the events surrounding amino acids, the commissioner of FDA has created a task force to develop options for regulating all dietary supplements. The report of that task force will soon be released for public comment as part of the agency's process of reviewing current policy for regulating these products (Food and Drug Administration, 1992).

The situation is perhaps different for other nutrients that are on the GRAS list as nutrient supplements, dietary supplements, or other functions. One could argue that a nutrient found to be effective for some function could be declared GRAS by a manufacturer or a distributor. As indicated earlier, such a position is not without risk. On the other hand, if the FDA has affirmed the substance as GRAS or has approved it as a food additive for one or more intended uses, there is assurance that the agency will not take action against the product. Furthermore, it stands to reason that an approval based on an independent review of the safety data will increase the chances of no harm.

A more interesting question will be whether the substance is a drug on the basis of its stated function. For example, if the function is described as preventing drowsiness or fatigue, then clearly the product is a drug. On the other hand, if the claim is that a substance maintains performance, alertness, or effectiveness, is it a drug claim? Perhaps an argument could be made that these are food claims, but the final determination may actually depend on other factors. Another important question is whether there is some element of risk of harm. If so, then the substance may fall in the category of a drug, which allows for some risk-benefit consideration. How will the product be administered? If the answer is by injection, then clearly the substance is a drug. Finally, what is the history of use? If the substance was consumed before 1958 as a food at the level found to satisfy some nutritional function and the manufacturer does not make drug claims, then it is likely a food.

CONCLUSIONS

In summary, the regulation of amino acids and other dietary components associated with maintaining or enhancing physical performance is dependent on the substance, the safety of the substance at the level of use, the way in which it is administered, its history of use, and the claims made for it. Approval for the use of a substance either as a drug or as a food will require data on its composition, toxicity, and function. In addition, drug approval requires data on effectiveness but allows for approval on the basis of a risk-benefit analysis, whereas food use does not. Self-declaration of GRAS status by a producer or a supplier, although practiced for some dietary supplements, places both the researcher and the subject at increased risk. Research conducted under an IND lowers the risk to the subject and the investigator and provides an atmosphere of trust.

REFERENCES

Code of Federal Regulations 1973 Food: Nutrition Labeling, 21CFR 38(49), 6959–6961.
Code of Federal Regulations. 1993 Amino Acids 21CFR 172.320, 38–40.
Federal Register. 1984 Rapeseed Oil. 49(31):5613.
Federal Register. 1961 Substances Generally Recognized as Safe. 26:1444.
Federal Register. 1972 Amino Acids in Food for Human Consumption. 37(67):6938–6940.
Federal Register. 1973 Amino Acids in Food for Human Comsumption. 38(143):20036–20057.
Federal Register 1993 Amino Acids. 58(116):33696.
Federation of the American Societies for Experimental Biology, Life Sciences Research Office 1992 Safety of amino acids used as dietary supplements. Center for Food Safety and Applied Nutrition. FDA Contract No. 223–88–2124, Task No. 8.
Food and Drug Administration. 1945 Statement Relating to the Use of Amino Acids in Foods and Drugs, FD&C Act Trade Correspondence. TC 2-A.
Food and Drug Administration. 1992 Task Force of Dietary Supplements, Final Report. FDA. The National Nutritional Foods Association and Solgar Co., Inc. vs. Food and Drug
1974 Administration, 491 F. 2d 1141 (2nd Cir.).
Nutriab, Inc. vs. Schweiker, 731 F. 2nd 335 (7th Cir.).
United States Code §321(f). 21 U.S.C. The Food, Drug, and Cosmetic Act of 1938 as amended. See §201(f).
United States Code §321(g). 21 U.S.C. The Food, Drug, and Cosmetic Act of 1938 as amended. See §201(g).
United States Code §321(s). 21 U.S.C. The Food, Drug, and Cosmetic Act of 1938 as amended. See §201(s).
United States Code §350. 21 U.S.C. The Food, Drug, and Cosmetic Act of 1938 as amended. See §411.
United States Congress. 1990 (Public Law 101–535) Nutrition Labeling and Education Act of 1990 104 STAT. 2353–2367.
United States Congress 1992 (Public Law 102–571). Dietary Supplement Act of 1992.

Varga, J., J.Uilto, and S.Jimenez. 1992 The Cause and Phaogenesis of Eosinophilia-Myalgia Syndrome. Annals of Internal Medicine 116:140–147.

DISCUSSION

ELDON ASKEW: Let me get to the heart of the issue: Say we take some applesauce, put some tyrosine in it, and give it to a soldier with instructions on the outside saying, "Take when exposed to cold or high-altitude stress." What problems are we running into there?

JOHN VANDERVEEN: If you want it to be recognized as a food, I would prefer you did not say "stress." I would prefer that you say, "This will maintain your performance," and then I can say it is a food. When you say "stress," I think that you are in a situation in which you may be making a drug claim. If it is a drug claim, FDA is going to ask you for an IND and will you have to go through that process. Not that I think that is a bad thing to do. If you are going to do research in this area, you may want to be in the IND category. Let me just say that you are taking a risk, by saying that applesauce with tyrosine was going to maintain performance without new safety data, you take the risk of the FDA determining that this was an unapproved use for tyrosine, and that should be made abundantly clear. Futhermore, if you look at the billions of dollars of lawsuits against the manufacturers and suppliers of L-tryptophan at the moment, it becomes evident that there is financial risk too. Even FDA becomes vulnerable by not providing consumer protection. It is a very serious situation. I do not know the answer to that.

DAVID SCHNAKENBERG: Who, in essence, when we talk about a scientist within a federal laboratory, is taking the risk: the individual scientist or the FDA? I presume it is the FDA.

JOHN VANDERVEEN: Some of that has changed, and you have to be very careful. Individuals now, at least civilians, can be sued along with the FDA. I do not know the real answers to that. I think you have to be very cautious and really ask your Inspector General (IG) where you are in that situation. I think that is very clear.

DAVID SCHNAKENBERG: Do you have the same thing with tyrosine? What if we had the same thing with glucose, which we used to enhance performance, and someone got hurt?

JOHN VANDERVEEN: I think you have more protection, because glucose is an approved food additive at any level. It is a carbohydrate, and we do not have a limit on the use of carbohydrates.

IRWIN TAUB: It becomes a semantics problem, and we have to deal with those semantics. You have clearly stated that as long as we are approving structured function of the body, we can use such ingredients. I am not going to say "amino acids"; I will say "ingredients." Furthermore, basically, if you also said in your definition that a food is used to support life (that is somehow included in the reply), part of life is to perform work. You determine your nutrients on the basis of what you have to do, and that becomes the required daily allowance, so we are saying here that performance of the kind of work that a soldier or anyone else has to do is simply going to require certain levels of ingredients, and again, I will use the word *ingredients.* As long as we stick to that and avoid words like *stress,* for example, I will say that under all conditions, we do not have to spell out what those conditions are; there is no longer a special case.

Just one last point about this, which is, we do not necessarily have to use the pure amino acid. We can use some natural ingredient that converts to those amino acids. There are many amino acids in soy protein and hydrolyzed vegetable protein. We use them for flavor and maybe we can use them for performance, as long as the distribution is right. By your definition, is it not true that we could be safe under the law?

JOHN VANDERVEEN: Approved ingredients can be used in it; there is no question there. The difficulty with amino acids, as Timothy Maher pointed out, is the fact that the FDA made a conscious decision in 1973 that they were not safe to be used individually. What data was used to arrive at this decision is not entirely clear. I tried to look back over the record, but unfortunately, the total record is no longer available. It has apparently been destroyed.

What we do have is what has been published in the *Federal Register,* and you can see that. We had a number of consultants. We had Dr. Alfred Harper and others who were knowledgeable about the metabolism of amino acids, and FDA decided that it was not appropriate to leave them on the GRAS list, so we took them off. And then FDA said that they could be used for a number of things but in very trivial amounts. Small amounts could be used for technological purposes, and then FDA said that larger amounts could be used to improve protein quality.

That is the difficulty we are in on the amino acids. On other things, of course, if you wanted to increase your omega-3 fatty acid level, you could buy an oil that has omega-3 fatty acid in it. As you say, you may even be able to get hydrolyzed vegetable protein, which is an ingredient that can be and is used.

One thing I did not say, of course, is that Good Manufacturing Practice is always implied in good manufacturing practices, and so as a consequence, you have to keep that in the general context. I think you are right, however, I think you could approach it in that manner, but you have to be cautious. It is a semantics problem.

ROBERT NESHEIM: How about a real simple one like caffeine? Two hundred milligrams in a tablet is a drug, and 600 milligrams in four or five cups of coffee would be a food.

JOHN VANDERVEEN: Caffeine is an approved food additive. It was obviously used in soft drink beverages.

ROBERT NESHEIM: But if we took it in a tablet like No-Doz, is that classified as a drug?

JOHN VANDERVEEN: Again, it depends on what you are taking it for.

ROBERT NESHEIM: It depends on the claim.

JOHN VANDERVEEN: The claim that it is being used for. Are you taking it to avoid drowsiness? That may be considered a drug.

HARRIS LIEBERMAN: How about what you said to maintain alertness?

UNIDENTIFIED SPEAKER: I have a question that relates to liability. If we made a product that, let's say, had peanuts in it and this individual was allergic to peanuts and died, can we be sued for that?

JOHN VANDERVEEN: Well, peanuts are clearly permitted in the food supply, and that is a food that has been around for a long time. By history of use, I doubt seriously if you could be considered liable. But now, you see, as part of the Nutrition Labeling and Education Act of 1990, you have to include all ingredients, regardless of the product, even if it is one ingredient. You have to tell the person that there is peanuts in it.

UNIDENTIFIED SPEAKER: I guess what I was driving at is the genetic variation that you see, that you mentioned, that somebody is going to be invariably susceptible to these products. How are you going to find out who is going to be susceptible, or are you liable?

JOANNA DWYER: Just one question, John. I am from a family of lawyers so I am familiar with weasel words. You know, every meal is something of semantics, but the thing I wonder about, you must forgive my ignorance, if the group here in the Army feeds soldiers substances, am I to understand that if it is considered a drug, that there has to be an IND? If I fed choline or something at New England Medical Center, is it pretty much the same situation?

JOHN VANDERVEEN: Actually, that is another point. The Army can do whatever it pleases because it is not subject to the Food, Drug, and Cosmetic Act per se. The problem they get into, as I understand it, is that their IG said, look, we are not going to take that risk; you are only going to use substances that are approved for use, and I think that is basically the philosophy that is now prevailing. But for years, when I was with DOD I ate irradiated food when it was not approved by the FDA. I was working for the Air Force and when the National Aeronautics and Space Administration (NASA) decided to use these same products for space flight. When they had the recent problem in NASA with the *Challenger,* their IG came out and said, you were feeding irradiated food and it was not approved by the FDA. As a result, the FDA got a letter from Richard Truly, the NASA administrator saying, wouldn't you approve the use of the irradiated food for use on board the shuttle, and we said "sure," and that took care of it.

DAVID SCHNAKENBERG: A related thing could come down the road: We could have a product intended for use just for military populations on the Meal Ready-to-Eat (MRE). However, when MREs get to the soldiers, it is now common practice through our Defense Personnel Subsistence Agency for those products to end up in the marketplace. They are given food relief; sometimes it is the Kurds, sometimes it is the Somali children, other times it is homeless people, and sometimes it is advertently or inadvertently resold, and then there we come into an issue.

JOHN VANDERVEEN: I do not think that this is an insurmountable problem. I think that you can go ahead and do what you want and need to do; it is just that you probably have to ask and get the agency to focus on your problem. We (FDA, CFSAN) have been reorganized as of last Monday and now there is an Office of Pre-Market Approval, which should help things to move smoothly.

FREDERICK MANNING: I was going to bring up by suggesting we really need to interact with the agency, but I was sort of taking off on your comment by the IG. I think we have to recognize as hard as we are working to be inside the law here that the military, at least in the eyes of the media, if not the general public, is somewhat suspect and that is why the IG says down here, if you are exempt or if you are not covered by the law, I want you to do it anyway. We have numerous examples here coming out of the Gulf. So that I think we need to think very carefully about whether we want to be ahead of the mainstream on this one. Even if it is legal, we may want to think about possible public relations disasters from pushing the envelope.

ELDON ASKEW: I tend to agree with John Vanderveen that the problem is not insurmountable with regard to the issue that David Schnakenberg raised. People do not go into the Army-Navy Surplus Store to buy a BD boost and then turn around and sue the Army because they get frozen toes. There is a precedent for that sort of thing, so I do not think we are getting in real deep trouble there, although it is certainly something to think about.

APPENDIXES

A. Scenarios that Illustrate Potential Usefulness of Food Components to Enhance Performance
B. Military Recommended Dietary Allowances, AR 40–25 (1985)
C. A Selected Bibliography on an Evaluation of Potential Performance-Enhancing Food Components for Operational Rations
D. Biographical Sketches

A

Scenarios that Illustrate Potential Usefulness of Food Components to Enhance Performance

Harris R.Lieberman[1]

and

Mary Z.Mays

On the following pages are seven scenarios, based on Army research experience, which illustrate possible applications of food components to enhance performance. These scenarios were developed at the request of the Committee on Military Nutrition Research (CMNR) during planning for the workshop, *An Evaluation of Potential Performance Enhancing Food Components for Operational Rations,* in order to provide a framework for the understanding of the committee members and speakers. These scenarios are presented to enable the reader to better understand the context within which this report was developed.

[1] Harris R.Lieberman, U.S. Army Research Institute of Environmental Medicine, ATTN: SGRD-UE-OPS, Natick, MA 01760–5007

How might nutrients be employed to enhance the mental performance of military forces? On occasion drugs have been effectively employed to enhance the mental performance of soldiers and other professionals performing similar duties. Therefore, in some instances, the effective use of drugs as performance enhancing agents may provide a model for the use of nutrients.

1. Scenario: Operations by all types of units during moderate and intensive combat or other continuous operations. Not only do combat soldiers engaged in combat operations need to continuously perform for many days with minimal rest, but critical support units (medical, supply, etc.) also need to work continuously. Severe sleep loss in inevitable. Virtually every form of cognitive and psychomotor performance deteriorates under such conditions. While impaired performance of combat troops would have severe consequences, the failure of support units to accomplish their duties could also be catastrophic.

   Amphetamine, and related compounds, are classic examples of performance-enhancing agents. Sleep deprivation studies lasting 60 hours have demonstrated that stimulant drugs, and caffeine to a lesser extent, clearly ameliorate the deficits in performance associated with significant sleep deprivation. This is an issue of great practical importance. For example, soldiers on long range patrols may require stimulants when they need to hastily return to base after completing a mission. Pilots may need stimulants when they are required to fly long missions. It is anticipated that continuous operations will be more likely in the future because technologic advances have made it easier to conduct nighttime operations.
2. Scenario: Sentry duty, watching a radar screen, listening to sonar and other military tasks that require sustained vigilance. It has been suggested that many critical mistakes occur as a result of boredom rather than excess operator workload. Routine day-to-day operations often require sustained vigilance and, even during wartime, crews can become bored and lose concentration. It was reported in the press that the crews of Patriot missile batteries in Saudi Arabia consumed large quantities of caffeine-containing beverages to maintain alertness when on duty. Simulator studies and laboratory research with caffeine support its utility in situations where vigilance must be maintained. Nutritional stimulants might be helpful when crew members must maintain vigilance for long periods of time.
3. Scenario: Intense and moderate combat where psychological stress leads to extreme fear and anxiety. Of special interest to the military would be agents that prevent acute combat stress syndrome, previously known as battle fatigue. In intense combat even highly motivated, well trained troops may suffer

significant attrition from this syndrome. Treatments that could prevent it would be invaluable.

4. Scenario: Impaired performance due to exposure to extreme environmental conditions. Treatments that reduce the adverse effects of environmental extremes on mental performance would be useful. Hypobaric hypoxia readily impairs performance. Soldiers may be rapidly deployed to high altitudes without time for acclimatization. Acetazolamide appears to enhance cognitive performance impaired by acute hypoxia. Temperature extremes can also affect brain function. Tyrosine, because it seems to reduce some of the adverse effects of acute stress, is a nutrient of interest for this application.
5. Scenario: Cognitive function, memory and judgement are clouded by information overload and stress. Virtually any task that is carried out by a soldier has a memory and cognitive component. They are especially critical at the command level. Although there are no compounds that reliably enhance memory or other higher level cognitive functions, a food constituent that sustains memory when soldiers are exposed to stress would be of great use to the military.
6. Scenario: In general, the unpredictability of combat means that soldiers may have to sleep whenever they have the opportunity, not necessarily when they are tired or relaxed. In addition, abrupt changes in duty hours are not uncommon. Conventional hypnotics, and also the nutrient tryptophan, have been tested as agents to speed reentrainment to new duty cycles. There are reports that British aircrews used benzodiazepines during the Falklands conflict, so that they could sleep during off-duty hours. Similar agents might be used to prevent jet lag and to speed entrainment to new work schedules. Agents that will assist soldiers to sleep are of great interest, however they must not impair performance, either after the designated sleep period, or if soldiers must be suddenly awakened. The hormone melatonin may be beneficial in such circumstances.
7. Scenario: Impaired fine motor performance due to acute stress. Snipers, tank gunners, and bombardiers are all required to maintain fine motor control under severely stressful conditions. Beta-adrenergic blockers have reportedly been used to enhance the performance of individuals engaged in a variety of situations including pistol marksmanship competitions, public speaking and concert performances, Presumably, such drugs reduce the peripheral consequences of acute stress, such as tremor, and therefore enhance performance and possibly reduce subjective perception of stress. They also may have direct central effects on higher level functions as well. Specialized units might employ nutrients with such effects; e.g. tank gunners, snipers.

B

Military Recommended Dietary Allowances, AR 40–25 (1985)

The most recent revision of the Military Recommended Dietary Allowances (MRDAs) are included in Army Regulation 40–25 (U.S. Army, 1985). The entire regulation has been included on the following pages for reference and comparison with existing RDAs. No changes other than page formatting were made to the text. Note that this regulation is a joint regulation and presents the nutrition responsibilities for the Army, Navy, and Air Force. As stated in Chapter 1, AR 40–25 is currently undergoing revision. Further information concerning this regulation can be obtained by writing to: Headquarters, Department of the Army (SGPS-CO-B), 5109 Leesburg Pike, Falls Church, VA 22041–2358. Copies of the original AR 40–25 can be obtained by writing to the address listed at the end of the regulation.

Headquarters Departments of the Army, the Navy, and the Air Force Washington, DC 15 May 1985	*Army Regulation 40–25/Naval Command Medical Instruction 10110.1/Air Force Regulation 160–95

Medical Services
Nutrition Allowances, Standards, and Education

Summary. This joint regulation on nutrition allowances, standards, and education has been revised. It defines the nutrition responsibilities of The Surgeons General of the Army, the Navy, and the Air Force. This regulation—

a. Provides a current statement of the military recommended dietary allowances.
b. Sets nutrient standards for packaged rations.
c. Provides a standardized nutrient density index for normal and reduced calorie menu planning.
d. Provides nutrition education guidance to assist the military in promoting a healthful diet.

Applicability. This regulation applies to all active elements of the Army, Navy, and Air Force. It also applies to the Reserve Components of these Services.

Impact on New Manning System. This regulation does not contain information that affects the New Manning System.

Supplementation. Supplementation of and exceptions to this regulation are prohibited without prior approval from HQDA (DASG-PSP), WASH DC 20310–2300; Department of the Navy, Naval Medical Command, WASH DC 20732; or HQ USAF/SGB, Bolling AFB, WASH DC 20332–6188, for each respective Service. Nutrient standards prescribed in table 2–3 for operational and restricted rations are not subject to exception.

Interim changes. Interim changes to this regulation are not official unless they are authenticated by The Adjutant General, Headquarters, Department of the Army (HQDA). Users will destroy interim changes on their expiration dates unless sooner superseded or rescinded.

Suggested improvements. The Army office of primary interest in this regulation is the Office of The Surgeon General, HQDA. Army users are invited to send comments and suggested improvements on DA Form 2028 (Recommended Changes to Publications and Blank Forms) directly to HQDA (DASG-PSP), WASH DC 20310–2300. Other users may send comments and recommendations through normal channels to their respective Surgeons General: Naval Medical Command, ATTN: MEDCOM-312, Navy Department, WASH DC 20372, for the NAVY; and HQ USAF/SGB, WASH DC 20332–6188, for the Air Force.

Contents

Chapter 1

1–1. Purpose

This regulation defines the nutrition responsibilities of The Surgeons General of the Army, Navy, and Air Force by—

a. Establishing dietary allowances for military feeding.
b. Prescribing nutrient standards for packaged rations.
c. Providing, basic guidelines for nutrition education as prescribed in DOD 1338.10-M.

1–2.References

a. Required Publications.

(1) DOD Manual 1338.10-M, Manual for the Department of Defense Food Service Program. (Cited in para 1–1.)
(2) TB MED 507/NAVMED P-5052–5/AFP 160–1, Occupational and Environmental Health: Prevention, Treatment, and Control of Heat Injury. (Cited in para 2–5*i*.)

b. Related publications. (A related publication is merely a source of additional information. The user does not have to read it to understand this regulation.)

(1) *Recommended Dietary Allowances,* ninth revised edition, 1980. (Copies may be obtained from the Office of Publications, National Academy of Sciences, 2101 Constitution Avenue, WASH DC 20418.)
(2) United States Department of Agriculture Handbook 8 Series, *Composition of Foods, Raw, Processed, and Prepared.* (Copies may be obtained from the Superintendent of Documents, US Government Printing Office, WASH DC 20402.)

1–3.Explanation of abbreviations and terms

Abbreviations and special terms used in this regulation are explained in the glossary.

1–4.Responsibilities

a. The Surgeon General, Department of the Army (TSG, DA). TSG, DA, will act as the Department of Defense (DOD) Executive Agent for Nutrition and will—

(1) Establish dietary allowances for military personnel subsisting under normal operating conditions.
(2) Establish nutrient standards for packaged rations.
(3) Adjust dietary allowances and nutrient standards to meet variations

in age, sex, body size, physical activity, climate, or other conditions that may influence nutritional requirements.

(4) Evaluate current and proposed operational rations. Recommend adjustments and other actions to ensure that the nutrient composition of the rations as offered for consumption meets the nutritional requirements of personnel in all operational environments.

(5) Coordinate the development of nutrition education programs for all Services.

(6) Provide qualified representatives to advise committees which support the DOD Food Service Program in matters that affect the nutritional quality of the military diet.

b. The Surgeons General of the Army, Navy, and Air Force. TSGs will—

(1) Review requests and make appropriate recommendations for deviations from established nutritional standards.

(2) Evaluate adjustments to planned diets (menus). Make recommendations to ensure that the nutrient composition of the diet as offered will promote and maintain health.

(3) Evaluate the nutritional status of personnel and report nutritional deficiencies or excesses.

(4) Recommend standard methods to assess body composition.

(5) Provide nutritional guidance to the Services' weight control and physical fitness programs.

(6) Develop and implement a Service-wide nutrition education program for military personnel and their dependents. Provide information to motivate the consumption of a nutritionally adequate diet that contains all of the macronutrients and micronutrients needed to promote health and to maintain desirable body weight.

(7) Assist in providing food service personnel with knowledge and skills of proper food preparation that will maintain the nutritional value of foods.

(8) Provide qualified representatives to—

(a) Advise local food service organizations, such as menu boards, on matters that affect the nutritional quality of meals prepared and consumed.

(b) Serve as consultants to installation commanders on the development and evaluation of nutritional aspects of the Services' weight control and physical fitness programs.

Chapter 2

2–1.Military recommended dietary allowances

a. Table 2–1 prescribes military recommended dietary allowances (MRDA) for military personnel. These allowances are adapted from the National Academy of Sciences/National Research Council publication *Recommended Dietary Allowances* (RDA), ninth revised edition, 1980. MRDA are the daily essential nutrient intake levels presently considered to meet the known nutritional needs of practically all 17- to 50-year old, moderately active military personnel.

b. MRDA are intended for use by professional personnel involved in menu planning, dietary evaluation on a population basis, nutrition education, nutrition research, and food research and development. MRDA are based on estimated nutritional requirements. They provide broad dietary guidelines for healthy military personnel.

c. MRDA represent recommended daily nutrient intake levels, which should meet the physiological requirements of nearly all healthy military personnel. The energy allowances shown in table 2–1 represent ranges of caloric intake reflecting wide variations in energy requirements among individuals at similar levels of activity. These energy allowances are designed to maintain desirable body weight for healthy service members under conditions of moderate physical activity in an environment compatible with thermal comfort. The allowances are not to be interpreted as individual requirements. Also, they may not apply to personnel requiring special dietary treatment for conditions such as infection, chronic disease, trauma, unusual stress, pregnancy, lactation, or weight reduction. The allowances are subject to adjustments as outlined in paragraphs 2–3 and 2–4.

d. MRDA refer to the nutrient concentrations of edible portions of food offered for consumption. Nutrient losses may occur during food processing and preparation. These nutrient losses must be considered when nutrient composition tables are used to compare menus or food products with these allowances. The most recent edition of the United States Department of Agriculture Handbook 8 series, *Composition of Foods, Raw, Processed, and Prepared,* will be used as the standard reference nutrient composition data base.

2–2.Estimated safe and adequate daily dietary intakes

Table 2–2 is based on the RDA and provides estimated safe and adequate adult dietary intake ranges for selected nutrients, which are known to be essential in the diet, but for which recommended levels of intake have not been established.

2–3. Nutrient standards for operational and restricted rations

Table 2–3 prescribes nutrient standards, which are the criteria for evaluating the nutritional adequacy of operational and restricted rations. Operational rations include the individual combat ration such as the meal, combat, individual (MCI); the meal, ready-to-eat (MRE); and other rations (A, B, or T) used to support operations in the field. A level of 3600 kilocalories (kcal) is required for operational rations to meet energy demands associated with extended field operations. (See para 2–4.) Total fat calories should not exceed 40 percent of the energy value of the operational ration or 160 grams (gm). It is essential that ration planners compensate for losses of nutrients, such as ascorbic acid, thiamin, riboflavin, niacin, and pyridoxine (vitamin B^6), which may occur during storage of operational and restricted rations.

a. Nutritionally complete, individual operational rations such as the MCI and MRE must be formulated so that the nutrient content of each day's ration satisfies these nutrient standards. It is desirable that each combat meal provides one-third of the nutrient standard.

b. Under certain operational scenarios such as long-range patrol, assault and reconnaissance, and other situations where resupply is unavailable, it may be necessary for troops to subsist for periods (up to 10 days) on a restricted ration. To minimize loss of performance, the restricted ration should provide 1100 to 1500 kilocalories, 50 to 70 grams of protein, and a minimum of 100 grams of carbohydrate on a daily basis. Vitamins and minerals should be provided at the levels prescribed in table 2–3. This restricted ration is not appropriate for use under extreme, cold climates.

c. The survival food packet is a packaged food bar of approximately 400 kilocalories derived from carbohydrates. The low protein content spares body water by reducing the obligatory water demand caused by consuming high protein foods. The nutrient standards for operational and restricted rations do not apply to the survival food packet. This packet is designed to be consumed for periods of less than 4 consecutive days.

2–4. Energy requirements

The following factors affect individual energy requirements:

a. *Age.* MRDA are intended for men and women 17 to 50 years of age. Upon completion of growth, energy requirements for adults gradually decline with age due to a reduced resting metabolic rate and curtailment in physical activity. Within the 17 to 50 year military age range, age-related differences in caloric allowances appear to be minimal under conditions of similar physical activity.

b. *Body size.* The energy allowances are established for average sized personnel, which represent approximately 70 percent of the military personnel between the ages of 17 and 50 years. (See table 2–1.) To maintain desirable body weight, caloric intake must be adjusted for variable energy requirements due to individual differences in lean body mass reflected by body size. Large individuals (such as those with greater height and appropriately higher weight) have slightly higher resting, basal metabolic rates. They, therefore, require more total energy per unit of time for activities that involve moving body mass over distance. Smaller sized individuals require fewer calories.

c. *Physical activity.* Differences in energy needs are largely due to differences in the amount of time an individual performs moderate and heavy work tasks in contrast to light or sedentary activities. MRDA for energy in table 2–1 are for military personnel who are moderately active and living in a temperate climate or in a thermally neutral environment. Total energy requirements are influenced by the intensity and duration of physical activity. For example, a day of moderate physical activity may include 8 hours of sleeping, 12 hours of light activity, and 4 hours of moderate to heavy activity. For military personnel doing heavy work or involved in prolonged, vigorous physical training, the recommended caloric allowance should be increased by at least 25 percent (approximately 500 to 900 kilocalories).

d. *Climate.* MRDA for energy intake are established for personnel in a temperate climate. (See table 2–1.) When there is prolonged exposure to cold or heat, energy allowances may need adjustment.

(1) *Cold environment.* In a cold environment (mean temperature less than 14°C (57.2°F), the energy cost of work for garrison troops is approximately 5 percent greater than in a warmer environment. There is an additional 2 to 5 percent increase in energy expenditure associated with carrying the extra weight of heavy, cold weather clothing and footgear (the "hobbling" effect). Garrison personnel may require an extra 150 to 350 kilocalories per day under these conditions. Energy allowances of 4500 calories for men and 3500 calories for women are required to support adequately clothed troops maneuvering for prolonged periods (several hours) with heavy gear on foot, snowshoes, and skis over snow- or ice-covered terrain. This increased energy allowance does not apply to troops stationed in cold climates who are engaged in moderate activity within a garrison setting.

(2) *Hot environment.* In a hot climate, loss of appetite may cause a voluntary but undesirable reduction in caloric intake below the level of need. This loss of appetite may be most noticeable after troops have arrived in a hot environment and before the process of acclimatization is completed. When personnel are required to perform the same amount of work in a hot environment as in a temperate environment, the caloric expenditure will be increased. Little adjustment appears to be necessary for a change in environmental temperature between 20°C (68°F) and 30°C (86°F). It is desirable under conditions of moderate physical activity to increase the caloric allowance by at least 0.7 percent for every degree centigrade rise in average ambient

temperature above 30°C (86°F). Daily energy requirements under extremely hot conditions (greater than 40°C (104°F), may reach 56 kcal/kilogram (kg) of body weight.

(3) *Nuclear, biochemical, and chemical environment.* Certain conditions will require special guidance and nutrient formulation not described in this regulation. One such condition is when troops are operating in contaminated environments for more than 6 hours while wearing protective clothing.

2–5. Nutrient discussion

a. *Protein.* MRDA for protein are based, in part, on an estimated nutritional requirement of 0.8 gm/day/kg of body weight. (See table 2–1.) For military personnel within the reference weight range, protein recommendations are set between 48 to 63 gm/day, for males and 37 to 50 gm/day for females. These computed protein levels have been further increased to 100 gm/day for male and 80 gm/day for female personnel. This increase reflects usual intake patterns and helps to maintain a high level of palatability and food acceptance among military personnel. These allowances are based on the consumption of a diet containing mixed proteins of animal and vegetable origin. A total day's protein intake of more than 100 gm/day has not been shown to improve heavy physical performance.

b. *Fat.* Fats are important in the diet to furnish energy, provide essential fatty acids, transport fat soluble vitamins and aid in their absorption, increase palatability, and give meal satisfaction. It is becoming increasingly clear that excessive amounts to total fat may lead to an increased risk of coronary heart and vascular disease. For this reason, it is recommended that the calories derived from total dietary fat should not exceed 35 percent under garrison feeding conditions. Higher proportions of fat calories are acceptable in combat, arctic, or other operational rations to increase caloric density. Emphasis should be placed on planning the military menu with lower fat concentrations while maintaining acceptability. A reduction of fat calories in the diet can be achieved by lowering added fats during food preparation and replacing foods high in fat with lean meats, fish, poultry, low fat milk, and other low fat dairy products in the military menu. As fat calories are reduced in the diet, it is recommended that the current level of about 7 percent of caloric intake as polyunsaturated fat be maintained to ensure an adequate intake of essential fatty acids.

c. *Carbohydrate.* Carbohydrates should contribute approximately 50 to 55 percent of the total dietary energy. It is recommended that simple, refined, and other processed sugars provide only about 10 percent of total dietary energy. The remaining carbohydrate calories should come from complex carbohydrates such as starches and naturally occurring sugars found in fruits, vegetables, and milk.

d. *Calcium and phosphorus.* MRDA are the same for both calcium (Ca) and phosphorus (P), although a wide variation in the Ca:P ratio is tolerated. In the presence of adequate vitamin D nutriture, a ratio of between 1:1 to 1.5:1 is nutritionally desirable.

e. *Iron, ascorbic acid, and animal protein.* The absorption of iron, a nutrient involved in maintaining optimal aerobic fitness, can be significantly affected by the composition of foods in a particular meal. Heme iron from animal protein sources is better absorbed (approximately 23 percent) than nonheme iron (approximately 3 to 8 percent) which is found in both animal and in many plant food sources. Certain cereal and legume proteins are known to reduce the bioavailability of nonheme iron. The nonheme iron absorption rate can be more than doubled when nonheme iron is consumed with a modest serving of meat, fish, poultry, or a source of ascorbic acid (vitamin C) at the same meal. The dietary iron allowance for females and 17- to 18-year old males is 18 milligrams (mg)/day, or 7.5 and 5.6 mg/1000 calories respectively. Moderately active female personnel consuming an average of 2400 calories per day may require supplemental iron to meet the recommended 18 mg/day. Issuing supplemental iron should be done on an individualized basis after a medical evaluation.

f. *Iodine.* Wide variation occurs in the amount of iodine present in food and water. All table and cooking salt used should be iodized to ensure an adequate intake of 150 micrograms (mcg) of iodine per day.

g. *Fluoride.* Fluoride is an essential nutrient which is found in the enamel of teeth and bone. This nutrient is an important factor in preventing tooth decay. Fluoride may confer some protection against certain degenerative bone diseases. Fluoride is found in varying amounts in most foods and water supplies. Maintaining a fluoride concentration of about 1 mg/liter (1 part per million) in water supplies has proven to be safe, economical, and efficient in reducing the incidence of dental caries.

h. *Sodium.* Sodium is the principal cation involved in maintaining osmotic equilibrium and extracellular fluid volume in the body.

(1) Under conditions of normal ambient temperature and humidity, the healthy adult can maintain sodium balance with an intake of as little as 150 mg/day (381 milligrams of salt). While daily intake below 2000 milligrams of sodium are generally considered upalatable, 3300 milligrams of sodium/day represents a lower acceptable limit to which the American population can adapt. The average young civilian male consumes approximately 5500 milligrams of sodium/day in food plus an additional 20 percent (1000 milligrams) as added salt. Although dietary levels of sodium for the military population are unknown, the average intake may well exceed the civilian level. The goal for the sodium content in foods as served within military dining facilities is 1700 milligrams of sodium/1000 kcal. (See table 3–1.)

(2) Hard physical work in a high ambient temperature greatly increases the amount of sodium lost in sweat. Sodium losses may reach levels as high as 8000 mg/day (20 grams of salt). Whenever more than 3 liters of water per day are required to replace sweat losses, extra salt intake may be required. The need for extra salt depends on the severity of sweat losses and the degree of acclimatization. Sodium should be replaced through food in both nondiscretionary form and as added salt.

i. *Water.* As caloric requirements are increased, water needs are also increased. During periods of light to moderate activity in a temperate climate, 1 milliliter of water per calorie expended is a reasonable intake goal. Water requirements may increase from 50 to 100 percent for personnel living in a hot climate expending similar energy levels. Water requirements may increase threefold above normal under conditions of heavy work in a hot environment. Even in cold climates sweat rates and, consequently, water needs may be quite high due to the hot microclimate that can develop under insulated clothing during heavy physical activity. Inadequate water intakes can be accompanied by a disturbance in electrolyte balance with a resultant performance decrement. (See TB MED 507/NAVMED P-5052–5/AFP 160–1.) Under conditions of normal dietary intake, the preferred fluid to replace losses is cool water. Electrolyte- and sugar-containing solutions are not necessary since glucose and electrolytes are adequately replenished in the normal diet. Under certain conditions, electrolyte and sugar solutions may actually impair rather than enhance performance.

Table 2–1 MRDA for selected nutrients1

Nutrient	Unit	Male	Female
Energy[2,3]	Kcal MJ	3200(2800–3600) 13.4(11.7–15.1)	2400(2000–2800 10.0(8.4–11.7)
Protein[4]	gm	100	80
Vitamin A[5]	mcg RE	1000	800
Vitamin D[6,7]	mcg	5–10	5–10
Vitamin E[8]	mg TE	10	8
Ascorbic Acid	mg	60	60
Thiamin (B_1)	mg	1.6	1.2
Riboflavin (B_2)	mg	1.9	1.4
Niacin[9]	mg NE	21	16
Vitamin B_6	mg	2.2	2.0
Folacin	mcg	400	400
Vitamin B_{12}	mcg	3.0	3.0
Calcium[7]	mg	800–1200	800–1200
Phosphorus[7]	mg	800–1200	800–1200
Magnesium[7]	mg	350–400	300
Iron[7]	mg	10–18	18
Zinc	mg	15	15
Iodine	mcg	150	150
Sodium	mg	See note[10]	See note[10]

[1]MRDA for moderately active military personnel, ages 17 to 50 years, are based on the *Recommended Dietary Allowances,* ninth revised edition, 1980.

[2]Energy allowance ranges are estimated to reflect the requirements of 70 percent of the moderately active military population. One megajoule (MJ) equals 239 kcals.

[3]Dietary fat calories should not contribute more than 35 percent of total energy intake.

[4]Protein allowance is based on an estimated protein requirement of 0.8 gm/kilograms (kg) desirable body weight. Using the reference body weight ranges for males of 60 to 79 kilograms and for females of 46 to 63 kilograms, the protein requirement is approximately 48 to 64 grams for males and 37 to 51 grams for females. These amounts have been approximately doubled to reflect the usual protein consumption levels of Americans and to enhance diet acceptability.

[5]One microgram of retinol equivalent (mcg RE) equals 1 microgram of retinol, or 6 micrograms betacarotene, or 5 international units (IU)

[6] As cholecalciferol, 10 micrograms of cholecalciferol equals 400 IU of vitamin D.

[7]High values reflect greater vitamin D, calcium, phosphorus, magnesium, and iron requirements for 17- to 18-year olds than for older ages.

[8]One milligram of alpha-tocopherol equivalent (mg TE) equals 1 milligram d-alphatocopherol.
[9]One milligram of niacin equivalent (mg NE) equals 1 milligram niacin or 60 milligrams dietary tryptophan.
[10]The safe and adequate levels for daily sodium intake of 1100 to 3300 mg published in the RDA are currently impractical and unattainable within military food service systems. However, an average of 1700 milligrams of sodium per 100 kilocalories of food served is the target for military food service systems. This level equates to a daily sodium intake of approximately 5500 milligrams for males and 4100 milligrams for females.

Table 2–2 Estimated safe and adequate daily dietary intake ranges of selected vitamins and minerals1

Nutrition	Unit	Amount
Vitamins		
Vitamins K	mcg	70–140
Biotin	mcg	100–200
Pantothenic Acid	mg	4–7
Trace Elements[2]		
Fluoride	mg	1.5–4.0
Selenium	mcg	50–200
Molybdenum	mg	0.15–0.50
Copper	mg	2–3
Manganese	mg	2.5–5.0
Chromium	mcg	50–200
Electrolytes		
Potassium	mg	1875–5625
Chloride	mg	1700–5100

[1]This table is based on the Recommended Dietary Allowances, ninth edition, 1980, table 10, "Estimated Safe and Adequate Daily Dietary Intakes of Selected Vitamins and Minerals." Estimated ranges are provided for these nutrients because sufficient information upon which to set a recommended allowance is not available. Values reflect a range of recommended intake over an extended period of time.
[2]Since toxic levels for many trace elements may only be several times the usual intakes, the upper levels for the trace elements given in this table should not be habitually exceeded.

Table 2–3 Nutritional standards for operational and restricted rations

Nutrient	Unit[1]	Operational rations	Restricted rations[2,4]
Energy	Kcal	3600	1100–1500
Protein	gm	100	50–70
Carbohydrate	gm	440	100–200
Fat	gm	160(maximum)	50–70
Vitamin A	mcg RE	1000	500
Vitamin D	mcg	10	5
Vitamin E	mg TE	10	5
Ascorbic Acid	mg	60	30
Thiamin	mg	1.8	1.0
Riboflavin	mg	2.2	1.2
Niacin	mg NE	24	13
Vitamin B_6	mg	2.2	1.2
Folacin	mcg	400	200
Vitamin B_{12}	mcg	3	1.5
Calcium	mg	800	400
Phosphorus	mg	800	400
Magnesium	mg	800	400
Iron	mg	18	9
Zinc	mg	15	7.5
Sodium	mg	5000–7000[5]	2500–3500[5]
Potassium	mg	1875–5625	950–2800

[1]See notes in table 2–1 for explanation of units.

[2]Values are minimum standards at the time of consumption unless shown as a range or a maximum level.

[3]The operational ration includes the MCI, MRE, A, B, and T rations.

[4]Restricted rations are for use under certain operational scenarios such as long-range patrol, assault, and reconnaissance when troops are required to subsist for short periods (up to 10 days) on an energy restricted ration.

[5]These values do not include salt packets.

Chapter 3

3–1. Nutrient density index

a. Table 3–1 lists selected nutrients from the MRDA (table 2–1) for which adequate food composition data are presently available on a nutrient density basis. A nutrient density index (NDI) is provided for both the general military diet and for the reduced calorie menu. (See para 3–2.) The NDI is a technique for evaluating the nutritional adequacy of individual foods, recipes, meals, and cycle menus.

b. The nutrient concentrations per 1000 calories in table 3–1 are based on the recommended calorie intake for healthy male and female personnel at moderate levels of activity. A single nutrient value is recommended for both sexes to simplify use. Because of lower caloric requirements for women, the NDI is generally higher for the female than for the male. Female nutrient values have been adopted for most nutrient densities except for iron and sodium.

c. The computed iron density represents an interpolation between the male and female MRDA for iron. Six milligrams of iron per 1000 calories is considered reasonable and consistent with the amounts of iron found in the usual food supply. This iron density may be inadequate for women. (See para 2–5*e*.)

d. The NDI for sodium is a target to be achieved in foods as served in military dining facilities.

e. The lower female MRDA for calcium and phosphorus were used to compute the NDI for calcium and phosphorus.

f. Personnel subsisting on a 1500-calorie meal plan require a diet that is nutritionally more dense. Guidance for this type of diet is in the column headed "Reduced calorie menu amount" in table 3–1.

g. It is emphasized that the purpose of representing the MRDA in terms of nutrient densities is for menu evaluation, not for calculating nutrient requirements.

h. The NDI may serve as an important basic tool for nutrition education within the military.

3–2. Reduced calorie menu (1500 kcal)

In support of the military physical fitness and weight control programs, each military dining facility will offer a nutritionally adequate reduced menu (1500 to 1600 kcal/day). Each meal should contain approximately 500 kilocalories except when serving line constraints or unique mission requirements make this impractical. The specified NDI for the reduced calorie menu in table 3–1 provides guidance for reviewing the nutritional quality of the menu. The calories derived from total dietary fat should not exceed 35 percent in the reduced calorie menu. Implementation procedures and exceptions to policy for a reduced calorie menu will be prescribed by each military service.

Table 3–1 Nutrient density index per 1000 calories for menu planning

Nutrient	Unit	Military diet amount	Reduced calorie menu amount
Protein	gm	33	53
Vitamin A	mcg RE	333	533
Ascorbic Acid	mg	25	40
Thiamin (B_1)	mg	0.5	0.7[1]
Riboflavin (B_2)	mg	0.6	0.8[2]
Niacin	mg	6.7	8.7[3]
Calcium	mg	333	533
Phosphorus	mg	333	533
Magnesium	mg	125	200
Iron	mg	6.0[4]	6.0[4]
Sodium	mg	1700	1700

[1]NDI for thiamin is based on a minimum recommended allowance of 1.0 mg/day.
[2]NDI for riboflavin is based on a minimum recommended allowance of 1.2 mg/day.
[3]NDI for niacin is based on a minimum recommended allowance of 13.0 mg/day.
[4]Iron supplementation is recommended for female personnel subsisting on a 1500 kilocalories diet. Levels higher than 6 mg/1000 calories are difficult to attain in a conventional US diet.

Chapter 4

4–1. Introduction

The following statements about a healthful diet are suggested guidelines to promote optimal fitness in the general military population. Each of the military services should incorporate these guidelines in their nutritional education programs. These statements should guide modification in food procurement policy, food preparation, recipe formulation, and menu development.

4–2. General guidelines for a healthful diet

a. *Eat a wide variety of nutritious foods.* A well-balanced diet must provide about 50 nutrients, including essential amino acids, carbohydrates, essential fatty acids, vitamins, minerals, water, and dietary fiber. No single food item supplies all the essential nutrients in the amounts required by the body. The greater the variety of foods consumed, the less likely is the chance of developing either a deficiency or an excess of any nutrient. Selection of a diet from a variety of food groups ensures a well-balanced intake of the numerous macronutrients and micronutrients. These groups include—

(1) Whole grains, enriched cereals, and breads.
(2) Fruits and vegetables.
(3) Dry peas and beans.
(4) Meats, poultry, fish, and eggs.
(5) Dairy products.

b. *Maintain ideal body weight.* Personnel should strive to maintain ideal body weight by consuming only as much energy as is expended. To lose weight, calorie intake should be reduced by decreasing total food intake, especially fats, oils, sugars, and alcohol. Also, physical activity should be increased.

c. *Avoid excessive dietary fat.* Consumption of fats and oils should be limited during weight reduction and weight maintenance because fats and oils have a high energy density. Military personnel who are identified as being "at risk" of heart disease should reduce saturated fats and cholesterol in their diet and proportionately increase their intake of polyunsaturated fats.

d. *Eat foods with adequate starch and fiber.* Complex carbohydrates should be increased to make up any calorie deficit due to reduction of fat and refined sugar calories. Emphasis should be placed on fiber-rich foods such as whole grain products, vegetables, and mature legumes.

e. *Avoid too much sugar.* The major health hazard from eating too much sugar is dental caries. Also, excessive intake of refined sugars may displace other foods that are important sources of essential nutrients.

f. *Avoid too much salt.* Under normal conditions, an adequate but safe daily intake ranges from 3 to 8 grams (.105 to .28 ounce) of salt (1100 to 3300 milligrams of sodium). Regular consumption of highly salted foods may result in excessive sodium intake. Personnel who are "at risk" of high blood pressure should avoid highly salted foods.

g. *Avoid excessive alcohol consumption.* Alcoholic beverages have a low nutrient density (that is, they are high in calories and low in other nutrients). Alcoholic beverages can displace valuable nutrient-rich foods in the diet. Impulsive alcohol consumption may lead to acute ethanol toxicity. Sustained, excessive alcohol consumption alters the way nutrients are utilized in the body and may contribute to liver disease and neurological disorders.

Glossary

Section I

Ca	calcium
DA	Department of the Army
DOD	Department of Defense
gm	gram (1 gm=.035 ounce)
IU	international unit
HQDA	Headquarters, Department of the Army
kcal	kilocalorie
kg	kilogram (2.2 pounds)
lb	pound
mcg	microgram (.000000035 ounce)
mg	milligram (.000035 ounce)
MCI	meal, combat, individual
MJ	megajoule (239 kilocalories)
MRDA	military recommended dietary allowances
MRE	meal, ready-to-eat
NDI	nutrient density index
NE	niacin equivalent
oz	ounce (28.571428 grams)
P	phosphorus
RDA	recommended dietary allowance
RE	retinol equivalent
TSG	The Surgeon General
TE	alpha-tocopherol equivalent

Section II

Kilocalorie

Energy provided to the body in the form of kilocalories—commonly called calories. One kcal is defined as the amount of heat necessary to raise 1 kg (liter) of water from 15°C to 16°C (59°F to 60.8°F). The joule is the accepted international unit of energy. To convert kcal to joules multiply by the factor of 4.2. (Example: 9 kcals=37.8 joules.)

Macronutrients

Nutrients essential for human nutrition in relatively large amounts; examples are carbohydrates, protein, calcium, phosphorus, and sodium.

Micronutrients

Nutrients essential for human nutrition in relatively small amounts; examples are the vitamins, iron, zinc, and copper.

Operational ration

A specialty designed ration normally composed of nonperishable items for use under actual or simulated combat conditions. This ration is used in peacetime for emergencies or contingencies, travel, and training.

Ration

The allowance of food for the subsistence of one person for 1 day.

Reference body weight range

A body weight range that covers the average weight for male (60 to 79 kg (132 to 173 lb)) and female (46 to 63 kg (101.2 to 138.6 lb)) military personnel based on average height data. This range is used in this regulation to estimate protein requirements which are computed on a per kilogram body weight basis.

Restricted ration

A light weight, operational ration requiring no further preparation, providing suboptimal levels of energy and nutrients, and intended for short-range patrols.

By Order of the Secretaries of the Army, the Navy, and the Air Force:

JOHN A.WICKHAM, JR

General, United States Army

Chief of Staff

Official:

DONALD J.DELANDRO

Brigadier General, United States Army

The Adjutant General

W.M.McDERMOTT, JR.

Rear Admiral, MC, United States Navy

Commander, Naval Medical Command

CHARLES A.GABRIEL

General, United States Air Force

Chief of Staff

Official:

JAMES H.DELANEY

Colonel, United States Air Force

Director of Administration

Distribution:

Army:

Active Army, ARNG, USAR: To be distributed in accordance with DA Form 12–9A, requirements for AR, Medical Services: Applicable to all Army elements—B.

Navy/Marine Corps:

Ships and stations having Medical Personnel; NAVSUP—CO, NAVFSSO (20); MARCORPS CODE IV plus 7000163 (10). Stocked: CO, NAVPUBFORMCEN, 5801 Tabor Ave., Philadelphia, PA 19120.

Air Force: F.

*U.S. GOVERNMENT PRINTING OFFICE: 1985–461–029:10199

C

Potential Food Components to Enhance Performance—A Selected Bibliography

On the following pages is a selection of references dealing with food components to enhance performance. This bibliography was compiled from the joint reference lists of the 23 chapters in this report, selected references from a computer-based literature search conducted in 1992, and references recommended by the invited speakers as background reading for the workshop participants. As a result, references that are historical in nature are included in this listing with the most current studies on food components to enhance performance.

AMAC American Medical Association's Council on Scientific Affairs 1984 Cafffeine labeling, a report on the safety of dietary caffeine. JAMA 252:803–806.

Anderson, S.A., and D.J.Raiten, eds. 1992 Safety of Amino Acids Used as Dietary Supplements. Bethesda, Md.: Life Sciences Research Office.

Arvedson, I., G.Sterky, and K.Tjernstrom 1969 Breakfast habits of Swedish schoolchildren: Effect of protein content. J. Am. Diet. Assoc. 55:257–261.

Askew, E.W., J.R.Claybaugh, S.A.Cucinell, A.J.Young, and E.G.Szeto 1987 Nutrient intakes and work performance of soldiers during seven days of exercise at 7,200 ft. altitude consuming the meal, Ready-to-Eat ration. Technical Report T3–87. Natick, Mass.: U.S. Army Research Institute of Environmental Medicine.

Askew, E.W., J.R.Claybaugh, G.M.Hashiro, W.S.Stokes, A.Sato, and S.A.Cucinell 1987 Mauna Kea III: Metabolic effects of dietary carbohydrate supplementation during exercise at 4,100 m altitude. Technical Report No. T12–87, AD A180 629 . Natick, Mass.: U.S. Army Research Institute of Environmental Medicine.

Banderet, L.E., and H.E.Lieberman. 1989 Treatment with tyrosine, a neurotransmitter precursor, reduces environmental stress in humans. Brain Res. Bull. 22:759–762.

Bartus, R.T., R.L.Dean, J.A.Goas, and A.S.Lippa 1980 Age-related changes in passive avoidance retention: Modulation with dietary choline. Science 209:301–303.

Battig, K., R.Buzzi, J.R.Martin, and J.M.Feierabend 1984 The effects of caffeine on physiological functions and mental performance. Experentia 40:1218–1223.

Beisel, W.R. 1991 Nutrition and infection. Pp. 507–542 in Nutritional Biochemistry and Metabolism, 2nd ed., M.C.Linder, ed. New York: Elsevier.

Benevenga, N.J., and R.D.Steele 1984 Adverse effects of excessive consumption of amino acids. Annu. Rev. Nutr. 4:157–181.

Bergman, J., and P.B.Dews 1987 Dietary cafeine and its toxicity. In J.Hathcock (ed.) Nutritional Toxicology. New York: Academic Press.

Bergström, J., L.Hermansen, E.Hultman and B.Saltin 1967 Diet, muscle glycogen and physical performance. Acta Physiol. Scand. 71:140–150.

Blom, P.C.S, A.T.Høstmark, O.Vaage, K.R.Kardel, and S.Maehlum 1987 Effect of different post-exercise sugar diets on the rate of muscle glycogen synthesis. Med. Sci. Sports Exerc. 19:491–496.

Blomstrand, E., F.Celsing, and E.A.Newsholme 1988 Changes in plasma concentrations of aromatic and branched-chain amino acids during sustained exercise in man and their possible role in fatigue. Acta Physiol. Scand. 133:115–121.

Blomstrand, E., P.Hassmén, B.Ekblom, and E.A.Newsholme 1991 Administration of branched-chain amino acids during sustained exercise—effects on performance and on plasma concentration of some amino acids. Eur. J. Appl. Physiol. 63:83–88.

Blundell, J.E. 1986 Serotonin manipulations and the structure of feeding behaviour. Appetite Supl. 7:39–56.

Boyd, W.D., W.J.Graham, G.Blackwood, I.Glen, and J.McQueen 1977 Clinical effects of choline in Alzheimer senile dementia. Letter. Lancet 2:711.

Bredle, D.L., J.M.Stager, W.F.Brechue, and M.O.Farber 1988 Phosphate supplementation, cardiovascular function, and exercise performance in humans. J. Appl. Physiol. 65:1821–1826.

Bruce, M., N.Scott, M.Lader, and V.Marks 1986 The psychopharmacological and electrophysiological effects of single doses of caffeine in healthy human subjects. Br. J. Clin. Pharmacol. 22:81–87.

Brzezinski, A.A., J.J.Wurtman, R.J.Wurtman, R.Gleason, T.Nader, and B.Laferrere 1990 D-fenfluramine suppresses the increased calorie and carbohydrate intakes and improves the mood of women with premenstrual syndrome. Obstet. Gynecol. 76:296–301.

Cade, R., M.Conte, C.Zauner, D.Mars, J.Peterson, D.Lunne, N.Hommen, and D.Parker 1984 Effects of phosphate loading on 2,3-diphosphoglycerate and maximal oxygen uptake. Med. Sci. Sports Exerc. 16:263–268.

Caputo, F.A., and R.D.Mattes 1992 Human dietary responses to covert manipulations of energy, fat, and carbohydrate in a midday meal. Am. J. Clin. Nutr. 56:36–43.

Childs, J.M. 1978 Caffeine consumption and target scanning performance. Hum. Factors 20:91–96.

Choi, O.H., M.T.Shamin, W.L.Padgett, and J.W.Daly 1988 Caffeine and theophylline analogues: Correlation of behavioral effects with activity as adenosine receptor antagonists and as phosphodiesterase inhibitors. Life Sci. 43:387–398.

Cohen, E.L., and R.J.Wurtman 1975 Brain acetylcholine: Increase after systemic choline administration. Life Sci. 16:1095–1102.

1976 Brain acetylcholine: Control by dietary choline. Science 191:561–562.

Conlay, L.A., R.J.Wurtman, K.Blusztajn, I.L.Coviella, T.J.Maher, and G.E.Evoniuk 1986 Decreased plasma choline concentrations inmarathon runners. Letter. N. Engl. J. Med. 315:892.

Cooper, C., E.J.Atkinson, H.W.Wahner, W.M.O'Fallon, B.L.Riggs, H.L. Judd, and L.J.Melton 1992 Is caffeine consumption a risk factor for osteoporosis? J. Bone & Min. Res. 7:465–471.

Costill, D.L. 1988 Carbohydrates for exercise: Dietary demands for optimal performance. Int. J. Sports Med. 9:1–18.

Costill, D.L., G.Dalsky, and W.Fink 1978 Effects of caffeine ingestion on metabolism and exercise performance. Med. Sci. Sports 10:155–158.

Costill, D.L., W.M.Sherman, W.J.Fink, C.Maresh, and M.Witten 1981 The role of dietary carbohydrate in muscle glycogen resynthesis after strenuous running. Am. J. Clin. Nutr. 34:1831–1836.

Coyle, E.F., J.M.Hagberg, B.R.Hurley, W.H.Martin, A.A.Ehsani, and J.O.Holloszy 1983 Carbohydrate feeding during prolonged strenuous exercise can delay fatigue. J. Appl. Physiol. 55:230–235.

Coyle, E.F., A.R.Coggan, M.K.Hemmert, and J.L.Ivy 1986 Muscle glycogen utilization during prolonged strenuous exercise when fed carbohydrate. J. Appl. Physiol. 61:165–172.

Craig, A. 1986 Acute effects of meals on perceptual and cognitive functioning. Nutr. Rev. 44 (Suppl):163–171.

Cromer, B.A., K.J.Tarnowski, A.M.Stein, P.Harton, and D.Thornton 1990 The school breakfast program and cognition in adolescents. Dev. Behav. Pediatr. 11:295–300.

Curatolo, P.W., and D.Robertson 1983 The health consequences of caffeine. Ann. Intern. Med. 98:641–653.

Curran, H.V. 1992 Antidepressant drugs, cognitive function and human performance. Pp. 319–336 in Handbook of Human Performance, Vol. 2, Health and Performance, A.P.Smith and D.M.Jones, eds. Boston: Academic Press.

Dews, P.B. 1984 Behavioral effects of caffeine. Pp. 86–103 in Caffeine, P.B.Dews, ed. New York: Springer-Verlag.

Diaz, E., G.R.Goldberg, M.Taylor, J.M.Savage, D.Sellen, W.A.Coward, and A.M.Prentice 1991 Effects of dietary supplementation on work performance in Gambian laborers. Am. J. Clin. Nutr. 53:803–811.

Dollins, A.B., L.P.Krock, W.F.Storm, and H.R.Lieberman 1990 Tyrosine decreases physiological stress caused by lower body negative pressure (LBNP). Aviat. Space Environ. Med. 61:491

Duffy, D.J., and R.K.Conlee 1986 Effects of phosphate loading on leg power and high intensity treadmill exercise. Med. Sci. Sports Exerc. 18:674–677.

Eskenazi, B. 1993 Caffeine during pregnancy: Grounds for concern? JAMA 270:2973– 2974.

Essig, D., D.L.Costill, and P.J.van Handel 1980 Effects of caffeine ingestion on utilization of muscle glycogen and lipid during leg ergometer cycling. Int. J. Sports Med. 1:86–90.

Federation of American Societies for Experimental Biology 1981 Effects of Consumption of Choline and Lecithin on Neurological and Cardiovascular Systems. PB82–133257. Springfield, Va.: National Technical Information Service.

Fernstrom, J.D., and R.J.Wurtman 1971 Brain serotonin content: Increase following ingestion of carbohydrate diet. Science 174:1023–1025.

Fogelholm, G.M., J.-J.Himberg, K.Alopaeus, C.-G.Gref, J.T.Laakso, J.J. Lehto, and H.Mussalo-Rauhamaa 1992 Dietary and biochemical indices of nutritional status in male athletes and controls. J. Am. Coll. Nutr. 11:181–191.

Food and Drug Administration 1982 Toxicological Principles for the Safety Assessment of Direct Food Additives and Color Additives Used in Food. Washington, D.C.: U.S. Department of Health and Human Services.

Friedman, M. 1991 Formation, nutritional value, and safety of D-amino acids. Pp. 447–81 in Nutritional and Toxicological Consequences of Food Processing. New York: Plenum Press.

Fulco, C.S., P.B.Rock, L.A.Trad, M.S.Rose, V.A.Forte, Jr., P.M. Young, and A.Cymerman 1989 Effect of caffeine on endurance time to exhaustion. Technical Report No. T17–89, AD A212 069. Natick, Mass.: U.S. Army Research Institute of Environmental Medicine.

Gelenberg, A.J., J.D.Wojcik, C.J.Gibson, and R.J.Wurtman 1983 Tyrosine for depression. J. Psychiatr. Res. 17(2):175.

Ghoneim, M.M., J.V.Hinrichs, C.K.Chiang, and W.H.Loke 1986 Pharmacokinetic and pharmacodynamic interactions between caffeine and diazepam. J. Clin. Psychopharmacol. 6:75–80.

Goldstein, A., R.Warren, and S.Kaizer 1965 Psychotropic effects of caffeine in man. I. Individual differences in sensitivity to caffeine-induced wakefulness. J. Clin. Pharmacol. Exp. Therapeutics 149:156–169.

Gonder-Frederick, L.A., J.L.Hall, J.Vogt, D.J.Cox, J.Green, and P.E.Gold 1987 Memory enhancement in elderly humans: Effects of glucose ingestion. Physiol. Behav. 41:503–504.

Gonder-Frederick, L.A., D.J.Cox, S.A.Bobbitt, and J.W.Pennebaker 1989 Mood changes associated with blood glucose fluctuations in insulin-dependent diabetes mellitus. Health Psychol. 8:45–59.

Gorostiaga, E.M., C.A.Maurer, and J.P.Eclache 1989 Decrease in respiratory quotient during exercise following L-carnitine supplementation. Int. J. Sports Med. 10:169–174.

Graham, D.M. 1978 Caffeine-Its identity, dietary sources, intake and biological effects. Nutr. Rev. 36:97–102.

Graham, T.E., and L.L.Spriet 1991 Performance and metabolic responses to a high caffeine dose during prolonged exercise. J. Appl. Physiol. 71:2292–2298.

Griffiths, R.R., and P.P.Woodson 1988 Reinforcing effects of caffeine in humans. J. Pharmacol. Exp. Ther. 246:21–29.

Hall, J.L., L.A.Gonder-Frederick, W.W.Chewning, J.Silveira, and P.E.Gold 1989 Glucose enhancement of memory in young and aged humans. Neuropsychologia 27:1129–1138.

Hartmann, E., and D.Greenwald 1984 Tryptophan and human sleep: An analysis of 43 studies. Pp. 297–304 in Progress in Tryptophan and Serotonin Research, H.G. Schlossberger, W.Kochen, B.Kinzen, and H.Steinhart, eds. New York: Walter de Gruyter.

Hartmann, E., C.L.Spinweber, and J.Fernstrom 1977 Diet, amino acids and sleep. Sleep Res. 6:61.

Heigenhauser, G.J.F., and N.L.Jones 1991 Bicarbonate loading. Pp. 183–212 in Ergogenics, Enhancement of Performance in Exercise and Sport, D.R.Lamb and M.H.Williams, eds. Ann Arbor, Mich.: William C.Brown.

Holder, M.D., and G.Huether 1990 Role of prefeedings, plasma amino acid ratios and brain serotonin levels in carbohydrate and protein selection. Physiol. Behav. 47:113–119.

Hughes, J.R., S.T.Higgins, W.K.Bickel, W.K.Hunt, J.W.Fenwick, S.B. Gulliver, and G.C.Mireault 1991 Caffeine self-administration, withdrawal, and adverse effects among coffee drinkers. Archives Gen. Psychiatr. 48:611–617.

Infante-Rivard, C., A.Fernandez, R.Gauthier, D.Michele, and G.E.Rivard 1993 Fetal loss associated with cafeine intake before and during pregnancy. JAMA 270:2940–2943.

Ivy, J.L., D.L.Costill, W.J.Fink, and R.W.Lower 1979 Influence of caffeine and carbohydrate feedings on endurance performance. Med. Sci. Sports 11:6–11.

Ivy, J.L., W.Miller, V.Dover, L.G.Goodyear, W.H.Sherman, S.Farrell, and H.Williams 1983 Endurance improved by ingestion of a glucose polymer supplement. Med. Sci. Sports Exerc. 15:466–471.

Jacobson, B.H., and B.M.Edgely 1987 Effects of caffeine on simple reaction time and movement time. Aviat. Space Environ. Med. 58:1153–1156.

Jarvis, M. 1993 Does caffeine intake enhance absolute levels of cognitive performance? Psychopharmacology 110:45–52.

Joesoef, M.R., V.Beral, R.T.Rolfs, S.O.Aral, and D.W.Cramer 1990 Are caffeinated beverages risk factors for delayed conception? The Lancet 335:136–137.

Johansson, C., D.Mellstrom, U.Lerner, and T.Osterberg 1992 Coffee drinking: a minor risk factor for bone loss and fractures. Age and Aging 21:20–26.

Johnson, W.R., and D.H.Black 1953 Comparison of effects of certain blood alkalinizers and glucose upon competitive endurance performance. J. Appl. Physiol. 5:577–578.

Kanarek, R., and R.Marks-Kaufman 1991 Nutrition and Behavior. New York: Van Nostrand.

Kinsella, J.E., B.Lokesh, S.Broughton, and J.Whelan 1990 Dietary polyunsaturated fatty acids and eicosanoids: Potential effects on the modulation of inflammatory and immune cells: An overview. Nutrition 6:24–44.

Kirk, S.J., and A.Barbul 1992 Arginine and Immunity. Pp. 160–161 in Encyclopedia of Immunology, I.M.Roitt and P.J.Delves, eds. London: Academic Press.

Kreider, R.B., G.W.Miller, M.H.Williams, C.T.Samma, and T.A.Nasser 1990 Effects of phosphate loading on oxygen uptake, ventilatory anaerobic threshold, and run performance . Med. Sci. Sports Exerc. 22:250–256.

Kruesi, M.J., and J.L.Rapaport 1986 Diet and human behavior: How much do they affect each other? Pp. 113–130 in Annual Review of Nutrition, R.E.Olson, E.Beutler, and H.P.Broquist, eds. Palo Alto, Calif.: Annual Reviews Inc.

Kuznicki, J.T., and L.S.Turner 1986 The effects of caffeine on caffeine users and non-users. Physiol. Behav. 37:397–408.

Lehnert, H.R., D.K.Reinstein, B.W.Strowbridge, and R.J.Wurtman 1984a Neurochemical and behavioral consequences of acute, uncontrollable stress: Effects of dietary tyrosine. Brain Res. 303:215–223.

Lieberman, H.R. 1989 Cognitive effects of various food constituents. Pp. 251–270 in Handbook of the Psychophysiology of Human Eating, R.Shepherd, ed. New York: John Wiley and Sons, Ltd.

1992 Caffeine. Pp. 49–72 in Factors Affecting Human Performance, Vol. 2: The Physical Environment, D.Jones and A.Smith, eds. London: Academic Press.

1992 Caffeine. Pp. 49–72 in Handbook of Human Performance, Vol. 2, Health and Performance, A.P.Smith and D.M.Jones, eds. Boston: Academic Press.

Lieberman, H.R., R.J.Wurtman, G.G.Emde, and I.L.G.Coviella 1987a The effects of caffeine and aspirin on mood and performance. J. Clin. Pharmacol. 7:315–320.

1987b The effects of low doses of caffeine on human performance and mood. Psychopharmacology 92:308–312.

Lieberman, H.R., S.Corkin, B.J.Spring, J.H.Growdon, and R.J.Wurtman 1983 Mood, performance, and pain sensitivity changes induced by food constituents. J. Psychiatr. Res. 17(2):135–145.

Lieberman, H.R., B.Spring, and G.S.Garfield 1986a The behavioral effects of food constituents: Strategies used in studies of amino acids, protein, carbohydrate and caffeine. Nutr. Rev. 44:61–69.

Lieberman, H.R., J.Wurtman, and B.Chew 1986b Changes in mood after carbohydrate consumption among obese individuals. Am. J. Clin. Nutr. 45:772–778.

Lieberman, H.R., L.E.Banderet, and B.Shukitt-Hale 1990 Tyrosine protects humans from the adverse effects of acute exposure to hypoxia and cold. Soc. Neurosci. Abstr. 16:272.

Lieberman, H.R., A.B.Dollins, and R.J.Wurtman 1991 Strategies to sustain and enhance performance in stressful environments: The effects of tyrosine pre-treatment on lower body negative pressure stress. Air Force Office of Scientific Research Report TR-90–0403, AD A221224. Bolling Air Force Base, Washington, D.C.: Air Force Office of Scientific Research.

Lieberman, H.R., B.J.Fine, J.L.Kobrick, and J.D.E.Gabrieli 1993 Effects of caffeine on mental performance and mood: Implications for aircrew members, in Nutrition and Metabolic Disorders and Lifestyle of Aircrew Advisory Group for Aerospace Research and Development Conference Proceedings, No. 533. Oslo, Norway. Loughton, U.K.: Specialized Printing Services (SPS).

Loke, W.H., J.V.Hinrichs, and M.M.Ghonheim 1985 Caffeine and diazepam: Separate and combined effects on mood, memory, psychomotor performance. Psychopharmacology 87:344–350.

Lumley, M., T.Roehrs, D.Asker, F.Zorick, and T.Roth 1987 Ethanol and caffeine effects on daytime sleepiness/alertness.Sleep 10:306–312.

Luo, S., L.Villamil, C.J.Watkins, and H.R.Lieberman 1992 Further evidence tyrosine reverses behavioral deficits caused by cold exposure. Soc. Neurosci. Abstr. 18:716.

Maher, T.J., and R.J.Wurtman 1980 L-threonine administration increases glycine concentrations in the rat central nervous system. Life Sci. 26:1283–1286.

Manning, C.A., J.L.Hall, and P.E.Gold 1990 Glucose effects on memory and other neuropsychological tests in elderly humans. Psychol. Sci. 1:307–311.

Mascioli, E.A., V.K.Babayan, B.R.Bistrian, and G.L.Blackburn 1988 Novel triglycerides for special medical purposes. J. Parenter. Enter. Nutr. 12:127S–132S.

McNair, D.M. 1973 Antianxiety drugs and human performance. Arch. Gen. Psychiatry 29:611.

Moore, R.J., J.F.Patton, E.W.Askew, and R.P.Mello 1991 Effects of dietary carbohydrate intake on perceptual responses to prolonged load carriage exercise. FASEB J. 5:A1657.

Myers, M.G. 1988 Effects of caffeine on blood pressure. Arch. Inter. Med. 148:1189–1193.

Newhouse, P.A., G.Belenky, M.Thomas, D.Thorne, H.C.Sing, and J.Fertig 1989 The effects of D-amphetamine on arousal, cognition, and mood after prolonged total sleep deprivation. Neuropsychopharmacology 2:153–164.

Opstad, P.K., and A.Aakvaag 1981 The effect of a high calorie diet on hormonal changes in young men during prolonged physical strain and sleep deprivation. Eur. J. Appl. Physiol. 46:31–39.

O'Rourke, D., J.Wurtman, R.Wurtman, R.Chebli, and R.Gleason 1989 Treatment of seasonal depression with D-fenfluramine. J. Clin. Psychiatry 50:343–347.

Owasoyo, J.O., D.F.Neri, and J.G.Lamberth 1992 Tyrosine and its potential use as a countermeasure to performance decrement in military sustained operations. Aviat. Space Environ. Med. 63:364–369.

Oyono-Enguelle, S., H.Freund, C.Ott, M.Gartner, A.Heitz, J.Marbach, F. Maccari, A.Frey, H.Bigot, and A.C.Bach 1988 Prolonged submaximal exercise and L-carnitine in humans. Eur. J. Appl. Physiol. 58:53–61.

Philen, R.M., D.I.Ortiz, S.B.Auerbach, and H.Falk 1991 Survey of advertising for nutritional supplements in health and bodybuilding magazines. J. Am. Med. Assoc. 268:1008–1010.

Rapoport, J.L., M.Jensvold, R.Elkins, M.S.Buchsbaum, H.Weingartner, C.Ludlow, T.P.Zahn, C.J.Berg, and A.H.Neims 1981 Behavioral and cognitive effects of caffeine in boys and adult males. J. Nervous Mental Dis. 169:726–732.

Rauch, T.M., and H.R.Lieberman 1990 Tyrosine pretreatment reverses hypothermia induced behavioral depression. Brain Res. Bull. 24:147–150.

Rosenthal, L., T.Roehrs, A.E.Zwyghuizen-Doorenbos, D.Plath, and T.Roth 1991 Alerting effects of caffeine after normal and restricted sleep. Neuropsychopharmacology 4:103–108.

Sandage, D.W., R.N.Sabounjian, R.White, and R.J.Wurtman 1992 Choline citrate may enhance athletic performance. Physiologist 35:236a.

Salter, C.A. 1989 Dietary tyrosine as an aid to stress resistance among troops. Milit. Med. 154:144–146.

Shurtleff, D., J.R.Thomas, J.Schrot, K.Kowalski, R.Harford, M.O.Thornton, P.A.Shea, and M.Malik 1992 Tyrosine reverses a cold-stress-induced memory deficit in humans. Soc. Neurosci. Abstr. 18:1210.

Siliprandi, N., F.Di Lisa, G.Pieralisi, P.Ripari, F.Maccari, R.Menabo, M.A. Giamberardino, and L.Vecchiet 1990 Metabolic changes induced by maximal exercise in human subjects following L-carnitine administration. Biochim. Biophys. Acta 1034:17–21.

Simon, E., G.Frenkel, and P.F.Kraicer 1972 Blockage of insulin secretion by mannoheptulose. Isr. J. Med. Sci. 8:743–752.

Simonson, E., J.Brozek, and A.Keys 1948 Effects of meals on visual performance and fatigue. J. Appl. Psychol. 1:270–278.

Simri, U. 1974 Assessment procedures for human performance. Pp. 362–379 in Fitness, Health, and Work Capacity—International Standards for Assessment, L.A.Larson, ed. New York: MacMillan.

Singh, A., B.A.Day, J.E.DeBolt, U.H.Trostmann, L.L.Bernier, and P.A. Deuster 1989 Magnesium, zinc, and copper status of U.S. Navy SEAL trainees. Am. J. Clin. Nutr.49:695–700.

Singh, A., B.L.Smoak, K.Y.Patterson, L.G.LeMay, C.Veillon, and P.A. Deuster 1991 Biochemical indices of selected trace minerals in men: Effect of stress. Am. J. Clin. Nutr. 53:126–131.

Sitaram, N., H.Weingartner, E.D.Caine, and J.C.Gillin 1978a Choline: Selective enhancement of serial learning and encoding of low imagery words in man. Life Sci. 22:1555–1560.

Sitaram, N., H.Weingartner, and J.C.Gillin 1978b Human serial learning: Enhancement with arecholine and choline impairment with scopolamine. Science 201:274–276.

Smith, A., S.Leekam, A.Ralph, and G.McNeill 1988 The influence of meal composition on post-lunch changes in performance efficiency and mood. Appetite 10:195–203.

Smith, A., A.Kendrick, and A.Maben 1994a Effects of breakfast and caffeine on cognitive performance, mood, and cardiovascular functioning. Appetite 22:39–55.

Smith, A., A.Maben, and P.Brockman 1994b Effects of evening meals and caffeine on cognitive performance, mood and cardiovascular functioning. Appetite 22:57–65.

Soblosky, J.S., and J.B.Thurmond 1986 Biochemical and behavioral correlates of chronic stress: Effects of tricyclic antidepressants. Pharmacol. Biochem. Behav. 24:1361–1368.

Soop, M., O.Bjorkman, G.Cederblad, L.Hagenfeldt, and J.Wahren 1988 Influence of carnitine supplementation on muscle substrate and carnitine metabolism during exercise. J. Appl. Physiol. 64:2394– 2399.

Spriet, L.L., D.A.MacLean, D.J.Dyck, E.Hultman, G.Cederblad, and T.E. Graham 1992 Caffeine ingestion and muscle metabolism during prolonged exercise in humans. Am. J. Physiol. 262:E891–E898.

Spring, B. 1984 Recent research on the behavioral effects of tryptophan and carbohydrate. Nutr. Health 3:55–67.

1986 Effects of foods and nutrients on the behavior of normal individuals. Pp. 1–47 in Nutrition and the Brain, Vol. 7, R.J.Wurtman and J. Wurtman, eds. New York: Raven Press.

Spring, B. , O.Maller, J.Wurtman, L.Digman, and L.Cozolino 1983 Effects of protein and carbohydrate meals on mood and performance: Interactions with sex and age. J. Psychiatric Res. 17:155–167.

Spring, B. , H.R.Lieberman, G.Swope, and G.S.Garfield 1986 Effects of carbohydrates on mood and behavior. Nutri. Rev. 44:51–60.

Spring, B. , J.Chiodo, and D.Bowen 1987 Carbohydrates, tryptophan and behavior: A methodological review. Psychol. Bull. 102:234–256.

Spring, B. , J.Chiodo, M.Harden, M.Bourgeois, J.Mason, and L.Lutherer, 1989 Psychobiological effects of carbohydrates. J. Clin. Psychiatry 50(5, Suppl.):274–333.

Spring, B., R.Pingitore, M.Bourgeois, K.Kessler, and E.Bruckner 1992 The effects and non-effects of skipping breakfast: The results of three studies. Paper presented at the Annual Meeting of the American Psychological Association, Washington, D.C.

Srzezinski, A.A. , J.J.Wurtman, R.Gleason, T.Nader, and B.Laferrere 1990 D-fenfluramine suppresses the increase calorie and carbohydrate intakes and improves the mood of women with premenstrual syndrome. Obstet. Gynecol 76:296–301.

Stanko, R.T. , R.J.Robertson, R.W.Galbreath, J.J.Reilly, Jr., K.D. Greenawalt, and F.L.Goss 1990b Enhanced leg exercise endurance with a high-carbohydrate diet and dihydroxyacetone and pyruvate. J. Appl. Physiol. 69:1651–1656.

Stewart, I., L.McNaughton, P.Davies, and S.Tristram 1990 Phosphate loading and the effects on in trained cyclists. Res. Q. Exerc. Sport 61:80–84.

Teff, K.L., S.N.Young, L.Marchand, and M.I.Botez. 1989 Acute effect of protein or carbohydrate breakfasts on human cerebrospinal fluid monoamine precursor and metabolite levels. J. Neurochem. 52:235–241.

Tharion, W.J., and R.J.Moore 1993 Effects of carbohydrate intake and load-bearing exercise on rifle marksmanship performance. Technical Report No. T5–93, AD A262 333. Natick, Mass.: U.S. Army Research Institute of Environmental Medicine.

Thayer, R.E. 1987 Energy, tiredness, and tension effects of a sugar snack versus moderate exercise. J. Personality Social Psychol. 52:119–125.

U.S. Food and Drug Administration 1990 Evaluation of the safety of amino acids and related products; announcement of study; request for scientific data and information; announcement of open meeting. Fed. Regist. 55:49141–49142.

Uziel, G., B.Garavaglia, and S.Di Donato 1988 Carnitine stimulation of pyruvate dehydrogenase complex (PDHC) in isolated human skeletal muscle mitochondria. Muscle Nerve 11:720–724.

Vecchiet, L., F.Di Lisa, G.Pieralisi, P.Ripari, R.Menabò, M.A. Giamberardino, and N.Siliprandi 1990 Influence of L-carnitine administration on maximal physical exercise. Eur. J. Appl. Physiol. 61:486–490.

Walsh, J.K., M.J.Muehlbach, T.Humm, Q.S.Dickens, J.L.Sugerman, and P.K.Schweitzer 1990 Effect of caffeine on physiological sleep tendency and ability to sustain wakefulness at night. Psychopharmacology 101:271–273.

Weiss, B., and V.G.Laties 1962 Enhancement of human performance by caffeine and the amphetamines. Pharmacol. Rev. 14:1–36.

Wenk, G.L. 1989 An hypothesis on the role of glucose in the mechanism of action of cognition enhancers. Psychopharmacology 99:431–138.

Wilson, P.W.F., R.J.Garrison, W.B.Kannel, D.L.McGee, and W.P.Castelli 1989 Is coffee consumption a contributor to cardiovascular disease? Insights from the Framingham Study . Arch. Int. Med. 149:1169– 1172.

Wurtman, R.J. 1983 Behavioral effects of nutrients. Lancet 1:145–147.

Wurtman, R.J., and J.J.Wurtman 1989 Carbohydrates and depression. Sci. Am. :68–75.

Wurtman, R.J., F.Larin, S.Mostafapour, and J.D.Fernstrom 1974 Brain catechol synthesis: Control by brain tyrosine concentration. Science 185:183–184.

Wurtman, R.J., F.Hefti, and E.Melamed 1980 Precursor control of neurotransmitter synthesis. Pharmacol. Rev. 32:315.

Wurtman, J.J., A.Brzezinski, R.J.Wurtman, and B.Laferrere 1989 Effect of nutrient intake on premenstrual depression. Am. J. Obstet. Gynecol. 161:1228–1234.

Yaspelkis, B.B., III, and J.L.Ivy 1991 Effect of carbohydrate supplements and water on exercise metabolism in the heat. J. Appl. Physiol. 71:680–687.

Yaspelkis, B.B., III, J.G.Patterson, P.A.Anderla, A.Ding, and J.L.Ivy 1993 Carbohydrate supplementation spares muscle glycogen press during variable intensity exercise. J. Appl. Physiol. 75:1477–1485.

Yokogoshi, H., and R.J.Wurtman 1986 Meal composition and plasma amino acid ratios: Effects of various proteins or carbohydrates, and of various protein concentrations. Metabolism 35:837–842.

Zeisel, S.H., K.A.daCosta, P.D.Franklin, E.A.Alexander, J.T.Lamont, N.F.Sheard, and A.Beiser 1991 Choline, an essential nutrient for humans. FASEB J. 5:2093–2098.

Zwyghuizen-Doorenbos, A., T.A.Roehrs, L.Lipschutz, V.Timms, and T.Roth 1990 Effects of caffeine on alertness. Psychopharmacology 100:36–39.

D

Biographical Sketches

COMMITTEE ON MILITARY NUTRITION RESEARCH

DONNA F.ALLEN ***(FNB Staff, Project Assistant)*** is the Project Assistant for the Committee on Military Nutrition Research. Mrs. Allen is a practiced meeting coordinator, and has acquired over twenty years of administrative, supervisory, and logistics experience in business administration, and computer science. Prior to coming to the Institute of Medicine, she was the Administration Assistant to the Computer Science and Telecommunications Board, National Research Council and has supported several other committees in her twelve years of service at the National Academy of Sciences. Mrs. Allen is working towards her degree in Business Administration.

RICHARD L.ATKINSON is Professor of Medicine and Nutritional Sciences; Chief, Section of Clinical Nutrition; and Director, Beers Clinical Nutrition Center at the University of Wisconsin, Madison. Prior to this appointment he was the Associate Chief of Staff for Research and Development at the Veterans Affairs Medical Center, Hampton, Virginia, and Chief, Division of Clinical Nutrition at the Eastern Virginia Medical School, Norfolk, Virginia. He also has been on the faculty of the University of Virginia and the

University of California, Davis. He served four years in the Army at Walter Reed Army Medical Center, in Washington, D.C., and at Fort Campbell, Kentucky, as Division Surgeon of the 101st Airborne Division and Chief of Medicine at the Fort Campbell Army Hospital. Dr. Atkinson is on the editorial board of the *International Journal of Obesity* and *Obesity Research.* He is a member of numerous professional societies, including the American Society for Clinical Nutrition (ASCN), American Institute of Nutrition, American College of Physicians, the Endocrine Society, and the North American Society for the Study of Obesity (NASSO). He was the President of NASSO (1990–1991) and is the current President of ASCN (1994–1995). In addition, he is Chair of the NIH Nutrition Study Section (1993–1995). After graduating from the Virginia Military Institute, Dr. Atkinson received his M.D. from the Medical College of Virginia, where he served a Medicine Internship. He served a Medicine Residency and an Endocrine-Metabolism Fellowship at Harbor General-UCLA Hospital in Torrance, California.

WILLIAM R.BEISEL for the past 8 years has been a semi-retired Adjunct Professor at The Johns Hopkins School of Hygiene and Public Health. He was initially a career Army physician. After specialty training in Internal Medicine, wartime service in Korea, and a tour as Chief of Medicine at Fort Leonard Wood, he joined Walter Reed Army Institute of Research (WRAIR) and Walter Reed Army Hospital. He became Chief of Enlisted Medicine and the Metabolic Research Department. In that capacity he led a WRAIR team to initiate cholera research in Thailand. He later joined U.S. Army Medical Research Institute of Infectious Diseases to study metabolic, endocrine and nutritional aspects of infection, work culminating in his discovery of Interleukin-1 and its metabolic actions. These efforts also allowed him to play a pioneering role in the field of nutritional immunology. He has been a long-term member (or chairman) of committees of the National Academy of Sciences/National Research Council, Federation of American Societies for Experimental Biology, the National Institutes of Health, the Veterans Administration, and the U.S. Department of Agriculture, and an editorial board member of three nutritional journals.

VALERIE McC.BREEN ***(FNB Staff, Research Assistant)*** is Research Assistant for the Committee on Military Nutrition Research, Food and Nutrition Board, Institute of Medicine, Washington, D.C. She received a bachelor of science degree with high scholastic achievement in biological and physical sciences from Indiana University. Before coming to the Institute of Medicine, she was on a three year diplomatic assignment in Paris, France.

GAIL E.BUTTERFIELD is the Director of Nutrition Studies at the Geriatric Research, Education, and Clinical Center of the Palo Alto Veterans Affairs Medical Center in California. Concurrently, she is a Lecturer in the Department of Medicine at Stanford University Medical School and a Consulting Assistant Professor in the Department of Human Biology at Stanford University. Her previous academic appointments were in the Department of Nutritional Sciences at the University of California-Berkeley, including Director of the Coordinated Program in Dietetics, and Assistant Professor and Assistant Nutritionist for the Agricultural Experiment Station. Dr. Butterfield belongs to the American Institute of Nutrition, American Dietetic Association, and American Physiological Society. As a fellow of the American College of Sports Medicine, she serves on the Position Stands Committee, the Editorial Board for Medicine and Science in Sports and Exercise, and the Board of Trustees. She also was the Past President and Executive Director of the Southwest Chapter of that organization and an Ad Hoc Member for the Respiratory and Applied Physiology Study Section of the National Institutes of Health. Dr. Butterfield received her A.B. in biological sciences, M.A. in anatomy, and M.S. and Ph.D. in nutrition from the University of California-Berkeley. She is also a registered dietitian and an active member of the Sports and Cardiovascular Nutritionists (SCAN) of the American Dietetic Association.

JOHANNA T.DWYER ***(Food and Nutrition Board, Liaison)*** is Professor of Medicine and Community Health at Tufts University School of Medicine and also at the Tufts School of Nutrition. She is also Senior Scientist at the U.S. Department of Agriculture (USDA) Human Nutrition Research Center on Aging at Tufts. She holds the D.Sc. from the Harvard School of Public Health. Research interests include energy balance, dietary aspects of disease, and special physiological stresses and diet.

JOHN D.FERNSTROM is Professor of Psychiatry, Pharmacology and Behavioral Neuroscience at the University of Pittsburgh School of Medicine; and Director, Basic Neuroendocrinology Program, Western Psychiatric Institute and Clinic.

Dr. Fernstrom graduated in 1969 from the Massachusetts Institute of Technology (M.I.T.), Cambridge Massachusetts, with an S.B. degree in biology, and obtained his Ph.D. degree in nutritional biochemistry in 1972, also from M.I.T. He was a post-doctoral fellow in neuroendocrinology at the Roche Institute for Molecular Biology (Nutley, New Jersey). Before coming to the University of Pittsburgh, Dr. Fernstrom was an Assistant and then Associate Professor in the Department of Nutrition and Food Science at M.I.T.

Dr. Fernstrom has served on numerous governmental advisory committees, and is presently a member of the National Advisory Council of the Monell Chemical Senses Center, and is chairman of the Neurosciences Section of the American Institute of Nutrition. He is a member of numerous professional societies, including the American Institute of Nutrition, the American Society for Clinical Nutrition, the American Physiological Society, the American Society for Pharmacology and Experimental Therapeutics, the American Society for Neurochemistry, the Society for Neuroscience, and the Endocrine Society.

Among other awards, Dr. Fernstrom received the Mead-Johnson Award of the American Institute of Nutrition, a Research Scientist Award from the National Institute of Mental Health, a Wellcome Visiting Professorship in the Basic Medical Sciences, and an Alfred P.Sloan Fellowship in Neurochemistry. His current major research interest concerns the influence of the diet and drugs on the synthesis of neurotransmitters in the central and peripheral nervous systems.

JOEL A.GRINKER is currently a Professor in the Human Nutrition Program, School of Public Health, a professor in Pediatrics at the Medical School, and a member of the Center for Human Growth and Development at the University of Michigan. She received a Ph.D. in experimental social psychology from New York University and was the recipient of a Russell Sage Foundation Fellowship at the Rockefeller University in biochemistry, biology, and behavior. After 15 years at Rockefeller University in the laboratory of Human Behavior and Metabolism, she moved to the University of Michigan to become Chair of the Program in Human Nutrition. Major areas of interest are in obesity, specifically the development and maintenance of obesity through the life span.

G.RICHARD JANSEN is Emeritus Professor of Nutritional Science and formerly Head of the Department of Food Science and Human Nutrition at Colorado State University. His Ph.D. in biochemistry was from Cornell University. His research interests deal primarily with protein nutrition, and he has co-authored a book on diet and health issues. Prior to his appointment at Colorado State, he was a research fellow at the Merck Institute. He served in the United States Air Force from 1950 to 1953.

ORVILLE A.LEVANDER is the Acting Research Leader for the U.S. Department of Agriculture's Nutrient Requirements and Functions Laboratory in Beltsville, Maryland. Previously, he was a Research Chemist at the USDA's Human Nutrition Research Center, a Resident Fellow in biochemistry at Columbia University's College of Physicians and Surgeons, and a Research

Associate at Harvard University's School of Public Health. Dr. Levander's prior Food and Nutrition Board involvement was on the Committee on the Dietary Allowances. He also served on the National Research Council's Committee on Animal Nutrition, the Committee on the Biological Effects of Environmental Pollutants, and the Safe Drinking Water Committee's Subcommittee on Nutrition. His was a member of the U.S. National Committee for the International Union of Nutrition Scientists and temporary advisor to the World Health Organization's Environmental Health Criteria Document on Selenium. Dr. Levander's former academic appointments include being a William Evans visiting fellow at the University of Otago in New Zealand, a traveling fellow for the Danish Medical Research Council, and a Burroughs Wellcome visiting professor of nutrition at Oregon State University. Additionally, he was awarded the Osborne and Mendel Award for the American Institute of Nutrition. His society memberships include the American Institute of Nutrition, American Chemical Society, and American Society for Clinical Nutrition. Dr. Levander received his B.A. from Cornell University and his M.S. and Ph.D. in biochemistry from the University of Wisconsin-Madison.

GILBERT A.LEVEILLE is Vice President of Research and Technical Services for Nabisco Brands, Inc. Prior to joining Nabisco in 1986 he was Director of Nutrition and Health for General Foods, and from 1971 to 1980 was Professor and Chairman of the Department of Food Science and Human Nutrition at Michigan State University. He holds a Ph.D. in nutrition and biochemistry from Rutgers University. His areas of research interest include carbohydrate and lipid metabolism, obesity, and metabolic adaptations to diet.

BERNADETTE M.MARRIOTT ***(FNB Staff, Program Director)*** is Program Director for the Committee on Military Nutrition Research, Food and Nutrition Board, Institute of Medicine. She has a Ph.D. degree in psychology from the University of Aberdeen, Scotland, and B.Sc. degree in biochemistry/immunology and post doctoral laboratory experience in trace mineral nutrition. Prior to joining the Institute of Medicine staff, she held university and medical school faculty positions at Johns Hopkins University and the University of Puerto Rico Schools of Medicine, and Goucher College. Her areas of research interest include bioenergetic modeling and social influences of food selection in human and nonhuman primates.

ROBERT O.NESHEIM ***(Committee Chairman)*** He retired as Vice President, Science and Technology, for the Quaker Oats Company, Chicago, Illinois, in 1983, and in 1991, as President of Advanced HealthCare, Monterey, California. He earned a Ph.D. degree in nutrition from the University of Illinois and has had extensive experience in research management. He has been involved in food and nutrition issues for many years, serving on many national committees, including the Food and Nutrition Board and the Food Advisory Committee, Office of Technology Assessment, U.S. Congress. He is a Fellow of the American Institute of Nutrition.

JOHN E.VANDERVEEN is the Director of the Food and Drug Administration's Office of Plant and Dairy Foods and Beverages in Washington, D.C. His previous position at the FDA was Director of the Division of Nutrition, at the Center for Food Safety and Applied Nutrition. He also served in various capacities at the United States Air Force School of Aerospace Medicine at Brooks Air Force Base, Texas. He has received accolades for service from the FDA and the USAF. Dr. Vanderveen is a member of the American Society for Clinical Nutrition, American Institute of Nutrition, Aerospace Medical Association, American Dairy Science Association, Institute of Food Technologists, and American Chemical Society. In the past, he was the treasurer of the American Society of Clinical Nutrition and a member of the Institute of Food Technology, National Academy of Science Advisory Committee. Dr. Vanderveen holds a B.S. in agriculture from Rutgers University, New Jersey and a Ph.D. in chemistry from the University of New Hampshire.

ALLISON A.YATES is Dean of the College of Health and Human Sciences at the University of Southern Mississippi and associate professor of foods and nutrition. She has a Ph.D. degree in nutrition from the University of California at Berkeley, and an M.S. in Public Health from UCLA, and is a registered dietitian. She currently serves as Project Director for the Division of Applied Research of the National Food Service Management Institute. Her areas of expertise are in food habits, diet composition, and protein and energy interrelationships.

AUTHORS

STEPHEN T.AHLERS is the Head of the Neurochemistry Division, Thermal Stress Adaptation Program of the Naval Medical Research Institute. He received his Ph.D. in physiological psychology from Kent State University in 1987 and has served as a Commissioned Naval Officer at the Institute since he obtained his doctorate degree. For the last ten years his research has focused on the effects of thermal stress on learning and memory. In addition to an extensive research effort on the behavioral effects of exposure to thermal stress and pharmacological strategies to alleviate stress-induced cognitive deficits, he has developed technologies to examine the affects of stress on neurochemical and neurophysiological changes in the central nervous system.

ELDON W.ASKEW is a U.S. Army Medical Service Corps Officer and Chief of the Military Nutrition Division of the Occupational Health and Performance Directorate, U.S. Army Research Institute of Environmental Medicine, Natick, Massachusetts. He received a Ph.D. in nutritional biochemistry from the Institute of Nutrition, Michigan State University, in 1970. He has spent most of his career in research assignments in the Army Medical Department; assignments include the U.S. Army Medical Research and Nutrition Laboratory, Denver, Colorado; Letterman Army Institute of Research, Presidio of San Francisco, California; Tripler Army Medical Center, Honolulu, Hawaii; and most recently to the U.S. Army Research Institute of Environmental Medicine, Natick, Massachusetts, where he is Chief of Military Nutrition Research. His research during his career in the U.S. Army Medical Department has involved the study of biochemical adaptations to exercise training, the role of nutrition in physical performance, assessment of nutritional status, and nutrition for environmental extremes. He and his staff have conducted cold weather and high altitude nutrition research studies in Alaska, and on Mt. Ranier, Mauna Kea, Pikes Peak, and the Bolivian Altiplano. He is a member of the American College of Sports Medicine, the American Institute of Nutrition, the Association of Military Surgeons, the International Society for Mountain Medicine, and the Wilderness Medical Society. He is a member of the Nutrition Advisory Panel to the United States Olympic Committee.

THOMAS BALKIN is the Chief of the Psychopharmacology Branch in the Department of Behavioral Biology at the Walter Reed Army Institute of Research. He earned his Ph.D. degree in Experimental Psychology from the Bowling Green State University. His research interests include sleep, the psychopharmacology of sleep-induction, and cerebral blood flow during sleep.

GREGORY BELENKY is Chief of the Department of Behavioral Biology at the Walter Reed Army Institute of Research. He earned his M.D. degree from Stanford University. He is clinically trained as a psychiatrist. His research interest include sleep and sleep deprivation, and combat psychiatry.

PEGGY R.BORUM is currently a Professor in the Department of Food Science and Human Nutrition and the Department of Pediatrics at the University of Florida. She received a Ph.D. in biochemistry from the University of Tennessee. After 11 years at Vanderbilt University School of Medicine in the Department of Biochemistry, she moved to the University of

Florida to continue her research in metabolic assessment and nutritional support of populations with special nutrient needs.

C.PATRICK DUNNE is a Senior Research Chemist in the Ration Systems Division, Sustainability Directorate, U.S. Army Natick Research, Development and Engineering Center in Natick, Massachusetts. He earned the Ph.D. degree in biochemistry at Brandeis University. His research specialties are vitamin chemistry, enzymology, and physical biochemistry. Current research is focused on the design and development of nutrient-dense rations and on mechanisms of new nonthermal food processing technologies.

CYNTHIA GALINSKI is a Post-Doctoral Fellow in the Department of Psychiatry at the University of Indiana School of Medicine. She was previously a Research Assistant in the Continuous Operations Branch in the Department of Behavioral Biology at the Walter Reed Army Institute of Research. She earned her Ph.D. in clinical psychology from The Catholic University. Her research interests include marital conflict and family dynamics.

CAROL E.GREENWOOD is an Associate Professor of Nutritional Sciences at the University of Toronto's Faculty of Medicine. She received her Ph.D. in 1980 from the University of Toronto and spent the next two years at the Laboratory for Neuroendocrine Control at MIT before returning to Toronto. She was a member of the Scientific Review Committee for Health and Welfare Canada that developed the recent Nutrition Recommendations. Her research interests focus on the inter-relationships among diet, brain biochemistry and behavior, especially as they relate to amino acid and fatty acid utilization in the brain and the impact of brain aging on these processes.

JOHN L.IVY is Professor and Director of the Exercise Science Laboratories, Department of Kinesiology and Health Education and Professor, Division of Pharmacology, College of Pharmacy, The University of Texas at Austin, Austin, Texas. He received his Ph.D. in exercise physiology from the University of Maryland and his post doctoral training at Ball State University and Washington University School of Medicine. His major research focus is on the acute and chronic effects of exercise on muscle metabolism, with special emphasis on carbohydrate regulation. Currently, Dr. Ivy is investigating the regulation of insulin- and contraction-stimulated muscle glucose transport, the etiology of muscle insulin resistance, and the mechanisms by which insulin resistance is reduced with exercise training. He is also investigating the regulation of muscle glucose utilization and glycogen synthesis during and immediately post exercise.

RONALD J.JANDACEK is a Principal Scientist at Procter and Gamble's Miami Valley Laboratories in Cincinnati. After receiving a Ph.D. in chemistry from the University of Texas in 1968, he joined Procter and Gamble where he has studied the physical properties and biological effects of lipids. His work has focused on the relationship of the phases of lipids with their absorption from the intestine.

F.MATTHEW KRAMER is currently a Research Psychologist at the U.S. Army Natick Research, Development and Engineering Center. He received a Ph.D. in Counseling Psychology from the Pennsylvania State University, and completed postdoctoral work at the University of Minnesota and the University of Pennsylvania. Dr. Kramer's interests focus on understanding human food habits, that is, the factors underlying food selection, intake, and acceptability.

JOHN LEU is a Staff Officer in the Headquarters of the United States Army Medical Research and Development Command. He was previously a Research Psychologist in the Special Studies Branch in the Department of Behavioral Biology at the Walter Reed Army Institute of Research. He earned his Ph.D. in Experimental Psychology from the University of Nebraska. His research interests include continuous operation, sleep and sleep deprivation, and biomedical monitoring.

HARRIS R.LIEBERMAN is currently a Research Psychologist in the Division of Military Performance and Neuroscience at the U.S. Army Research Institute of Environmental Medicine (USARIEM) in Natick, Massachusetts. He directs a research program that examines the effects of various food constituents, drugs, hormones and environmental variables on brain function and behavior. Dr. Lieberman is an internationally recognized expert in the area of nutrition and behavior and has published over 60 original, full length scientific papers in scientific journals and edited books. He has been an invited lecturer at numerous national and international conferences, government research laboratories and universities.

Dr. Lieberman received his Ph.D. in physiological psychology in 1977 from the University of Florida. Upon completing his graduate training he was awarded a National Eye Institute fellowship to conduct postdoctoral research at the Department of Psychology and Brain Science at the Massachusetts Institute of Technology (MIT).

In 1980 Dr. Lieberman established an interdisciplinary research program at the MIT Department of Brain and Cognitive Sciences to examine the effects of various food constituents on human behavior and brain function. Key accomplishments of the laboratory included the development of appropriate methods for assessing the effects of food constituents and other subtle environmental factors on human brain function and the determination that specific foods and hormones reliably altered human behavior. In 1990 Dr. Lieberman joined the civilian research staff of USARIEM where he has continued his work in nutrition and behavior as well as several other related areas.

TIMOTHY J.MAHER is Professor of Pharmacology at the Massachusetts College of Pharmacy and Allied Health Sciences. He is also on the faculty at the Massachusetts Institute of Technology in Cambridge, Massachusetts. His area of research involves the ability of amino acids to serve as precursors for neurotransmitters, and their utility as pharmacologic agents in the treatment of disease. He served as a member of the Federation of American Societies for Experimental Biology Life Sciences Research Office's ad hoc Expert Panel which investigated the safety of amino acids as dietary supplements for the Food and Drug Administration.

UNA MCCANN is a Research Psychiatrist in the Section on Anxiety and Affective Disorders in the National Institute of Mental Health. She earned her M.D. degree from Duke University. She is clinically trained as a psychiatrist. Her research interests include affective disorders, sleep, and human psychopharmacology.

HERBERT L.MEISELMAN is Senior Research Scientist (Behavior and Performance) at the U.S. Army Natick Research, Development and Engineering Center. His research interests include consumer and sensory research related to product development, field research, food habits and nutrition, and human factors, with emphasis on individual performance and product/system design. Dr. Meiselman served previously as Special Assistant for the Department of Defense Food Program and as Chief, Behavioral Sciences Division. He is Editor of the journal *Food Quality and Preference.* He earned his doctorate from the University of Massachusetts (1967, psychology) and worked as a postdoctoral fellow at Cornell University (1967–69, neurobiology/psychology) under National Science Foundation fellowships.

DAVID M.PENETAR is a Research Psychologist in the U.S. Army. He received his Ph.D. in psychopharmacology from the University of Minnesota in 1977 and has been involved in the assessment of sleep deprivation effects at the Walter Reed Army Institute of Research since 1987.

REGINA PINGITORE is Health Science Officer at the Veterans Affairs Medical Center, North Chicago and an adjunct faculty member in the

Department of Psychology at University of Health Sciences/The Chicago Medical School. She earned her Ph.D. in social psychology from Loyola University of Chicago and her M.A. in clinical psychology from Edinboro University of Pennsylvania. She is a member of the American Psychological Association and the Society of Behavioral Medicine. Her research focuses on two primary interests: obesity and smoking cessation.

KATHRYN POPP is a Research Psychologist in the Continuous Operations Branch in the Department of Behavioral Biology at the Walter Reed Army Institute of Research. She earned her Ph.D. in psychology from the Uniformed Services University of the Health Sciences. Her research interests include continuous operations, sleep and sleep deprivation, and biomedical monitoring.

DANIEL REDMOND is Chief of the Special Studies Branch in the Department of Behavioral Biology at the Walter Reed Army Institute of Research. He earned his M.D. degree from University of Texas, Southwestern Medical School. He is clinically trained as an internist. His research interests include continuous operations and biomedical engineering.

ALINE SCHELLING is a Research Assistant with Health Information Designs, Inc., Fairfax, Virginia. She was previously a Research Assistant in the Continuous Operations Branch in the Department of Behavioral Biology at the Walter Reed Army Institute of Research. She earned her B.A. degree from Chatham College.

JEN SCHOENFELD is a Graduate Student in the clinical psychology Ph.D. program at the University of Health Sciences/The Chicago Medical School. She earned a B.A. with high honors from Emory University. She is a graduate student member of the American Psychological Association. Her research interests include nutrition and behavior.

JOHN SCHROT is a Research Psychologist and Head, of the Behavioral Neuroscience Branch, Thermal Stress Adaptation Program of the Naval Medical Research Institute, Bethesda, Maryland. His areas of specialty include operant conditioning, behavioral effects of thermal stress and the pathophysiology of non-freezing cold injury.

DAVID SHURTLEFF is a Research Psychologist at the Naval Medical Research Institute. He received his Ph.D. in experimental psychology from The American University in 1989. His areas of expertise include the experimental analysis of behavior and behavioral pharmacology. His current research focuses on the effects of thermal stressors on behavior and cognitive performance.

HELEN SING is a Statistician in the Continuous Operations Branch in the Department of Behavioral Biology at the Walter Reed Army Institute of Research. She earned her M.S. in physical chemistry from the University of Maryland, College Park. Her research interests include sleep, sleep deprivation, continuous operations, circadian rhythms, and cerebral metabolism during sleep deprivation.

BONNIE J.SPRING is Professor of Psychology at University of Health Sciences/The Chicago Medical School and Health Sciences Officer at Veterans Affairs Medical Center, North Chicago. She earned her Ph.D. in psychology from Harvard University, completed a clinical internship at the Massachusetts Mental Health Center, served as Director of Clinical Training at Texas Tech University, and has held faculty appointments at Harvard University, Columbia University, University of Maryland, and M.I.T. An elected Fellow of the American Psychological Association in Clinical Psychology and Health Psychology, she also holds the Diplomate in Health Psychology, awarded by the American Board of Professional Psychology, and serves as Field Editor for the international journal, *Psychopharmacology*. Her research has been concentrated in two primary areas: psychopathology, and nutrition and behavior.

IRWIN A.TAUB is a Senior Research Scientist at the U.S. Army Natick Research Development and Engineering Center. He received his Ph.D. in chemistry from the University of Minnesota in 1961, and was a Resident Research Associate at Argonne National Laboratory and a Research Fellow at the Mellon Institute of Carnegie-Mellon University before becoming involved in food research at Natick. His broad range of scientific experience covers radiation phenomena, chemical kinetics, food chemistry, preservation technologies, food structure, and nutritional tailoring. He is currently coordinating efforts to formulate ration components to contain performance-enhancing natural ingredients.

JOHN R.THOMAS is Director of the Thermal Adaptation Stress program, Naval Medical Research Institute. He earned his Ph.D. degree in physiological psychology and pharmacology at the University of Maryland. He has over thirty years of experience in research concerned with the effects of pharmacological agents on behavior and physiology and effects of extreme environmental influences, such as hypobaric, hyperbaric, electromagnetic, toxicological, and thermal environments, on performance. Research efforts in cold weather medicine over the last several years have focussed on the study and understanding of the impact of cold environments on degradation of performance and the development of technologies, such as pharmacological and nutritional supplementation, for the prevention of performance degradations.

MARIA THOMAS is the Chief of the Continuous Operations Branch in the Department of Behavioral Biology at the Walter Reed Army Institute of Research. She is earning her Ph.D. in psychology at George Mason University and has completed all but her dissertation. Her research interests include sleep, sleep deprivation, continuous operations, and cerebral metabolism during sleep deprivation.

DAVID THORNE is a Research Psychologist in the Continuous Operations Branch in the Department of Behavioral Biology at the Walter Reed Army Institute of Research. He earned his Ph.D. degree in Psychology at Arizona State University. His research interests include sleep, sleep deprivation, and the measurement of human performance.

JAMES A.VOGEL is Director of Occupational Health and Performance, U.S. Army Research Institute of Environmental Medicine, which encompasses research programs in occupational medicine, occupational physiology, nutrition and behavioral performance-neuroscience. He earned a Ph.D. degree in physiology from Rutgers University. He is the principal consultant to the Department of the Army in the biomedical aspects of physical fitness and exercise physiology and chairs a NATO Research Study Group on the Biomedical Aspects of Military Physical Training.

NANCY WESENSTEN is a Research Psychologist in the Psychopharmacology Branch in the Department of Behavioral Biology at the Walter Reed Army Institute of Research. She earned her Ph.D. degree in experimental psychology from Bowling Green State University. Her research interests include sleep, the psychopharmacology of sleep induction, and cerebral blood flow during sleep.

RICHARD J.WURTMAN is Professor of Neuroscience at the Massachusetts Institute of Technology, and Director of MIT's Clinical Research center. His laboratory initially demonstrated that the rates at which neurons in the brain and elsewhere synthesize such neurotransmitters as serotonin, acetylcholine, and the catecholamines dopamine and norepinephrine normally depend on the concentrations of their precursors (tryptophan; choline; tyrosine) that happen to be available. Since brain levels of these precursors can be affected by eating, food consumption can thus influence neurotransmission. These relationships, and their implications in health and disease, are considered in an eight-volume series, *Nutrition and the Brain,* edited by Drs. Richard and Judith Wurtman, and in perhaps half of his laboratory's output of approximately 850 research publications. Other topics explored by this laboratory have included melatonin and biologic rhythms; neuroendocrinology; Alzheimer's Disease; and phospholipid metabolism.

STEVEN H.ZEISEL is Professor and Chair, Department of Nutrition; and Professor, Department of Pediatrics, University of North Carolina at Chapel Hill. He received his M.D. from Harvard University, and his Ph.D. in Neuroendocrine Regulation/Nutrition from the Massachusetts Institute of Technology. Dr. Zeisel's research focuses on nutrient metabolism, with special emphasis on establishing human nutrient requirements and on identifying cancer-causing agents which are produced within our bodies. His work has focused on the nutrient choline as it relates to: a) transmembrane signal transduction (diacylglycerol and protein kinase) and carcinogenesis in liver, b) perinatal brain development, c) human nutrient requirements, and d) choline and secretion of components of milk by isolated mammary epithelial cells.

Dr. Zeisel is a member of the American Institute of Nutrition, American Society for Clinical Nutrition, American Society for Biochemistry and Molecular Biology, American College of Nutrition, Society for Pediatric Research, and American Public Health Association. He serves on the governing council of the American Society for Clinical Nutrition, on the Medical Education Committee and the Joint Membership Committee of the American Institute of Nutrition/ American Society for Clinical Nutrition. Dr. Zeisel is the Editor-in-Chief of *The Journal of Nutritional Biochemistry.*

Index

N

R

S